Neuroradiology - Expect the Unexpected

Martina Špero • Hrvoje Vavro

Neuroradiology - Expect the Unexpected

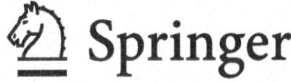 Springer

Martina Špero
University Hospital Dubrava
Department of Diagnostic and
Interventional Radiology
Zagreb
Croatia

Hrvoje Vavro
University Hospital Dubrava
Department of Diagnostic and
Interventional Radiology
Zagreb
Croatia

ISBN 978-3-030-08796-8   ISBN 978-3-319-73482-8   (eBook)
https://doi.org/10.1007/978-3-319-73482-8

This Springer imprint is published by the registered company Springer International Publishing
AG part of Springer Nature.
The registered company address is: Gewerbestrasse 11, 6330 Cham, Switzerland

Acknowledgements

Although we know each other from the time when we were both medical students, this book is a result of our mutual work as neuroradiologists for the past nine years. All cases presented in this book are cases from our daily work at the Department of Diagnostic and Interventional Radiology, University Hospital Dubrava in Zagreb. These cases are small but important and interesting part of our busy and fruitful work. We have more cases to present and maybe we will have another chance to do it in the future.

We would like to thank Antonella Cerri from Springer Milan who invited us and gave us a chance to prepare this book and Corinna Parravicini for assisting us in the process.

We wish to thank Boris Brkljačić, Professor of Radiology and Chairman of our Department, who gave us the chance to become neuroradiologists and always supported our work.

Special thanks to Majda Thurnher, Professor of Radiology at the University Hospital Vienna, Austria, for always being our friend and teacher and supporting us and our work.

We are deeply grateful to the closest members of our families, to our closest friends and colleagues, who always stood by us, helping us and supporting us in our private and professional life.

Contents

Abbreviations

ABC	Aneurysmal bone cyst
ADC	Apparent diffusion coefficient
AQP4	Aquaporin-4
AVM	Arteriovenous malformation
CBV	Cerebral blood volume
CFD	Cranial fibrous dysplasia
CISS	Constructive interference in steady-state
CO	Carbon monoxide
CPA	Cystic pituitary adenoma
CS	Crouzon syndrome
CSF	Cerebrospinal fluid
CT	Computed tomography
CTA	Computed tomography angiography
DSA	Digital subtraction angiography
DWI	Diffusion weighted imaging
EHD	Emergency hospital department
EMG	Electromyography
FD	Fibrous dysplasia
FLAIR	Fluid attenuation inversion recovery
FNA	Fine needle aspiration
FS	Fat suppressed
GCT	Giant cell tumour
IDH	Isocitrate dehydrogenase
IE	Intradiploic encephalocele
LMC	Leptomeningeal carcinomatosis
MRA	Magnetic resonance angiography
MRI	Magnetic resonance imaging
MRS	Magnetic resonance spectroscopy
NAA	N-acetylaspartate
NMO	Neuromyelitis optica
PAVF	Pulmonary arteriovenous fistula
PCNSL	Primary central nervous system lymphoma
PDL	Primary dural lymphoma
PTC	Papillary thyroid carcinoma
PVS	Perivascular space
RCC	Rathke's cleft cyst

R-CHOP	Rituximab-cyclophosphamide, doxorubicin, vincristine, prednisone
SLSC	Sphenoid lateral spontaneous cephalocele
STIR	Short tau inversion recovery
SWI	Susceptibility weighted imaging
TDL	Tumefactive demyelinating lesion
TIRM	Turbo inversion recovery magnitude
TOF	Time-of-flight
VBD	Van Buchem disease
VRT	Volume rendering technique
WHO	World Health Organisation

Part I

Most Likely Differential Diagnosis

Cerebrovascular Infarction: Oligodendroglioma

One morning in November 2009, a 73-year-old female was referred to the brain computed tomography scanning from emergency hospital department (EHD) due to motoric dysphasia lasting for 5 days and subjective right-sided weakness (Fig. 1.1).

It was reported as an acute ischaemic lesion by a referring radiologist, and the patient was hospitalised: during hospitalisation MRI of the brain or control brain CT has not been ordered by neurologist.

During following 16 months, patient has developed spasms of the right arm, and due to a present mild motoric dysphasia, she has again started with speech therapy. Therefore, in February 2011, neurologist referred her to the brain CT scanning as an out-hospital patient (Fig. 1.2).

At that time, it was obvious that the lesion is primary brain tumour, and MRI of the brain was performed (Fig. 1.3).

According to the described morphological characteristics on CT and MRI, we concluded it could be the case of low-grade oligodendroglioma which was confirmed histologically by stereotactic biopsy: low-grade oligodendroglioma WHO grade II.

I could say this is a case of oligodendroglioma mimicking an acute ischaemic lesion in an early tumour stage, or I could say it is obviously a case of misdiagnosed primary brain tumour. The basic CT examination was performed using old single-slice CT scanner without possibility of making adequate coronal and sagittal reconstructions that could help analysing the lesion. Patient age, clinical presentation and duration of symptoms matched together with CT finding of subcortical ill-defined hypodense lesion with narrow overlying sulci in the vascular territory of the left middle cerebral artery and therefore have probably led radiologist to report an acute ischaemic lesion. This diagnosis has also matched neurologist suspicion of an acute stroke as a working diagnosis. Probably that was the reason why neurologist did not order a MRI or a follow-up CT of the brain during the hospitalisation. The absence of restricted diffusion on the MRI, as well as the absence of changes in size, shape, density and sharpness of the lesion edges on follow-up CT scans, would alert radiologist to report that the lesion in question is not an acute ischaemic lesion, but a brain tumour.

1.1 Oligodendroglioma

Different conditions may mimic stroke; tumours may be one of the mimickers, usually gliomas and meningiomas. Anaplastic oligodendroglioma is prone to haemorrhage; therefore, those tumours may mimic haemorrhagic stroke [1]. Ischaemic stroke does not present a "great mimicker" of oligodendroglioma due to features like involvement of a specific vascular territory, diffusion

© Springer International Publishing AG, part of Springer Nature 2018
M. Špero, H. Vavro, *Neuroradiology - Expect the Unexpected*,
https://doi.org/10.1007/978-3-319-73482-8_1

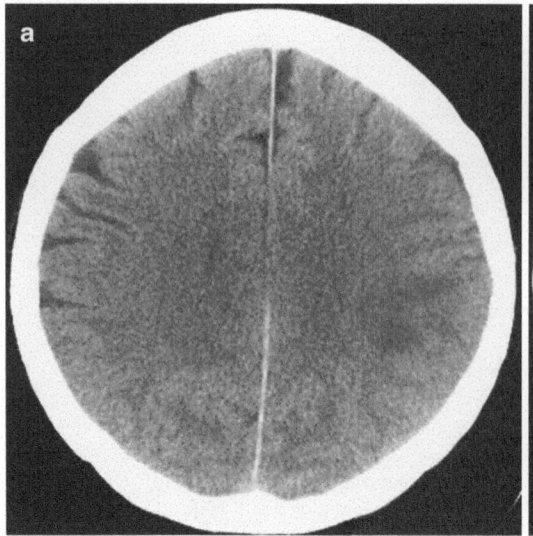 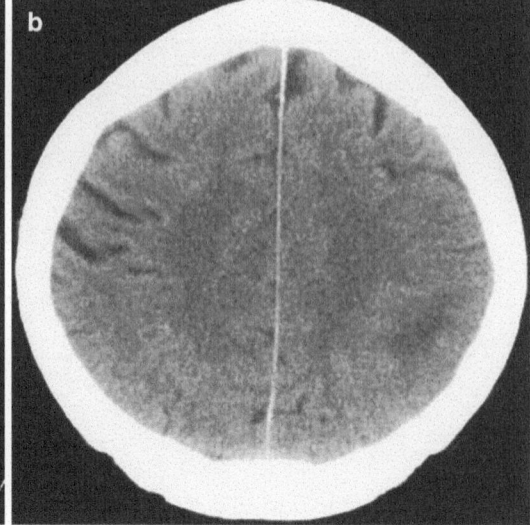

Fig. 1.1 Computed tomography of the brain, axial scan (**a**, **b**), performed at the emergency admission, revealed supratentorial subcortical hypodense lesion in the left hemisphere, involving parenchyma around the central sul-cus, involving left frontal and parietal lobes. Lesion was irregularly shaped with ill-defined borders and narrowed overlying sulci

restriction or typical gyriform contrast enhance-ment in case of subacute ischaemia. In early stage of oligodendroglioma, if an ischaemic stroke is suspected and radiologist is not completely con-vinced in vascular aetiology of a lesion, MRI is mandatory to exclude one and confirm other diagnosis. It is important to reach the correct diagnosis as early as possible, due to a prompt medical treatment and subsequent better prognosis.

Oligodendrogliomas are typically slow-growing glial tumours (5–18% of all glial tumours) composed predominantly of neoplastic oligodendrocytes, most common in adults with a peak incidence in ages 35–44. Anaplastic oligo-dendrogliomas tend to occur in slightly older adults, ages 45–74. Although these tumours are found in both sexes, they tend to occur more often in men [2].

Genotyping of these tumours has revealed chromosomal loss of the short arm of chromo-some 1 (1p) and the long arm of chromosome 19 (19q) as a genetic signature in about 60–90% of all oligodendrogliomas which has diagnostic, prognostic and predictive relevance: tumours with codeletion demonstrate improved disease-free survival and median survival and may respond better to alkylating chemotherapeutics [2, 3]. The 2016 WHO classification uses "inte-grated" phenotypic and genotypic parameters for CNS tumour classification and now divides oli-godendrogliomas into oligodendroglioma, IDH-mutant and 1p/19q-codeleted, oligodendroglioma NOS (not otherwise specified), anaplastic oligo-dendroglioma IDH-mutant and 1p/19q-codeleted, anaplastic oligodendroglioma NOS, oligoastro-cytoma NOS and anaplastic oligoastrocytoma NOS. In case of oligodendrogliomas, NOS cate-gories should be rendered only in the absence of diagnostic molecular testing or in the very rare instance of a dual-genotype oligoastrocytoma [4].

The most common symptoms in oligodendro-glioma clinical presentation are seizures, head-aches and personality changes. Other symptoms vary due to location and size of a tumour and may include weakness, numbness or visual symptoms.

The majority of oligodendrogliomas are located supratentorially: codeleted tumours are most commonly located in the frontal, parietal and occipital lobes; intact tumours are more

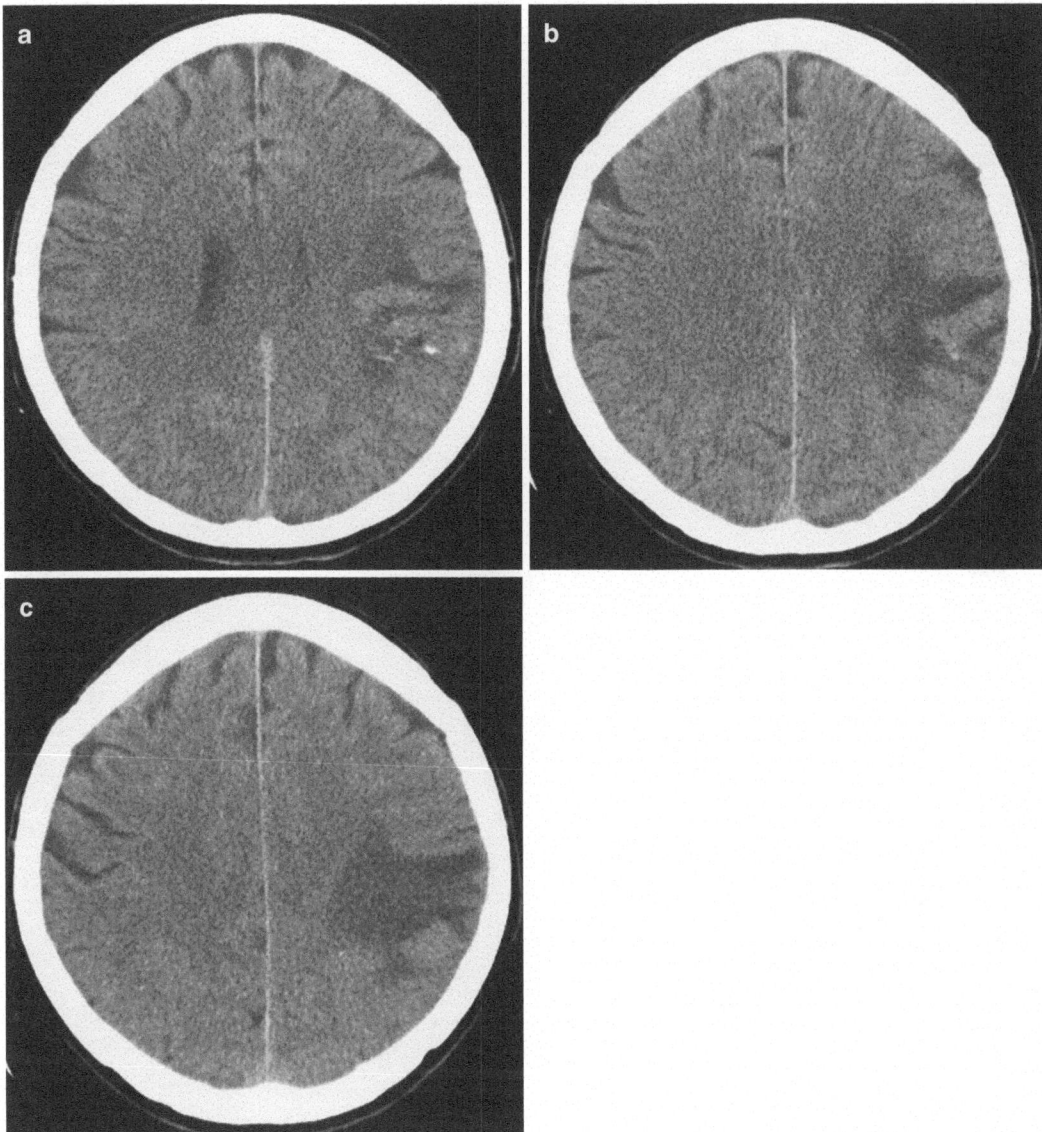

Fig. 1.2 Follow-up non-contrast computed tomography of the brain, axial scan (**a–c**), performed 16 months after the initial one, revealed enlargement in the size of the left frontoparietal lesion around the central sulcus, lesion involved cortical-subcortical parenchyma (**b, c**), it was more irregular in shape, well-circumscribed, more hypodense, with a few coarse, linear calcifications (**a**). Overlying left frontoparietal sulci were more reduced and narrowed, while adjacent part of the left lateral ventricle was compressed

likely found in the temporal, insular or temporo-insular locations. In frontal location, tumours may extend through the corpus callosum producing a "butterfly" pattern. Infratentorial involvement is very rare, but possible [2, 5].

Oligodendrogliomas are relatively well-circumscribed masses resembling low-grade diffuse astrocytoma in shape. They typically involve cortex and subcortical white matter and due to peripheral location may involve overlying skull causing focal thinning or remodelling of the bone [2, 5].

On CT scans, oligodendrogliomas are usually hypodense with coarse calcifications but, due to

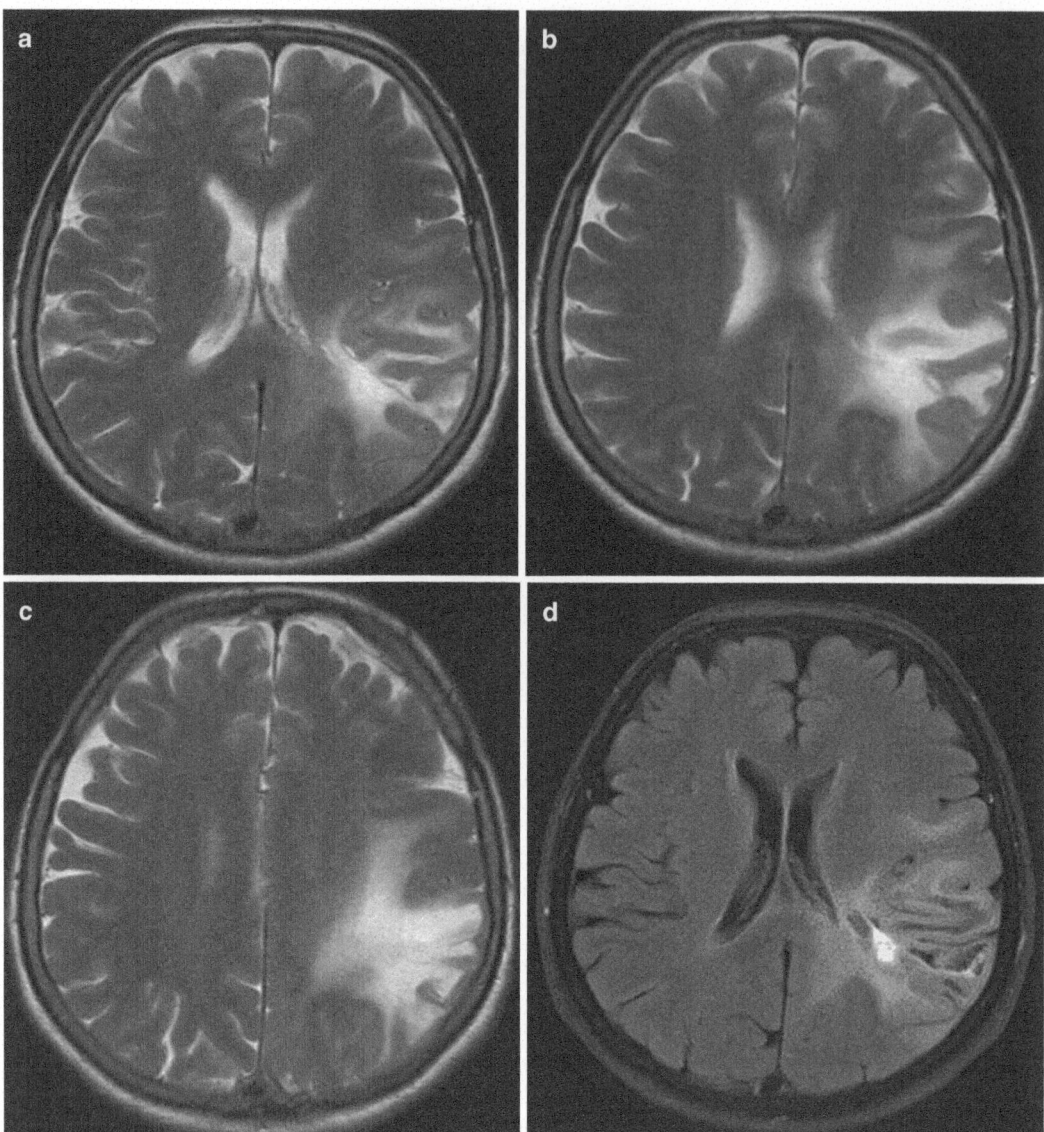

Fig. 1.3 Magnetic resonance imaging confirmed all morphological characteristics of the tumour described on CT scans: axial T2WI (**a–c**), axial FLAIR (**d–f**), axial DWI (**g**), ADC (**h**), T2*WI (**i**), axial post-contrast T1WI (**j–l**), and MR spectroscopy (MRS). Infiltrating, expansile tumour hyperintense on T2WI and FLAIR with moderate cystic degeneration, without restricted diffusion (**g**, **h**). Few linear calcifications were visible on T2*WI, there was no sign of haemorrhage (**i**), as well there was no surrounding vasogenic oedema. After intravenous administration of gadolinium contrast media, there was no contrast enhancement (**j–l**). MR spectroscopy (MRS) revealed elevated choline (Cho) and decreased n-acetylaspartate (NAA), without lactate peak (**m**)

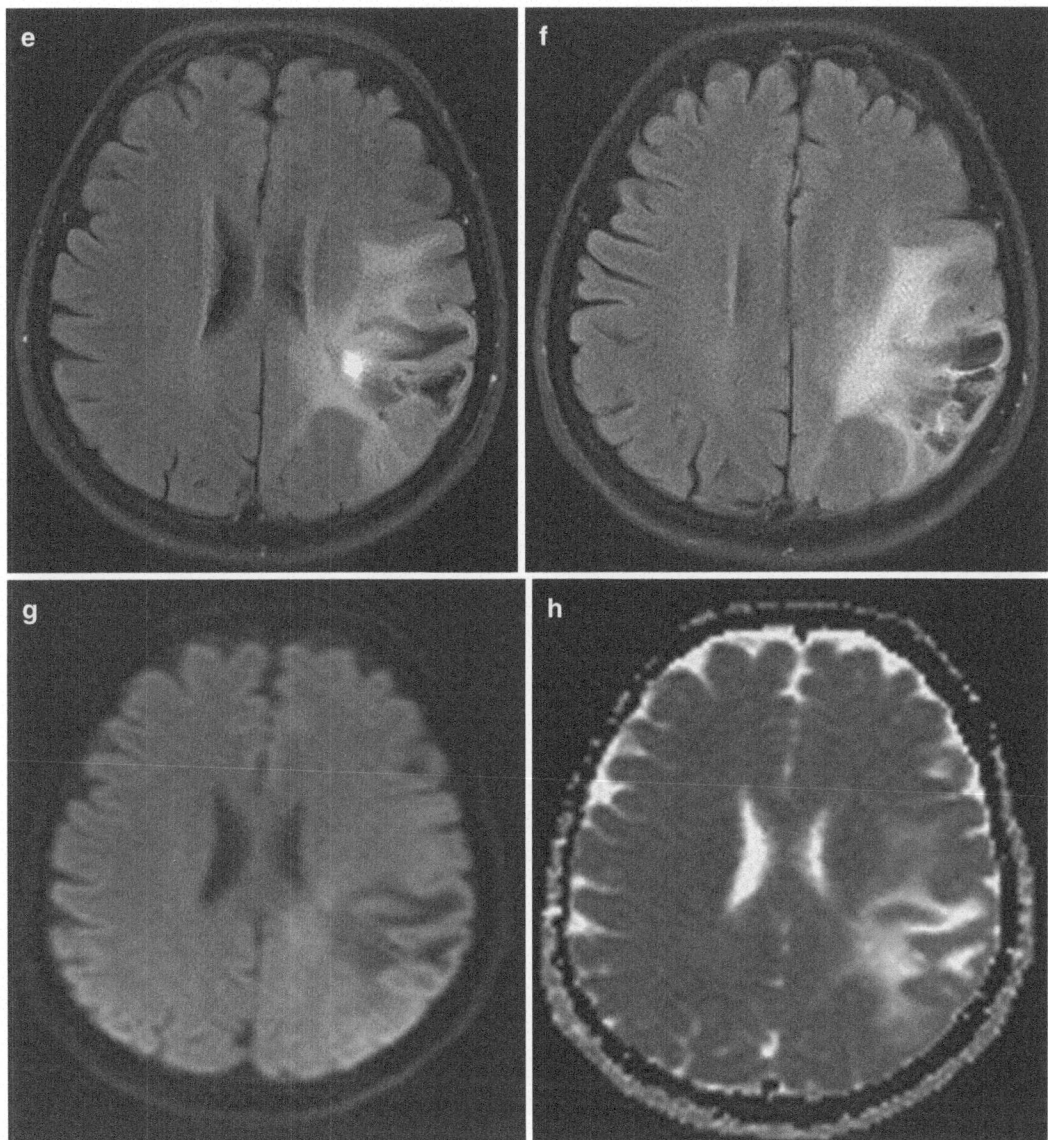

Fig. 1.3 (continued)

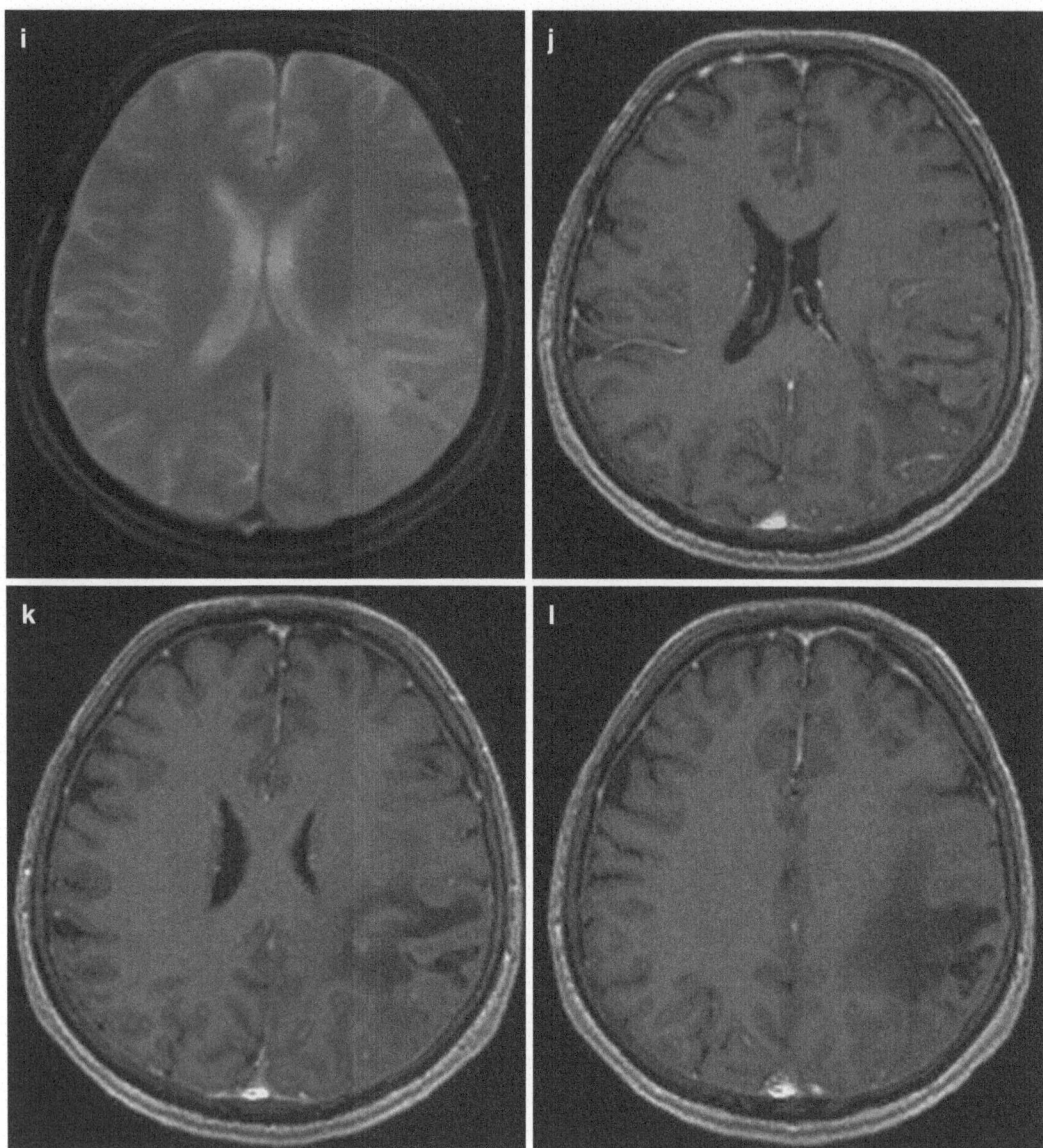

Fig. 1.3 (continued)

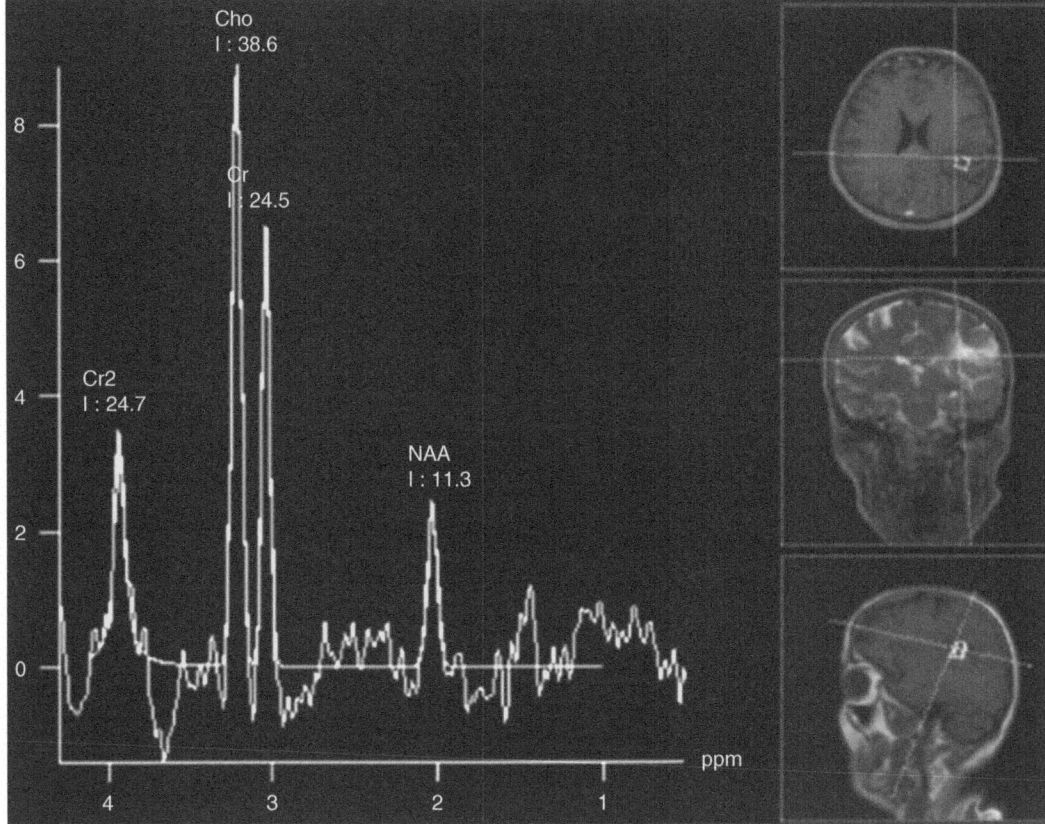

Fig. 1.3 (continued)

possible cystic degeneration or haemorrhage, could have mixed density. On MRI, these tumours are hypointense on T1WI compared to the grey matter and hyperintense on T2WI and FLAIR; calcifications may be less prominent or not visible at all. Cystic degeneration and haemorrhage may occur but are not frequent findings. Codeleted oligodendrogliomas commonly have indistinct margins, calcification and heterogeneous signal intensity in comparison to intact oligodendrogliomas [6–8]. After intravenous administration of a contrast media, oligodendroglioma generally does not enhance, but there are studies which reported "dot-like" or lacy contrast enhancement accounted to delicate branching network of capillaries producing a "honeycomb" or "chicken-wire" pattern on histopathologic evaluation [2, 5, 9]. Although anaplastic tumours tend to enhance somewhat more frequently, the presence of contrast enhancement is not a reli-

able imaging feature to grade oligodendroglioma.

Diffusion restriction is typically absent in oligodendroglioma, while perfusion may be moderately increased: rCBV (cerebral blood volume) is increased due to the increased microvascular density and numerous slow-flowing collateral vessels [10–12]. MR spectroscopy in oligodendroglioma shows typical spectrum with moderately elevated Cho and decreased NAA without lactate peak: the absence of lipid/lactate peak aids in differentiating oligodendroglioma from its anaplastic form, while Cho/Cr ratio threshold of 2.33 was found to distinguish high- from low-grade oligodendroglioma [5, 13].

Differential diagnosis of oligodendrogliomas includes anaplastic form or other tumours like low-grade diffuse astrocytoma; in case of intraventricular location, central neurocytoma is a differential diagnosis: distinction relies only on immunohistochemistry or ultrastructural examination. Cerebritis and cerebral ischaemia in case of cortically located lesions, and entirely thrombosed arteriovenous malformation due to typical flow void absence and prominent gyriform calcifications, are included as possible differential diagnosis [2, 5, 13].

Surgical resection is the main form of therapy. Combination of procarbazine, lomustine and vincristine (PLC) in combination with radiotherapy is remarkable in patients with codeleted tumours.

References

1. Hatzitolios A et al (2008) Stroke and conditions that mimic it: a protocol secures a safe early recognition. Hippokratia 12(2):98–102
2. Koeller KK et al (2005) From the archives and its variants: oligodendroglioma and its variants: radiologic-pathologic correlation. Radiographics 25:1669–1688
3. Sonnen JA et al (2010) Molecular pathology: neuropathology. In: Coleman WB, Tsongalis GJ (eds) Essential Concepts in molecular pathology. Elsevier, San Diego, pp 373–398
4. Louis DN et al (2016) The 2016 World Health Organization classification of tumors of the Central Nervous System: a summary. Acta Neuropathol 131:803–820
5. Smits M (2016) Imaging of oligodendroglioma. Br J Radiol 89(1060):20150857
6. Kim JW et al (2011) Relationship between radiological characteristics and combined 1p adn 19q deletion in World Health Organization grade III oligodendroglial tumours. J Neurol Neurosurg Psyshiatry 82:224–227
7. Meyesi JF et al (2004) Imaging correlates of molecular signatures in oligodendrogliomas. Clin Cancer Res 10:4303–4306
8. Jenkinson MD et al (2006) Histological growth patterns and genotype in oligodendroglial tumours: correlation with MRI features. Brain 129(Pt 7):1884–1889
9. White ML et al (2005) Can tumor contrast enhancement be used as a criterion for differentiating tumor grades of oligodendrogliomas? AJNR Am J Neuroradiol 26:784–790
10. Law M et al (2003) Glioma grading: sensitivity, specificity, and predictive values of perfusion MR imaging and proton MR spectroscopic imaging compared with conventional MR imaging. AJNR Am J Neuroradiol 24:1989–1998
11. Khalid L et al (2012) Imaging characteristics of oligodendrogliomas that predict grade. AJNR Am J Neuroradiol 33:852–857
12. Jenkinson MD et al (2006) Cerebral blood volume, genotype and chemosensitivity in oligodendroglial tumours. Neuroradiology 48:703–713
13. Osborn A (2013) Osborn's brain imaging pathology anatomy. Amirsys, Salt Lake City, pp 494–497

Cerebrovascular Infarction: Primary Brain Lymphoma

A 65-year-old lady suddenly developed speech difficulties and numbness in the left arm and leg which progressed to limb weakness. She did not have any other symptoms. She was rushed to the emergency hospital unit. On examination there was no limb weakness, only central left-sided facial palsy; during examination she developed left-sided facial myoclonus, as well as myoclonus of the first and second finger of her left hand which was felt to be an epileptic seizure and promptly resolved on intravenous antiepileptic therapy. A brain CT examination was done (Fig. 2.1).

The CT report stated this was a subacute ischaemic stroke but morphologically it might differentially be in keeping with a tumour. A brain MRI exam was done the very next day (Fig. 2.2).

No carotid or vertebral artery abnormalities were found on the duplex Doppler examination.

The patient was referred to a rehabilitation facility several days later, with improved neurological status and residual mild left-sided supranuclear facial nerve paresis, mild speech impairment and a very mild left-sided hemiparesis.

There was further improvement of the patient's neurological status until it suddenly deteriorated 3 weeks later, at the rehabilitation facility. The patient was transferred back to the hospital, and a follow-up CT exam was done (Fig. 2.3).

A sample of the lesion tissue was obtained by stereotactic biopsy. The histopathology reported non-Hodgkin lymphoma of the brain, with perivascular infiltration.

The patient was transferred to the haematology department, and additional workup was done, including CT scans of the thorax, abdomen and pelvis and bone marrow biopsy, which did not reveal any other lymphoma foci.

It was concluded that the lesion was a primary brain lymphoma and chemotherapy protocol was started (Fig. 2.4).

© Springer International Publishing AG, part of Springer Nature 2018
M. Špero, H. Vavro, *Neuroradiology - Expect the Unexpected*,
https://doi.org/10.1007/978-3-319-73482-8_2

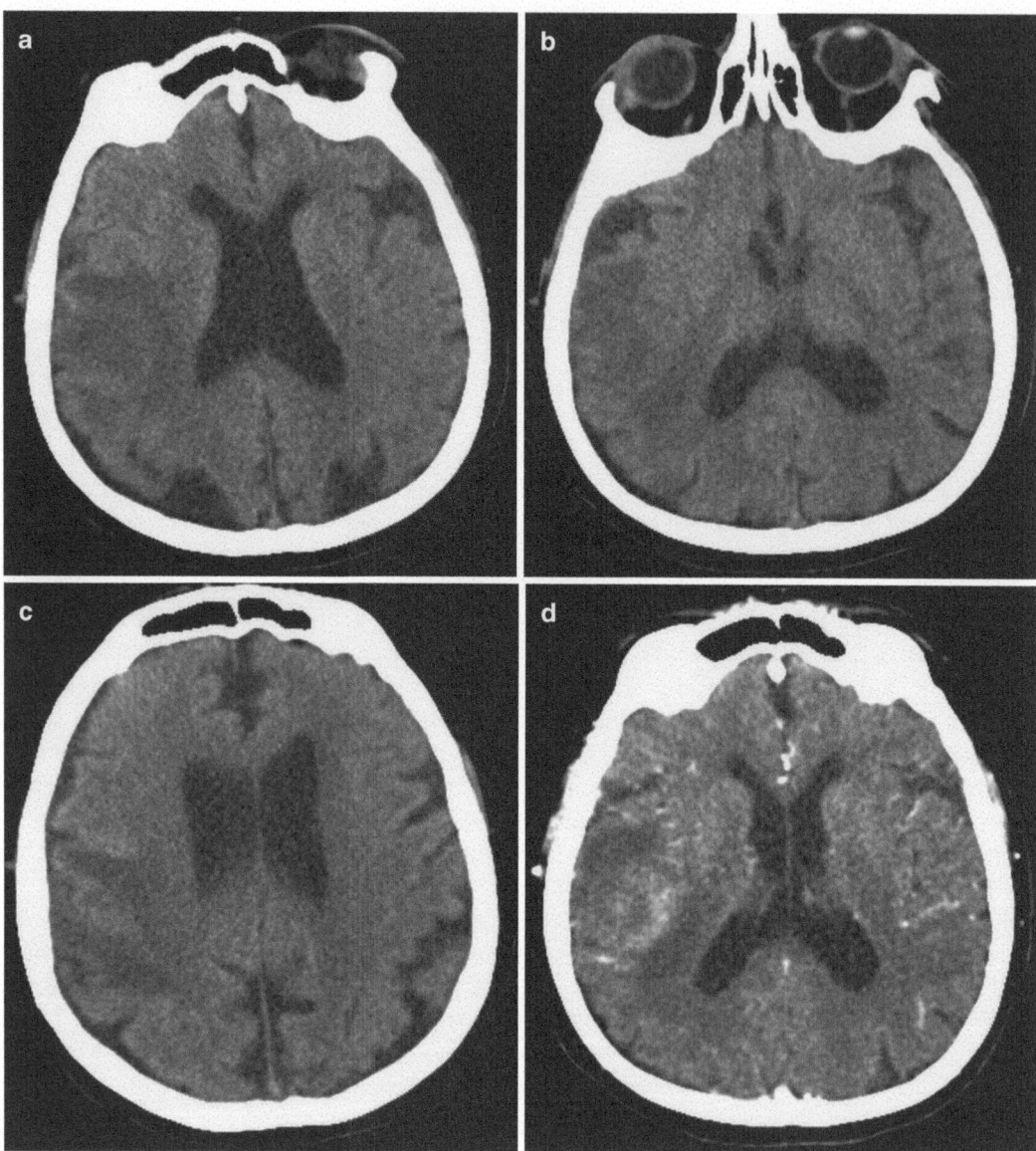

Fig. 2.1 Non-contrast- (**a–c**) and contrast-enhanced (**d–i**) CT scan of the brain showing cortical-subcortical irregular hypodensity with sulcal effacement and gyriform contrast enhancement in the right frontoparietal operculum

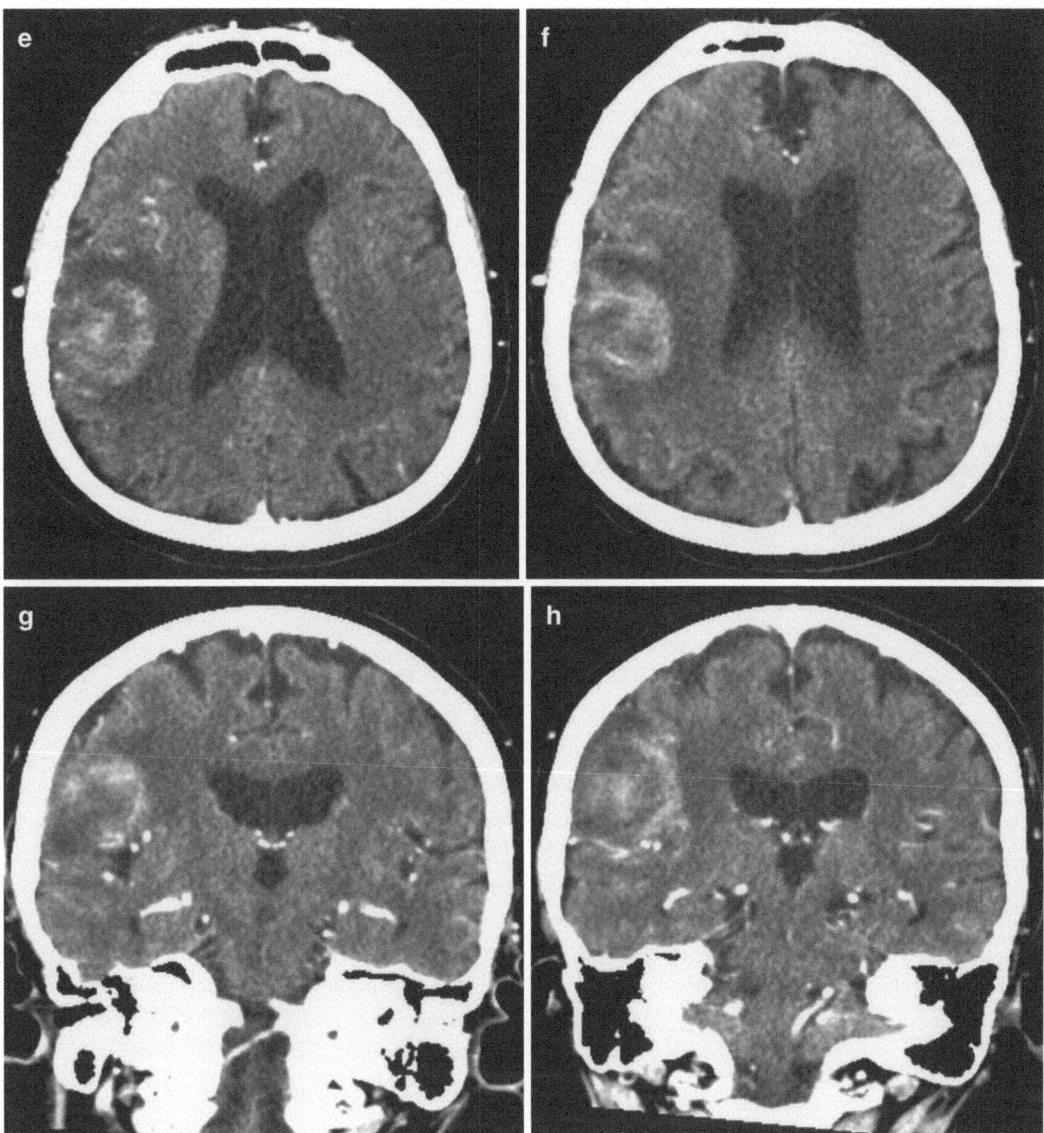

Fig. 2.1 (continued)

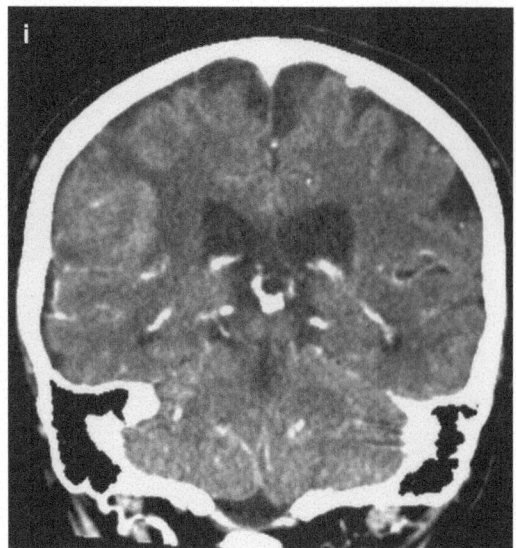

Fig. 2.1   (continued)

2.1   Primary Central Nervous System Lymphoma

Primary central nervous system lymphoma (PCNSL) is a presentation of extranodal lymphoma confined to the central nervous system. It is a relatively uncommon entity, accounting for only 1–2% of all lymphoma cases and 3–6% of all primary brain tumours. The prevalence of PCNSL is higher in immunocompromised patients—a PCNSL in an HIV-seropositive patient is an AIDS-defining condition [1]. Transplant patients are another group at risk for a PCNSL. Additionally, congenital deficiency syndromes and prolonged immunosuppressive therapy, as well as some autoimmune diseases such as Sjogren's syndrome and systemic lupus erythematosus, are reported to be risks for PCNSL development. Histologically, over 90% of PCNSL are high-grade non-Hodgkin B-cell lymphoma. Malignant cells accumulate around and within blood vessels. They mostly present as solitary (60–70%) supratentorial periventricular white matter lesions, although occurrence is possible in the cortex or deep grey matter.

In immunocompetent patients, CT appearance of a PCNSL is that of a hyperdense mass. MR imaging reveals a T1 hypointense, T2 hypointense to isointense lesion with a very low diffusion coupled with characteristic dark appearance on ADC maps—it is a hypercellular tumour with high nucleus-to-cytoplasm ratio. Both CT and MR post-contrast enhancements are typically avid and homogeneous, indicating breakdown of the blood-brain barrier. Linear enhancement along perivascular spaces is highly suggestive of PCNSL [2]. Most lesions occur in the central hemispheric or in periventricular white matter [2]. There is a propensity of PCNSL to spread through subependymal white matter, involving the periventricular regions, corpus callosum and septum pellucidum. Crossing of the corpus cal-

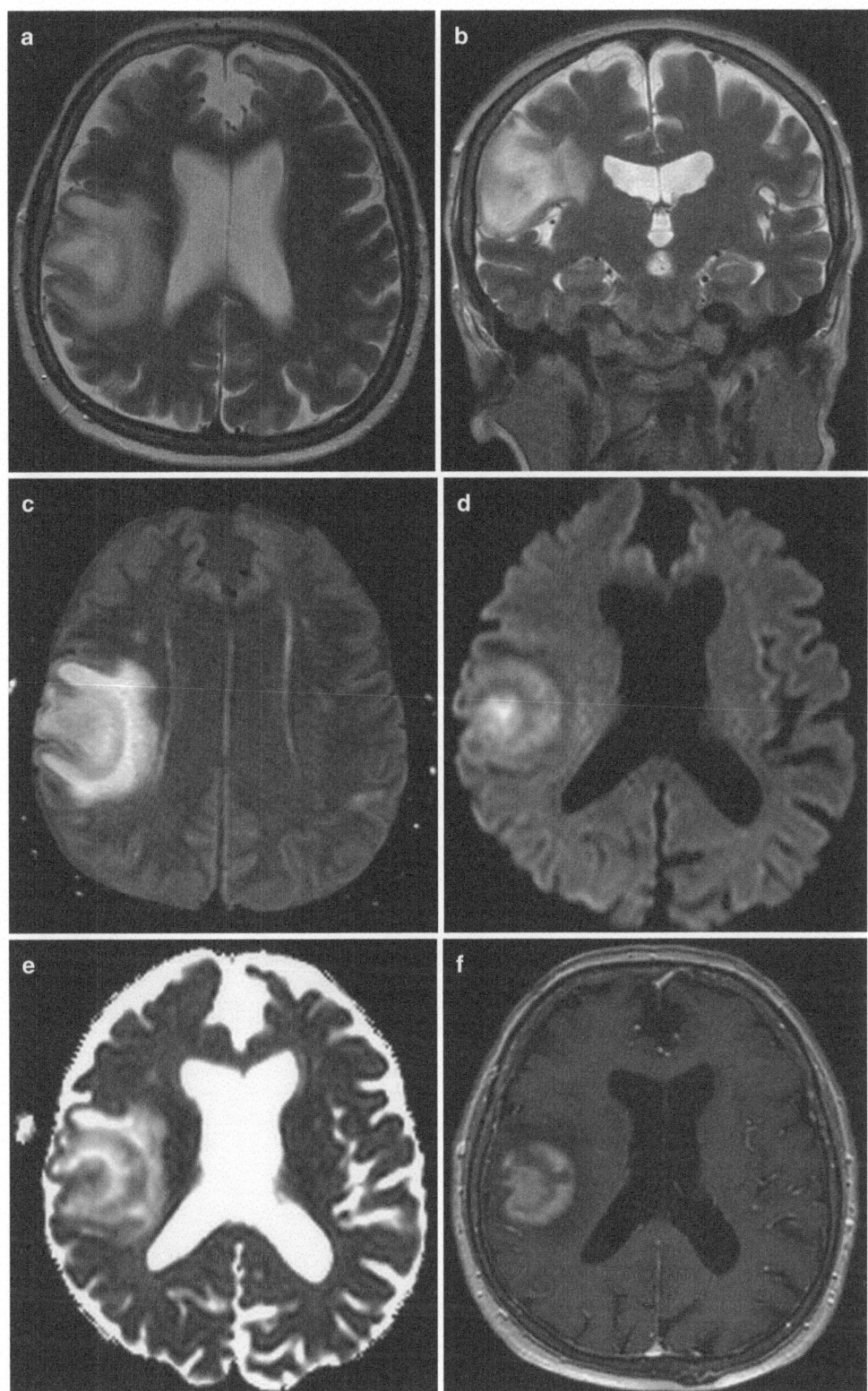

Fig. 2.2 Brain MRI exam—axial (**a**) and coronal (**b**) T2WI, axial T2-FLAIR image (**c**), axial DWI (**d**) and ADC map (**e**), post-contrast axial T1WI (**f**). The report described right-sided frontal cytotoxic cortical oedema and gyriform enhancement which was probably in keeping with acute or subacute ischaemic lesion

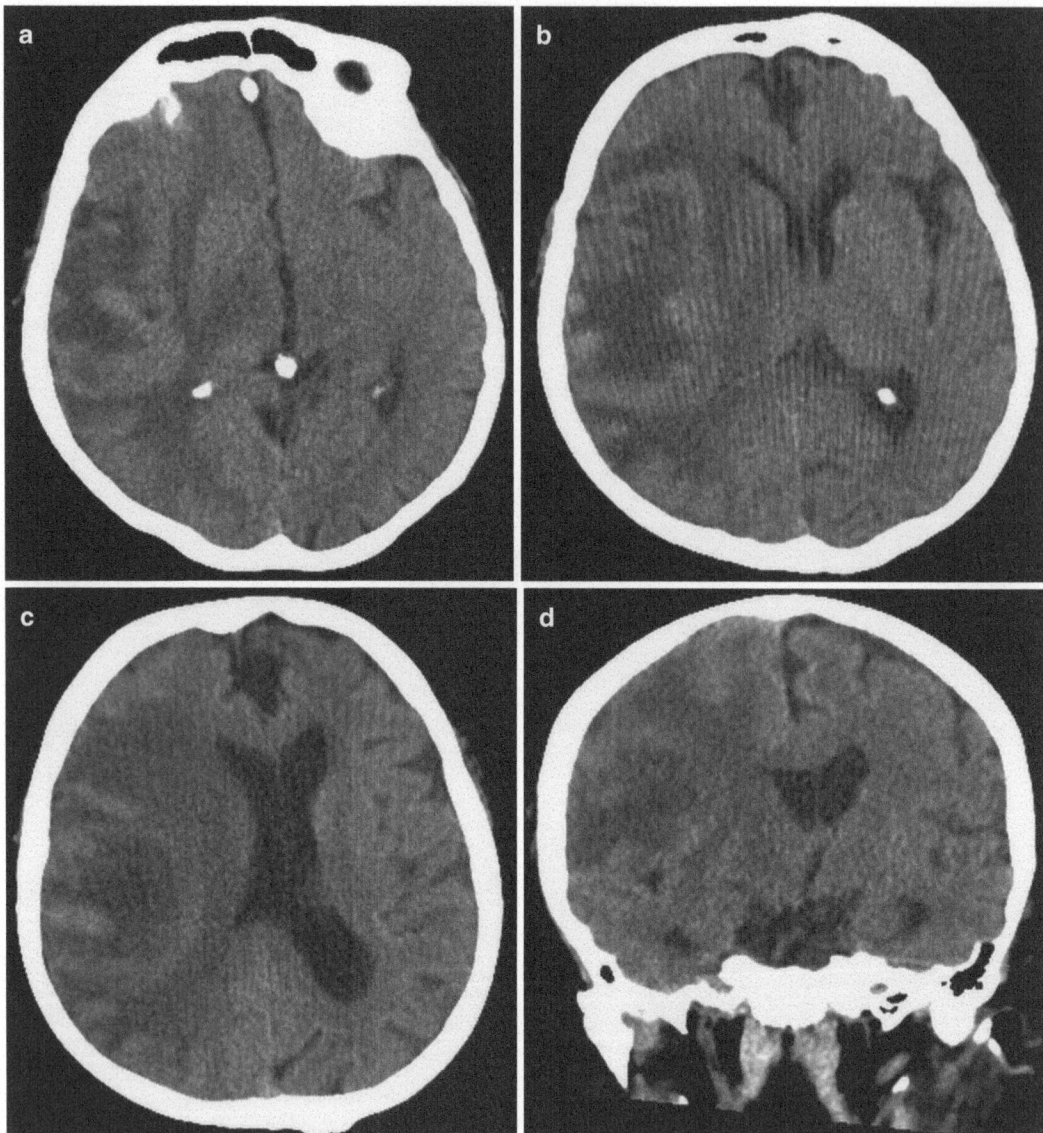

Fig. 2.3 Non-contrast and contrast-enhanced CT exam of the brain—non-contrast axial (**a**–**c**) and coronal reformatted (**d**–**f**) images. Contrast-enhanced axial (**g**, **h**) and coronal reformatted (**i**) images. There has been enlarge-ment of the irregular intra-axial lesion in the right-sided frontal lobe, with progression of the perifocal oedema and mass effect. The findings were suggestive of a space-occupying lesion

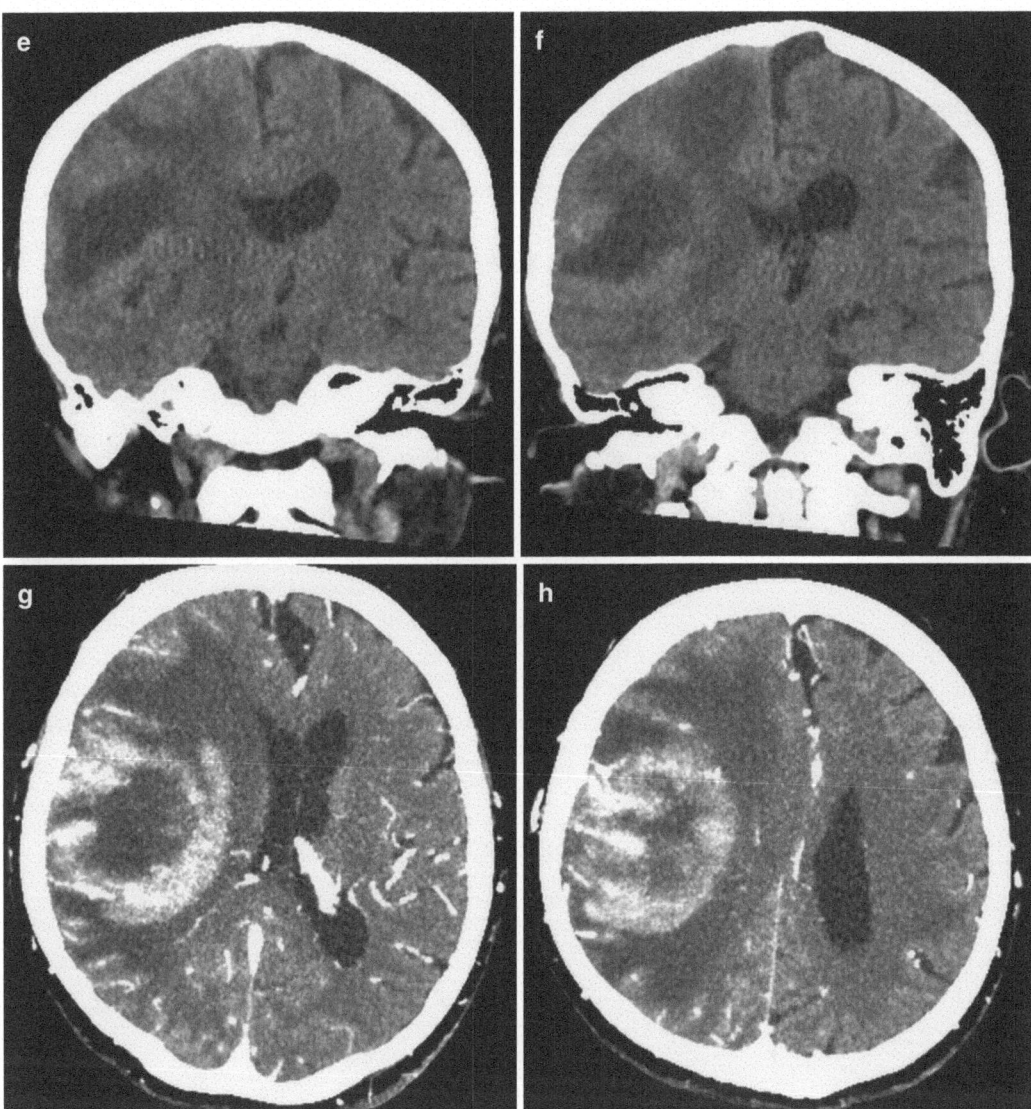

Fig. 2.3 (continued)

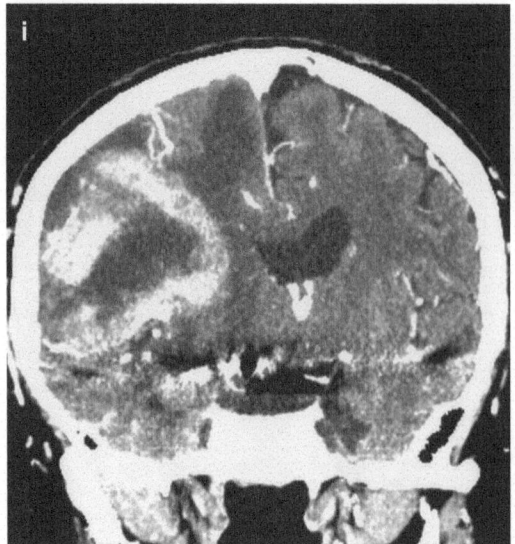

Fig. 2.3 (continued)

losum is not uncommon. Usually there is associated vasogenic oedema and mass effect, less prominent than in malignant gliomas or metastases. On perfusion studies, there is a very mild or absent increase in rCBV, as opposed to a very high rCBV in malignant gliomas.

Pretherapeutic ADC measurement within the contrast-enhancing tumour tissue is predictive of the clinical tumour behaviour—lower ADC values mean shorter progression-free survival and overall survival. Under treatment, ADC increase indicates favourable response to therapy [2].

In immunocompromised patients, the appearances are more of necrotic and haemorrhagic lesions, and contrast enhancement may vary or be completely absent, especially after steroid treatment [3].

Differential diagnoses include glioblastoma (usually necrotic, heterogeneous, irregularly enhancing, with very high rCBV on perfusion studies and not as low ADC values of the solid enhancing tumour), tumefactive demyelination (specific contrast enhancement pattern, minimal oedema, low rCBV), toxoplasmosis, metastatic tumour, abscess [2, 3] and stroke [2]. It is often difficult to uniequivocally differentiate PCNSL from these lesions based on characteristic MR imaging appearance only [2].

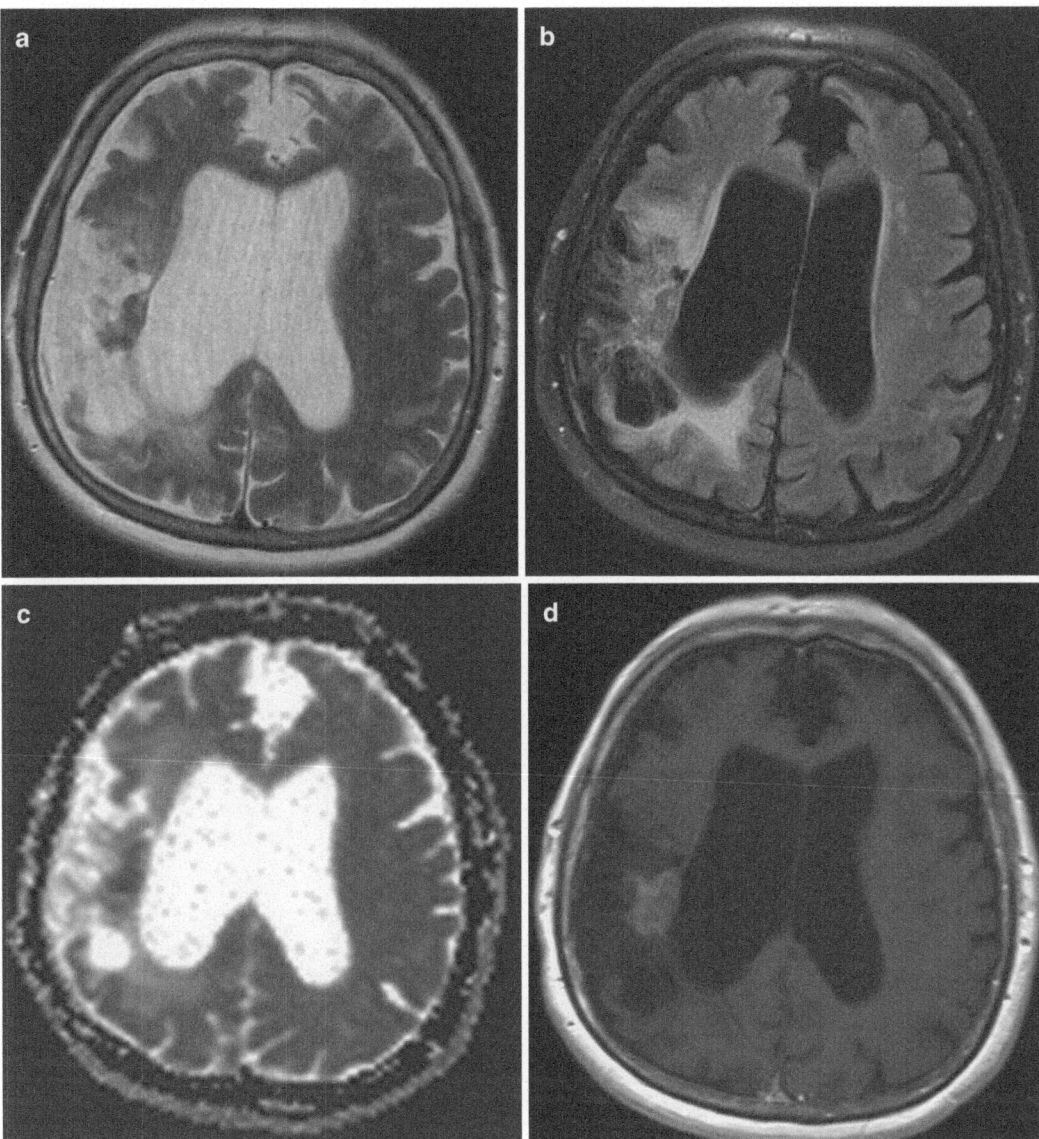

Fig. 2.4 Follow-up MRI of the brain 1 year into therapy – axial T2WI (**a**), axial T2-FLAIR (**b**), axial ADC map (**c**) and axial post-contrast T1WI (**d**). There is a residual/recurrent lymphoma adjacent to the right-sided lateral ventricle. Note the low ADC signal (**c**) of the enhancing tumour (**d**)

References

1. Newton HB, Jolesz FA (2008) Handbook of neuro-oncology neuroimaging. Academic Press, Amsterdam
2. Haldorsen IS et al (2011) Central nervous system lymphoma: characteristic findings on traditional and advanced imaging. Am J Neuroradiol 32(6):984–992. https://doi.org/10.3174/ajnr.A2171
3. Rumboldt Z et al (2010) Brain imaging with MRI and CT: an image pattern approach. Cambridge University Press, New York. https://doi.org/10.1017/CBO9781139030854

Cerebrovascular Infarction: Enlarged Perivascular Spaces

In November 2011, a 64-year-old male patient was referred from his neurologist, as an out-hospital patient, to perform MRI of the brain, due to general weakness with nausea lasting for a year on a daily basis. He worked as a captain of merchant overseas ships and, back then he was retired for a year, had a mild arterial hypertension in anamnesis.

Patient has enclosed MRI of the brain which he performed 5 years before in a private clinic—in year 2006, an experienced neuroradiologist reported those lesions as multiple chronic lacunar infarcts in the left cerebral peduncle. There were no changes in number, size and signal intensities of those lesions comparing two brain MRIs performed in 2006 and 2011 (Fig. 3.1). Lacunar infarctions are differential diagnosis of enlarged PVSs, but in this particular case, the diagnosis of chronic lacunar infarction reported in 2006 is a misdiagnosis. Although our patient had a mild arterial hypertension, the following facts, together with typical PVS imaging features, exclude chronic lacunar infarction as the diagnosis: there were no other vascular lesions in the rest of the brain parenchyma, cerebral peduncles are not pre-dilection site for lacunar infarcts which are usually larger than PVSs, and chronic lacunar infarction has signal intensities that reflect gliosis.

3.1 Enlarged or Giant Perivascular Spaces

It is important not to mistake enlarged perivascular spaces (PVSs) with cerebral pathologies like cystic neoplasms or lacunar infarcts, because such diagnosis will burden a patient and probably initiate unnecessary diagnostic procedures. PVSs are "do not touch lesions" which require regular timely follow-up MR examinations, for example, the first follow-up MRI about 6 months after the basic one and, if needed, the third follow-up MRI a year after the second one, to detect any increase in size.

Perivascular spaces (PVSs) or Virchow-Robin spaces surround the walls of arteries, arterioles, veins and venules as they course from the sub-arachnoid space through the brain parenchyma. Those spaces represent the lymphatic drainage pathways of the brain and do not communicate directly with subarachnoid spaces [1]. Small perivascular or Virchow-Robin spaces, up to 2 mm in diameter, are common finding in the inferior basal ganglia clustering around the anterior commissure, in the centrum semiovale and in the cerebral peduncle [2].

Perivascular spaces can be moderately enlarged from 2 to 5 mm, but when measure more

© Springer International Publishing AG, part of Springer Nature 2018
M. Špero, H. Vavro, *Neuroradiology - Expect the Unexpected*,
https://doi.org/10.1007/978-3-319-73482-8_3

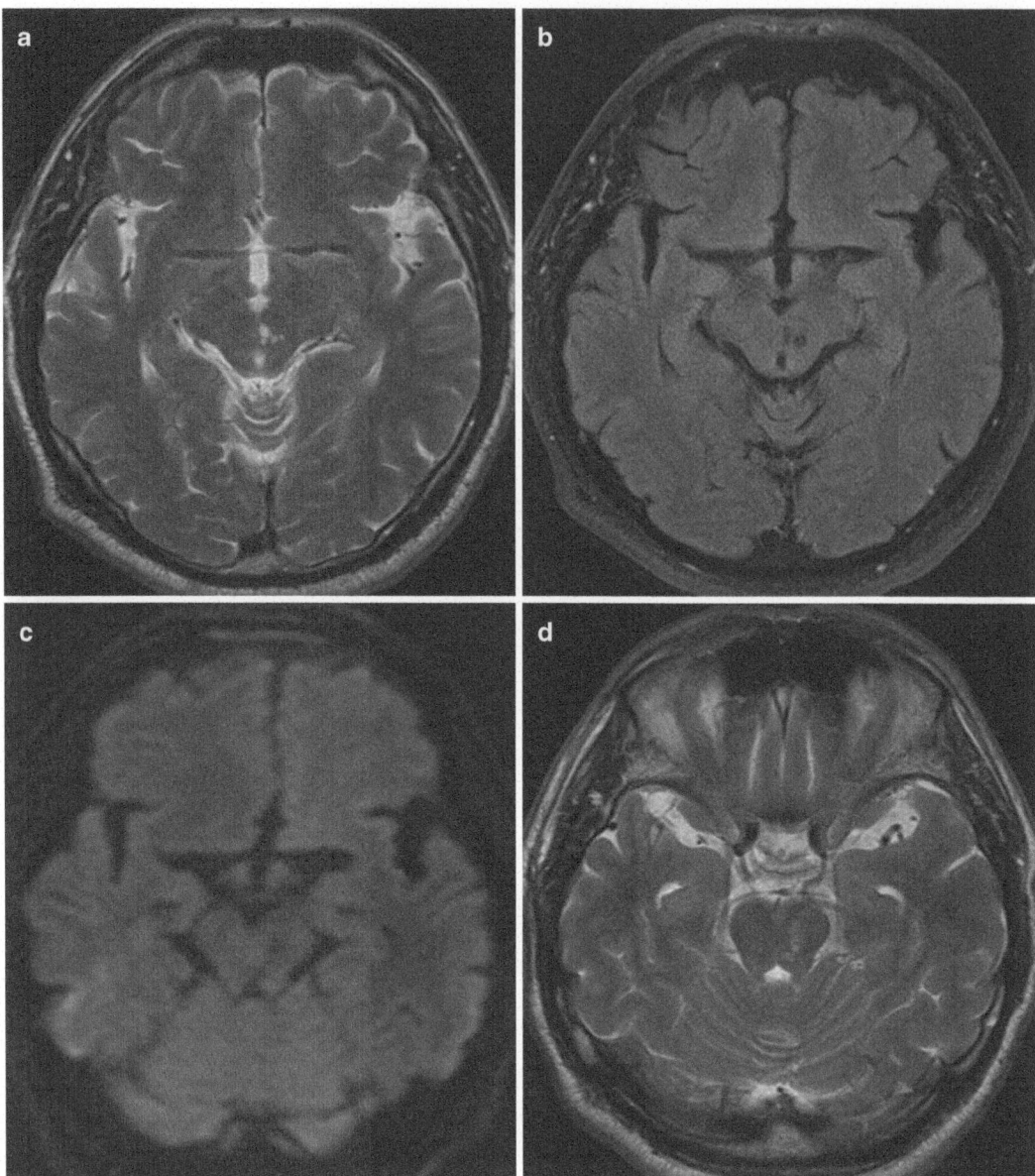

Fig. 3.1 Magnetic resonance imaging of the brain: axial (**a**, **d**) and coronal (**g**, **h**) T2WI, axial FLAIR (**b**, **e**), axial DWI (**c**) and ADC (**f**), axial T2*WI (**i**), post-contrast T1WI (**j**–**l**), revealed multiple, well defined, oval and round lesions in the left cerebral peduncle and two in the right cerebral peduncle, without mass effect. Lesion signal intensities were similar to the CSF on all sequences; there were no restricted diffusion and no contrast enhancement, while the surrounding parenchyma showed normal signal intensities on all sequences. According to the described morphological characteristics, those were reported as enlarged type III perivascular spaces (PVSs)

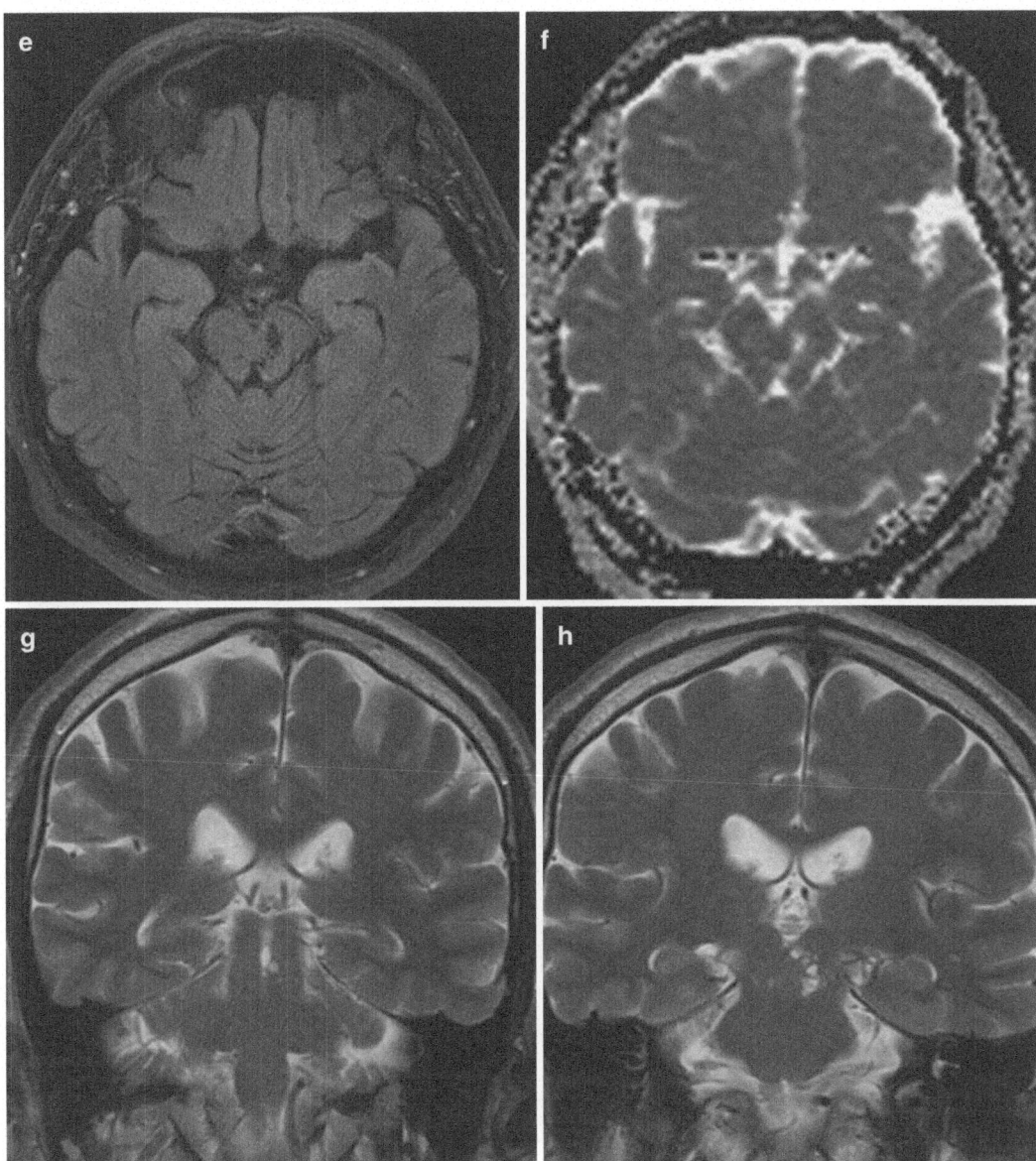

Fig. 3.1 (continued)

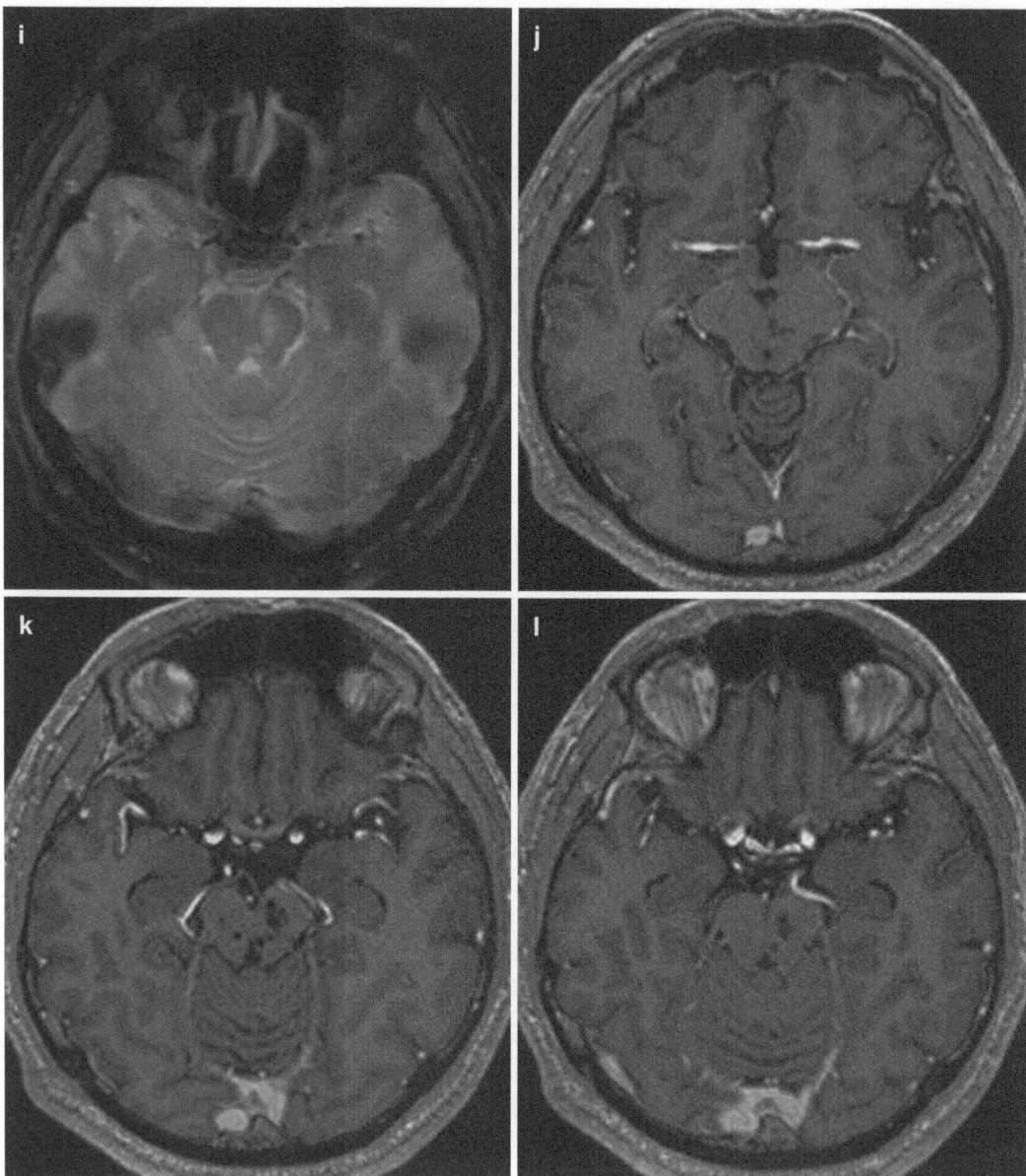

Fig. 3.1 (continued)

than 5 mm, sometimes up to 2 or 3 cm, these are termed giant PV spaces. According to typical locations, there are three types of dilated PVSs: type I appear along the lenticulostriate arteries entering the basal ganglia through the anterior perforated substance, type II are located along the paths of the perforating medullary arteries as they enter the cortical grey matter over the high convexities and extend into the white matter and the third type (III) of dilated PVSs are located in the midbrain—in the lower midbrain at the pontomesencephalic junction and in the upper midbrain at the mesencephalodiencephalic junction [1, 3]. The exact mechanism of PV spaces dilatation is still not defined, but several mechanisms are postulated.

Perivascular spaces are typically oval, round or curvilinear, with well-defined, smooth margin, and on CT are isodense to the CSF, and on MRI they visually follow signal intensities of CSF on all sequences, without contrast enhancement after its administration. When small or moderately enlarged, PVSs do not demonstrate any mass effect, and the surrounding parenchyma is of normal signal intensity [1, 3, 4]. Giant or markedly enlarged PVSs may assume bizarre cystic shapes and cause mass effect, while the surrounding parenchyma may reveal discrete T2 and FLAIR hyperintensities secondary due to gliosis or spongiosis in younger patients or due to advanced chronic ischaemic changes related to mass effect in elderly patients [3]. Alternatively, those signal intensity changes may be related to multiple tiny tightly clustered PVSs that are too small to be discriminated on the basis of current MRI findings [3].

Small or dilated PVSs are asymptomatic and are usually accidental finding on MRI of the brain performed due to symptoms which are not attributable to dilated PVSs, like headache, dizziness, dementia, visual changes, syncope, post-trauma, scizures, memory problems and poor concentration. Giant PVSs may be symptomatic when they are located at the mesencephalothalamic region

where they may compress the adjacent third ventricle or Sylvian aqueduct causing hydrocephalus that requires surgical shunt surgery [1, 3].

It is important to distinguish dilated PVSs not only from cystic neoplasms or lacunar infarcts but also from other cerebral pathologies such as non-neoplastic neuroepithelial cyst, parasitic cysts, periventricular leukomalacia and mucopolysaccharidosis. Cystic neoplasms do not demonstrate signal intensity of the CSF; parasitic cysts like neurocysticercosis usually have a small scolex and enhancing cyst walls. Lacunar infarcts have clinical symptoms of stroke, on MRI have restricted diffusion if acute or show T2 and FLAIR hyperintensities in adjacent parenchyma if chronic. Differentiation between neuroepithelial cysts and enlarged PVSs can be made with certainty only by pathologic study. Patients with mucopolysaccharidosis have typical clinical features, while periventricular leukomalacia occurs in premature infants and shows loss of periventricular, predominantly periatrial white mater [1, 5].

I will end this chapter with several CT and MR images revealing giant PVSs in the right midbrain and right cerebellar hemisphere (Fig. 3.2).

In these two cases, the possibility of enlarged PVSs was not considered as possible differential diagnosis at all. Maybe it is because radiologists sometimes forget about this simple pathology or do not even take it into consideration because they think more often of other, possibly ominous, cerebral pathologies. Therefore, when you find a lesion on brain CT or MRI looking like cystic space with smooth regular margins and normal adjacent parenchyma, located along the course of cerebral vessels, isodense with CSF on CT, having similar signal intensity to CSF in all MR sequences, without contrast enhancement, with or without mass effect, recall this simple diagnosis of enlarged or giant perivascular Virchow-Robin spaces and take it into consideration as differential diagnosis; it will help you in decision-making and solving a case you have in front of you and maybe sweat about.

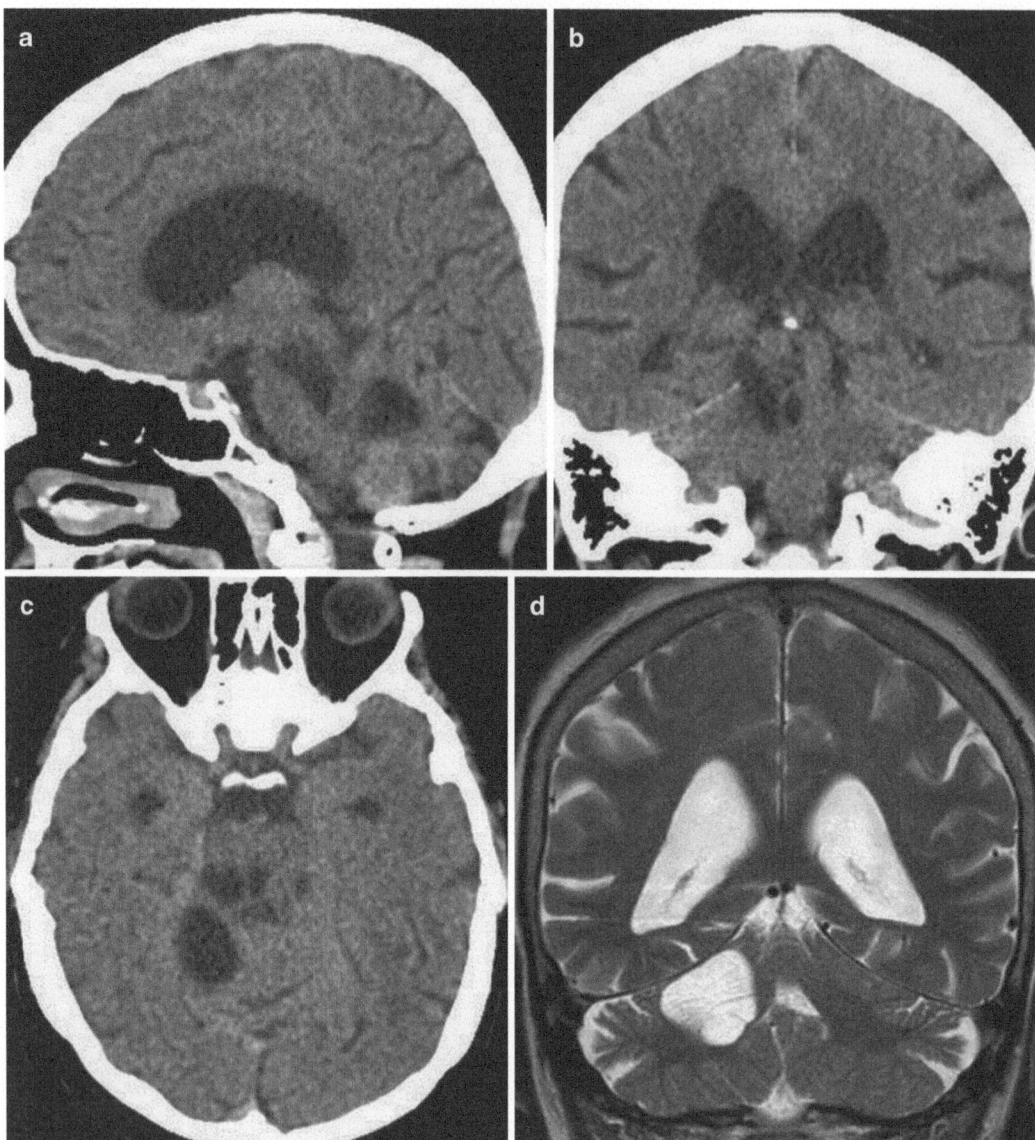

Fig. 3.2 A 75-year-old female with blurred vision on both eyes during several years. Computed tomography (axial **a–c**) and magnetic resonance imaging of the brain: coronal (**d, e**) and axial (**f**) T2WI, axial FLAIR (**g**), DWI (**h**) and ADC (**i**), pre-contrast sagittal T1WI (**j**) and post-contrast axial T1WI (**k, l**), revealed oval and round, well-demarcated cystic lesions in the right cerebral peduncle and upper cerebellar hemisphere showing mild mass effect, isodense with the CSF on CT scans, following signal intensities of the CSF on all MRI sequences, without restricted diffu-sion, without contrast enhancement on post-contrast T1 sequence, without signal intensity changes in adjacent parenchyma. She had several MRIs performed in other hospitals during the past 5 years: cystic lesions and possible cystic neoplasm without changes in size, number and radiological features on follow-up examinations were reported by radiologist in enclosed previous reports—giant perivascular spaces were never mentioned in those reports but were reported in our report due to typical location, size and described radiological features

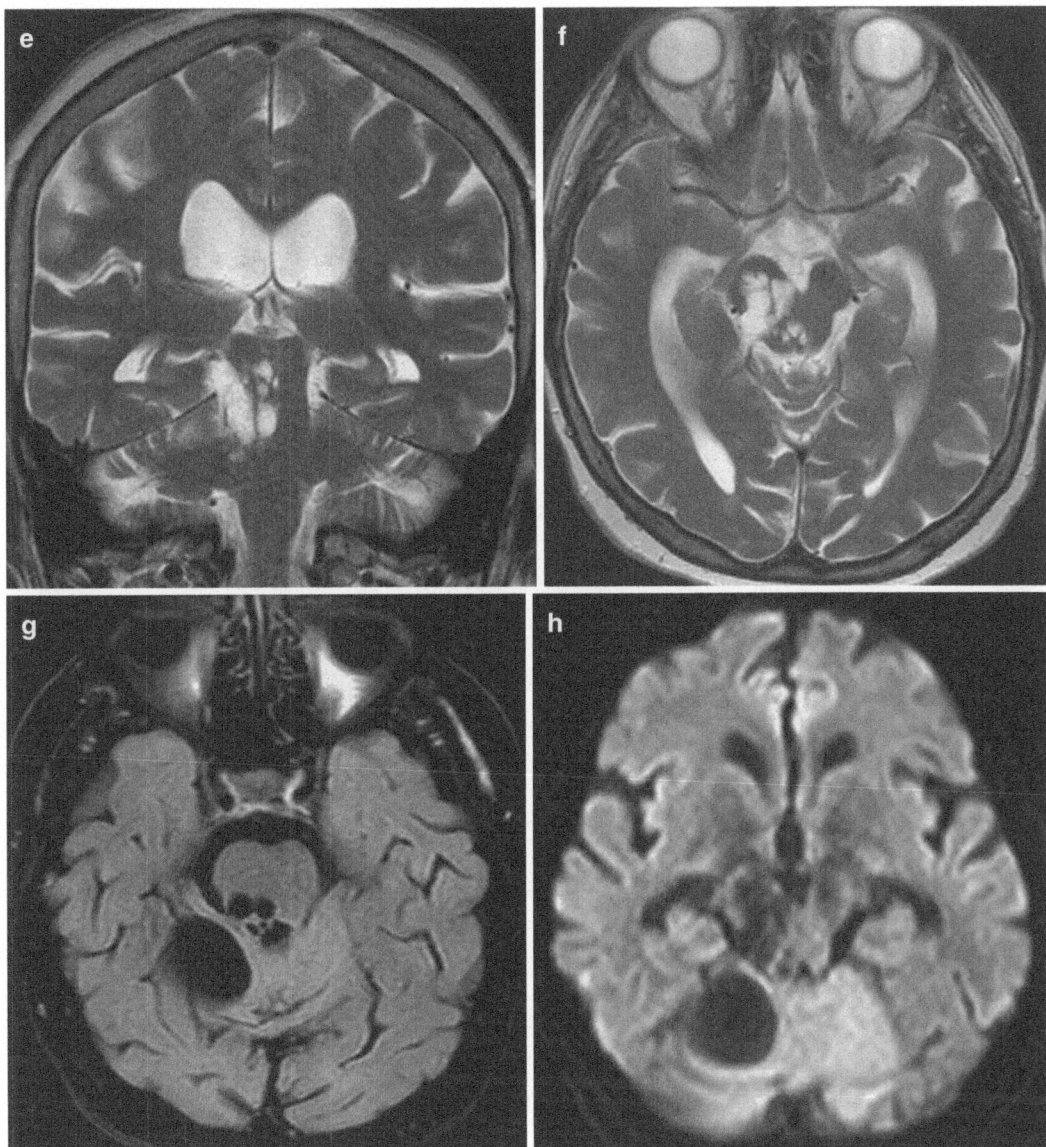

Fig. 3.2 (continued)

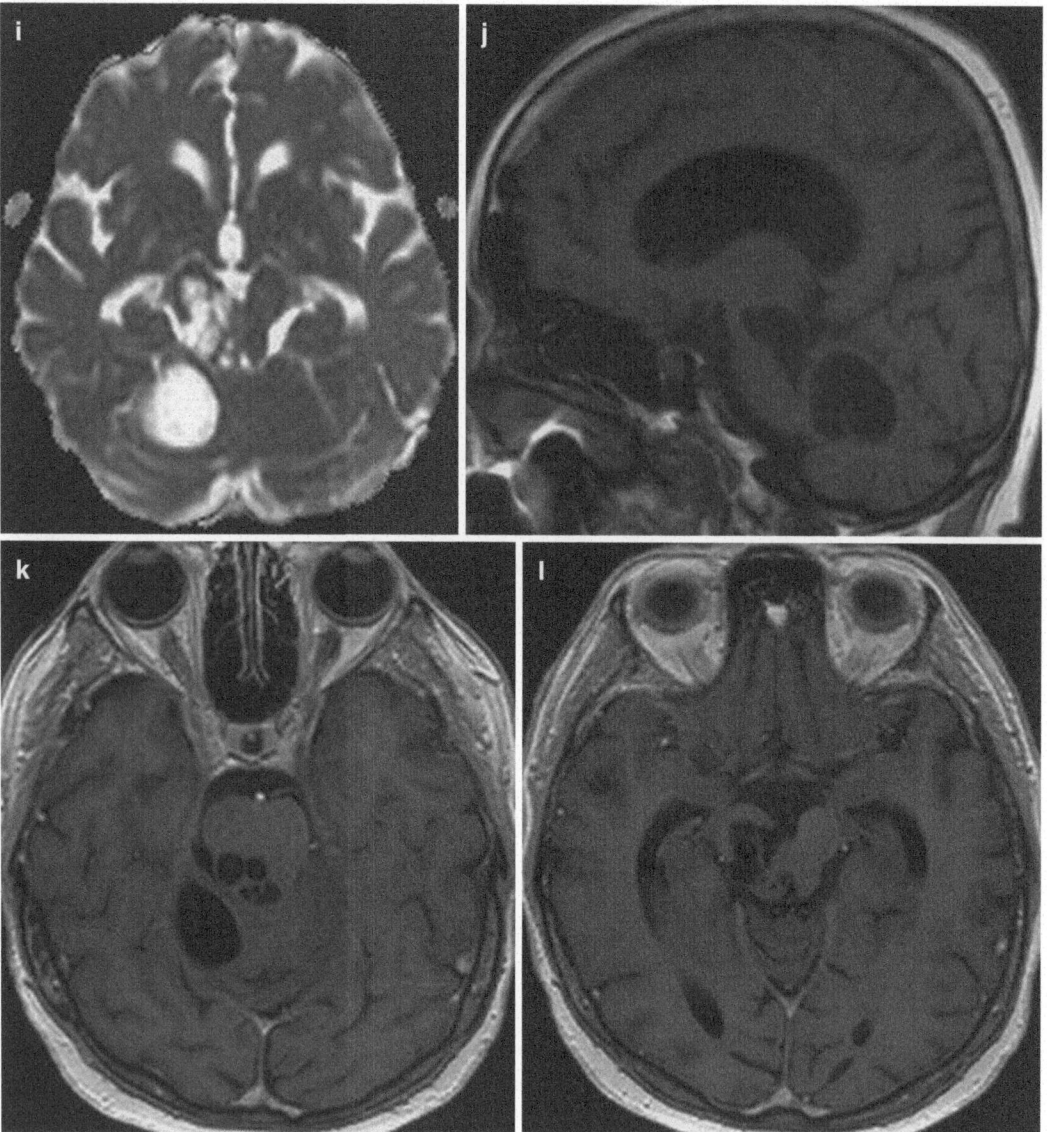

Fig. 3.2 (continued)

References

1. Kwee RM, Kvee TC (2007) Virchow-Robin spaces at MR imaging. Radiographics 27:1071–1086
2. Boukobza M, Laissy JP (2016) Unusual unilateral dilated VR spaces in the basal ganglia with mass effect: diagnosis and follow-up. Glob Imaging Insights 2(1):1–2
3. Salzman KL et al (2005) Giant tumefactive perivascular spaces. Am J Neuroradiol 26:298–305
4. Wani NA et al (2011) Giant cystic Virchow-Robin spaces with adjacent white matter signal alteration. Turk Neurosurg 21(2):235–238
5. Ahmad A et al (2014) Giant perivascular spaces: utility of MR in differentiation from other cystic lesions of the brain. JBR-BTR 97:364–365

Tumefactive Demyelination: Glioblastoma

At the end of November 2014, a 55-year-old male patient woke up in the morning with, as he described, face slightly distorted towards right and discrete speech disorder. During next few days, he noticed he was slightly clumsy with left hand and leg but without more pronounced motor difficulties. He was afebrile, without headache or nausea, and without previous head trauma.

He was admitted to an emergency room at a local hospital: brain CT was performed, but it was unremarkable; there were no signs of stroke, haemorrhage or tumour. Therefore, he was released from the hospital with recommendation for brain MRI. On the first day of December, brain MRI was performed in a private clinic: contrast medium was not applied for unknown reason (Fig. 4.1).

Described expansile lesion was reported as possible tumefactive demyelination lesion (TDL) or tumour, and further diagnostic work-up was recommended. Because weakness of the inferior right half of the face, right hand and leg has progressed during next 2–3 weeks, patient was admitted to a hospital, and wide diagnostic work-up has been commenced, including lumbar puncture and CT of the thorax and abdomen that did not reveal malignant process. CSF analysis did not reveal autoimmune intrathecal process; it demonstrated blood-brain barrier disruption, typical in intrathecal primary or secondary tumours. Follow-up MRI of the brain was performed at the end of December 2014, during hospitalisation (Fig. 4.2).

According to CSF analysis and described imaging features, including enlargement in short time period with development of central necrosis with hemosiderin deposits, distribution of oedema involving corticospinal tract and contrast enhancement pattern, we have reported the lesion was a primary brain tumour. Stereotactic biopsy was performed, and glioblastoma (grade IV) was confirmed. Oncologic therapy, including chemotherapy and irradiation, was conducted, but a patient died about a year after beginning of the symptoms.

4.1 Tumefactive Demyelination or Glioblastoma

Isolated cerebral mass with clinical features including acute or subacute onset, neurologic deficits and contrast enhancement, particularly ring-like or open-ring enhancement, with little mass effect and surrounding oedema should alert radiologist of possible diagnosis: TDL, brain tumour or glioblastoma?

Tumefactive demyelinating lesions (TDLs) are large (2–6 cm or larger) demyelinating lesions that usually appear as solitary supratentorial lesions with little mass effect and surrounding vasogenic oedema which are usually less conspicuous than malignancy but increase with larger lesions. They have predilection for white matter of frontal and parietal lobes but may

M. Špero, H. Vavro, *Neuroradiology - Expect the Unexpected*,
https://doi.org/10.1007/978-3-319-73482-8_4

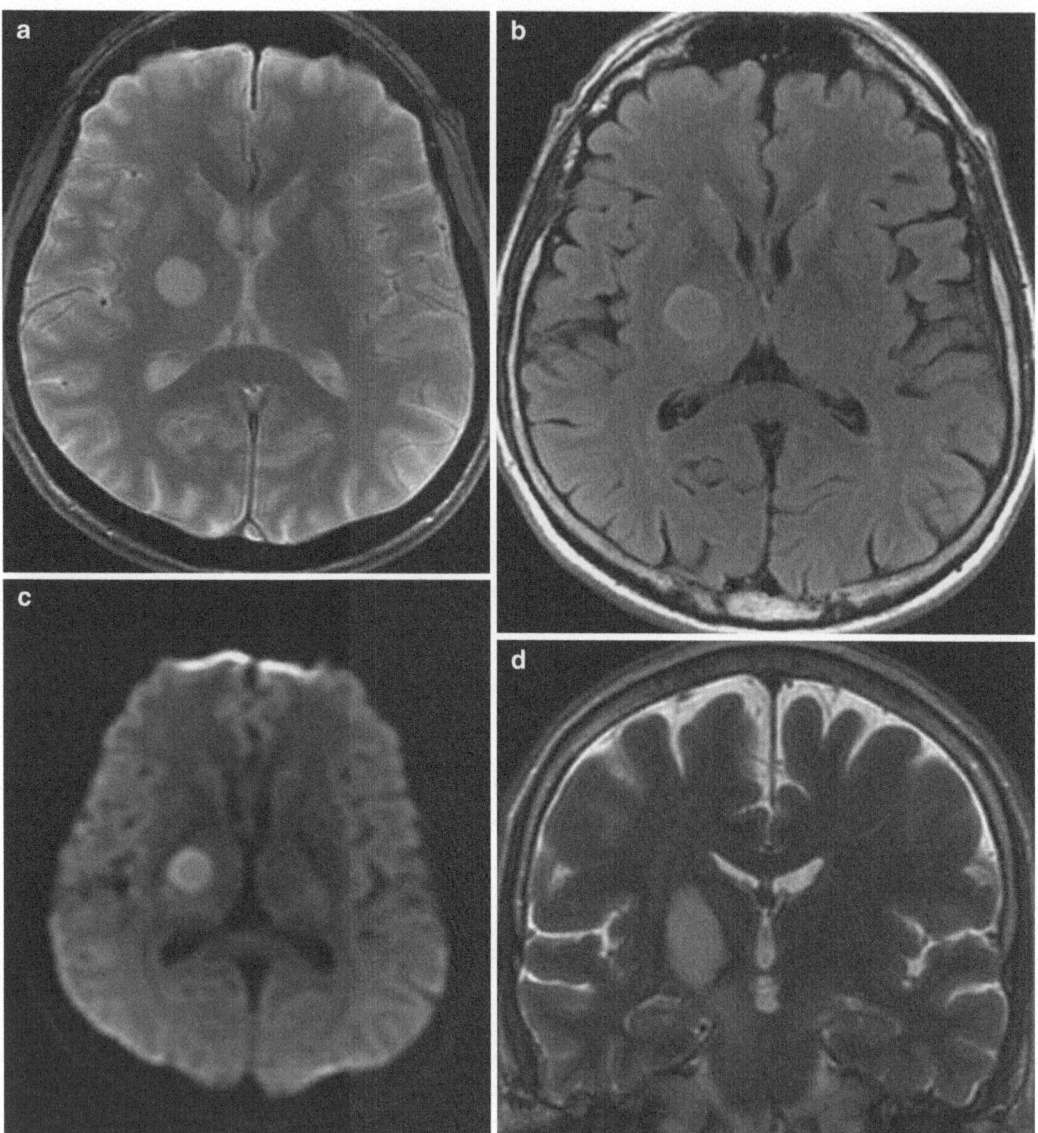

Fig. 4.1 Non-contrast MRI of the brain, axial greT2*WI (**a**), FLAIR (**b**), DWI (**c**), coronal T2WI (**d**), sagittal T1WI (**e**), axial ADC (**f**), revealed supratentorial expansile lesion, oval and well-circumscribed (16 × 16 × 27 mm) in the globus pallidus and genu of internal capsule, without surrounding vasogenic oedema, except a mild oedema coming from the inferior rim of the lesion to the right cerebral peduncle. It was hypointense on T1WI, moderately hyperintense on T2WI and FLAIR, did not show restricted diffusion. There was no central dilated vascular structure within the lesion on T2WI and greT2*WI

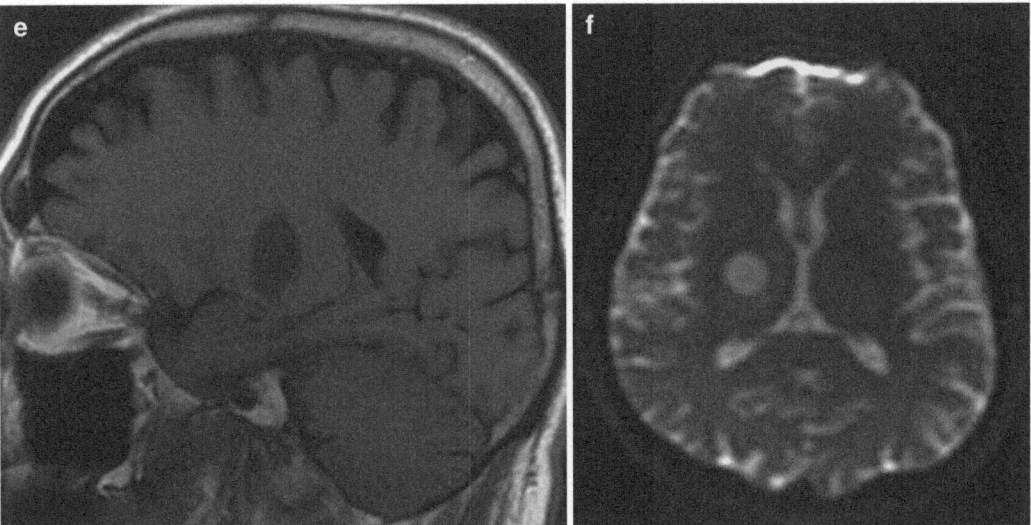

Fig. 4.1 (continued)

involve corpus callosum or basal ganglia as well [1]. Glioblastoma is the most common and most malignant brain tumour: the mortality and disability rates are among the highest. Therefore, early diagnosis and surgical treatment followed by radiation and chemotherapy are key to prolonging patient life and improving their life quality.

Clinical presentation of TDL and brain tumours includes symptoms of an increased intracranial pressure (headache and vomiting), local neurological deficits and seizures [2]. In gliomas, symptoms usually have longer duration between onset and admission (weeks to months), while in TDLs have more acute onset and shorter duration [3]. Clinical presentation and imaging characteristics of TDL overlap with brain tumours; therefore, it is not rare to misdiagnose TDL with intracranial tumours, especially gliomas. Primary brain lymphoma and metastases are other possibilities. To avoid misdiagnosis and consequently unnecessary surgery or even radiotherapy, it is important to try to distinguish TDL and brain tumour. Differentiation of TDL and brain tumours presents a diagnostic challenge; sometimes it is not possible only according to imaging features and clinical presentation—CSF analysis is more than helpful, but correct diagnosis is often made after biopsy.

Both TDL and glioblastoma may present as a well-circumscribed or ill-defined lesion. Central necrosis and cystic degeneration are typical for glioblastoma but are present in cases of severe demyelination, while signs of haemorrhage of different age are seen in glioblastoma. Peripheral diffusion restriction is present in TDL due to intramyelinic oedema in acute or subacute phase and due to hypercellular part of a tumour. Low-grade gliomas usually present as subcortical mass with little mass effect and surrounding vasogenic oedema, without contrast enhancement, while high-grade gliomas enhance and demonstrate pronounced mass effect and vasogenic oedema [2].

TDLs demonstrate ring-like or open-ring pattern of contrast enhancement: enhancing periphery represents advancing area of active inflammation, while non-enhancing core represents more chronic phase of the inflammatory process. Metastases and gliomas in certain cases may show ring-like contrast enhancement [1, 2].

Dilated vascular structure running centrally within the lesion on T2W and T2*W images probably represents dilated vein draining towards the distended subependymal veins, and is specific for TDLs, and may be used to distinguish it from gliomas [2, 4]. Perfusion studies showed decreased relative cerebral blood volume (rCBV)

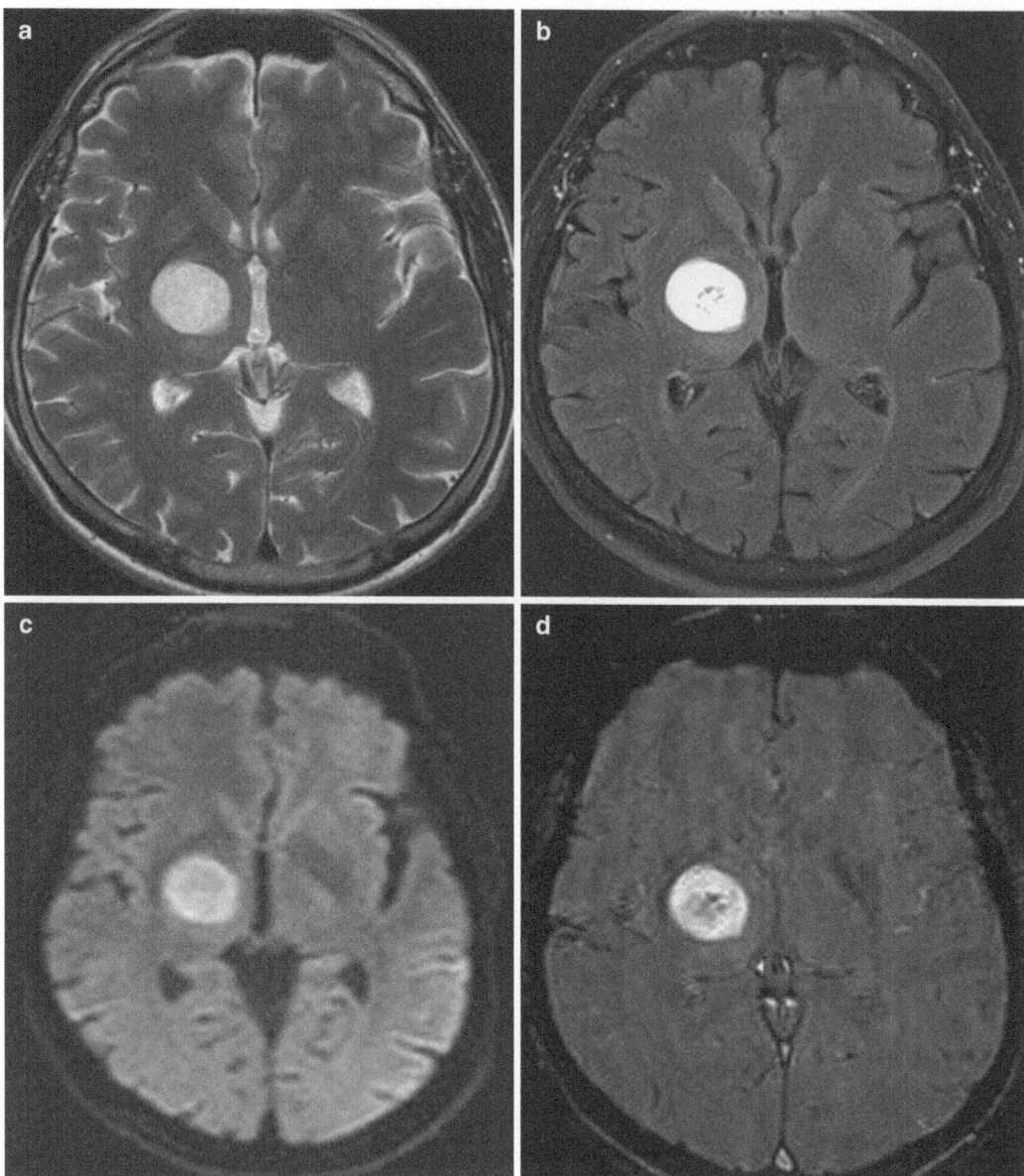

Fig. 4.2 Follow-up brain MRI performed about 4 weeks after the initial one, axial T2WI (**a**), FLAIR (**b**), DWI (**c**), axial SWI (**d**), coronal T2WI (**e**), axial ADC (**f**), sagittal T1WI (**g**), post-contrast axial T1WI (**h**), single-voxel MR spectroscopy (**i**): during 4 weeks expansile lesion (25 × 25 × 34 mm) in the right globus pallidus and genu of the internal capsule had enlarged, with central necrosis (**b**, **h**) and hemosiderin deposits (**c**). It showed intensive contrast enhancement in the rest of the lesion (**h**). Oedema in the right cerebral peduncle was more pronounced involving anterior right half of the pons (**e**). MR spectroscopy demonstrated elevated choline and moderately decreased NAA levels, and inverted lactate/lipids peak at 1.3 ppm

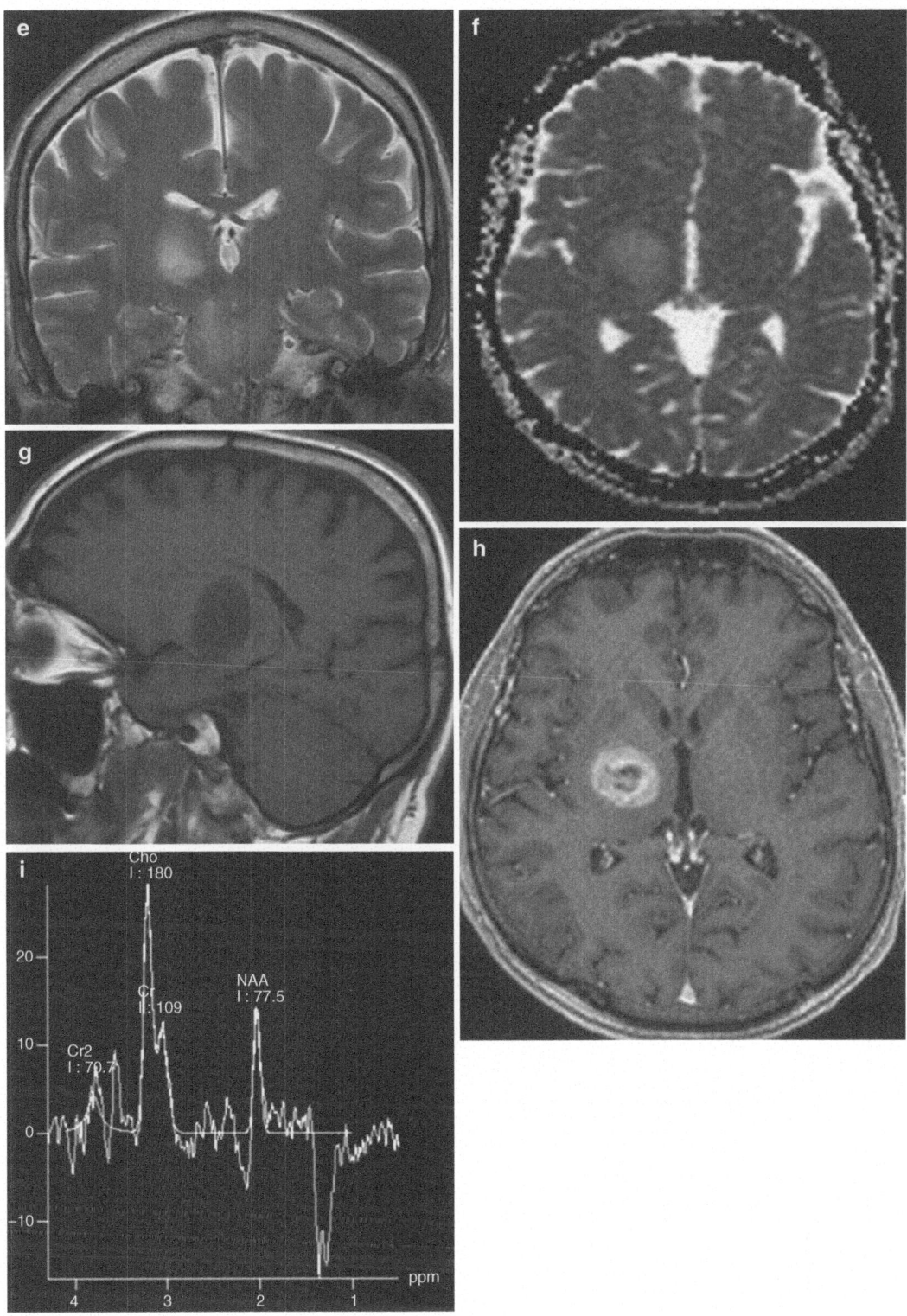

Fig. 4.2 (continued)

in TDL, while, due to vascular proliferation and tumour angiogenesis, rCBV is increased in glioblastoma compared to TDL [5].

Elevated choline level and decreased NAA levels on MR spectroscopy are typically regarded as diagnostic feature of brain tumours, with lactate/lipid signal at 1.3 ppm. In active demyelination, MRS shows increased choline and lactate levels and decreased NAA levels as well, allowing inflammatory demyelinating process to mimic malignant glioma: NAA/Cr ratios are normal or decreased due to neuronal or axonal loss concomitant with increased choline levels corresponding to glial proliferation that occurs in demyelinating plaques [6, 7].

Toh and his team suggested diffusion tensor imaging (DTI) could be helpful in differentiating TDL from high-grade gliomas by using visual inspections and quantitative analysis [8].

In our case it was important to distinguish between TDL and primary brain tumour. It was not easy: clinical presentation, lesion location and brain CT finding, together with the initial brain MRI, were more in favour of secondary TDL, although there was no central vein sing on greT2*WI or restricted diffusion due to possible intramyelinic oedema. Follow-up MRI was more in favour of tumour due to enlargement in size in short time, development of central necrosis with hemosiderin deposits. CSF analysis was more than helpful in decision making: no obvious oligoclonal band or pleocytosis confirmed our suspicion. Final confirmation was done by lesion biopsy.

References

1. Abdoli M, Freedman MS (2015) Neuro-oncology dilemma: tumour or tumefactive demyelinating lesion. Mult Scler Relat Disord 4:555–566
2. Qi W et al (2015) Cerebral tumefactive demyelinating lesions. Oncol Lett 10:1763–1768
3. Kim DS et al (2009) Distinguishing tumefactive demyelinating lesions from glioma or central nervous system lymphoma: added value of unenhanced CT compared with conventional contrast-enhanced MR imaging. Radiology 251:467–475
4. Fallah A et al (2010) Tumefactive demyelinating lesions: a diagnostic challenge. Can J Surg 53(1):69–70
5. Wang S et al (2011) Differentiation between glioblastomas, solitary brain metastases, and primary cerebral lymphomas using diffusion tensor and dynamic susceptibility contrast-enhanced MR imaging. AJNR Am J Neuroradiol 32(3):507–514
6. Oz P et al (2014) Clinical proton MR spectroscopy in central nervous system disorders. Radiology 270(3):658–679
7. Hayashi T et al (2003) Inflammatory demyelinating disease mimicking malignant glioma. J Nucl Med 44:565–569
8. Toh CH et al (2012) Differentiation of tumefactive demyelinating lesions from high-grade gliomas with the use of diffusion tensor imaging. AJNR Am J Neuroradiol 33:846–851

Cerebrovascular Infarction: Glioblastoma

5

While sitting in front of TV with his family on a calm Sunday evening, a 63-year-old man suddenly experienced what looked like tonic seizures of his left arm and face and became unresponsive for a moment or two. Afterwards he had speech difficulties and left facial droop. The patient had no previous health issues. He was immediately brought to an emergency hospital department, and a CT exam of the brain was done (Fig. 5.1).

However, the second reader was not convinced this was an ischaemic lesion, in spite of abrupt onset of symptoms. A brain MRI exam was recommended (Fig. 5.2).

The patient was immediately scheduled for a neurosurgical stereotactic tumour biopsy. The histopathological examination revealed a glioblastoma (WHO grade IV).

5.1 Glioblastoma

Glioblastoma (GB) is the most common malignant primary brain tumour in adults. It represents about 15% of all primary brain tumours and 60–75% of all astrocytomas. The most common type is IDH wild-type form, which corresponds to clinically defined primary GB [1], occurring without evidence of a lower-grade precursor tumour, with a short clinical course of approximately 3 months; mean patient age is 55 years [2, 3]. IDH-mutant type, clinically defined as secondary, is less frequent, arises from a lower-grade astrocytoma, has a longer clinical course and affects younger patients (mean age 40 years) [2, 3].

GB is frequently hypodense on CT and hyperintense in T2 MRI images. Thus, it is often difficult to assess its size on non-contrast-enhanced CT, due to the similar appearance of the perifocal vasogenic oedema. The oedema is generally infiltrative, containing tumour cells beyond the enhancement borders [4]. Post-contrast imaging almost always demonstrates thick, irregular peripheral enhancement and unenhanced central necrotic part of the lesion. Solid, enhanced portions of the tumour often show increased DWI signal and ADC hypointensity. Large haemorrhage is uncommon, but there are often T2* or SWI hypointensities representing small haemorrhagic foci. MRS features elevated choline and decreased NAA, in necrotic areas also elevated lipid and lactate peaks. A characteristic of glioblastoma perfusion imaging is markedly elevated rCBV.

In 10–20% of cases, the initial imaging studies show multifocal lesions. Spread along white matter tracts is common. True multicentric tumours are uncommon.

Seizures are not as common at presentation as in low-grade gliomas. Typically patients present with a focal neurological deficit or symptoms of increased intracranial pressure, rarely with stroke-like symptoms. However, in rare cases a sudden alteration of neurological status is caused by haemorrhage or direct vascular infiltration and subsequent acute cerebral infarct [4].

M. Špero, H. Vavro, *Neuroradiology - Expect the Unexpected*,
https://doi.org/10.1007/978-3-319-73482-8_5

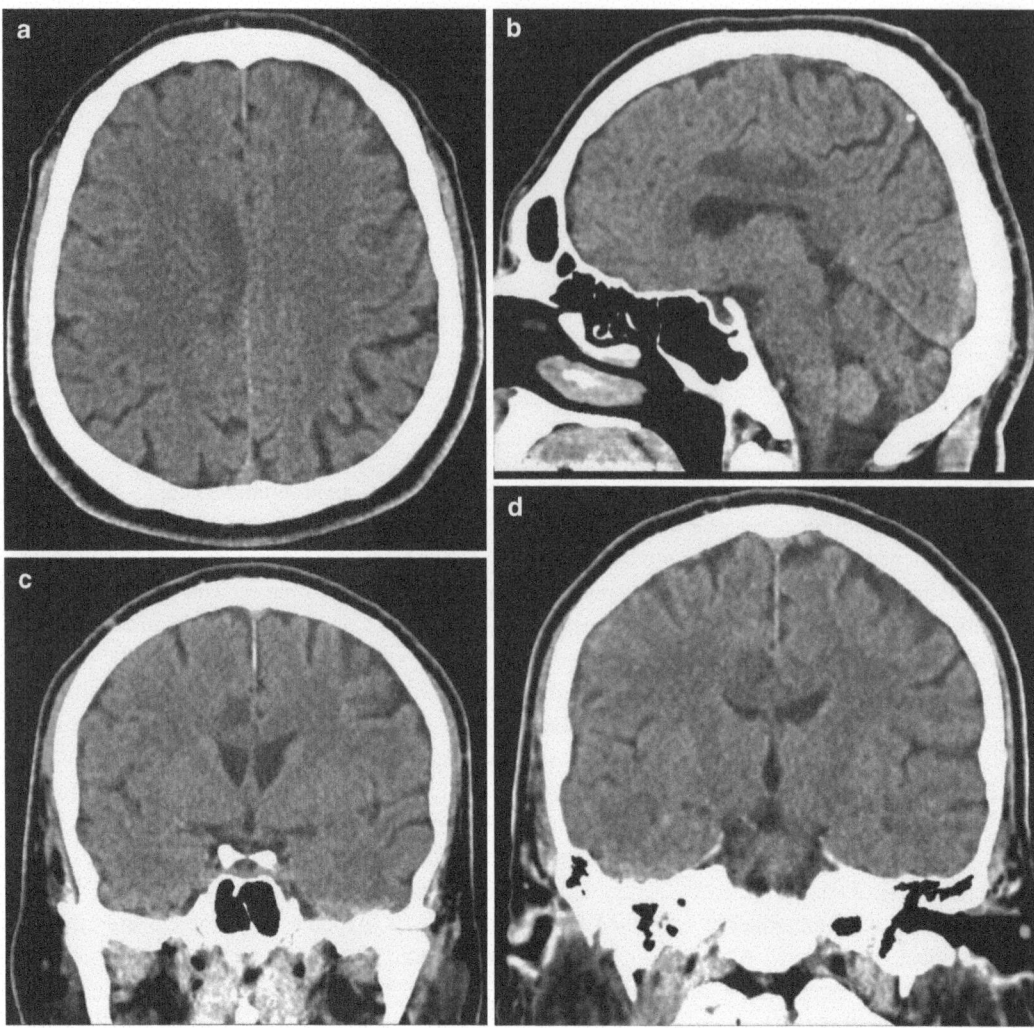

Fig. 5.1 Initial CT exam of the brain—axial image (**a**) with sagittal (**b**) and coronal (**c**, **d**) reformatted images done in an emergency setting. A hypodense lesion adjacent to the body of corpus callosum on the right (in the right cingulate gyrus) in keeping with an acute ischaemic lesion was reported

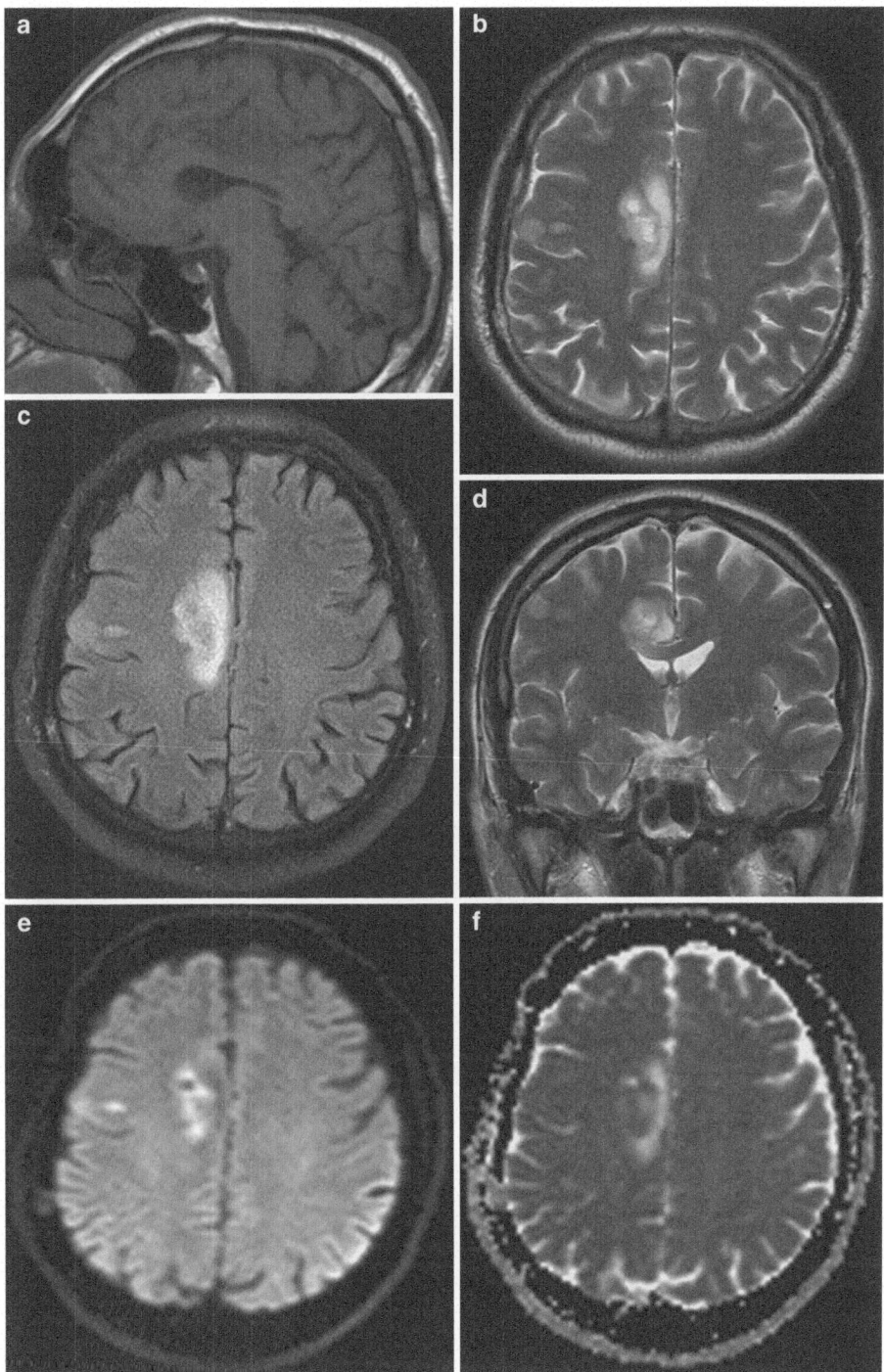

Fig. 5.2 MRI exam of the brain—sagittal T1WI (**a**), axial T2WI (**b**), axial T2-FLAIR (**c**), axial DWI (**d**), axial ADC (**e**), coronal T2WI (**f**) and post gadolinium coronal (**g**), axial (**h**) and sagittal (**i**) T1WI demonstrate a peripherally enhancing lesion within the right-sided cingulate gyrus, with perifocal oedema and mild compression of the corpus callosum. Additionally, there are two smaller enhancing lesions in the lateral basal aspect of the right precentral gyrus. The findings are suggestive of a space-occupying lesion (glioma) with two smaller satellite lesions. No features of acute ischaemia were found—the DWI and ADC signal abnormalities are subtle—in the core of the biggest lesion they are actually opposite of what would be expected in an ischaemic lesion. The peripheral DWI hyperintensities reveal the hypercellular segments of the tumour, which also enhance the most

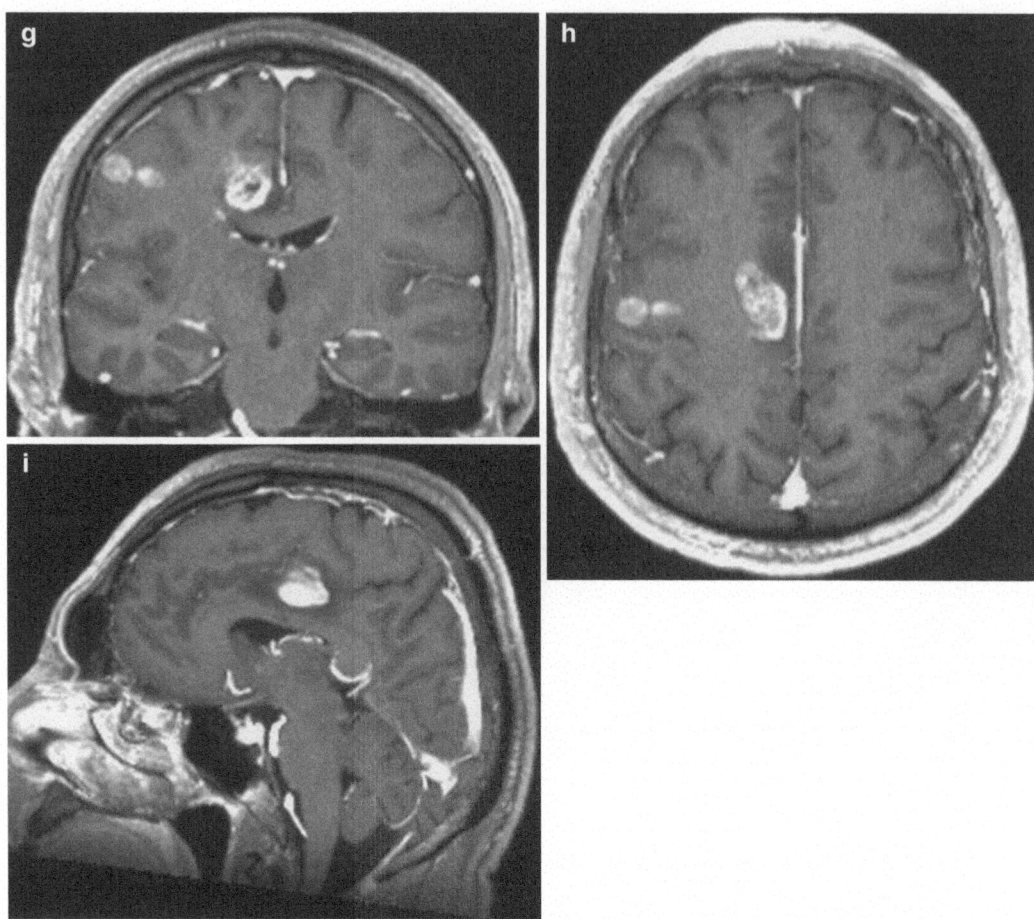

Fig. 5.2 (continued)

Differential diagnoses include metastasis, primary CNS lymphoma, tumefactive demyelinating lesion (see Chap. 4), abscess and subacute infarction.

References

1. Komori T (2017) The 2016 WHO classification of tumours of the central nervous system: the major points of revision. Neurol Med Chir 57(7):301–311. https://doi.org/10.2176/nmc.ra.2017-0010

2. Altman DA et al (2007) Best cases from the AFIP: glioblastoma multiforme. Radiographics 27(3):883–888

3. Eidel O et al (2017) Tumor infiltration in enhancing and non-enhancing parts of glioblastoma: a correlation with histopathology. PLoS One 12(1):e0169292. https://doi.org/10.1371/journal.pone.0169292

4. Pina S et al (2014) Acute ischemic stroke secondary to glioblastoma. A case report. Neuroradiol J 27(1): 85–90. https://doi.org/10.15274/NRJ-2014-10009

Cystic Pituitary Macroadenoma: Rathke's Cleft Cyst with Intracystic Nodule

6

During the spring of 2014, a 22-year-old female patient was admitted to Department of Neurology for a diagnostic work-up of right-sided headaches and menstrual cycle disturbance. Headaches occurred almost every evening for several months, while menstrual cycle was regular until June 2013: from that time periods were irregular and finally were missed. She has attributed headaches and menstrual cycle disturbance to a stress she was exposed to daily. A patient also gained weight, 6 kg in 4 months, and did not have visual field loss, and later on we found out she did not have galactorrhea.

Pituitary MRI was performed before pituitary hormone level report was finished by a biochemical laboratory (Figs. 6.1, 6.2, and 6.3).

According to the described imaging features, cystic pituitary macroadenoma (CPA) or Rathke's cleft cyst (RCC) with intracystic nodule was reported as possible diagnosis, and further endocrine work-up was recommended. Pituitary hormone level report revealed high prolactin levels, 4237 mIU/L (normal levels for women, 127–637 mIU/L). Since Rathke's cleft cyst symptoms do not include high pituitary hormone levels, it was confirmed that the lesion was a cystic pituitary macroadenoma, not a RCC with intracystic nodule. A committee of endocrinologist, neuroradiologist and neurosurgeon has chosen a medicamentous treatment as a therapeutic approach.

6.1 Cystic Pituitary Adenoma or Rathke's Cleft Cyst with Intracystic Nodule

Pituitary adenoma is a benign neoplasm that arises from the adenohypophysis and represents the most common intrasellar pathology. Imaging findings of an uncomplicated adenoma are typical, but intratumoural haemorrhage and ischemic changes in larger pituitary adenomas result in haemorrhagic and cystic changes or both, leading to various signal intensities and imaging features, wherefore it may be difficult to differentiate CPA from large RCC [1–5]. Therefore, pretreatment differentiation between these two entities remains a common issue but is important for treatment planning.

Rathke's cleft cyst is a benign epithelial cyst that originates from the embryonic remnants of Rathke's pouch and is located mainly in the midline of the pituitary gland. Typical imaging findings include intrasellar and/or suprasellar cyst of various signal intensities depending on the content of the intracystic fluid: it may follow CSF signal intensities on T1WI and T2WI, but it may be iso- to hyperintense on T1WI (Figs. 6.4c and 6.5a, b, e) due to protein, mucopolysaccharides and/or high cholesterol content [4]. It usually does not enhance, but in case of larger RCCs enhancing thin rim of compressed pituitary

© Springer International Publishing AG, part of Springer Nature 2018
M. Špero, H. Vavro, *Neuroradiology - Expect the Unexpected*,
https://doi.org/10.1007/978-3-319-73482-8_6

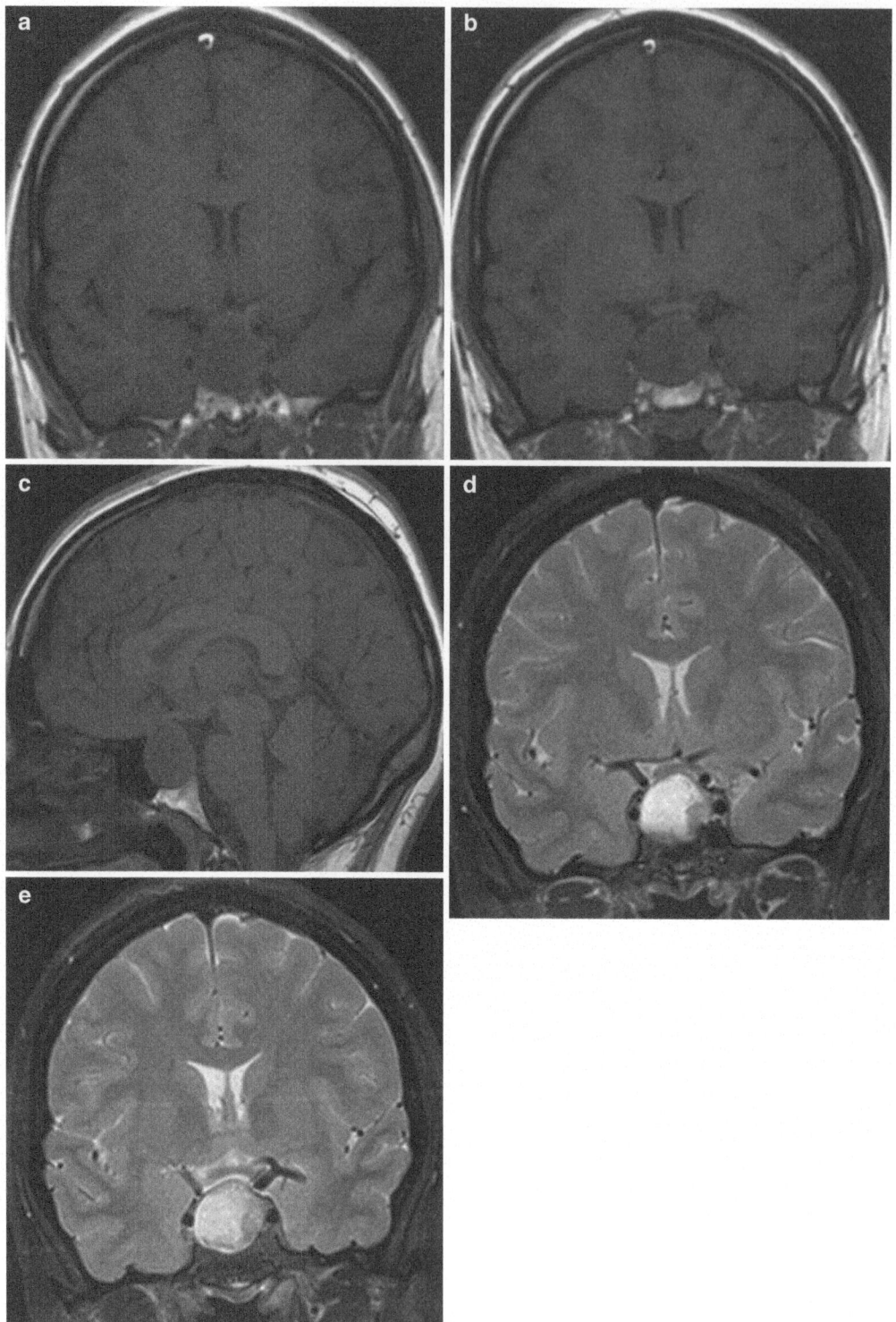

Fig. 6.1 Non-contrast pituitary MRI, coronal (**a**, **b**) and sagittal (**c**) T1WI, coronal FST2WI (**d**, **e**), revealed enlarged sella turcica due to intrasellar and suprasellar cystic lesion reaching and slightly stretching optic chiasm. The cystic lesion was hypointense on T1WI and hyperintense on T2WI: irregular structure extended inside the cystic lesion, along the inferior and left lateral cystic wall, almost isointense with the grey matter on T1WI and T2WI

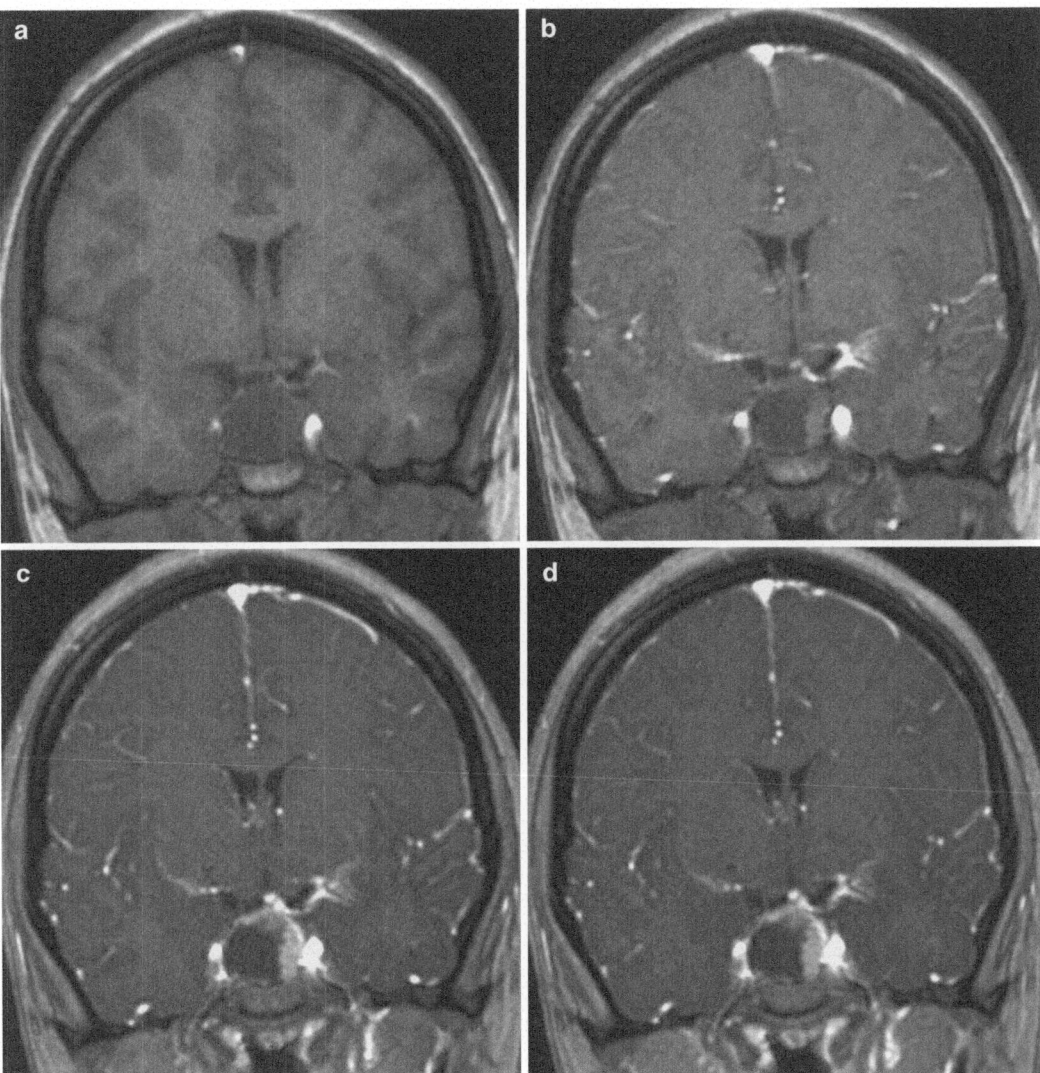

Fig. 6.2 Post-contrast pituitary MRI, dynamic post-contrast coronal T1WI (**a–d**): cystic lesion revealed rim enhancement, as well as the enhancement of the intracystic nodule along the inferior and left lateral cyst wall (**c, d**)

gland, surrounding non-enhancing cyst, mimics cyst wall enhancement (Fig. 6.4a, b). Intracystic nodule may be present (up to 75%), freely floating inside a cyst or adherent to a cyst wall, consisting of cholesterol and protein. It may be hyperintense on T1WI and iso- or hypointense on T2WI and does not enhance on post-contrast T1WI (Fig. 6.5) [1, 3, 4]. Wen et al. have reported RCC with markedly enhanced intracystic nodule: histology revealed squamous metaplasia cell debris as the main component of the enhanced nodule [4].

Functioning pituitary adenomas can cause a variety of signs and symptoms depending on the hormone they produce. Signs and symptoms of non-functioning pituitary tumours are related to their growth and the pressure they put on surrounding structures. Pituitary adenomas usually enlarge slowly over years and exhibit size change, while RCCs remain stable in dimension with time and no neoplastic transformation is reported in the literature. The majority of RCCs are asymptomatic, while symptomatic patients present with headache, pituitary dysfunction (hypopituitarism) and visual impairment [1, 3, 4].

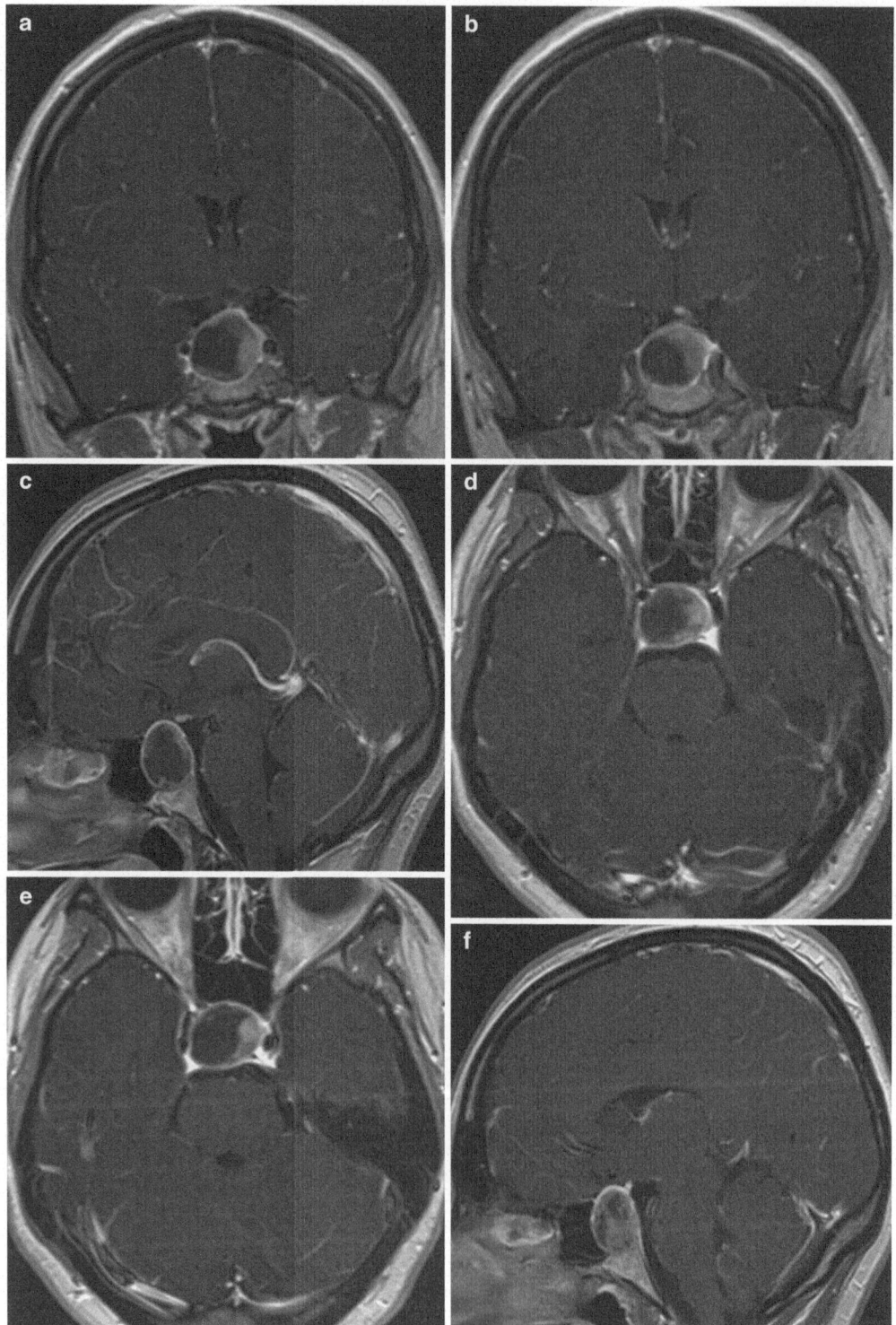

Fig. 6.3 Post-contrast pituitary MRI: post-contrast T1WI in coronal (**a**, **b**), sagittal (**c**, **f**) and axial (**d**, **e**) planes. Midline cystic pituitary lesion revealed rim enhancement, homogeneous enhancement of the intracystic nodule. Infundibulum was slightly tilted towards left. Sellar floor bulged into the sphenoid sinus. Lesion did not involve cavernous sinuses

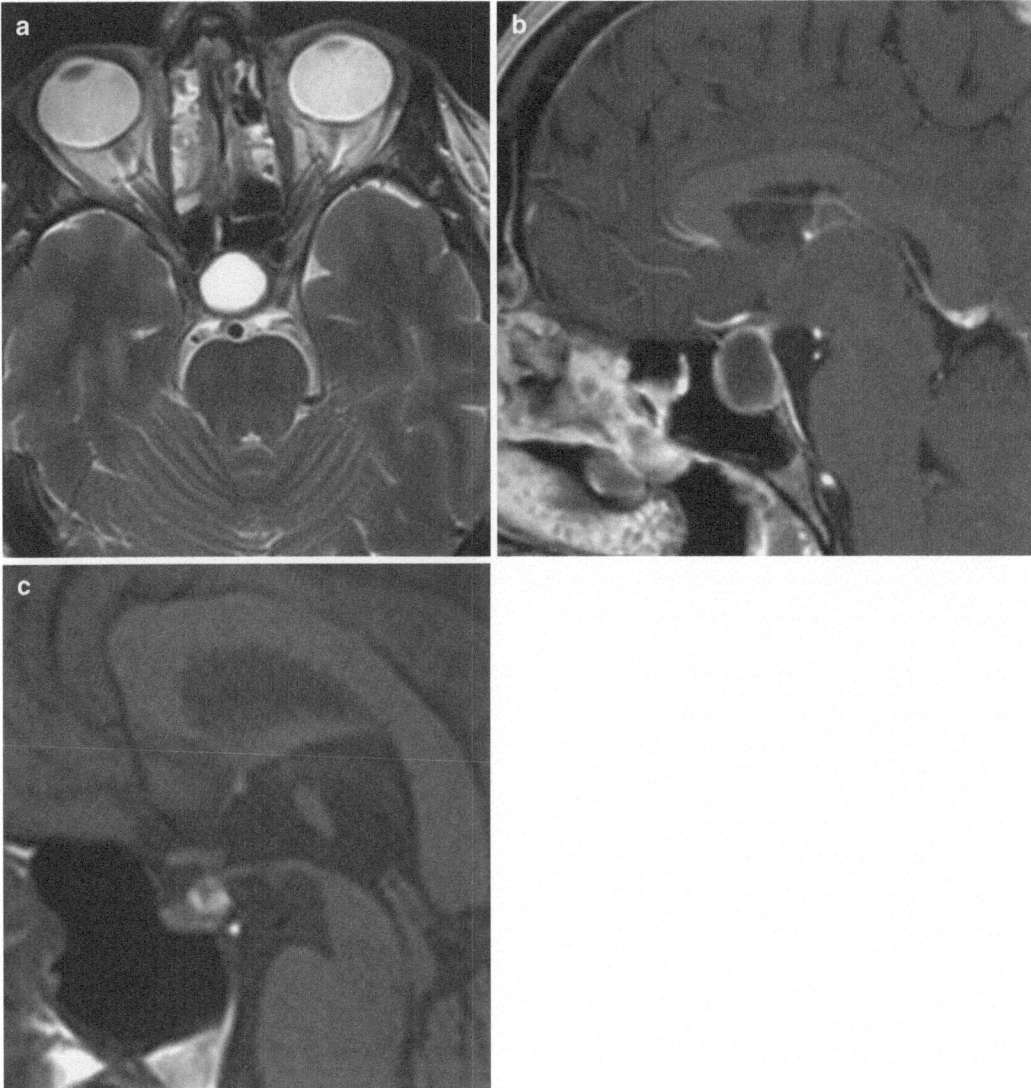

Fig. 6.4 Pituitary MRI, axial T2WI (**a**), post-contrast sagittal T1WI (**b**), pre-contrast sagittal T1WI (**c**): large Rathke's cleft cyst with enhancing thin rim of compressed pituitary gland, surrounding non-enhancing cyst, mimics cyst wall enhancement (**a**, **b**). Small Rathke's cleft cyst hyperintense on pre-contrast T1WI (**c**)

To help differentiate CPA and large RCC, different authors have developed their own models for differentiation between these two entities on the basis of MR imaging findings. For example, according to the diagnostic model reported by Park et al., the presence of fluid-fluid level, a hypointense rim on T2WI, septation and an off-midline location favoured CPA, whereas the presence of an intracystic nodule was more common with RCC [1]. Bonneville JF suggested those imaging features might be helpful, but are not strictly typical because pituitary adenomas may be on the midline, as well as RCC may be rarely in an off-midline location, while fluid-fluid level and septations are inconstant. Bonneville proposed ancillary signs for differentiating RCC and CPA: intrasellar adenomas give rise to more mass effect compared to less or even no mass effect of RCC; strict midline location, regular convex symmetric anterior surface and close contact with the posterior lobe are characteristic T1WI features of a RCC [5].

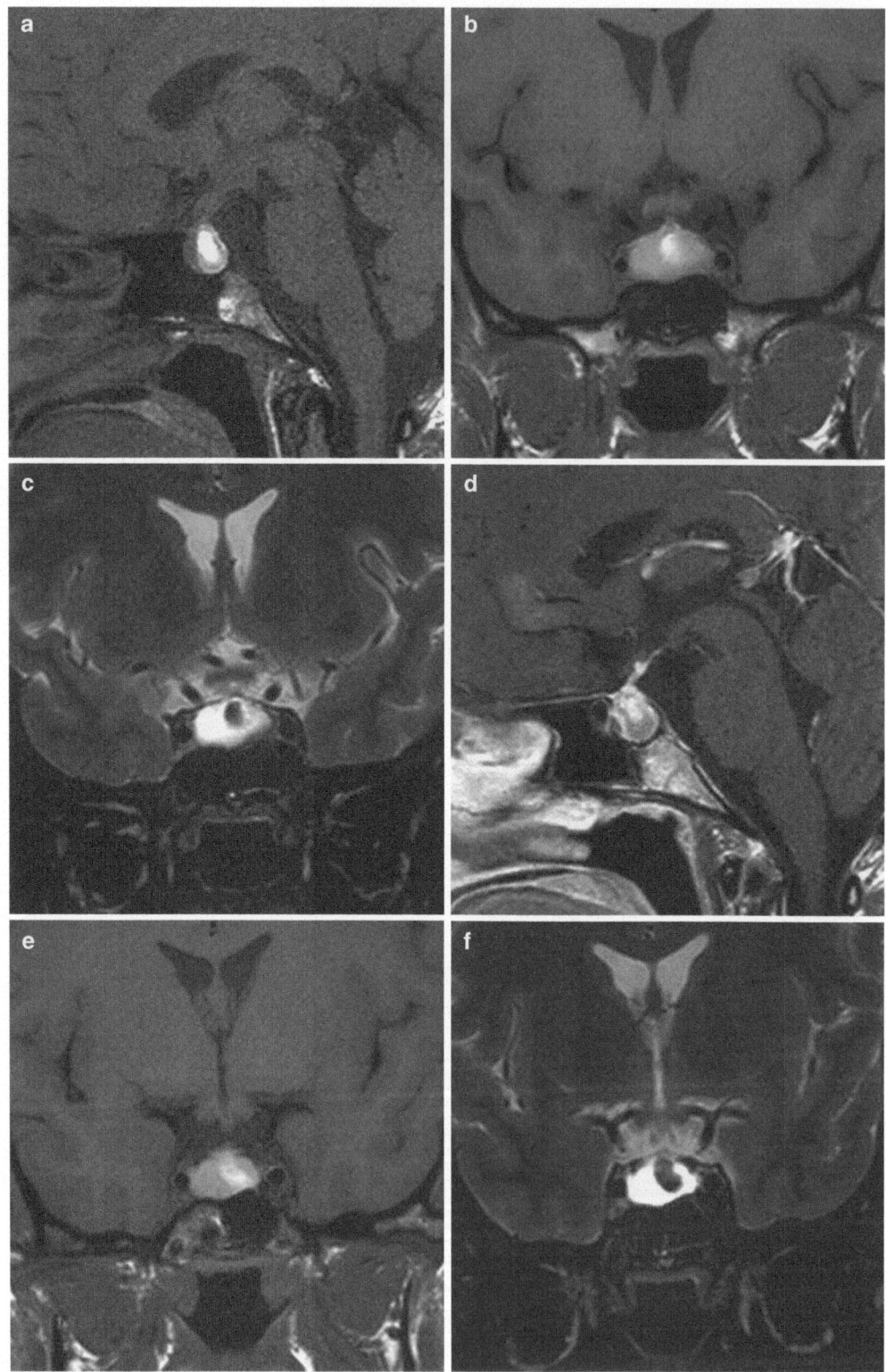

Fig. 6.5 Pituitary MRI pre-contrast sagittal T1WI (**a**), coronal T1WI (**b**, **e**), coronal T2WI (**c**, **f**), post-contrast sagittal T1WI (**d**): intrasellar Rathke's cleft cyst with intracystic nodule adherent from a cyst roof, hyperintense on T1WI (**a**, **b**, **e**), hypointense on T2WI (**c**, **f**). On post-contrast T1WI thin rim of compressed pituitary gland enhanced, intracystic nodule did not enhance. RCC content was slightly hyperintense on pre-contrast T1WI (**a**, **b**, **e**)

In case of our patient, symptoms were not specific for pituitary adenoma but have pointed out to a possible female sex hormone imbalance. Pituitary MRI was a proper choice for imaging work-up: large intrasellar and suprasellar cystic lesion, with rim enhancement and enhancing intracystic nodule, definitely pointed out to a possible RCC with atypical enhancing intracystic nodule. In such case, especially if pituitary hormone level report is not available, the best is to report RCC and CPA as differential diagnosis. Hypopituitarism is typical for symptomatic RCC as well as headache, but hyperprolactinemia is not: pituitary hormone levels have helped us make final, pretreatment, diagnosis. Therefore, if you have a patient with an intrasellar and/or suprasellar expansile cystic pituitary lesion and, according to previously mentioned MRI features, you are not sure if it is a RCC or CPA, look for a pituitary hormone levels to help you decide and report which of those two differential diagnosis is more favoured.

References

1. Park M et al (2015) Differentiation between cystic pituitary adenomas and Rathke cleft cysts: a diagnostic model using MRI. AJNR Am J Neuroradiol 36(10):1866–1873
2. Bonneville JF et al (2005) Magnetic resonance imaging of pituitary adenomas. Eur Radiol 15:543–548
3. Gaddikeri S et al (2013) Rathke cleft cyst: MRI criteria for presumptive diagnosis. Neuroscience 18(3):258–263
4. Wen L et al (2010) Rathke's cleft cyst: clinicopathological and MRI findings in 22 patients. Clin Radiol 65:47–55
5. Bonneville JF (2016) Hemorrhagic pituitary adenoma versus Rathke cleft cyst: a frequent dilemma. http://www.ajnrblog.org. Accessed 01 Apr 2016

Part II

Vascular

Cerebral Proliferative Angiopathy: AVM

A 32-year-old female patient, in 8 months of pregnancy, had to perform MRI of the brain as a part of neurological evaluation of ataxia she had suffered from the childhood and never been evaluated before. According to anamnestic data, from a childhood she was motorically clumsy and had problems with coordination, mild degree of hearing loss and a slow rate of speech. During the last 3 years, she described occasional headaches, visual disturbance in the form of oscillopsia while watching television and occasional tremor in right hand. All the symptoms have become pronounced during pregnancy.

In September 2016, MRI of the brain revealed large infratentorial arteriovenous malformation without sign of previous haemorrhage (Figs. 7.1 and 7.2).

I have reported a large arteriovenous malformation of the posterior cerebral fossa, possible cerebral proliferative angiopathy, and recommend consultation of an interventional neuroradiologist regarding digital subtraction angiography after a scheduled caesarean section, to differentiate this vascular malformation as CPA or classical brain AVM. Interventional neuroradiologist appraised this large AVM, according to the Spetzler-Martin scale, as grade V arteriovenous malformation, incurable regarding possible surgery or interventional procedure, but also recommended DSA after delivery.

Caesarean section was scheduled for the beginning of October 2016 and was performed without complications. A patient underwent a recommended DSA at the end of August 2017, which differentiated this large arteriovenous malformation as a classical brain AVM, grade V (Fig. 7.3).

7.1 Cerebral Proliferative Angiopathy or AVM?

When a patient entered MRI machine and examination was commenced, after the first two sequences, sagittal T1WI and axial T2WI were completed, I was a bit astonished by the large infratentorial vascular malformation I saw. It reminded me of "something" I have already seen during lectures on different courses and in the literature but never had a chance to see it in my patients: did I have a patient with cerebral proliferative angiopathy in MRI machine or is it just a large, peculiar classical cerebral arteriovenous malformation?

Cerebral proliferative angiopathy (CPA) is a rare subgroup of AVMs, different from classical brain AVMs, first suggested by Pierre Lasjaunias and his group in 2008. It is congenital condition that differs significantly from classical brain AVMs in terms of epidemiology, clinical presentation, angiographic and histopathological features, natural history and treatment considerations. Classical AVMs consist of a tangle of abnormal arteries and veins without intervening capillary bed [1].

© Springer International Publishing AG, part of Springer Nature 2018
M. Špero, H. Vavro, *Neuroradiology - Expect the Unexpected*,
https://doi.org/10.1007/978-3-319-73482-8_7

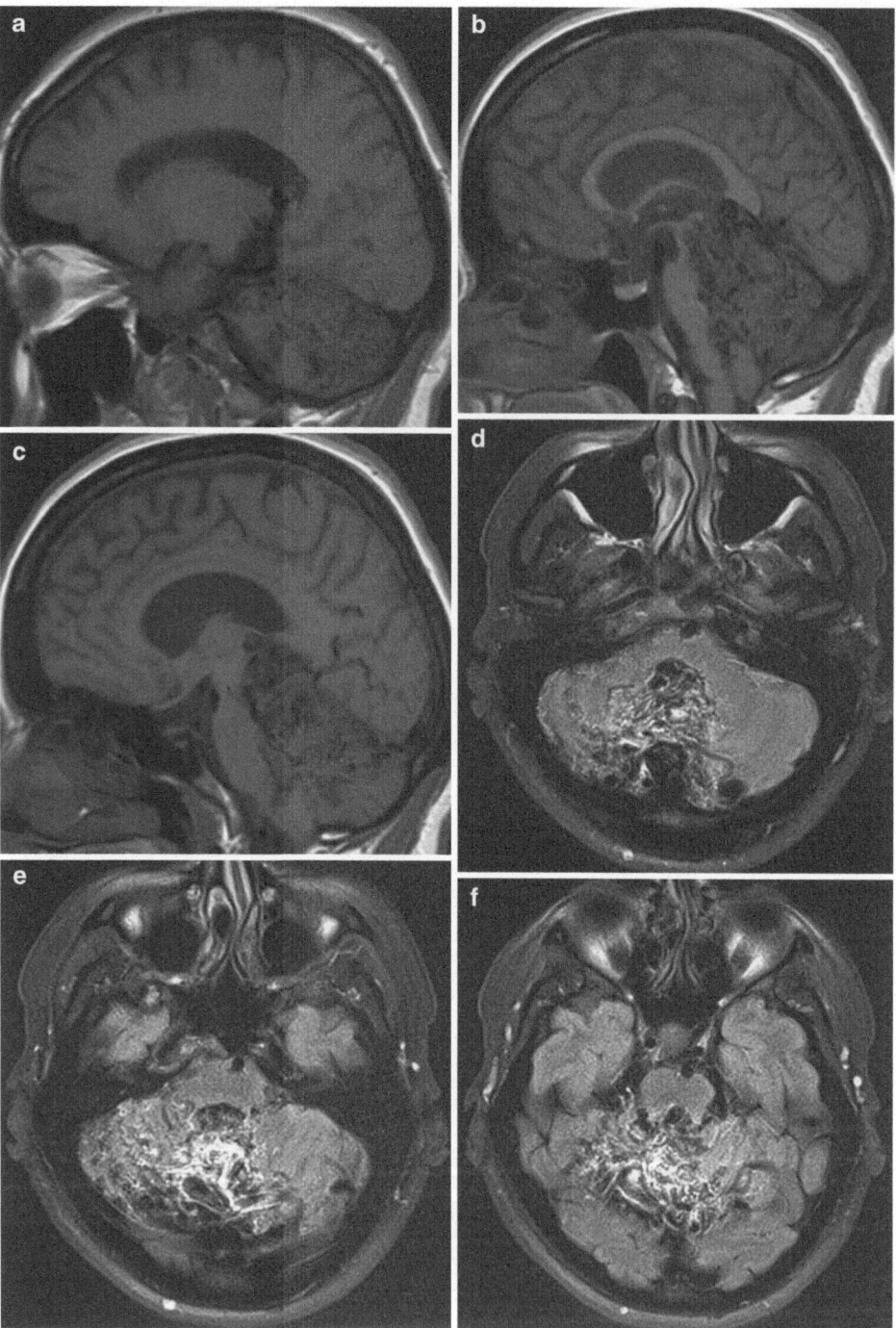

Fig. 7.1 Non-contrast magnetic resonance imaging of the brain, sagittal T1 (**a–c**), axial FLAIR (**d–f**) and T2WI (**g–i**), coronal (**j–l**) and sagittal (**m–o**) T2WI, axial T2*WI (**p–r**), revealed large infratentorial AVM in vermis and predominantly in right cerebellar hemisphere, extending cranially up to mesencephalic tectum and caudally up to foramen magnum. It filled up the fourth ventricle, anteriorly compressed structures of the brainstem, pons and medulla oblongata, while cerebellar tonsils protruded through foramen magnum. AVM consisted of a diffuse network of vascular channels and dilated veins between different vascular territories. Normal brain parenchyma appeared to intermingle between vascular structures of the AVM, with mild reactive marginal gliosis. There were no signs of previous haemorrhage. Cerebral proliferative angiopathy (CPA) or large classical brain arteriovenous malformation

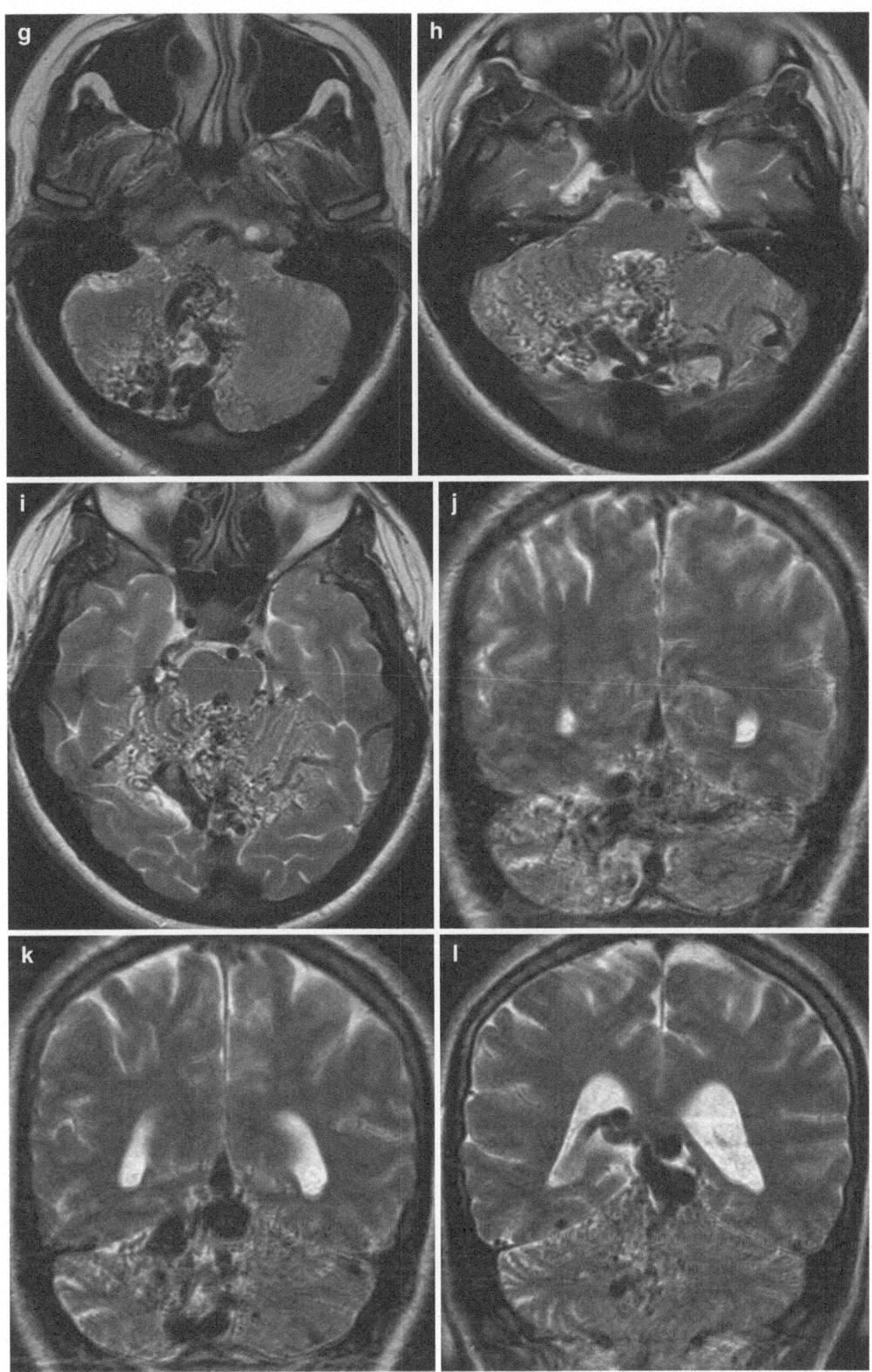

Fig. 7.1 (continued)

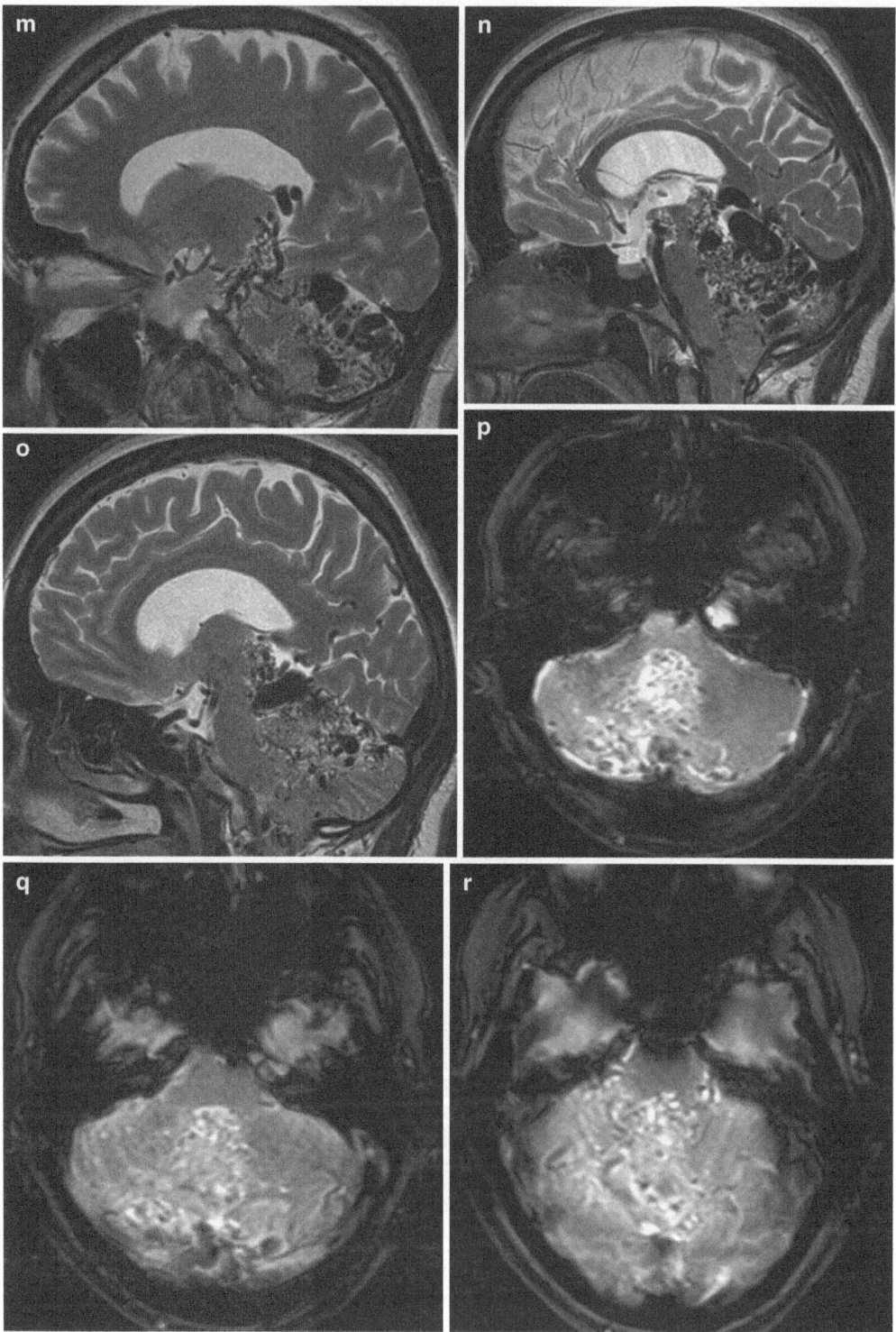

Fig. 7.1 (continued)

Most commonly CPAs present in adolescent and middle-aged females with symptoms depending on the site of CPA, usually headaches, seizures and progressive neurological deficits [1–3]. CPAs are associated with low risk of haemorrhage compared to classical brain AVM, but if presented with haemorrhage, CPAs have a high chance (12%) of recurrent bleeding. CPAs usually have supratentorial location, most commonly in the right hemisphere, while infratentorial location is found in 22% of cases [1, 3].

The pathogenesis of CPA remains unclear; presumably progressive and uncontrolled angiogenesis is induced as a response to cortical ischaemia with the feeding arteries having altered internal elastic lamina and smooth muscle cells and collagenous thickening of the veins. Normal functioning brain is interspersed between anomalous vessels and may present reactive gliosis [1, 2, 4].

Angiographic features of CPA reveal the absence of dominant feeders or flow-related aneurysms: multiple feeding arteries, not or moderately enlarged, contribute equally to a malformation. Nidus is usually large, 3–6 cm, or larger, ill-defined, with scattered "puddling" of contrast persisting into the late arterial and early venous phase within capillary ectasia. Veins are moderately enlarged compared to the size of nidus [1–3]. Perfusion-weighted MRI demonstrates increased blood volume within the nidus with an increased mean transit time which is indicative of capillary and venous ectasias and area of hypoperfusion that could be seen throughout the affected hemisphere [1].

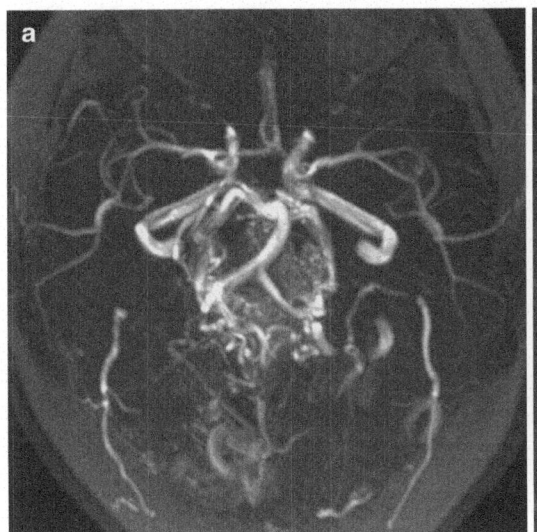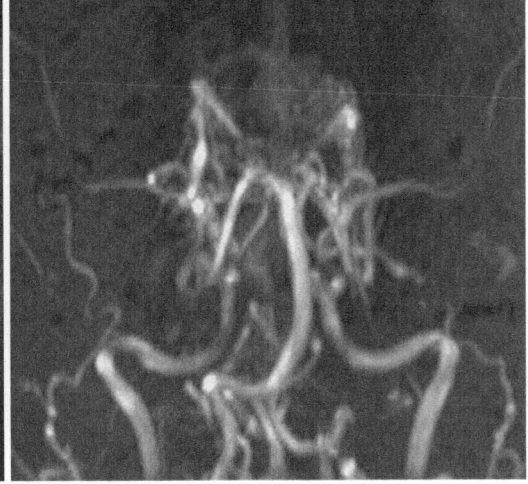

Fig. 7.2 Magnetic resonance angiography, 3D TOF technique (**a–c**) and magnetic resonance venography, 3D PC technique (**d–f**) revealed dense diffuse network of vascular channels and dilated veins in the midline and predominantly right part of the posterior fossa. There were no dominant arterial feeders and arterial supply came from both posterior cerebral arteries, basilar artery branches and thalamoperforating arteries. Venous drainage was to the straight sinus and to both transverse sinuses, draining veins were enlarged

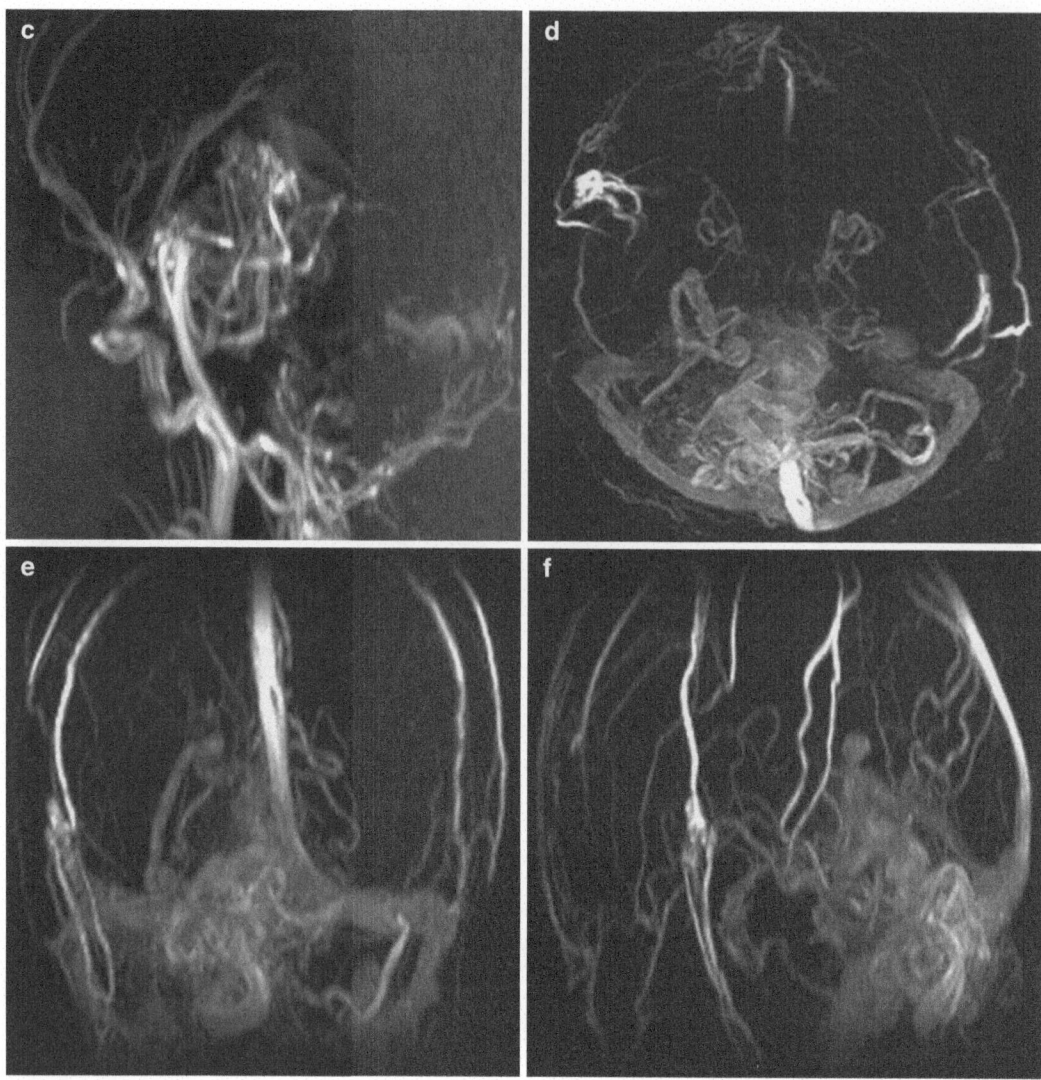

Fig. 7.2 (continued)

MRI features of CPA are described previously. Chronic haemorrhage, gliosis or both may be found in adjacent parenchyma; post-contrast T1W sequences demonstrate enlarged serpiginous vessels.

I have presumed I have a case of CPA in front of me due to patient sex, age and clinical presentation, described MRI features with normal intermingled brain parenchyma in-between vascular structures and absence of large arterial feeders, although veins were remarkably dilated. Case report published by Kumar et al. in 2015,

described infratentorial haemorrhagic CPA, led me to suspect that maybe I could be on a right track regarding MRI features [3]. CPA may be diagnosed using MRI and MRA, but DSA remains the "gold standard" to confirm or exclude the diagnosis, because it allows direct vessel visualisation, shunt estimation and possibility of intervention if required. In the case, DSA was performed about 11 months after the brain MRI, confirming angiographic features in terms of classical brain AVM. DSA assessed arterial supply more accurately in comparison to MRA:

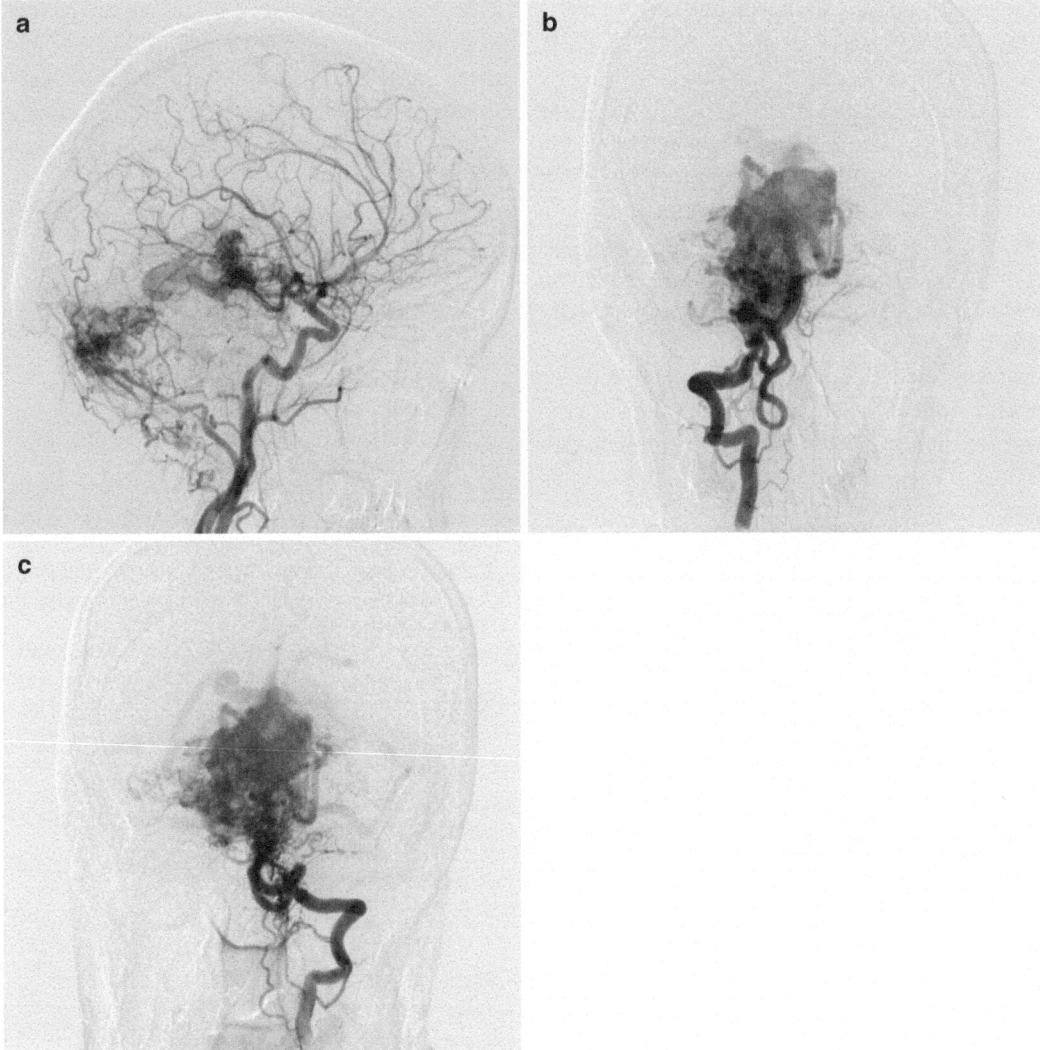

Fig. 7.3 Cerebral digital subtraction angiography (courtesy of assisted professor David Ozretić and professor Marko Radoš), right internal carotid artery lateral view (**a**), right (**b**) and left (**c**) vertebral artery frontal view: confirmed large predominantly infratentorial, plexiform arteriovenous malformation with numerous short feeding arteries that vascularised the greatest part of the nidus in the posterior cerebral fossa. Catheterisation of the right common carotid artery showed vascularisation of the greatest part of the nidus through feeders coming from posterior choroidal arteries over the posterior communicating artery. Catheterisation of the left common carotid artery and vertebral artery showed vascularisation of the nidal segments through the posterior inferior cerebellar artery, superior cerebellar artery and choroidal group of arteries coming from the P1 segment of the posterior cerebral artery. The greatest part of the nidus was drained over deep venous system, dilated draining veins had developed venous ectasias. There were no capillary ectasias and scattered "puddling" of contrast within them, and there were no transdural supply. Therefore, large classical brain arteriovenous malformation, grade V, was reported

there were no dominant arterial feeders but numerous short feeders coming from different arterial territories. The method also confirmed there was no capillary bed and its ectasias with scattered "puddling" of contrast within them, and there were no transdural supply as well. Cerebral DSA was performed by an interventional neuroradiologist and described angiographic features confirmed vascular malformation not to be a CPA. Therefore large incurable AVM, grade V, was reported at the end.

It is important to differ classical brain AVM and CPA because of different treatment options. Unfortunately, primary treatment in CPA is nor surgery, radiation therapy or embolization because those treatment options carry risk of permanent neurological deficit due to intervening normal brain parenchyma between vascular channels in CPA. Symptomatic medication therapy, including analgesic and antiepileptic drugs, is usually offered to such patients. Limited arterial embolization in non-eloquent areas may be performed for patients presenting with uncontrolled seizures and headaches [1–3, 5].

In case of this patient, MRI features have led me to suspect this large malformation to be CPA, but DSA has confirmed large classical brain AVM. Cerebral DSA did not change treatment options, since this large vascular malformation is considered incurable. Infratentorial CPAs are difficult to manage because critical vessels that originate in the posterior vascular territory ultimately perfuse both the vital structures of posterior fossa and CPA; therefore, any mentioned treatment procedure may be fatal [3].

References

1. Lasjaunias PL et al (2008) Cerebral proliferative angiopathy clinical and angiographic description of and entity different from cerebral AVMs. Stroke 39:878–885
2. Rohit PSG (2015) Diffuse proliferative cerebral angiopathy: a case report and review of the literature. J Radiol Case Rep 9(9):1–10
3. Kumar S et al (2015) Infratentorial haemorrhagic cerebral proliferative angiopathy: a rare presentation of a rare disease. Asian J Neurosurg 10(3):240–242
4. Radalle Biasi P et al (2015) Cerebral proliferative angiopathy – description of a rare clinical entity. Arq Bras Neurocir 34:82–85
5. Liu P et al (2016) Cerebral proliferative angiopathy: clinical, angiographic features and literature review. Interv Neuroradiol 22(1):101–107

Part III

Infections/Metabolic/Toxic

Pulmonary Arteriovenous Fistulas and Nocardial Brain Abscess in Close Relatives

8

This is a story about a 63-year-old female patient, a mother, and a 41-year-old male patient, a son, who were both previously operated because of pulmonary arteriovenous fistulas (PAVFs): mother in 1996 and a son in 1995. In 2013, they were both admitted to our emergency hospital department (EHD) due to neurological symptoms.

On December 19, 2012, mother had a sudden onset of left-sided weakness, but she was admitted to the EHD in 2013 on January 3: during a two-week period, weakness did not progress or improve. At the admission total leukocyte count and C-reactive protein levels were normal; lumbar puncture was not performed.

Patient was hospitalised and diagnostic work-up commenced (Figs. 8.1, 8.2, and 8.3). MRI of the brain (Fig. 8.2) followed the CT performed at the admission (Fig. 8.1) confirming imaging features of brain abscesses.

Seven days after the admission, 63-year-old patient was operated and brain abscesses evacuated.

On September 9, 2013, her son developed tension headache which mildly progressed during the day: he also had difficulties pronouncing some words. Therefore, he looked for a help in the EHD of our hospital. At the admission total leukocyte count was normal, while C-reactive protein level was elevated, measuring 15.5 mg/L (normal level <5 mg/L), lumbar puncture revealed slightly elevated protein level, normal glucose level and 50 white blood cells/μL.

Due to the CT report, patient was hospitalised: MRI of the brain followed the CT examination confirming two brain abscesses in the right temporal lobe (Figs. 8.4 and 8.5).

Neurosurgeon did not trust neuroradiologist report; he has suspected described lesion was a tumour, not an abscess. Three days after the admittance, patient was operated, lesions were evacuated and abscess was confirmed on pathohistology.

Microbiology of abscesses revealed *Nocardia* species as a causative microorganism, both in mother and son. Medicamentous therapy with trimethoprim and sulfamethoxazole followed surgery in both cases.

8.1 Pulmonary Arteriovenous Fistulas and Nocardial Abscess

If you have a patient with a brain abscess and cannot find usual source of infection from the ear, nose, orbits or throat, look further for possible source from the heart, or like in our case, from the lung. Pulmonary arteriovenous fistulas (PAVFs) or malformations are caused by abnormal communications between pulmonary arteries and pulmonary veins, without an intervening

© Springer International Publishing AG, part of Springer Nature 2018
M. Špero, H. Vavro, *Neuroradiology - Expect the Unexpected*,
https://doi.org/10.1007/978-3-319-73482-8_8

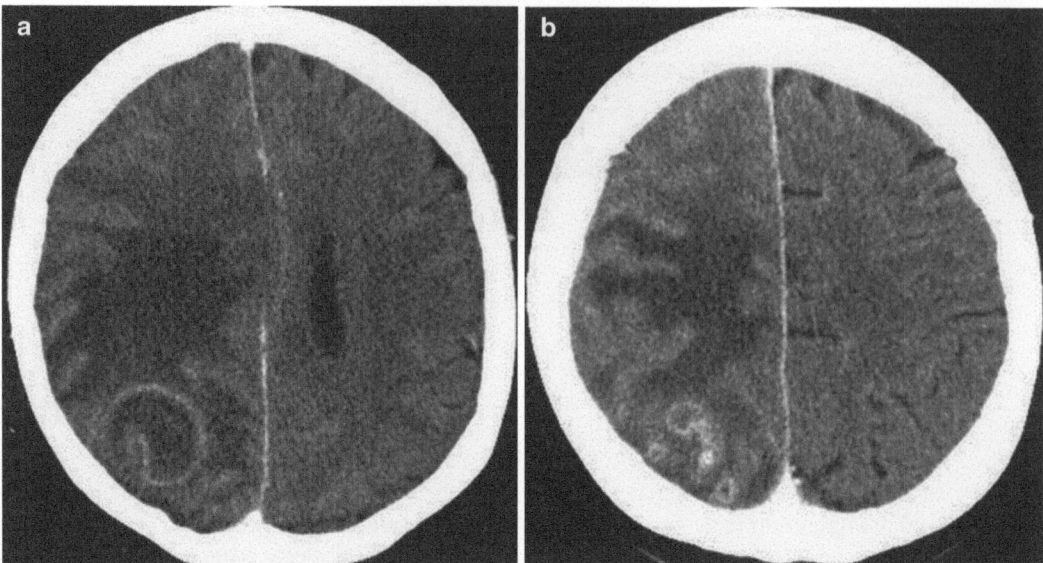

Fig. 8.1 Post-contrast computed tomography of the brain, axial scans (**a**, **b**), performed at the emergency admission revealed subcortical expansile ring-enhancing, hypodense lesion in the right parietal lobe with marked vasogenic oedema. At the upper rim of the lesion, there were several smaller ring-enhancing lesions

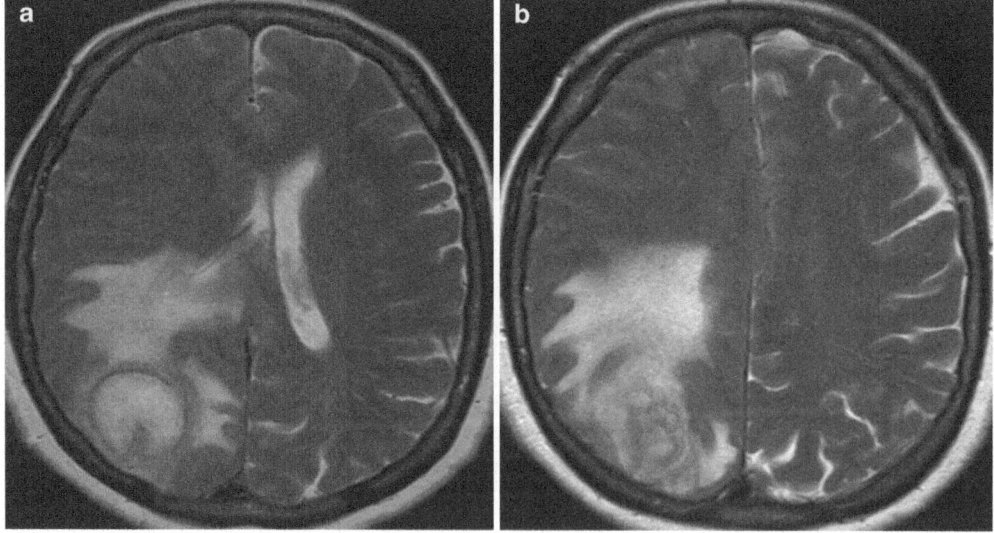

Fig. 8.2 Magnetic resonance imaging of the brain showed brain abscess subcortical in the right parietal lobe parenchyma with several smaller daughter abscesses flourishing from the large parent abscess, surrounded with marked vasogenic oedema: axial (**a**, **b**) and coronal (**g**) T2WI, axial FLAIR (**d**, **e**), axial DWI (**c**), ADC (**f**), sagittal pre-contrast T1WI (**h**), sagittal (**i**), coronal (**j**, **k**) and axial (**l**) post-contrast T1WI. Well-defined oval and round expansile lesions of different size, hyperintense with hypointense collagen capsule on T2WI which were mildly hyperintense on pre-contrast T1WI, showing ring contrast enhancement on post-contrast T1WI. Diffusion was restricted in the abscess wall and cavity

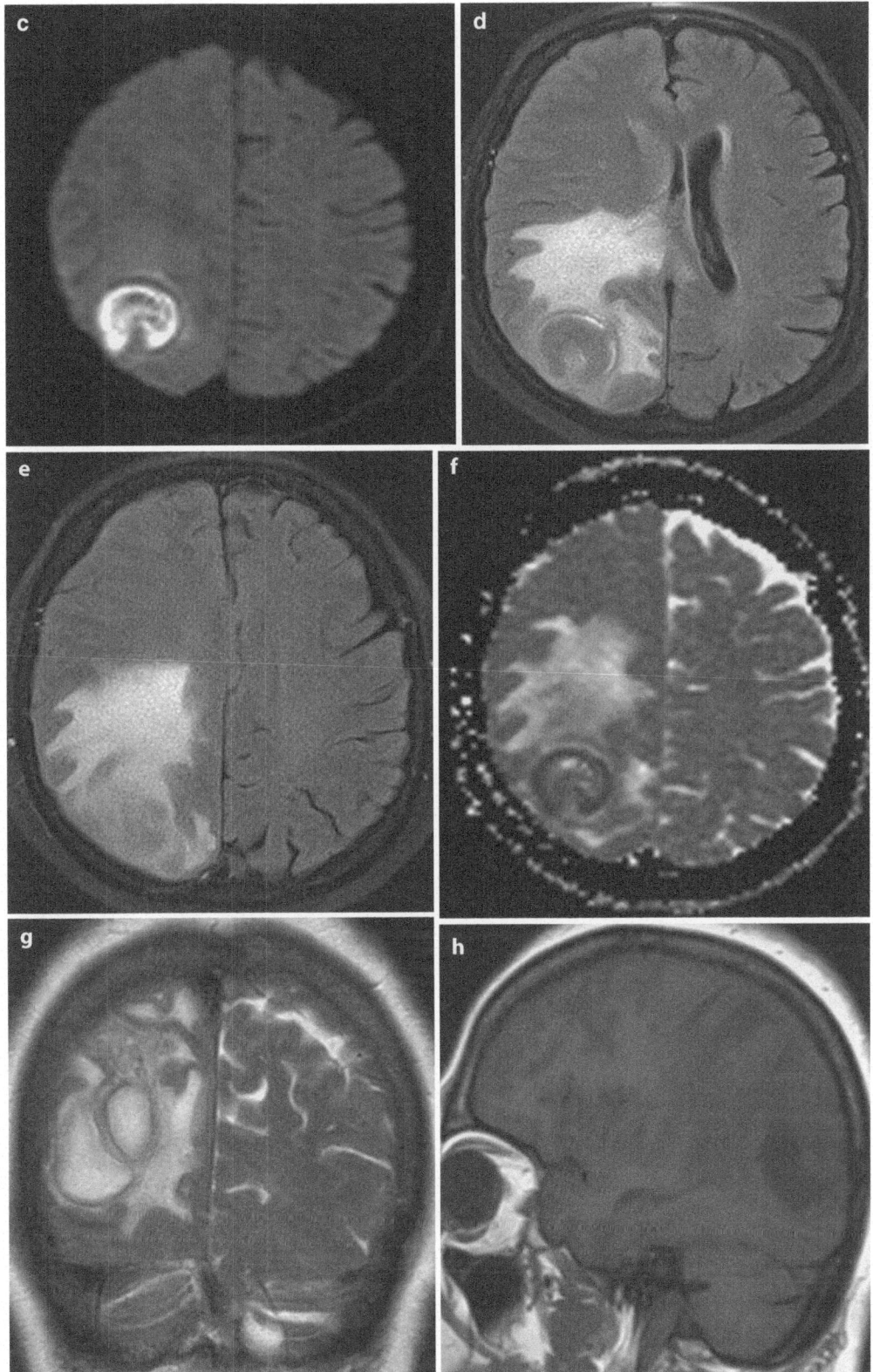

Fig. 8.2 (contineud)

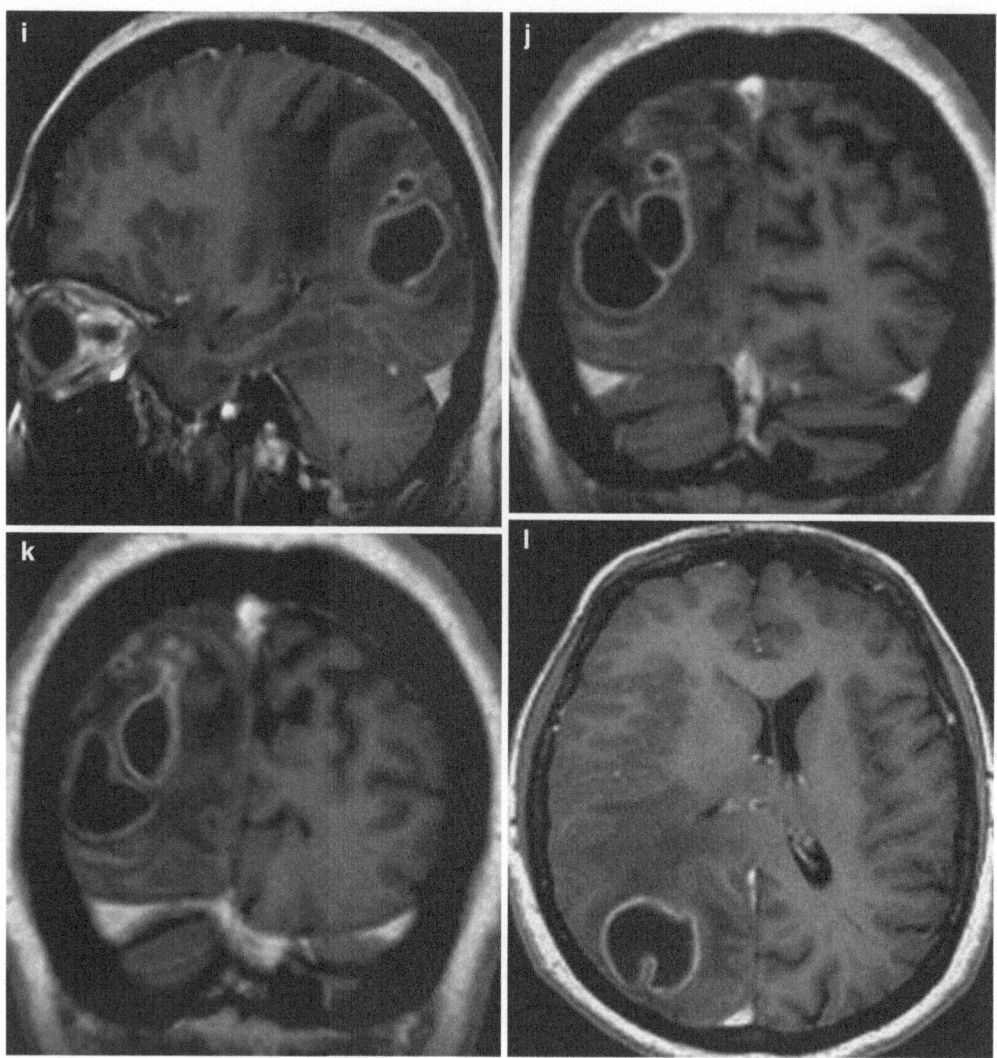

Fig. 8.2 (contineud)

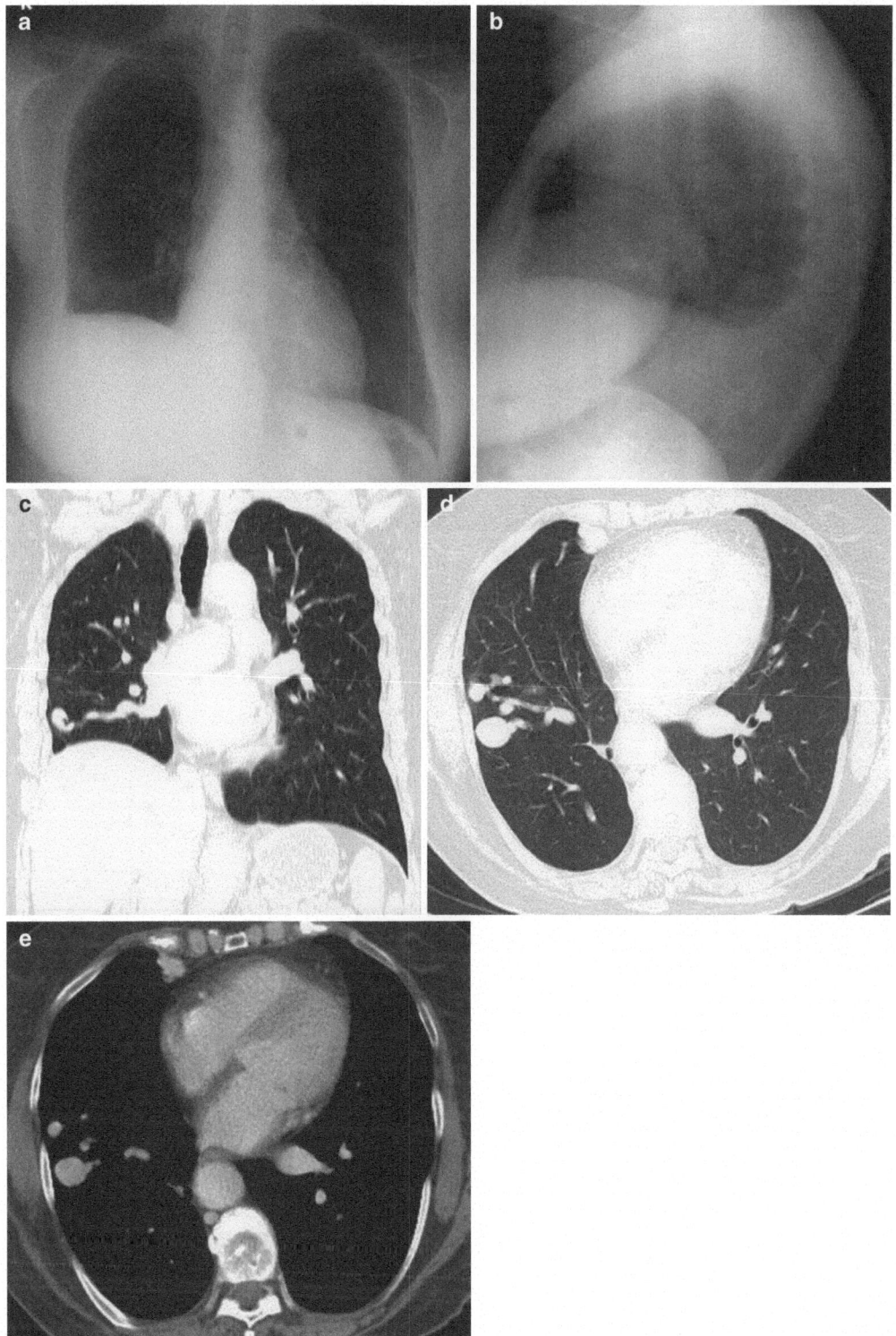

Fig. 8.3 Plain (**a**) and right lateral (**b**) chest radiograph at the admission, coronal (**c**) and axial (**d**, **e**) post-contrast chest computed tomography performed during hospitalisation as a part of diagnostic work-up of a 63-year-old female patient. Chest radiographs and computed tomography revealed postoperative changes after right inferior lobectomy (1996) and fistulous vascular abnormality in the middle pulmonary lobe

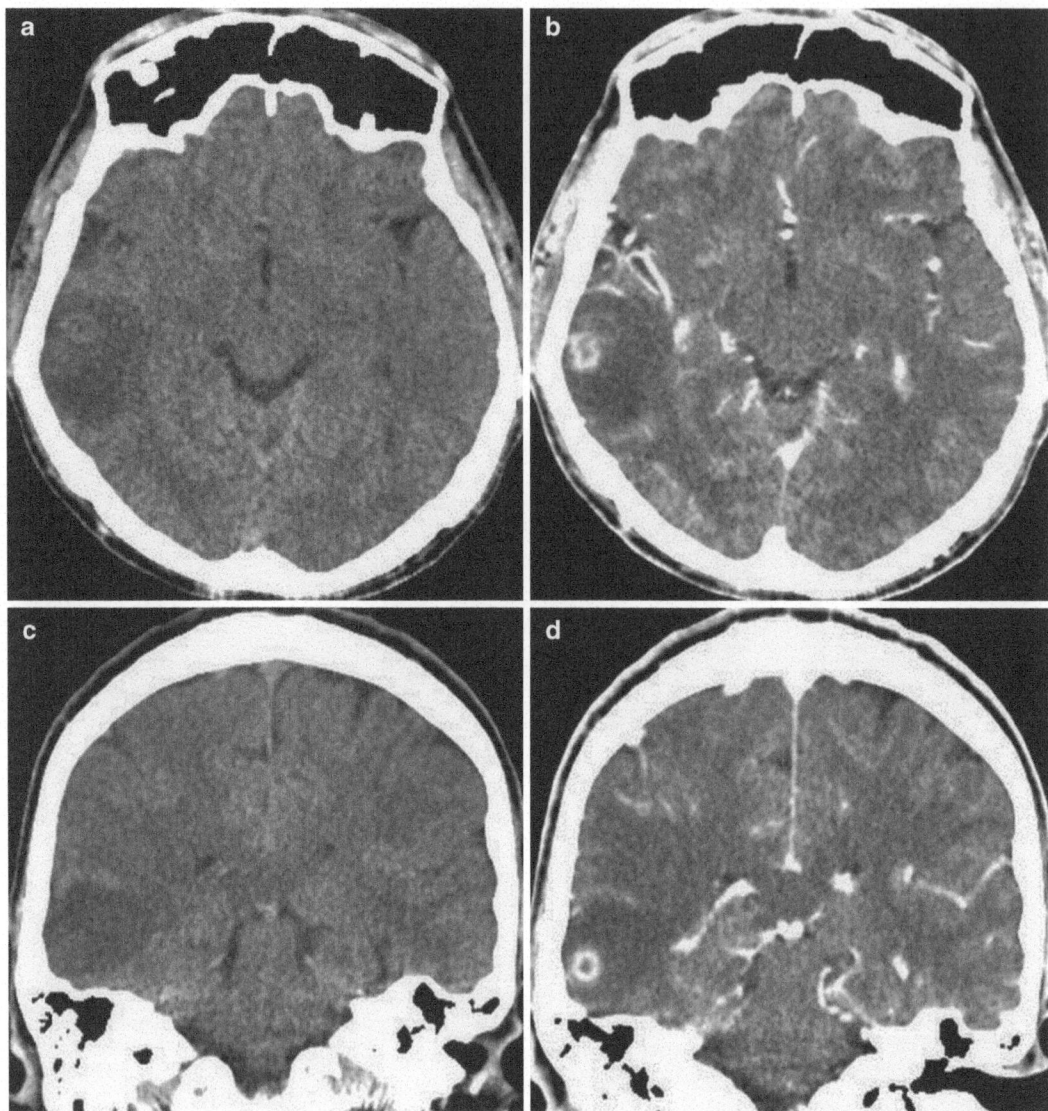

Fig. 8.4 Computed tomography of the brain performed at the emergency admission revealed two subcortical expansile lesions in the right temporal lobe, iso- and hypodense on pre-contrast axial (**a**) and coronal (**c**) scans, showing ring enhancement on post-contrast axial (**b**) and coronal (**d**) scans, surrounded with moderate vasogenic oedema. Radiologist who was on call reported primary or secondary neoplasm

capillary bed, resulting in pulmonary right to left shunt. Most commonly are congenital, but could be acquired in hepatic cirrhosis, mitral stenosis, trauma or chronic infections [1].

Congenital PAVFs are twice as common in female. Up to 70% of PAVFs are unilateral and found in lower lobes. They are classified as simple or complex: simple (about 80%) have a single feeding segmental artery leading to a single drain-ing pulmonary vein, while complex have two or more feeding arteries or draining veins. About 95% PAVFs are supplied by pulmonary arteries, less frequently by systemic arteries, while drainage is usu-ally to left atrium. Individual PAVF measures from 1 to 5 cm in size: usually a single PAVF less than 2 cm in diameter does not cause symptoms [1].

Abnormal vascular connections in PAVFs result in bypassing filtering effect of pulmonary capillaries and right to left shunting [2, 3]. When feeding arteries are larger than 3 mm in diameter, consequent paradoxical septic or non-septic embolisms result in the most frequently reported central nervous system complications including strokes (18%), transient ischaemic attacks (43%), brain abscesses (9%), migraine headaches (43%) and seizures (8%) [1, 2]. The most serious neurological complication is a brain abscess occurring in about 5 to 10% of patients with PAVFs [3].

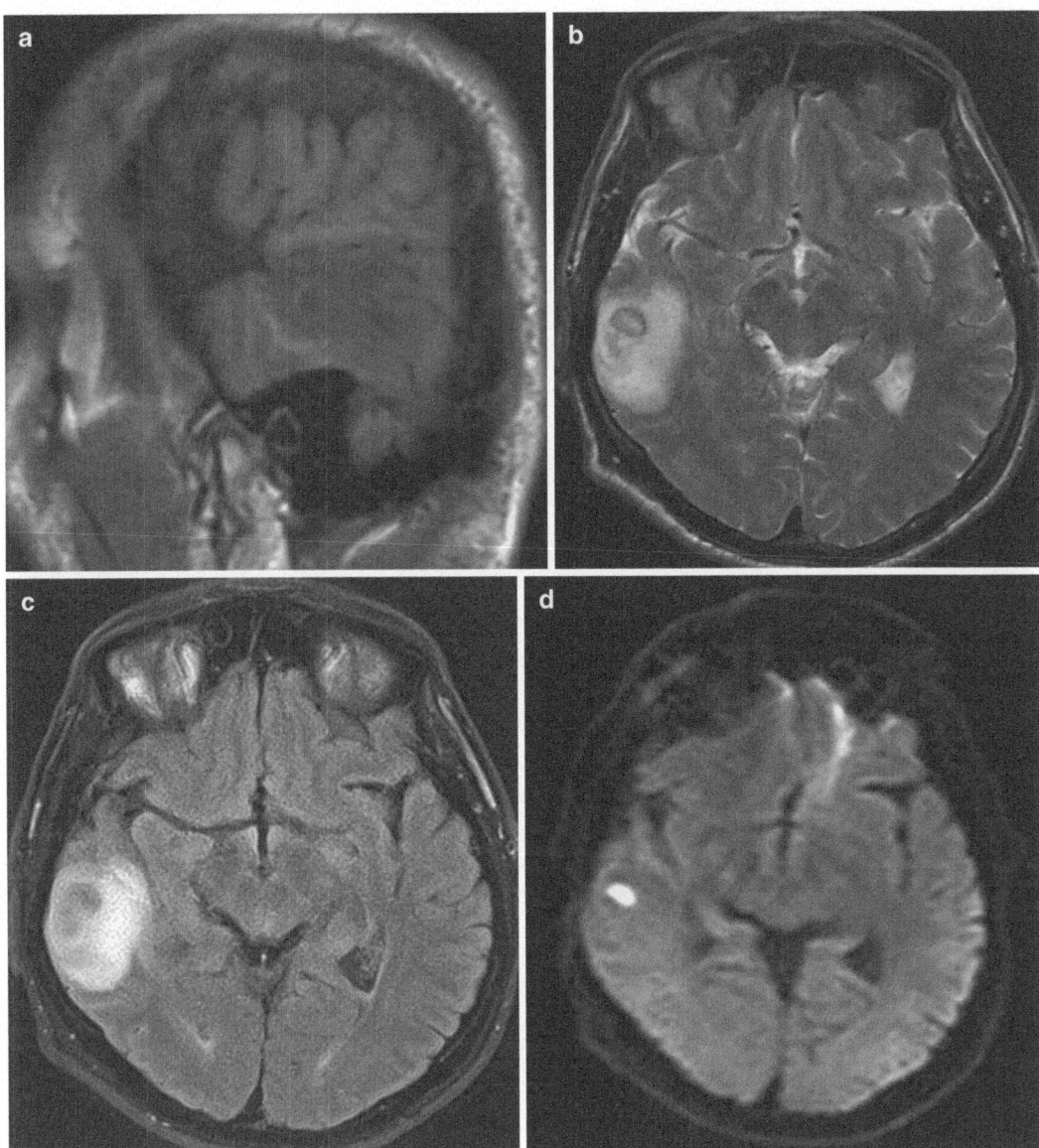

Fig. 8.5 Magnetic resonance imaging of the brain demonstrated two small subcortical brain abscesses in the right temporal lobe surrounded with moderate vasogenic oedema which was not finger-like: pre-contrast sagittal T1WI (**a**), axial T2WI (**b**) and FLAIR (**c**), axial DWI (**d**) and ADC (**e**), axial (**f**), coronal (**g**, **h**) and sagittal (**i**) post-contrast T1WI. Two small, oval, well-circumscribed expansile lesions located one behind the other: anterior lesion had typical imaging features of frank abscess, while posterior lesion did not revealed T2WI hypointense signal of collagen capsule neither restricted diffusion, while on post-contrast T1WI revealed irregular contrast enhancement. On sagittal post-contrast T1WI, it seemed like one lesion was "coming out" from the other

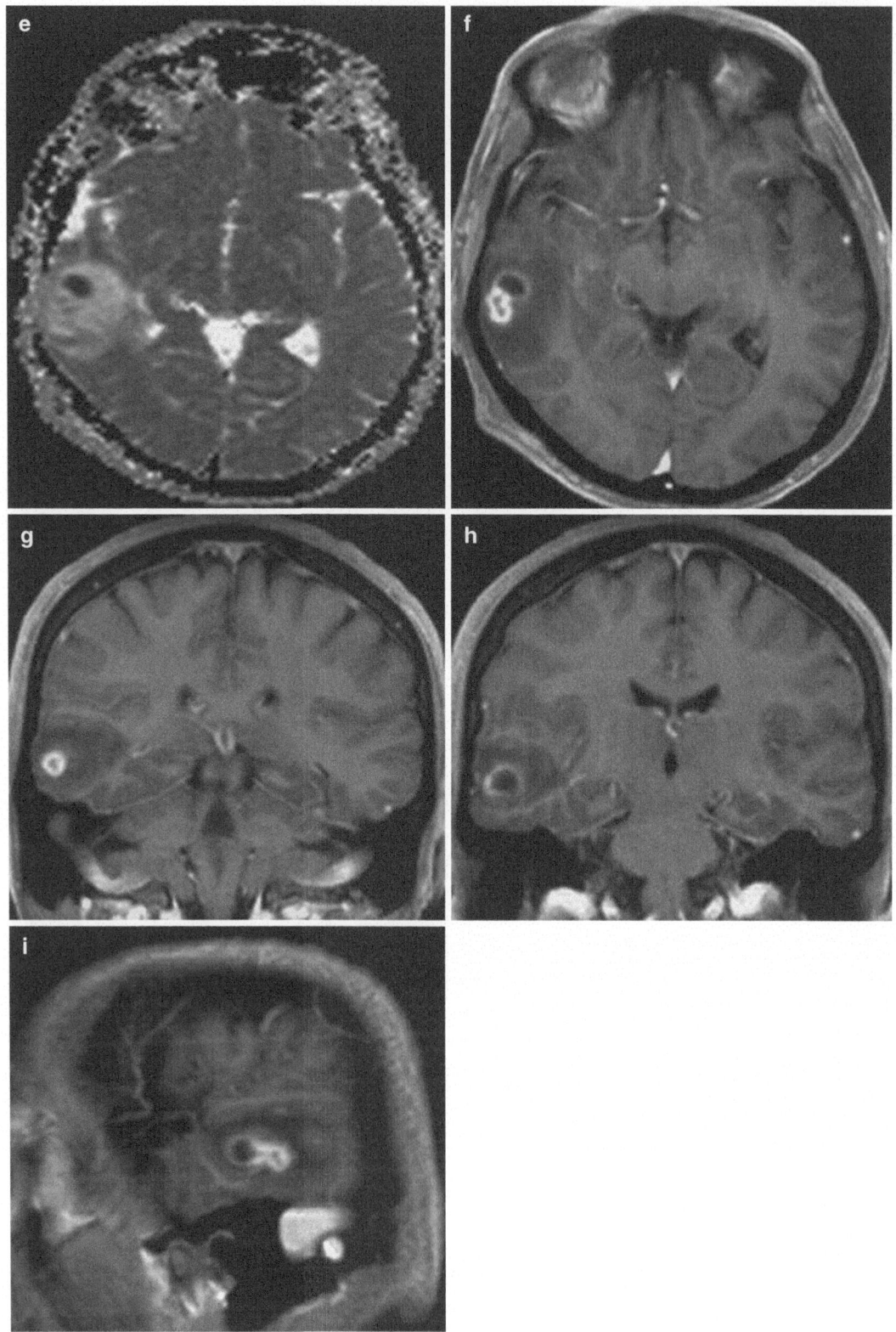

Fig. 8.5 (continud)

Nocardia is a genus of weakly staining Gram-positive, rod-shaped bacteria that forms partially acid-fast beaded branching filaments acting as fungi but being truly bacteria. Those organisms are mostly isolated from plants and soil, while infection usually occurs after inhalation or direct skin inoculation [4]. Nocardial brain abscesses are relatively uncommon (2% of all abscesses) and are usually secondary sequels of haematogenous dissemination from the lungs, as the most common primary site, in immunocompromised patients with predisposing factors such as malignancy, diabetes mellitus, malnutrition and uraemia. But it may also appear in immunocompetent patients [5]. Clinical presentation of this insidious brain infection is not specific and includes headaches, focal neurological deficits and seizures.

It is important not to misdiagnose brain abscess for a metastatic tumour which unfortunately is not uncommon, especially with radiologists who are inexperienced in the field of neuroradiology. On brain CT, it usually presents as round or oval hypodense expansile lesion with thin and ring-enhancing wall, surrounded by vasogenic oedema which may not be present around small abscesses. Surrounding oedema may extend through white matter in finger-like fashion, and in case of a solitary abscess, it may be misdiagnosed for a metastatic tumour, especially if a pulmonary nocardiosis is presented with multifocal nodules or mass. MRI of the brain is the method of choice to distinguish metastasis from brain abscess and possibly refer to it as a pyogenic or fungal abscess.

Pyogenic abscesses of haematogenous origin are usually located at the grey-white matter junction in the distribution of the anterior or middle cerebral arteries [6]. In brain abscess, necrotic debris accumulates centrally, while collagenous capsule is formed around it. Capsule of a brain abscess has isointense to slightly hyperintense rim on T1WI, while on T2WI rim is hypointense due to the presence of paramagnetic free radicals within the activated microglia, collagen and haemorrhage [6–8]. On SWI, pyogenic abscess demonstrates the dual-rim sign as its distinctive feature, and it is not present in fungal abscess.

Dual-rim sign consists of two concentric rims surrounding the central cavity at lesion margins: the outer one is hypointense and inner one hyperintense compared with the cavity content on SWI [8]. Pyogenic abscess demonstrates restricted diffusion on DWI with low ADC values in the abscess cavity due to restricted motion of water molecules in the organised purulent setting of microorganisms, macromolecules and intact inflammatory cells. The ring enhancement on post-contrast T1WI is attributed to the disrupted blood-brain barrier and may persist for up to 8 months after medication treatment: reliable signs of good response to medication treatment are shrinkage of the necrotic centre and decrease in capsular hypointensity on T2WI [9]. MR spectroscopy in pyogenic abscess wall reveals amino acids, lipid and lactate and acetate and succinate which are usually seen only in pyogenic abscesses [6].

Nocardial brain abscesses can progress rapidly and have significant morbidity and mortality rates (31%) [5]. Therefore, prompt diagnosis followed by aggressive surgical management and antibiotics treatment according to the drug sensitivity test is necessary. The low specificity of CNS nocardiosis imaging features is a problem, but it is important to recognise abscess as an inflammatory process, not a metastatic tumour or even tuberculosis; therefore, the accurate diagnosis will not be delayed and prompt treatment may commence on time.

References

1. Gossage JR, Kanj G (1998) Pulmonary arteriovenous malformations a state of the art review. Am J Respir Crit Care Med 158:643–661
2. Moradi M, Adeli M (2014) Brain abscess as the first manifestation of pulmonary arteriovenous malformation: a case report. Adv Biomed Res 3:28
3. Nam TK et al (2017) Brain abscesses associated with asymptomatic pulmonary arteriovenous fistulas. J Korean Neurosurg Soc 60(1):118–124
4. Lyu X et al (2017) Radiological findings in patients with nocardiosis: a case series and literature review. Radiol Infect Dis 4:64–69
5. Zhang Y et al (2016) Nocardial brain abscess in an immunocompetent patient and review of the literature. Chin Neurosurg J 2:26

6. Luthra G et al (2007) Comparative evaluation of fungal, tubercular, and pyogenic brain abscesses with conventional and diffusion MR imaging and proton MR spectroscopy. Am J Neuroradiol 28:1332–1338

7. Nandhagopal R et al (2014) Nocardia brain abscess. Q J Med 107:1041–1042

8. Antulov R et al (2014) Differentiation of pyogenic and fungal abscesses with susceptibility-weighted MR sequence. Neuroradiology 56:937–945

9. Sud S et al (2008) Case series: Nocardiosis of the brain and lungs. Indian J Radiol Imaging 18(3):218–221

Cysticercosis: Multiple Metastases

Headache and dizziness lasting for 3 weeks made this 55-year-old lady seek medical help at the neurological clinic. Her initial neurological status was normal; personal medical history was unremarkable. The neurologist referred her to a brain CT examination (Fig. 9.1).

A MRI examination of the brain was requested for further differentiation of the lesions (Fig. 9.2).

Further radiologic and serologic work-up was done, and a detailed medical history obtained. The patient remembered consuming uncertified pork meat of dubious quality approximately a year ago.

Immunofluorescent and immunosorbent (ELISA) serology test came positive for cysticercosis.

CT examination of thorax, abdomen and pelvis did not reveal convincing evidence of a possible primary tumour; there were two mediastinal peripherally calcified cystic lesions along the right tracheal wall, of uncertain aetiology. There were also several mildly enlarged paratracheal lymph nodes (Fig. 9.3).

The patient was treated with albendazole for 8 days, but during the course of therapy, her clinical status deteriorated. Meanwhile, the tumour markers serology report came in positive for CA 15.3 and CEA

She was subjected to stereotactic brain biopsy—histopathology reported metastatic brain carcinoma, positive for CK-7 (cytokeratin 7) and TTF-1 (thyroid transcription factor 1).

Ultrasound and CT exams of the neck revealed a nodular lesion in the inferior pole of the left thyroid gland lobe, as well as multiple enlarged lymph nodes. Cytology obtained by FNA of the biggest lymph node revealed a papillary thyroid carcinoma (Fig. 9.4).

Further deterioration of patient's status prompted thoracotomy and removal of the peripherally calcific masses next to the trachea. Histologically, the mass was in keeping with a papillary carcinoma of the thyroid gland.

9.1 Papillary Thyroid Carcinoma

Papillary thyroid carcinoma (PTC) is the most common neoplasm of the thyroid gland, accounting for approximately 70% of thyroid neoplasms and 85% of thyroid malignancies. Approximately 50% of patients have a nodal involvement at presentation, usually of the ipsilateral lymph nodes. The incidence of distant metastasis at the time of diagnosis is generally low. The usual metastatic sites are lung and bone, while brain metastases are extremely rare, with a relatively short time of survival after diagnosis of approximately 12 months [1]. Higher incidence of distant metastasis with a serious impact on survival is found in patients younger than 20 and older than 60 years of age, harbouring higher-grade tumours measuring more than 4 cm and having an extra-thyroid tumour focus at the time of initial examination [2].

© Springer International Publishing AG, part of Springer Nature 2018
M. Špero, H. Vavro, *Neuroradiology - Expect the Unexpected*,
https://doi.org/10.1007/978-3-319-73482-8_9

The presentation of PTC brain metastasis varies from solitary, homogenously enhancing nodular lesions to multiple cystic foci. When multiple cystic, as in this case, the differential diagnoses include multiple microabscesses, fungal infections and cysticercosis.

9.2   Neurocysticercosis

Neurocysticercosis (NC) is a brain infection caused by the pork tapeworm (*Taenia solium*). The time interval between the infection and onset of symptoms is very variable, ranging from 1 to

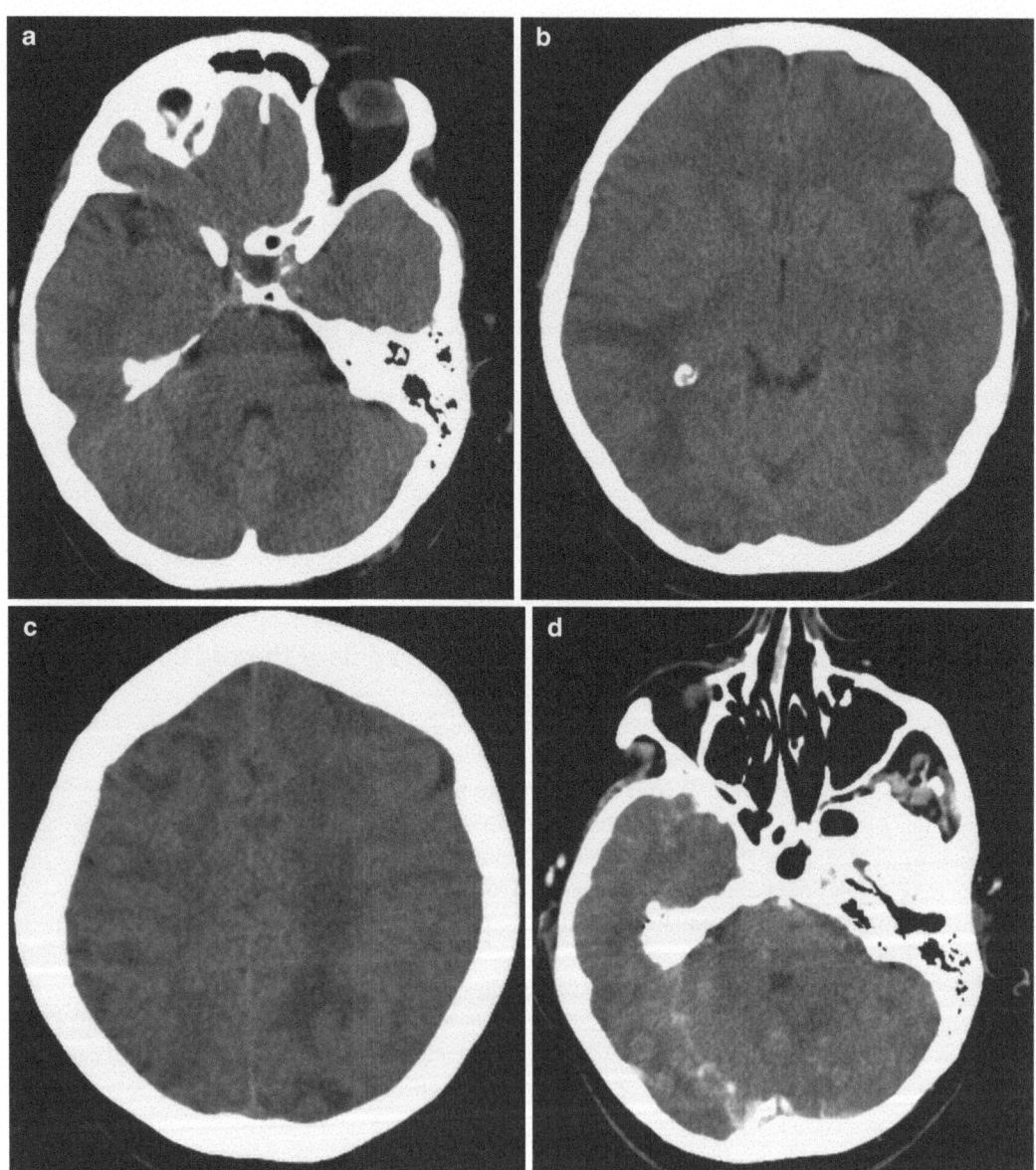

Fig. 9.1 CT examination of the brain. Axial non-enhanced (**a–c**) and contrast-enhanced (**d–f**) images. The report described numerous infratentorial and supratentorial ring-enhancing lesions up to 10 mm in diameter, some with perifocal oedema, which represent metastases. Differential diagnosis included multiple abscesses

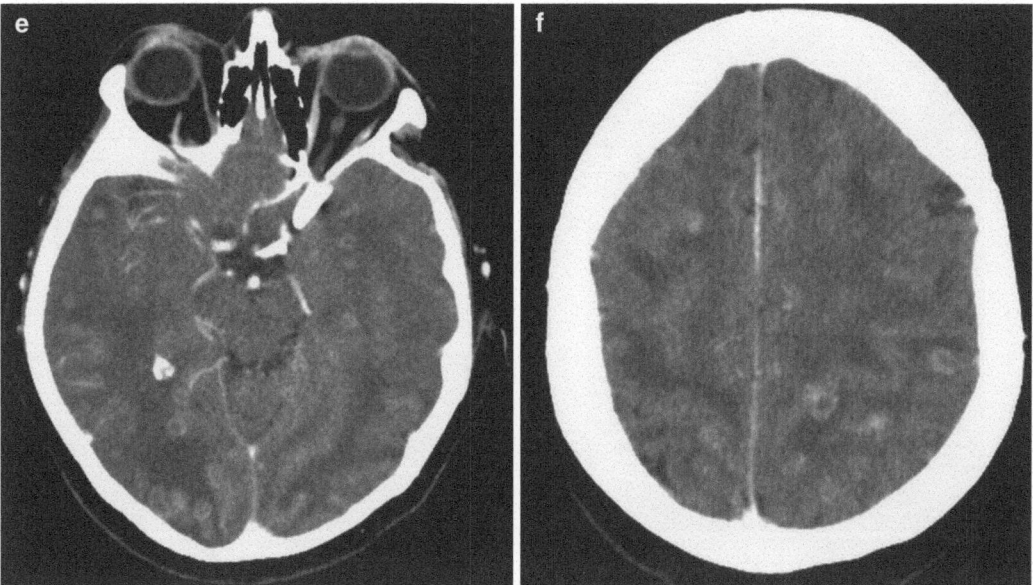

Fig. 9.1 (continued)

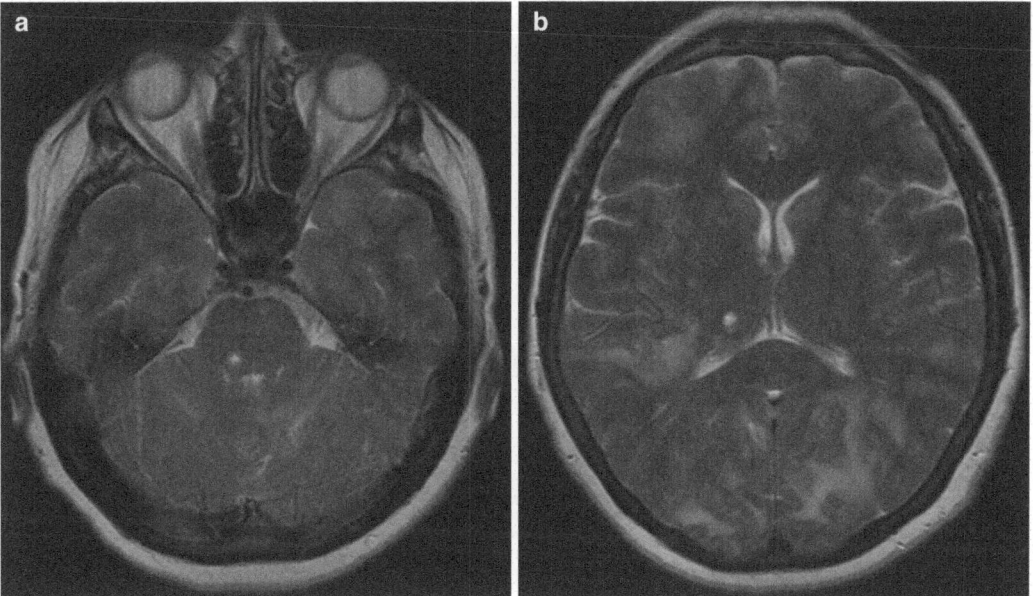

Fig. 9.2 MRI examination of the brain. Axial T2WI (**a–c**), DWI (**d**), T2-FLAIR (**e, f**), post-contrast axial T1WI (**g–i**). Multiple infratentorial and supratentorial parenchymal and subarachnoid cystic lesions, some of them with a tiny solid central nodule, which enhance peripherally and demonstrate perifocal oedema, were thought to represent neurocysticercosis, with most of the lesions in vesicular and colloidal vesicular stage

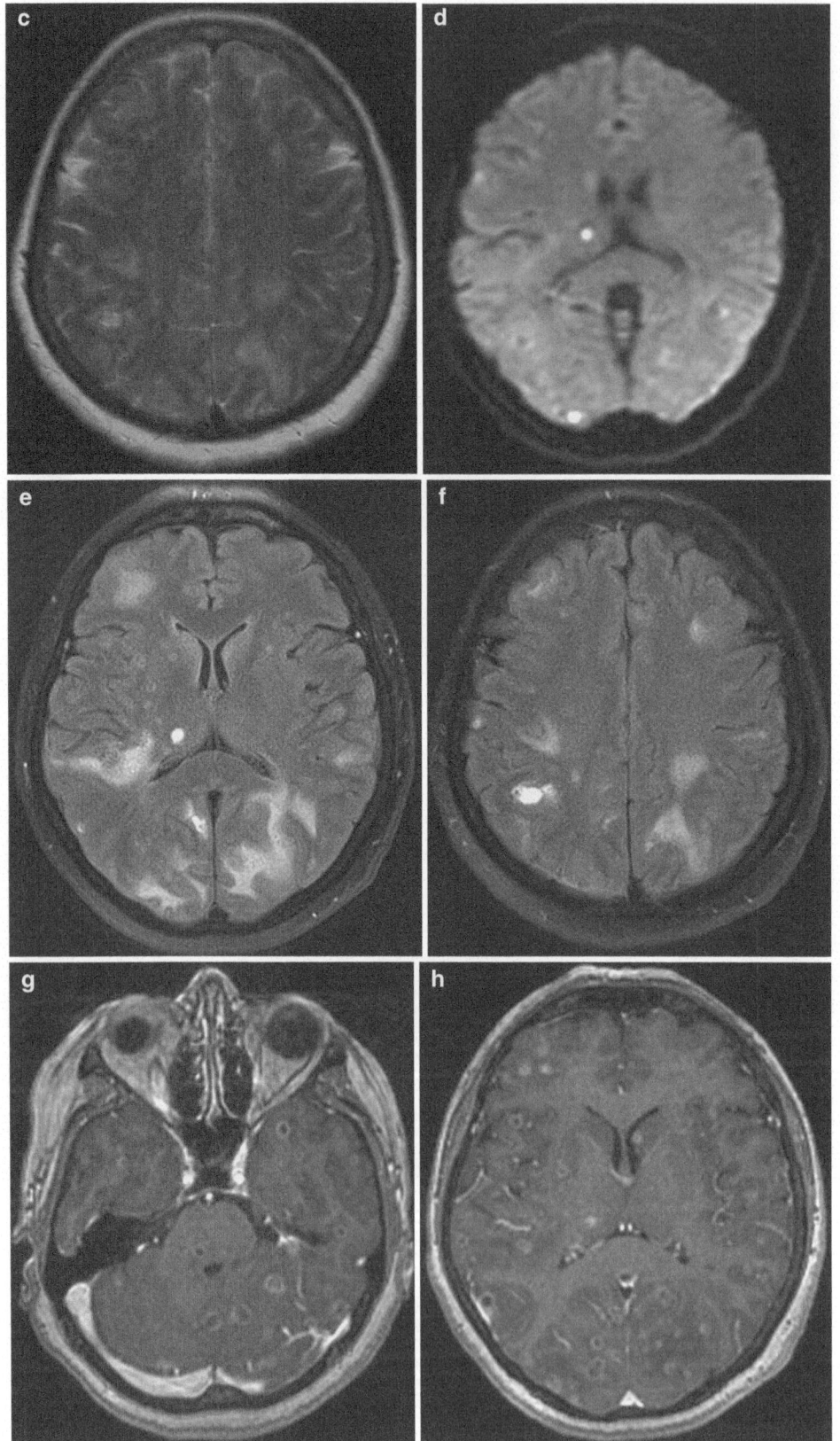

Fig. 9.2 (continued)

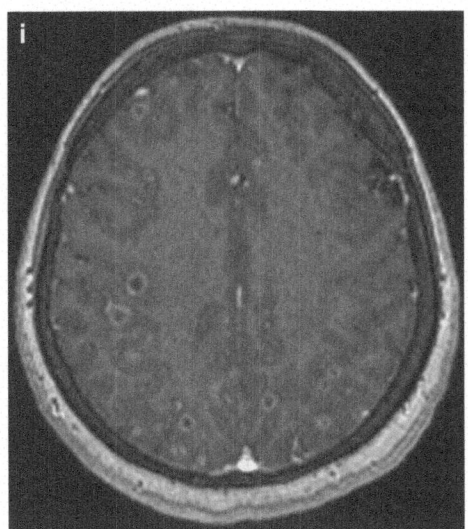

Fig. 9.2 (continued)

30 years. Symptoms may include seizures, headaches, hydrocephalus, neurological deficits and altered mental status. NC represents a leading cause of seizures and epilepsy in the developing world [3]. The radiological appearance of parenchymal NC varies depending on the stage of disease:

1. Vesicular stage is seen as CSF-like cysts with a small eccentric scolex, usually without perifocal oedema and contrast enhancement, although mild peripheral enhancement is possible [4]. The scolex is pathognomonic hallmark of this stage and presents as a bright dot on T2 FLAIR images.
2. Colloidal vesicular stage is represented by a cyst whose wall becomes thicker and enhances with contrast; there is also perifocal oedema.

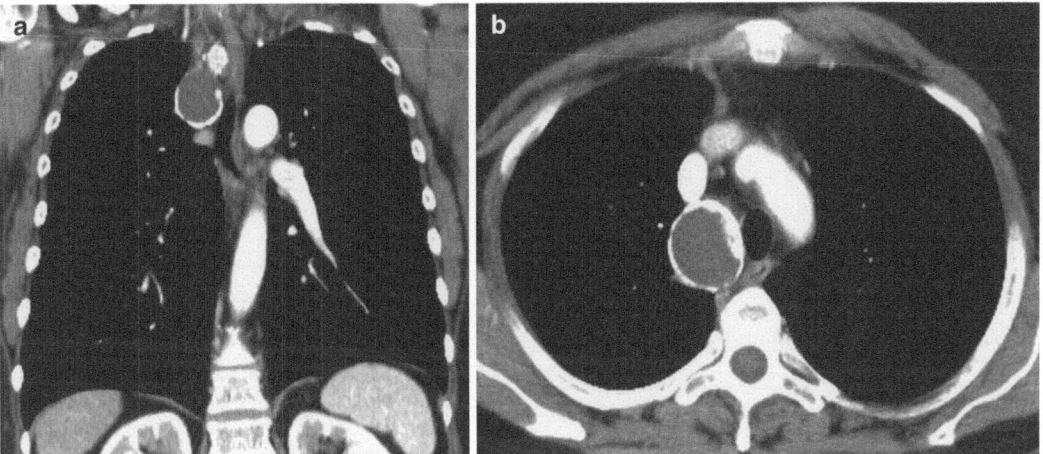

Fig. 9.3 Coronal (**a**) and axial (**b**) contrast-enhanced CT images of the thorax

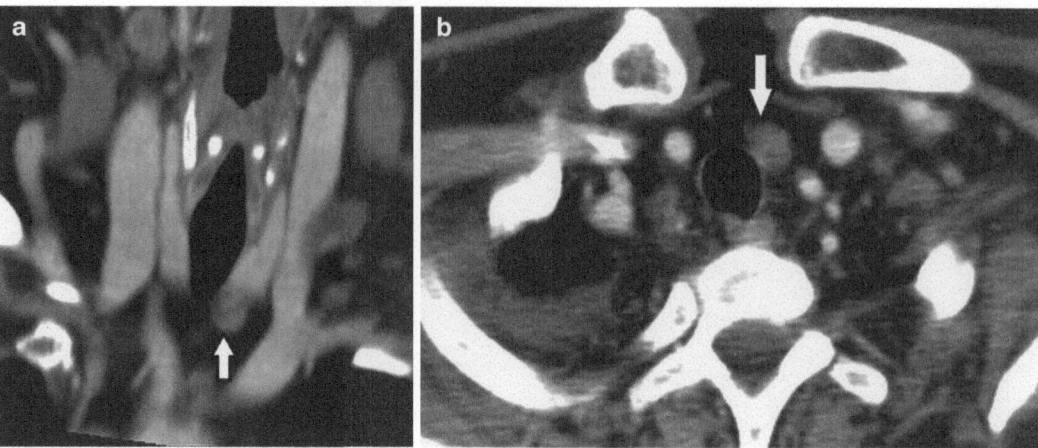

Fig. 9.4 Coronal (**a**) and axial (**b**) contrast-enhanced CT images of the neck showing a 12 mm node protruding caudally from the inferior pole of the left thyroid lobe

The appearance of the intracystic fluid is different from CSF due to an increase in proteinaceous content—hyperdense on CT, slightly hyperintense on T1-weighted images and markedly hyperintense on T2-weighted images and T2-FLAIR images. The scolex decreases in size. In this stage multiple lesions may generate marked immune response of the post, causing diffuse brain oedema and collapse of the ventricular system without midline shift—this is called acute cysticercosis encephalitis and is more often seen in children [5].

3. Granular nodular stage occurs with cyst retraction, while nodular or ring enhancement persists. The surrounding oedema decreases gradually. Pericystic gliosis is a common finding.

4. Nodular calcified stage represents an inactive, final stage—the lesion has shrunk for more than 50% of its original size; it is almost completely mineralised. There is no surrounding oedema. There may be mild peripheral contrast enhancement on MRI, sometimes with minimal oedema [5].

The imaging appearances are heterogenous, as most patients harbour parasites in all four evolution stages.

Neurocysticercosis is the most common parasitic disease of the central nervous system, and it should be considered as a differential diagnosis of multiple brain metastases, especially in endemic areas. In cases with clear peripheral lesion enhancement, metastatic disease must be ruled out in the first place, even though the appearances may suggest neurocysticercosis—several cases of initial misdiagnosis have been reported [6, 7].

References

1. Miranda ER et al (2010) Papillary thyroid carcinoma with brain metastases: an unusual 10-year-survival case. Thyroid 20(6):657–661. https://doi.org/10.1089/thy.2009.0442

2. Hoie J et al (1988) Distant metastases in papillary thyroid cancer: a review of 91 patients. Cancer 61:1–6

3. DeGiorgio CM et al (2004) Neurocysticercosis. Epilepsy Curr 4(3):107–111

4. Rumboldt Z et al (2010) Brain imaging with MRI and CT: an image pattern approach. Cambridge University Press, New York. https://doi.org/10.1017/CBO9781139030854

5. Zhao J-L et al (2015) Imaging spectrum of neurocysticercosis. Radiol Infect Dis 1(2):94–102. https://doi.org/10.1016/j.jrid.2014.12.001

6. Mota PC et al (2011) Lung cancer: atypical brain metastases mimicking neurocysticercosis. Int J Clin Oncol 16:746. https://doi.org/10.1007/s10147-011-0221-7

7. Troiani C et al (2011) Cystic brain metastases radiologically simulating neurocysticercosis. Sao Paulo Med J 129(5):352–356

Ethylene Glycol Poisoning

One evening in December 2015, a 34-year-old male came home from a night out with his friend. His mother claimed, at the time he retuned home that evening, her son was sorber, physical and mental status were not altered. Next morning she found him in a living room agitated, restless and disoriented. Ambulance transported him to a hospital: on an emergency admission, he was soporous and had metabolic acidosis with an anion gap, hypercalcemia and slightly increased urea (5.3 mmol/L) and creatinine (126 µmol/L) levels, while CT of the brain was unremarkable (Fig. 10.1).

During next 24-h he became comatose; urea (14 mmol/L) and creatinine (324 µmol/L) levels were rising. Due to the clinical course and status, haemodialysis was performed during following days.

Eight days after the admission, patient restored consciousness and has told doctors he suspected somebody had poured an antifreeze into his drink during a night out. All drug tests, toxins as well as ethylene glycol (EG) derivatives were negative, but those tests were performed after haemodialysis.

Brain MRI was performed 10 days after the admission (Figs. 10.2 and 10.3), without contrast media administration (creatinine 911 µmol/L).

Due to a patient information about possible poisoning, laboratory data and MRI findings that revealed lesions compatible with the acute EG toxicity, kidney biopsy was performed revealing diffuse acute tubular injury with calcium oxalate crystal depositions in tubular lumen and about 30% interstitial inflammation proving acute kidney injury due to the EG toxicity.

Two months after the poisoning, his neurologist reported almost complete neurological recovery, while 4 months after the poisoning, urea (6.3 mmol/L) and creatinine (101 µmol/L) levels were normal.

10.1 Ethylene Glycol Poisoning

Ethylene glycol is a colourless, sweet tasting and nearly odourless fluid, a poisonous form of alcohol. As an organic solvent, it is found in a variety of common household products including antifreeze, de-icing fluids, cleaners, paints, dyes, etc. It may be ingested intentionally in an attempt of suicide, or accidentally by alcoholics, or because of its sweet taste and the ease of access, by children and animals.

Ingestion of small quantity, as little as 100 mL in adult, will result in toxicity [1]. EG poisoning is characterised with development of successive presenting stages including an initial latency phase followed by the onset of severe metabolic acidosis and severe systemic and neurological complications leading to renal insufficiency, cardiorespiratory symptoms and brain oedema with coma within 12–24 h of ingestion. EG poisoning has produced cranial nerve deficits (usually VII nerve dysfunction) after a delay of 5–20 days [2].

© Springer International Publishing AG, part of Springer Nature 2018
M. Špero, H. Vavro, *Neuroradiology - Expect the Unexpected*,
https://doi.org/10.1007/978-3-319-73482-8_10

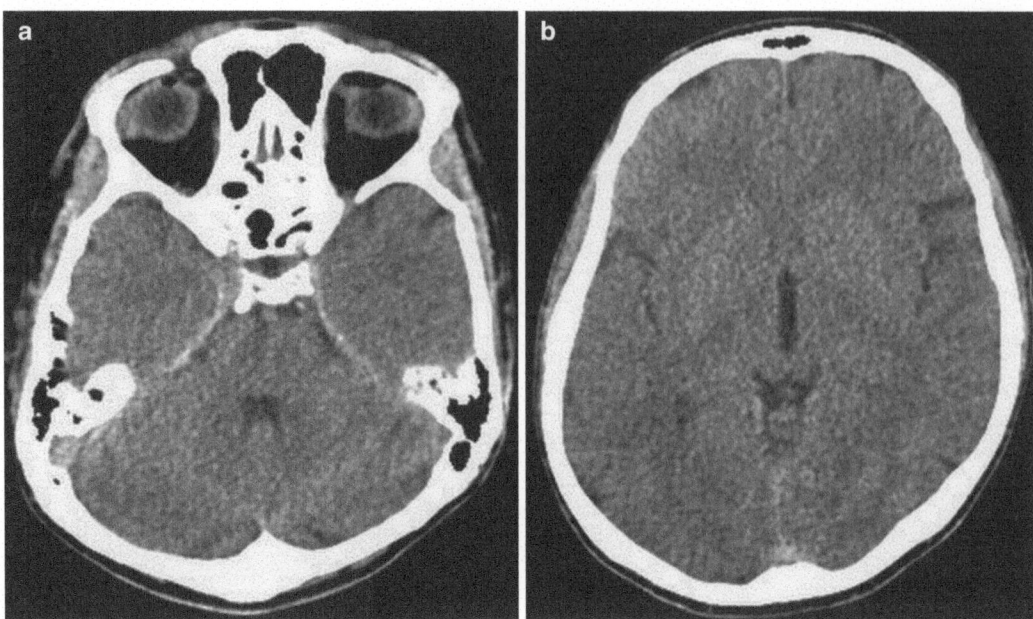

Fig. 10.1 Computed tomography of the brain, axial scan (**a**, **b**), performed on admission: both thalamus and lentiform nuclei were of normal density as well as pons

Except the initial EG-related transient inebriation, central nervous system impairment is usually delayed, evidencing that EG toxicity results from its conversion to toxic metabolites, thus explaining the lack of correlation between symptoms and EG concentrations. It is metabolised in the liver through a series of enzymes into intermediate metabolites: glycolaldehyde, glycolic acid and glyoxylic acid. Those toxic metabolites are cellular poisons. Glycolic acid is mainly responsible for the metabolic acidosis. Glyoxylic acid is converted to oxalic acid which precipitates with calcium into calcium oxalate crystals which are deposited in various tissues. Calcium oxalate crystals deposits in the cerebral vessel walls are responsible for cerebral oedema and ischaemia, as well as in the brain parenchyma having direct toxic effect at the cellular level within the basal ganglia and surrounding white matter [3–5].

In the first 24–48 h after the ingestion, CT and MRI of the brain reveal bilateral basal ganglia oedema or diffuse brain oedema, while 2–3 days after the ingestion, MRI reveals bilateral lesions of basal ganglia, thalami, amygdala, hippocampi, midbrain and upper pons consistent with vasogenic oedema (Figs. 10.2 and 10.3), cytotoxic oedema

and ischaemia involving frontal white matter, and haemorrhagic lesions in lentiform nuclei—putamen—could disappear after 5–35 days [5–10]. Lesions with vasogenic oedema are likely reversible [8]. Restricted diffusion within the white matter tracts of the corona radiata was reported with EG toxicity [5]. Putaminal necrosis may be found in subacute and chronic stages. Midbrain, sparing the red nuclei and the corticospinal tracts, as well as medulla oblongata and cerebellum may be involved in case of EG poisoning [8].

The basal ganglia are one of the most metabolically active regions in the brain due to its high energy demand, increased blood flow and richness in neurotransmitters and, therefore, are sensitive to toxic and metabolic disorders, hypoxia and acidosis. Differential diagnosis of EG poisoning therefore includes lesions due to hypoxic ischaemic encephalopathy, carbon monoxide poisoning, toxic encephalopathy, hepatic encephalopathy and hypoglycaemia and possible deep venous cerebral thrombosis (Fig. 10.3).

Making the exact diagnosis may be problematic in the absence of an appropriate history of EG ingestion, but if you are presented a comatose patient with metabolic acidosis with an increased anion gap, normal chloride level and elevated serum osmolarity, EG poisoning should be strongly suspected [7].

Early treatment with an alcohol dehydrogenase inhibitor fomepizole is very effective: it prevents toxic metabolites formation, metabolic acidosis and injury to the brain and kidneys. Other treatments include alkali to combat acidosis, ethanol as an EG antimetabolite and haemodialysis.

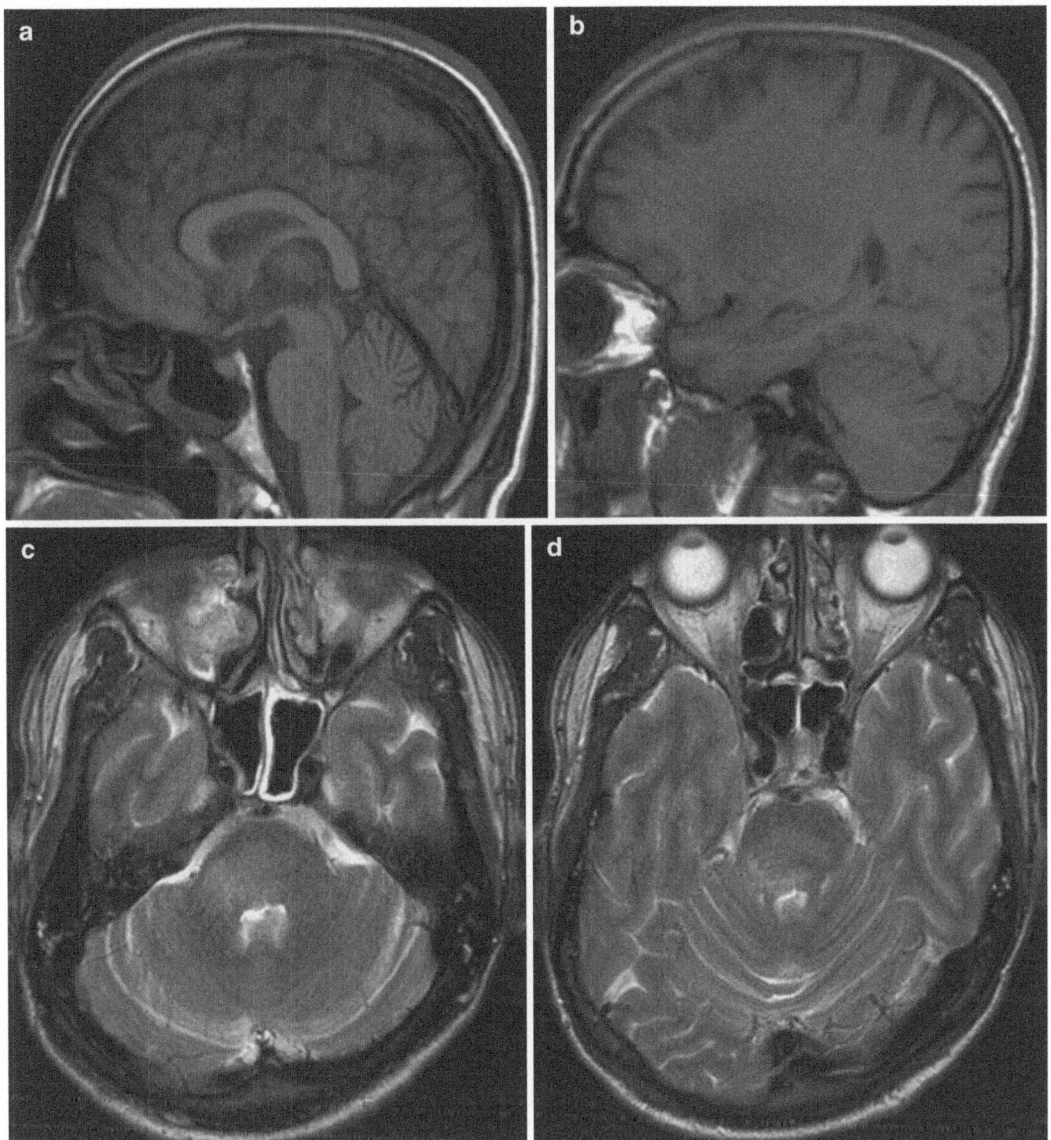

Fig. 10.2 Magnetic resonance imaging, sagittal T1WI (**a, b**), axial T2WI (**c–e**) and FLAIR (**f–h**), revealed symmetrical extensive heterogeneous T2 and FLAIR hyperintensities of slightly voluminous putamen, globus pallidus and external capsule, hyperintensities in both thalami. Asymmetrical T2 and FLAIR hyperintensities in pons, predominantly in the dorsal part which was slightly voluminous with mild compression of the IV ventricle. Involved supratentorial and infratentorial parenchyma was hypointense on T1WI, without sign of haemorrhage

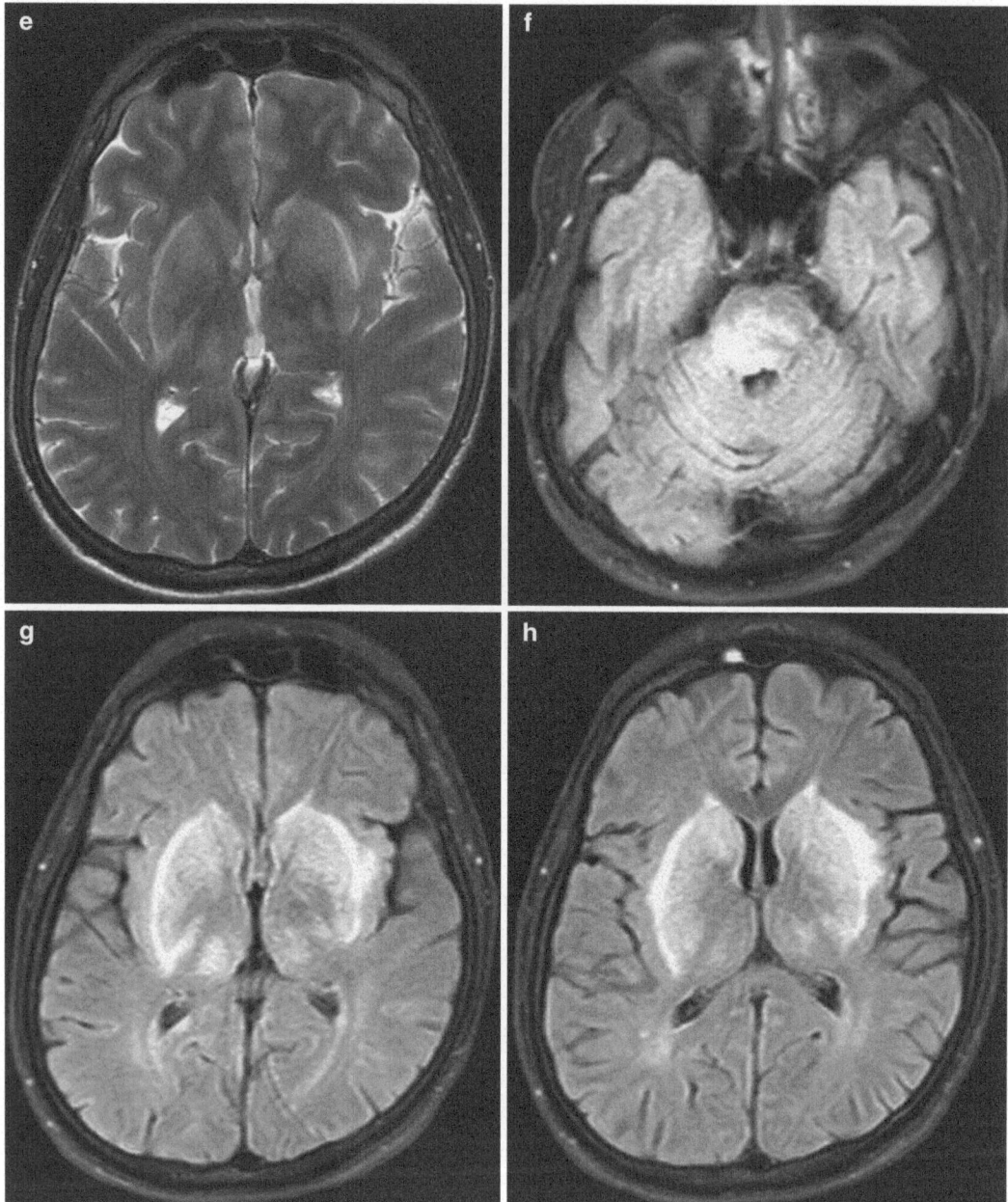

Fig. 10.2 (continued)

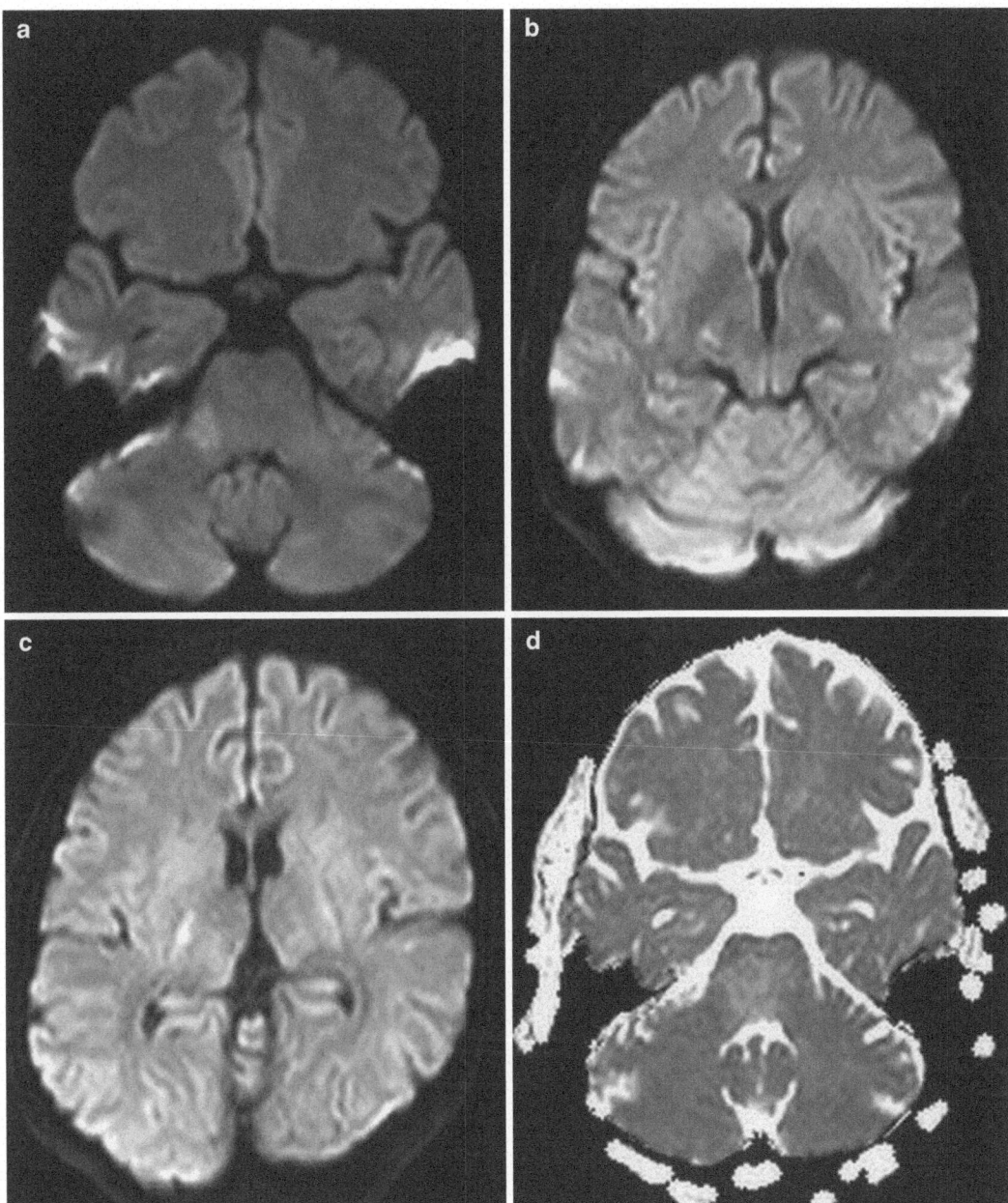

Fig. 10.3 Magnetic resonance imaging, axial DWI (**a–c**) and ADC (**d–f**): without restricted diffusion of the involved brain parenchyma—lesions were related to vasogenic oedema

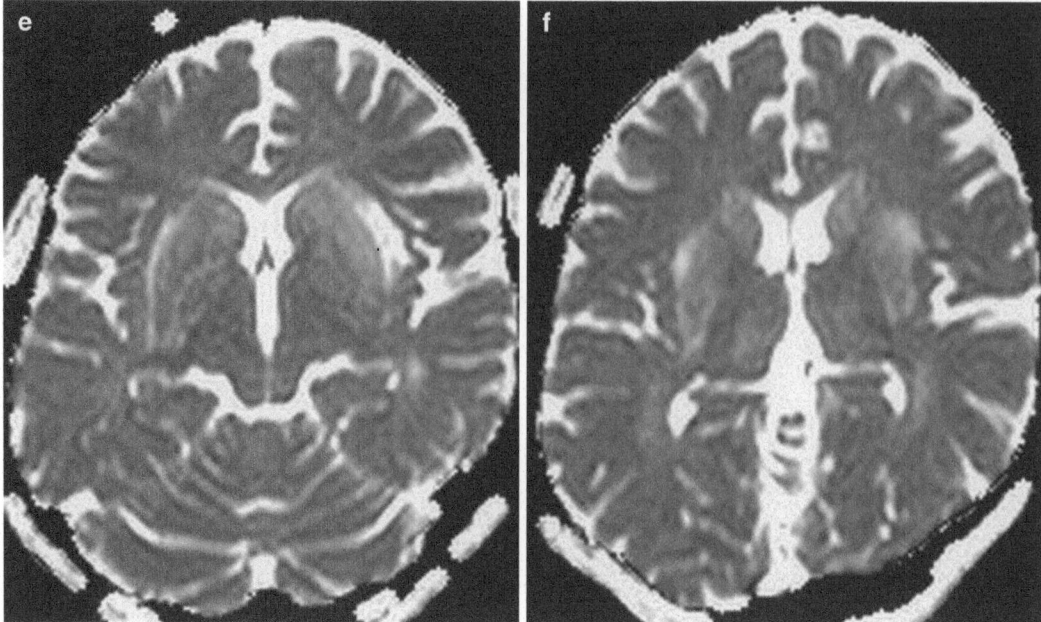

Fig. 10.3 (continued)

References

1. Scally R et al (2002) Treatment of ethylene glycol poisoning. Am Fam Physician 66:807–812
2. Readdy N et al (2010) Delayed neurological sequelae from ethylene glycol, diethylene glycol and methanol poisonings. Clin Toxicol (Phila) 48(10):967–973
3. Davis DP et al (1997) Ethylene glycol poisoning: case report of a record-high level and a review. J Emerg Med 15(5):653–667
4. Gabow PA et al (1986) Organic acids in ethylene glycol intoxication. Ann Intern Med 105(1):16–20
5. Moore MM et al (2008) Ethylene glycol toxicity: chemistry, pathogenesis, and imaging. Radiol Case Rep 3:122. https://doi.org/10.2484/rcr.v3i1.122
6. Zeiss J et al (1989) Cerebral CT of lethal ethylene glycol intoxication with pathologic correlation. AJNR Am J Neuroradiol 10:440–442
7. Corr P, Szolics M (2012) Neuroimaging findings in acute ethylene glycol poisoning. J Med Imaging Radiat Oncol 56:442–444
8. Boukobza M et al (2015) Neuroimaging findings and follow-up in two cases of severe ethylene glycol intoxication with full recovery. J Neurol Sci 359:343–346
9. Maekawa N et al (2015) Brain magnetic resonance image changes following acute ethylene glycol poisoning. Neurol India 63:998–1000
10. Santana-Cabrera L et al (2013) Ethylene glycol toxic encephalopathy. J Neurosci Rural Pract 4(4):477–478

Carbon Monoxide Poisoning Sequelae

11

Two days before being admitted to our university hospital, a young lady (28) was urgently hospitalised at a regional hospital after she had been found unresponsive on the bathroom floor. Carbon monoxide poisoning caused by malfunctioning gas-powered water boiler was suspected. The initial CT exam was reported as normal. Upon waking from coma, she had left-sided hemiparesis. During the next several days, her neurological status became completely normal, but ventricular extrasystolia was noticed, so a suspicion of cardiogenic loss of consciousness arose. A MRI exam of the brain was requested (Fig. 11.1).

The imaging findings were compatible with carbon monoxide poisoning, but not very dramatic since the MRI exam was done 6 days after carbon monoxide inhalation and the patient recovered completely.

An example of CT and MRI findings in the setting of acute carbon monoxide poisoning (in a different patient) is shown in Fig. 11.2:

11.1 Carbon Monoxide Poisoning

Carbon monoxide (CO) is a colourless, odourless, tasteless, non-irritant gas produced by incomplete combustion of carbon-based fuels and substances. It is produced by common household appliances, heating equipment and internal combustion engine motors.

Carbon monoxide poisoning is the most frequent cause of accidental poisoning and can be fatal; it is frequently unrecognised due to its non-specific clinical presentation, unless typical history of CO exposure is provided. The patient is often unresponsive; the clinical findings are highly variable and non-specific. The symptoms may vary from headache, nausea and vomiting to confusion, ataxia, seizures, coma, myocardial infarction and death. Long-term low-level CO exposure may be the cause of chronic fatigue, memory deficits, vertigo, neuropathy, diarrhoea and abdominal pain. There may be a delayed encephalopathy of carbon monoxide intoxication, characterised by a recurrence of neurological or psychiatric symptoms [1]. The lucid interval between acute and recurrent symptoms usually lasts 2–3 weeks. The delayed encephalopathy may end with full recovery but also with progressive deterioration ending in coma or death, which depends on the severity of the initial carbon monoxide intoxication.

The affinity of the CO for heme protein is approximately 250 times that of oxygen—such formation of carboxyhaemoglobin reduces the oxygen-carrying capacity of the blood and the off load of oxygen to tissues is greatly reduced. This causes tissue hypoxia/anoxia. There is also a direct toxic effect of the CO on mitochondria, interfering with oxidative phosphorylation. These lead to anoxic-ischaemic encephalopathy.

© Springer International Publishing AG, part of Springer Nature 2018
M. Špero, H. Vavro, *Neuroradiology - Expect the Unexpected*,
https://doi.org/10.1007/978-3-319-73482-8_11

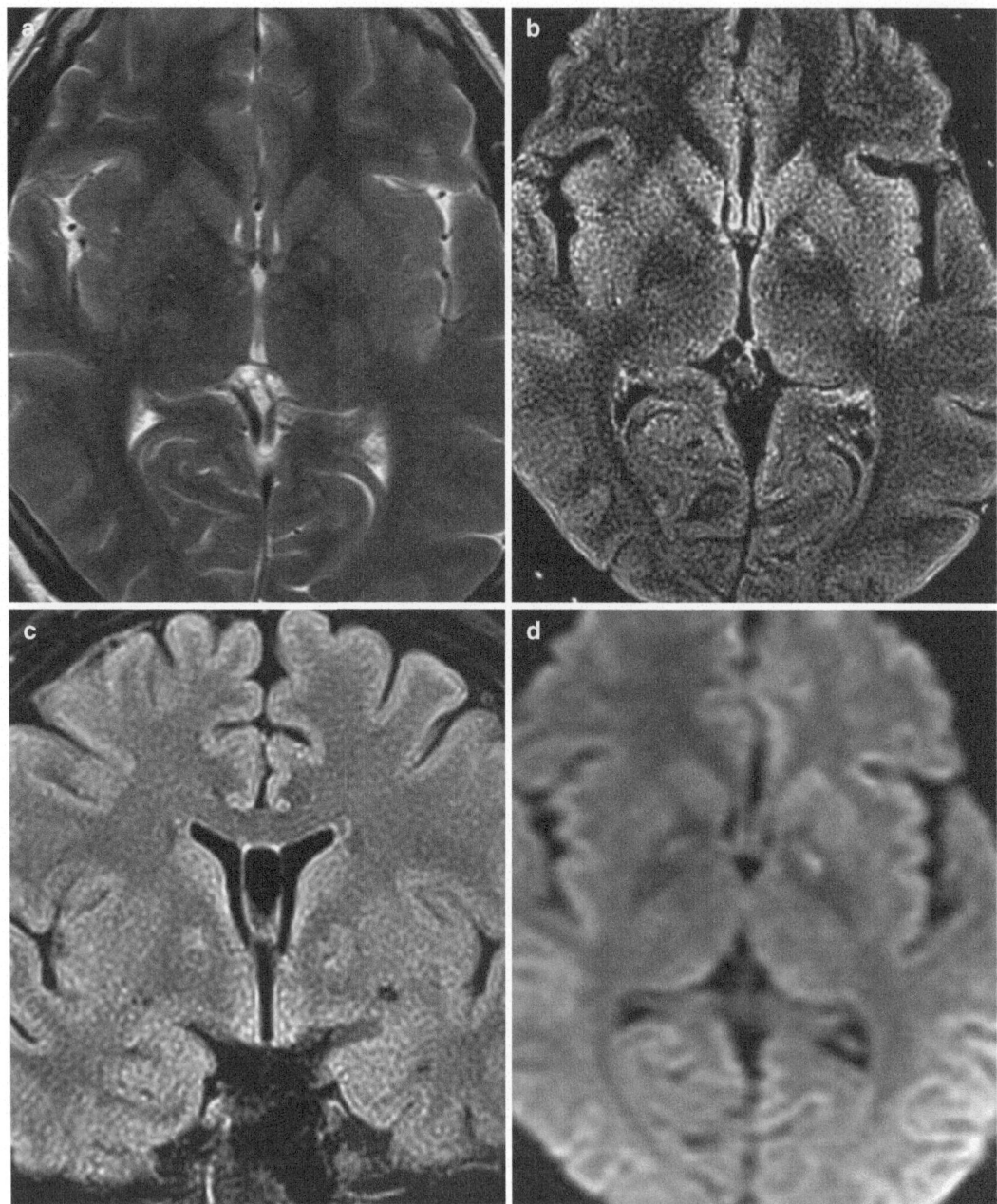

Fig. 11.1 MRI exam of the brain, 6 days after the incident. Axial T2WI (**a**) and axial and coronal T2-FLAIR images (**b, c**) show a focal hyperintensity bilaterally in the globus pallidus, best appreciated in the T2-FLAIR images. A mild hyperintensity on the diffusion-weighted image (**d**) in the same areas may be attributed to mild residual cytotoxic oedema or to T2 shine-through—the ADC map (**e**) is normal. There is mild hypointensity in the left globus pallidus shown on the sagittal T1WI (**f**)

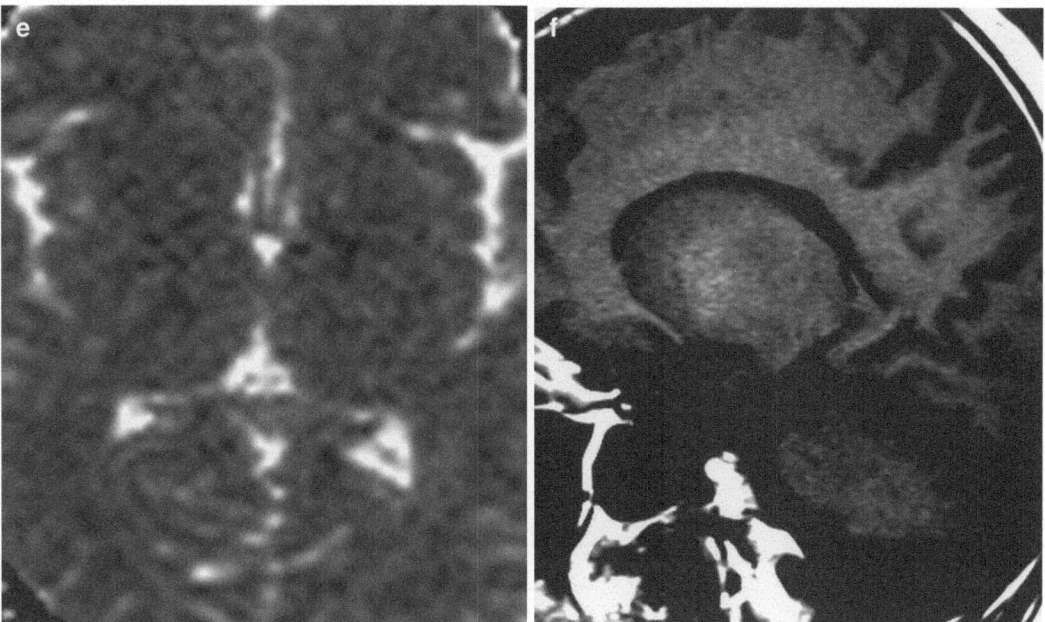

Fig. 11.1 (continued)

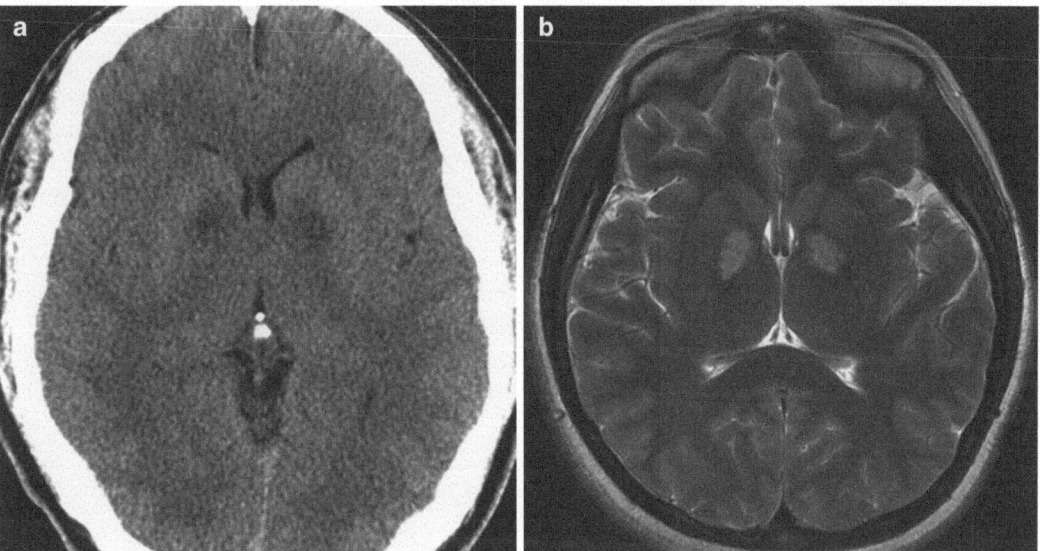

Fig. 11.2 CT and MRI findings in acute carbon monoxide poisoning (images courtesy of Prof. Z. Rumboldt). Non-enhanced CT image (**a**) shows a hypodense area in the globus pallidus bilaterally, compatible with hyperin tense areas on MRI T2WI image (**b**). There is also high DWI signal within the lesions (**c**), indicating low diffusivity due to cytotoxic oedema

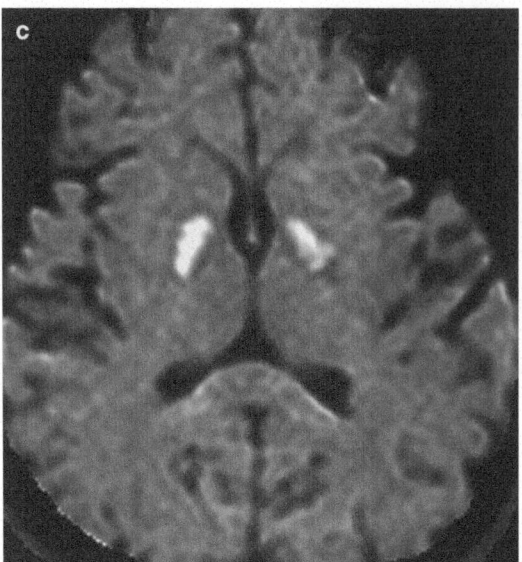

Fig. 11.2 (continued)

Normal blood levels of carboxyhaemoglobin are up to 3% in non-smokers and up to 10% in smokers. A note is made that the standard two-wavelength pulse oximetry cannot differentiate between carboxyhaemoglobin and oxyhaemoglobin [2].

The treatment of CO poisoning consists of administering 100% oxygen, preferably in a hyperbaric setting.

Standard imaging findings in acute CO poisoning include symmetric CT hypodensity in globus pallidus, which is seen as low T1 and high T2 and DWI signal on MRI. There may be a T1 hyperintensity and a rim of low T2 signal, reflecting haemorrhagic necrosis [3]. Patchy peripheral enhancement is possible in the acute phase. There may also be similar abnormalities in the cerebral cortex, hippocampus, and substantia nigra, and cerebellar abnormalities have also been described [2]. In patients who develop a delayed leukoencephalopathy, there are confluent T2 hyperintense areas in the periventricular white matter with mild temporary decrease of diffusivity; the extent and degree of low ADC values are correlated with the clinical course and severity of CO intoxication [1].

Differential diagnoses include other toxic encephalopathies such as cyanide neurotoxicity which may be indistinguishable from carbon monoxide poisoning. Methanol poisoning typically affects the putamina, sparring the globi pallidi. Ethylene glycol (antifreeze) poisoning involves globi pallidi, other basal ganglia and thalami (see Chap. 10). Leigh disease usually presents in infancy or early childhood, with lesions in bilateral basal ganglia, thalami and brainstem. Pantothenate kinase-associated neurodegeneration (PKAN) presents as symmetric T2 hyperintensity within iron-laden hypointense globi pallidi ("eye of the tiger").

References

1. Ji-hoon K et al (2003) Delayed encephalopathy of acute carbon monoxide intoxication: diffusivity of cerebral white matter lesions. Am J Neuroradiol 24(8):1592–1597
2. Ryan AS et al (2012) Carbon monoxide poisoning: novel magnetic resonance imaging pattern in the acute setting. Int J Emerg Med 5:30
3. Rumboldt Z et al (2010) Brain imaging with MRI and CT: an image pattern approach. Cambridge University Press, New York. https://doi.org/10.1017/CBO9781139030854

CLIPPERS: Infiltrative Brainstem Lymphoma

12

In November 2016, an 80-year-old female patient has fallen while walking: after a fall, she could not move her right leg; therefore she searched for a medical help. The patient described she had mild walking problems due to discrete occasional weakness of a right leg, during a month or two before a fall. According to patient medical data, she was taking antihypertensive medications due to arterial hypertension.

The patient was hospitalised: bone X-rays did not reveal fracture of a right femur or bones of a right lower leg. MRI of the brain was performed and revealed a process in pons and midbrain (Figs. 12.1 and 12.2).

Neuroradiologist who first reviewed the MRI examination has reported possible chronic lymphocytic inflammation with pontine perivascular enhancement responsive to steroids (CLIPPERS) or primary neoplastic process. We have revised the MRI examination and, due to clinical presentation and imaging features (Figs. 12.1 and 12.2), have reported primary neoplastic process infiltrating part of the pons, left cerebral peduncle and part of the thalamus possible lymphoma or glioma. Brain biopsy was performed and revealed primary brain lymphoma. The patient died just before the onset of oncological treatment.

12.1 CLIPPERS or Primary Brain Lymphoma

First described in 2010 by Pittock and his colleagues, CLIPPERS is a relatively new and rare CNS inflammatory disorder, defined as a distinct form of brainstem encephalitis centred on the pons, which is characterized by a predominant T-cell pathology and responsive to immunosuppression with glucocorticosteroids [1]. Histopathology after brain biopsy demonstrated predominantly T-cell infiltration with perivascular predominance in the involved white matter, accompanied by a moderate number of histiocytes and activated microglia [1–3].

There is no definitive sex predilection, and the age of onset ranges between 13 and 86 years: in large series a mean age of onset was in the fifth or sixth decade of life. Clinical course is subacute with progressive gait disorders, ataxia, dysarthria and diplopia as main symptoms [2, 3].

The hallmark of the brain MRI is punctate and curvilinear bilateral symmetrical perivascular enhancement peppering the pons with variable superior extension to the midbrain, inferior extension to the medulla and posterior extension to the middle cerebellar peduncles and cerebellum. Similar type of contrast enhancement may

© Springer International Publishing AG, part of Springer Nature 2018
M. Špero, H. Vavro, *Neuroradiology - Expect the Unexpected*,
https://doi.org/10.1007/978-3-319-73482-8_12

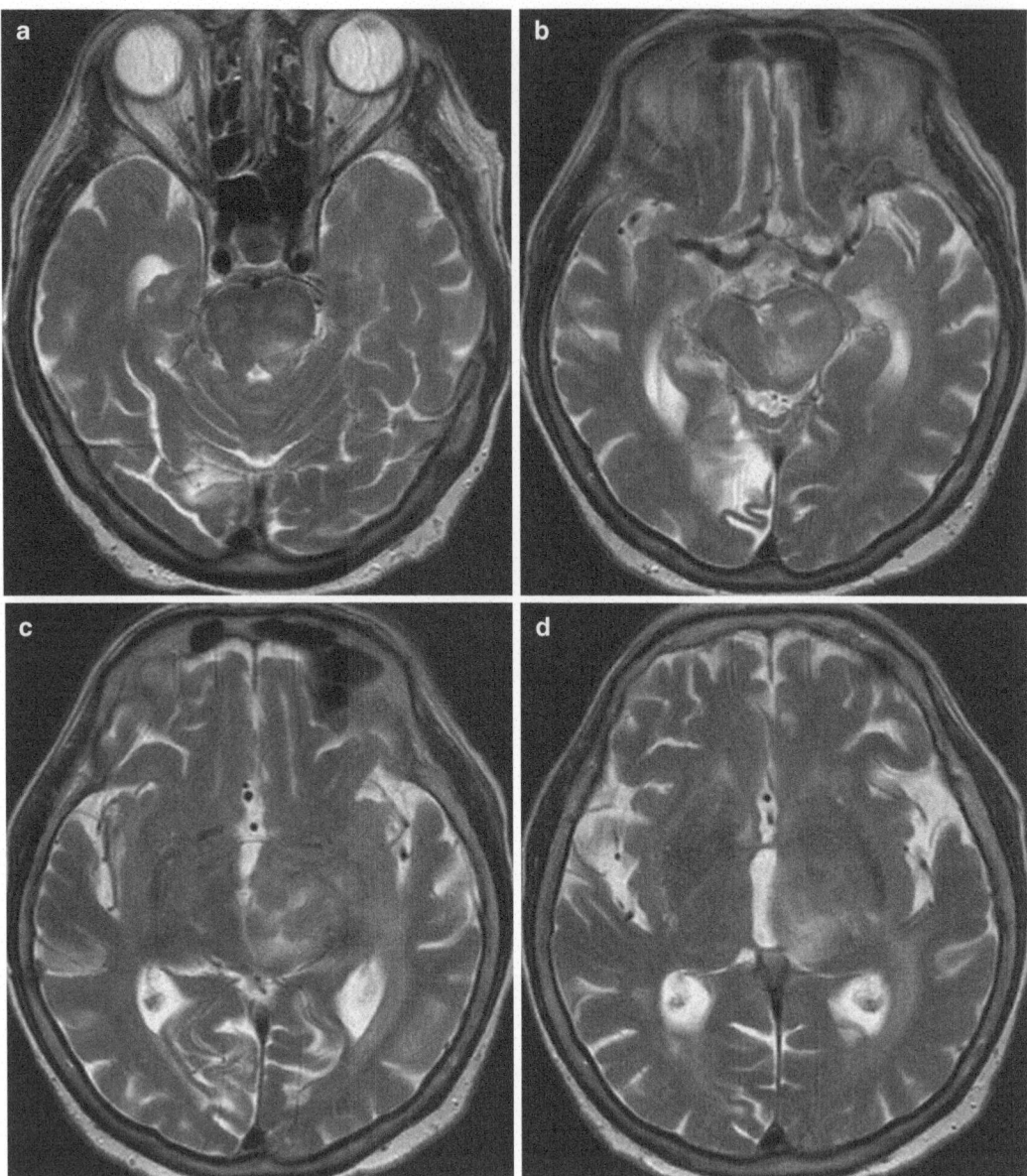

Fig. 12.1 Magnetic resonance of the brain, axial T2WI (**a–d**), FLAIR (**e–h**) and DWI (**i**) revealed lesion involving posterior and upper part of the left pons, left cerebral peduncle of the midbrain and part of the thalamus. Lesion had an expansive effect and involved parts of the midbrain were more voluminous: it was inhomogeneous, slightly hyperintense on T2WI and FLAIR, diffusion was not resticted

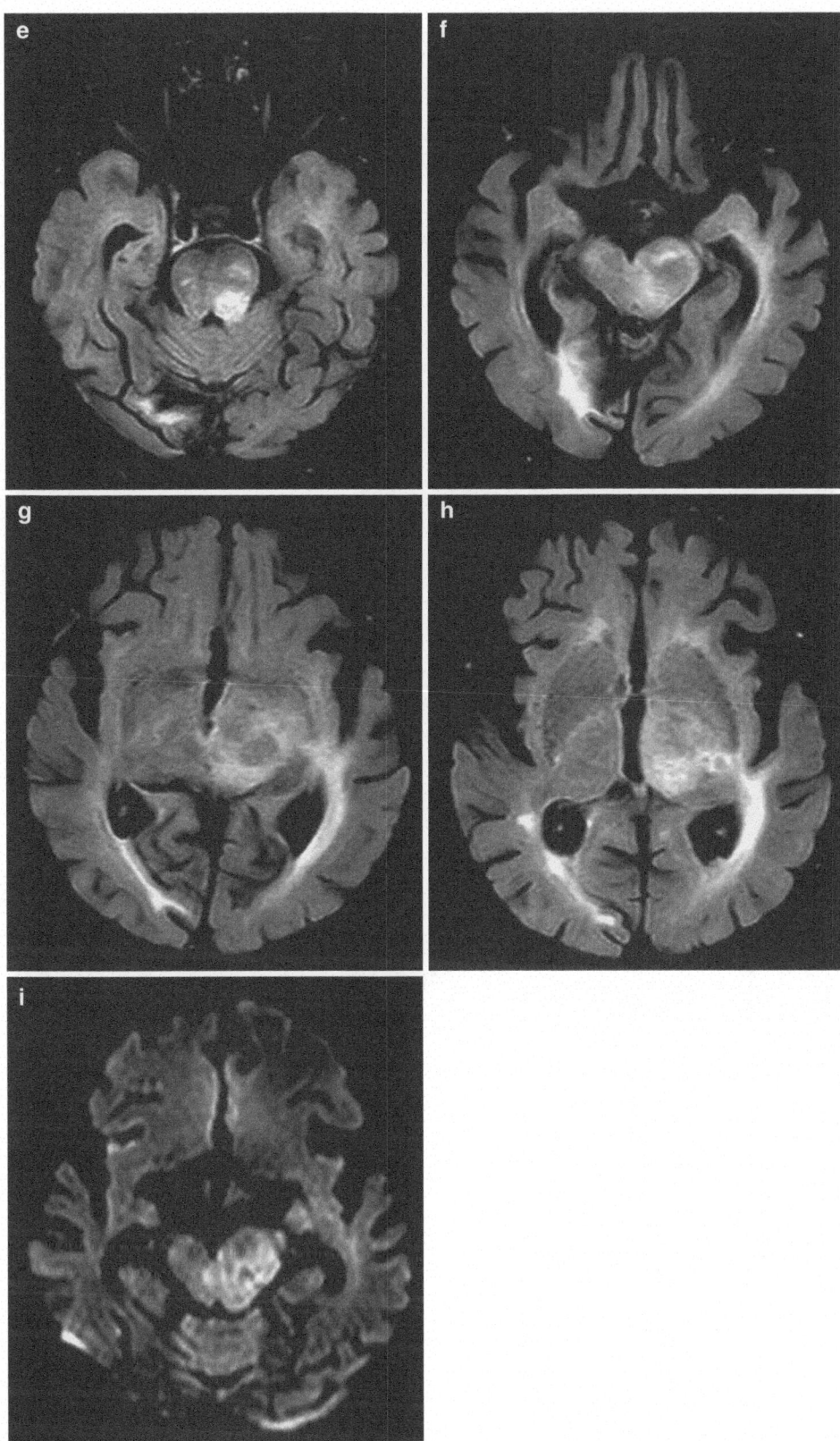

Fig. 12.1 (continued)

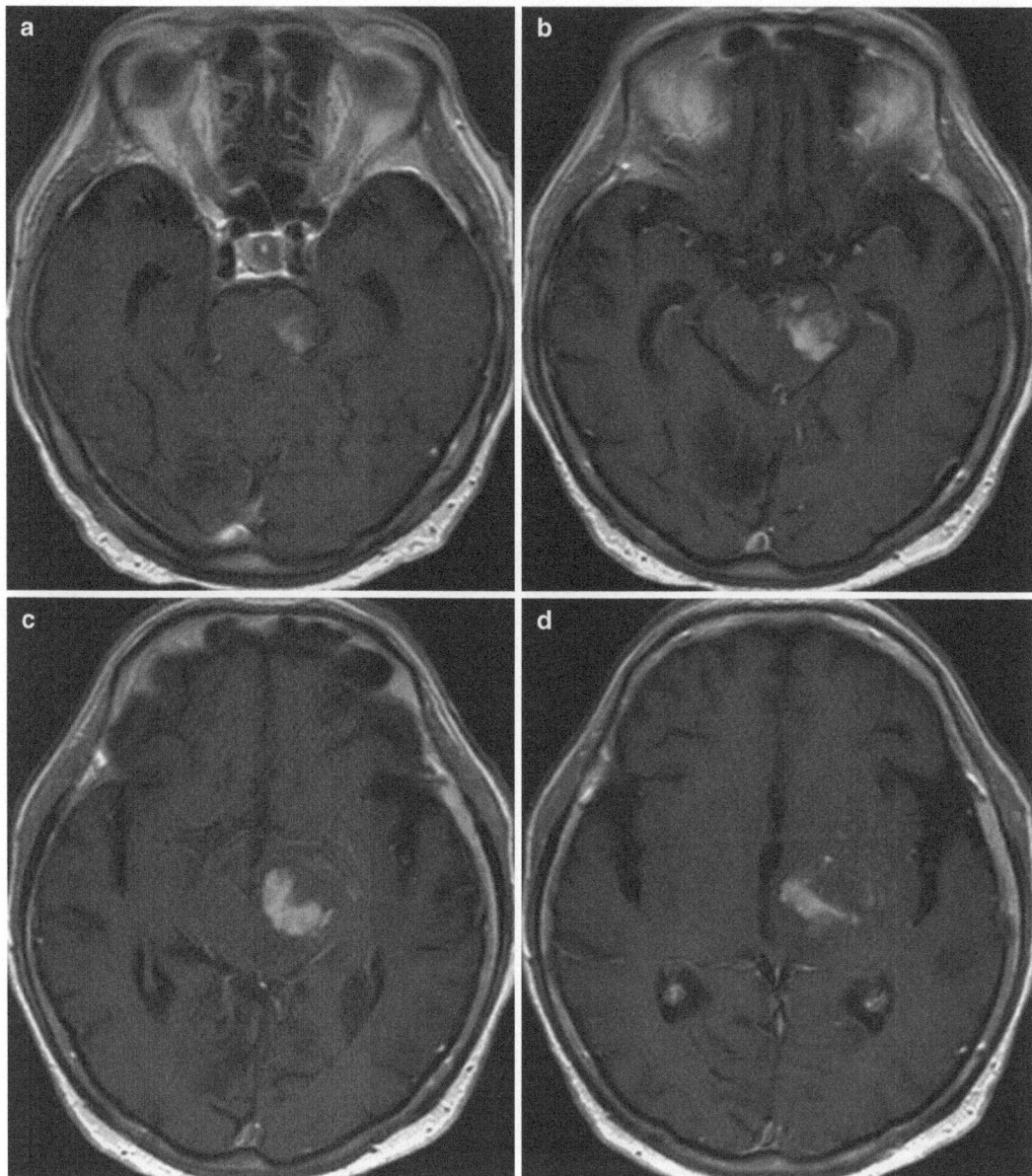

Fig. 12.1 (continued)

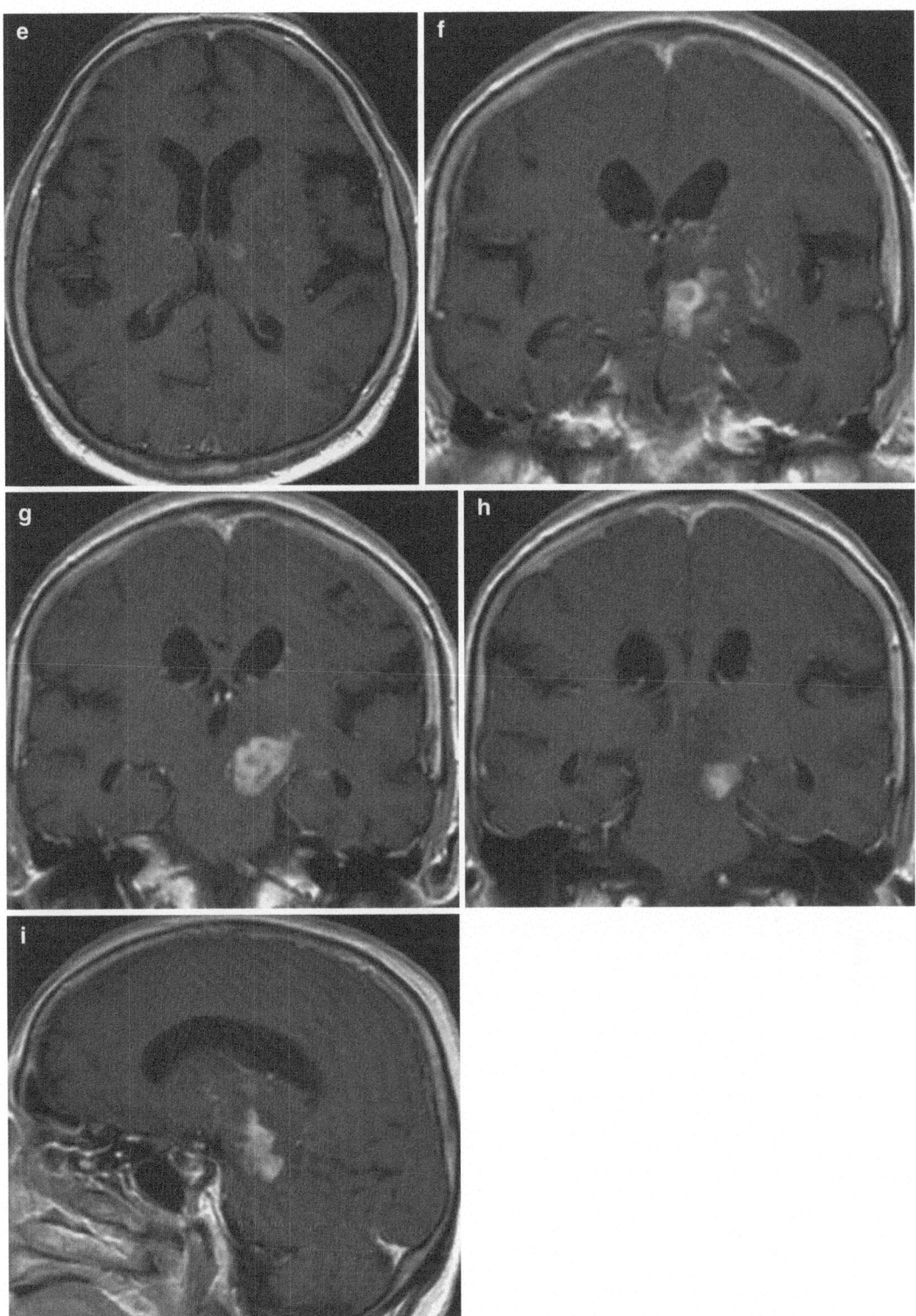

Fig. 12.2 Post-contrast MRI of the brain, axial (**a–e**), coronal (**f–h**) and sagittal (**i**) T1WI, demonstrated irregular expansile lesion that enhanced inhomogeneously, with punctate and curvilinear contrast enhancement in the left basal ganglia. Gyri around left central sulcus were mildly enlarged, with slightly reduced sulci, probably due to infiltration of the involved tracts (**f–h**)

involve the basal ganglia, thalami, internal capsule, corpus callosum and spinal cord, while a cerebral cortex is usually spared. Punctate enhancing foci range in size between 1 and 3 mm, when larger than 3 mm typically have nodular appearance. There are patchy T2WI and FLAIR hyperintensities in areas of contrast enhancement. Usually there is no mass effect or vasogenic oedema which can be minimal as well. Contrast enhancement responds to the lymphocytic perivascular inflammatory pattern and decreases as the patient responds to immunosuppressive therapy [1–3].

Pathogenesis is poorly understood and unknown: according to histopathology after a brain biopsy and clinico-radiological response to immunosuppressive therapies, it suggests an autoimmune or other inflammatory-mediated pathogenesis, while the targeted autoantigen could be located in perivascular regions, probably in pons [1, 3]. Laboratory investigation is usually unrevealing: the most common CSF anomaly is an elevated protein level, while occasional presence of oligoclonal band has been described [1–3].

Although age, subacute onset, involved brain parenchyma and curvilinear contrast enhancement in the basal ganglia may fit into described characteristics of CLIPPERS, clinical symptom of leg weakness; unilateral involvement of the pons, midbrain and thalamus; contrast enhancing irregular process causing mass effect fit into favour of primary brain neoplasms. Differential diagnosis of CLIPPERS includes, among other diagnosis, primary brain lymphoma and glioma as well.

Primary CNS lymphomas nearly are diffuse large B-cell lymphomas. Imaging findings vary with the immune status of a patient. Typical CNS lymphoma neuroimaging features include supratentorial white matter and corpus callosum involvement but may also involve midbrain and cerebellum. CNS lymphomas are hypercellular tumours causing mass effect and marked post-contrast enhancement. Due to its hypercellularity, those are hypointense on T2WI and show restricted diffusion, although, if tumour is atypical, like in immunodeficient and immunocompetent patients, diffusion may not be restricted. On FLAIR sequence those tumours are hyperintense. Primary CNS lymphomas demonstrate marked perivascular or intravascular tumour infiltration that, together with a lack of neoangiogenesis, results in low rCBV but, on post-contrast T1WI, may reveal punctate or curvilinear contrast enhancement as well. Similar type of contrast enhancement may be present in parenchyma around glioma as satellite lesions. In this case it was difficult to decide what kind of tumour process it was, lymphoma or glioma, but due to lack of necrosis in the tumour mass and curvilinear contrast enhancement in the surrounding parenchyma, it made us decide CNS lymphoma as the first differential diagnosis, which was proved by stereotactic brain biopsy [4–6].

References

1. Pittock SJ et al (2010) Chronic lymphocytic inflammation with pontine perivascular enhancement responsive to steroids (CLIPPERS). Brain 133:2626–2634
2. Dudesek A et al (2014) CLIPPERS: chronic lymphocytic inflammation with pontine perivascular enhancement responsive to steroids. Review of an increasingly recognized entity within the spectrum of inflammatory central nervous system disorder. Clin Exp Immunol 175:425–438
3. Bag AK et al (2014) Case 212: chronic lymphocytic inflammation with pontine perivascular enhancement responsive to steroids. Radiology 273:940–947
4. Kickingereder P et al (2014) Primary central nervous system lymphoma and atypical glioblastoma: multiparametric differentiation by using diffusion-, perfusion-, and susceptibility-weighted MR imaging. Radiology 272:843–850
5. Mansour A et al (2014) MR imaging features of intracranial primary CNS lymphoma in immune competent patients. Cancer Imaging 14:22–30
6. Da Rocha AJ et al (2016) Modern techniques of magnetic resonance in the evaluation of primary central nervous system lymphoma: contributions to the diagnosis and differential diagnosis. Rev Bras Hematol Hemoter 38(1):44–54

Part IV

Skull and Orbit Anomalies

Crouzon Syndrome

13

After having several surgeries performed by neurosurgeons and maxillofacial surgeons (at the age of 2, 3 and 8), a 17-year-old girl with an established diagnosis of Crouzon syndrome (craniofacial dysostosis) visited a maxillofacial surgery referral centre for a second opinion on further treatment options (Fig. 13.1).

13.1 Crouzon Syndrome

Crouzon syndrome (CS) is a rare genetic disorder producing characteristic craniofacial features and other associated abnormalities, caused by premature closure of cranial sutures. The premature fusion of skull base causes midface hypoplasia, maxillary hyperplasia, shallow orbits and subsequent vision problems. It may be associated with hydrocephalus, stylohyoid ligament calcification, Chiari I malformation, cervical spine abnormalities and airway obstruction. Other clinical features include hypertelorism, beaked nose, short upper lip and relative mandibular prognathism. The hands and feet are usually normal which is a feature that can be used to distinguish CS from other craniosynostoses [1]. It is caused by a FGFR2 gene mutation on chromosomal locus 10q 25.3-q26 and inherited in the autosomal dominant pattern. The expressivity is variable [2].

CS accounts for approximately 4.8% of all craniosynostosis cases [2]. The prevalence rate is 1 in 25,000 live births. There is no race or sex predilection, but frequency of sagittal or metopic craniosynostosis is higher in boys, whereas coronal craniosynostosis is more frequent in girls.

Differential diagnosis includes other syndromes which feature similar craniofacial abnormalities, such as Pfeiffer syndrome, apert syndrome, Saethre-Chotzen syndrome, Carpenter syndrome and Jackson-Weiss syndrome.

Early diagnosis is crucial, as CS should be managed as early as possible by a multidisciplinary approach. Treatment usually begins during the first year of life with cranial decompression and correction of midfacial hypoplasia. Early craniectomy treats increased intracranial pressure. A technique of craniofacial disjunction followed by gradual bone distraction may correct exophthalmos and improve aesthetics of the middle face [3].

Crouzon syndrome was named after L.E. Octave Crouzon, a French physician who first described the condition in 1912.

© Springer International Publishing AG, part of Springer Nature 2018
M. Špero, H. Vavro, *Neuroradiology - Expect the Unexpected*,
https://doi.org/10.1007/978-3-319-73482-8_13

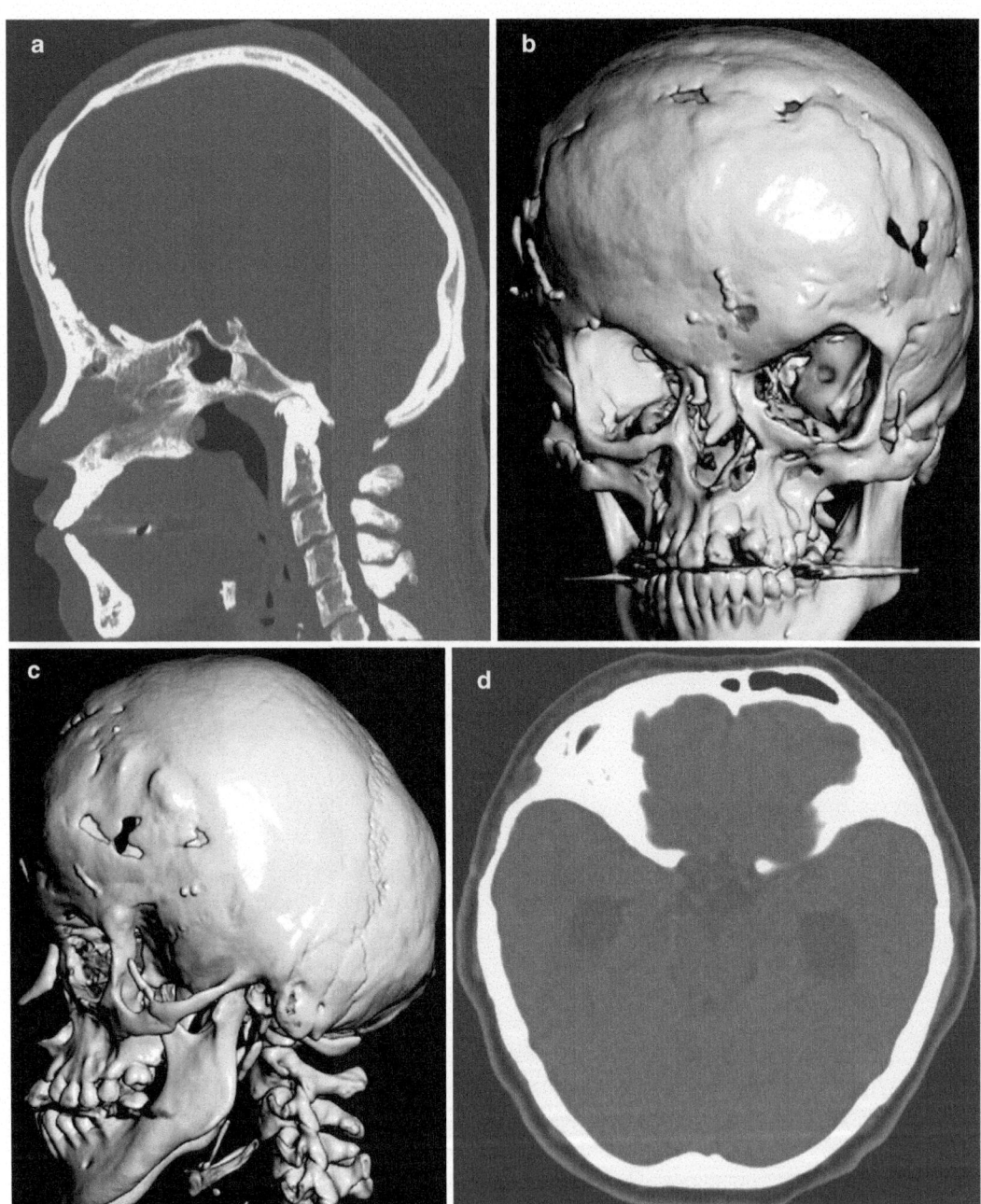

Fig. 13.1 Low-dose CT exam of the head revealed abnormal calvarial shape (**a–c**) with small anterior cranial fossa (**d**), shallow orbits with exophthalmos (**e**), mild mid-facial hypoplasia, beak-shaped nose (**f**) deviated to the right with a right nasal bone defect (**g**), significant left convexity nasal septum deviation and several calvarial bone defects (**b, c, i**) in keeping with previous surgical procedures. No significant mandibular prognathia was detected. Additionally, there was a left-sided stylohyoid ligament calcification (**f, h**—marked by an *arrow*). Intracranially, corpus callosum agenesis with subsequent specifically shaped lateral ventricles was seen (**i**). Chiari malformation was not evident. No evidence of upper cervical spine fusion was seen

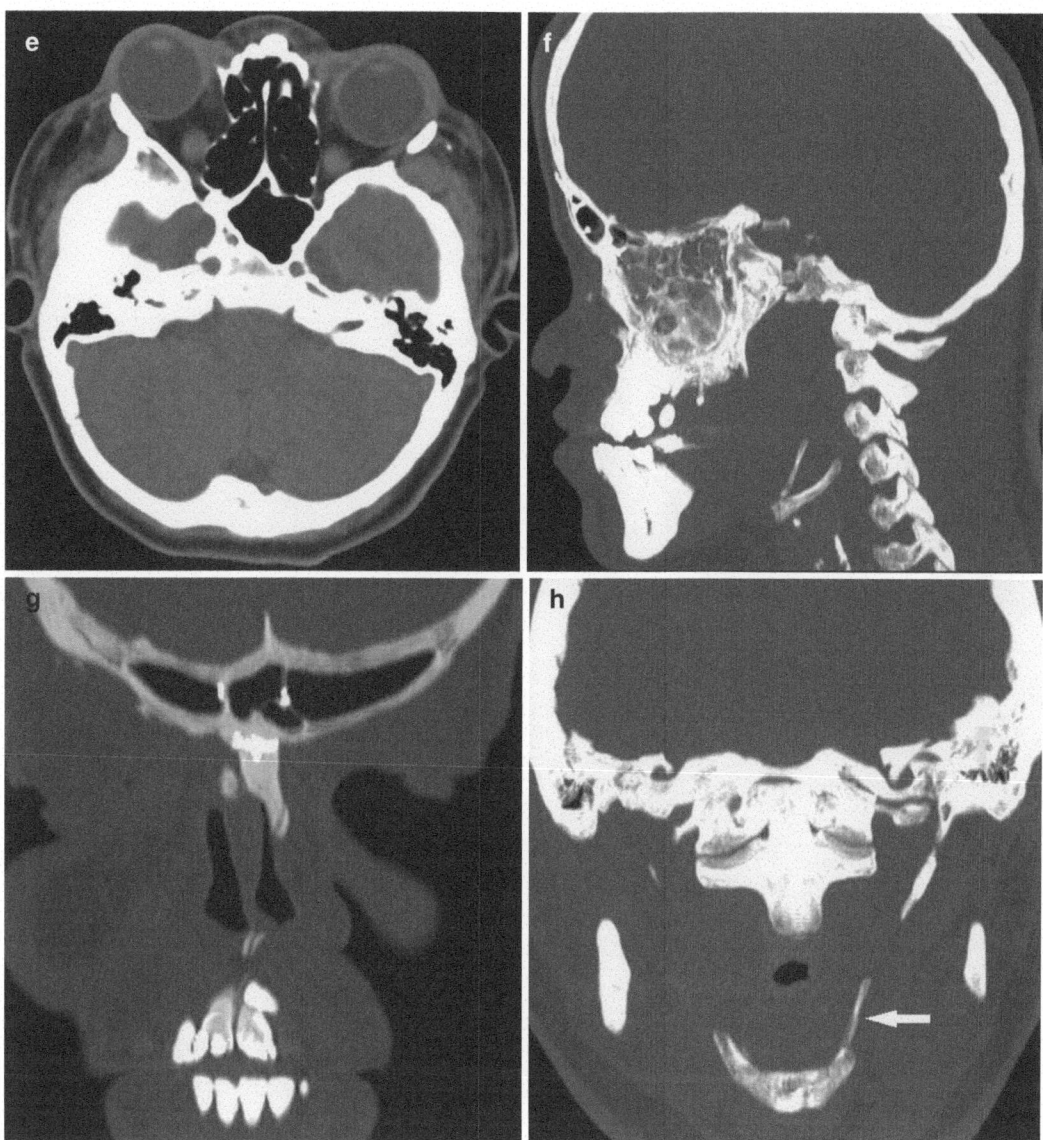

Fig. 13.1 (continued)

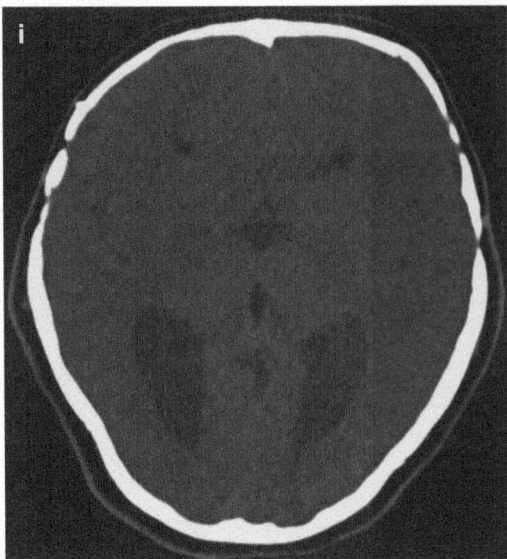

Fig. 13.1 (continued)

References

1. Pournima G et al (2011) Crouzon syndrome: a case report. Eur J Dent Med 10:1–5
2. Padmanabhan V et al (2011) Crouzon's syndrome: a review of literature and case report. Contemp Clin Dent 2(3):211–214. https://doi.org/10.4103/0976-237X.86464
3. Mohan RS et al (2012) Crouzon syndrome: clinico-radiological illustration of a case. J Clin Imaging Sci 2:70. https://doi.org/10.4103/2156-7514.104303

Primary Intraosseous Haemangioma of the Skull Base

An ophthalmologist had noticed a mild right eye exophthalmos on a 42-year-old female patient during a regular vision check-up. The patient was referred to a CT exam of orbits in her hometown (Fig. 14.1).

The CT report stated a bony tumour involving the right-sided greater wing of sphenoid bone, orbital wall and temporal bone. Differentially, the findings were felt to be in keeping with fibrous dysplasia or spongious osteoma.

The patient was further referred to a maxillo-facial surgery referral centre where consultants were worried about a potentially missed malignant diagnosis—osteosarcoma, in particular.

They had performed tumour biopsy and requested a subsequent MRI exam in order to obtain more imaging data on the lesion and exact locations of the tissue sampling (Fig. 14.2).

The MRI findings were compatible with an intraosseous haemangioma of the skull base.

Please note a small occipital meningioma (arrow in image e) on the right and a choroid plexus xanthogranuloma (arrowhead in image e) in the posterior horn of the left lateral ventricle—both represent incidental findings.

The biopsy results were available after MRI exam had been done; histopathological analysis did not reveal any malignant tumour tissue, just bony material with some myxoid stroma and endothelium—the findings were in keeping with an intraosseous haemangioma and compatible with the MRI report findings.

Two months later, the patient started complaining of right-sided facial and cervical pain. The local clinical status was unchanged. The repeat MRI findings were stable. A decision was made that a joint maxillofacial and neurosurgical team would perform surgery (Fig. 14.3).

Histopathology report: torn bone pieces, normal in structure, fatty bone marrow and vascular spaces with variable wall thickness, most of them capillary in appearance. Impression: intraosseous haemangioma.

The patient recovered normally, and there was resolution of exophthalmos.

14.1 Primary Intraosseous Haemangioma

Primary intraosseous haemangioma is a benign vascular tumour, often found in the vertebral column but less frequently within the skull vault, the most common sites being frontal and parietal bone. Its occurrence in the skull base, such as in this case, is extremely rare [1]. When multiple bones of the orbit are involved, it is called primary intraosseous orbital haemangioma. It accounts for 0.7–1% of all bone tumours. It is slow-growing and predominantly asymptomatic, except in cases of compression of the adjacent soft tissue structures or producing a lump by expanding the outer bony table. Neurological symptoms are uncommon as the tumour tends to

© Springer International Publishing AG, part of Springer Nature 2018
M. Špero, H. Vavro, *Neuroradiology - Expect the Unexpected*,
https://doi.org/10.1007/978-3-319-73482-8_14

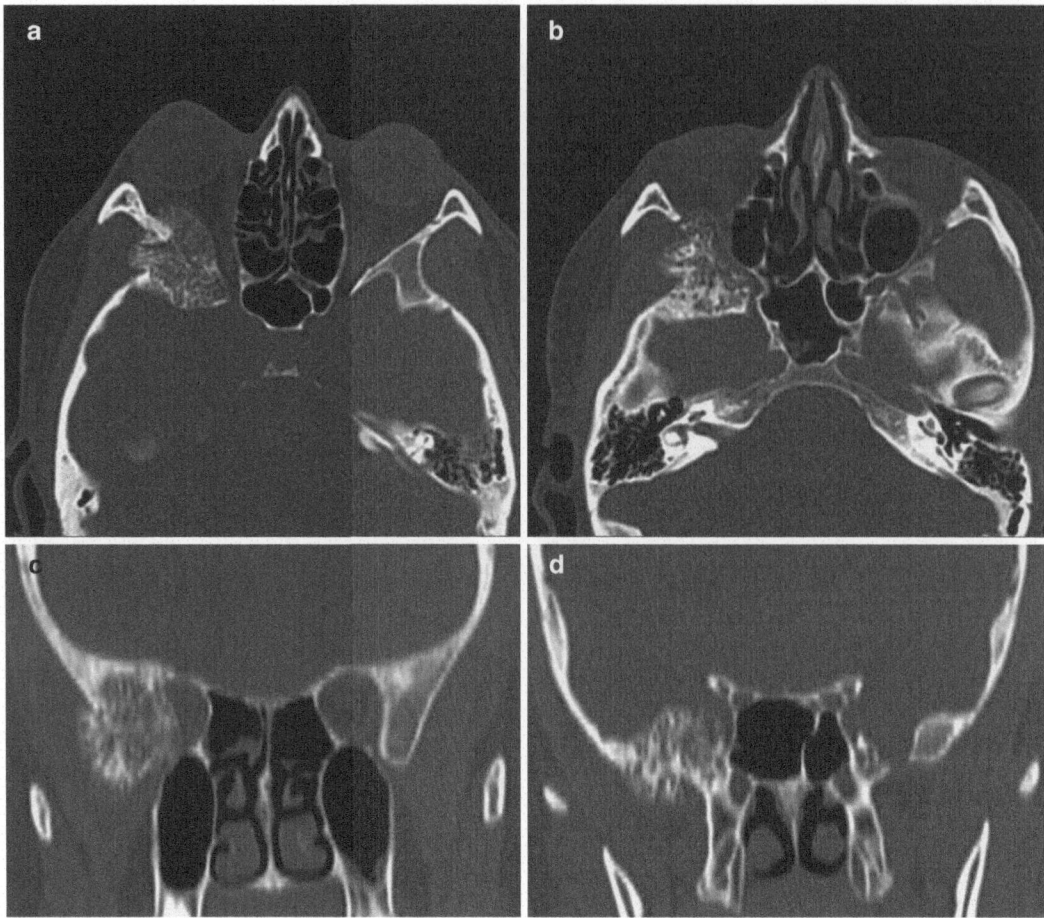

Fig. 14.1 CT exam of the orbits—axial scans (**a**, **b**) and coronal reformats (**c**, **d**)—shows a well-delineated bony expansile lesion within the right greater sphenoid wing which demonstrates spongy, trabecular, "honeycomb" structure. There is compression of the right-sided lateral rectus muscle and right eye proptosis

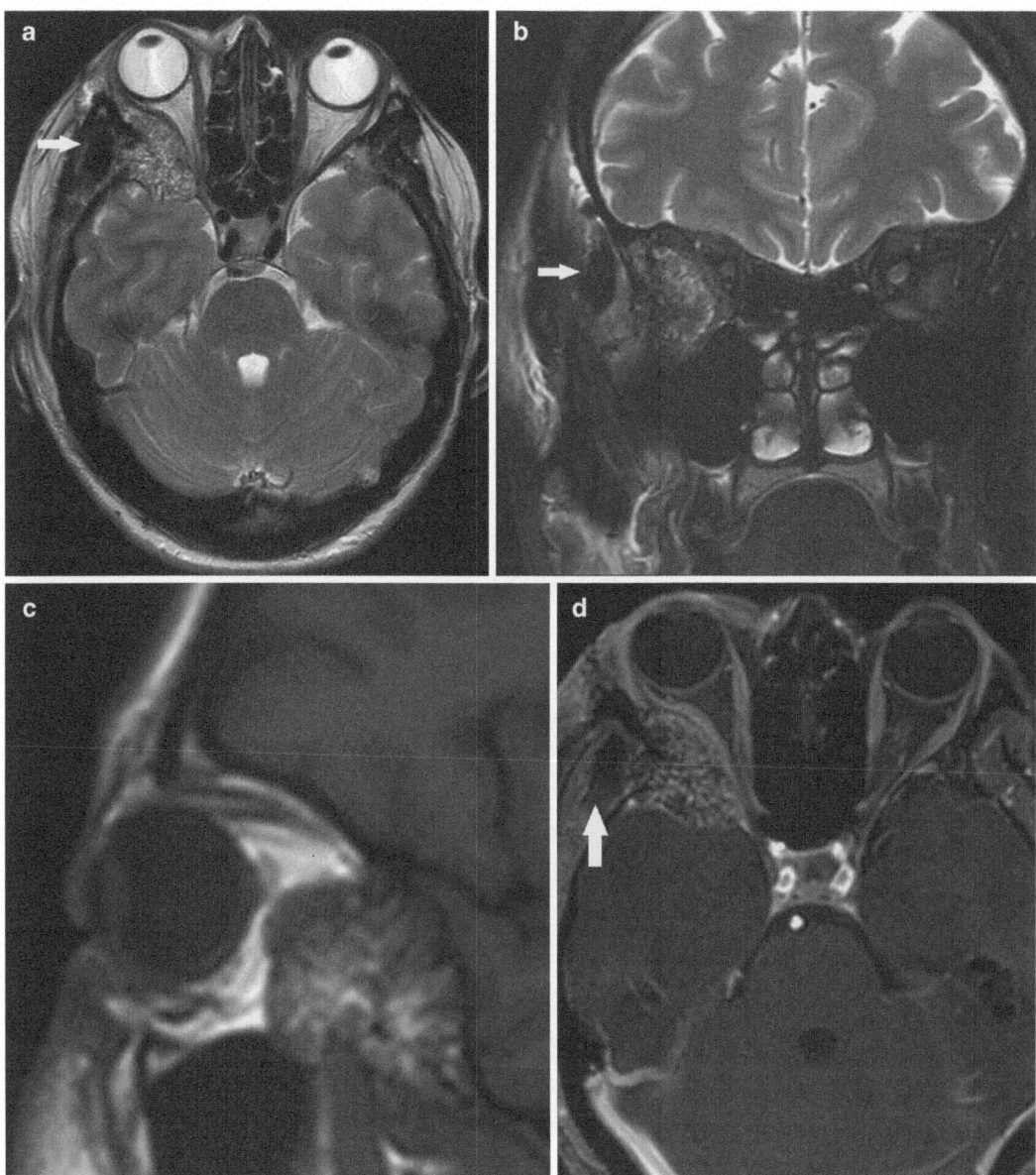

Fig. 14.2 MRI exam of the brain and orbits—axial T2WI (**a**), coronal T2 FS (**b**), sagittal T1WI (**c**), post gadolinium axial T1WI (**d**, **e**). There is a right-sided, large, trabecular expansile lesion of the greater sphenoid wing, peripherally also involving the lesser sphenoid wing, protruding into the right orbit and anterior aspect of the middle cranial fossa, causing proptosis of the right eye. There is moderate contrast enhancement. A small post biopsy defect is evident in the lateral half of the tumour (*arrow* in images **a**, **b** and **d**). There is no evidence of dural infiltration

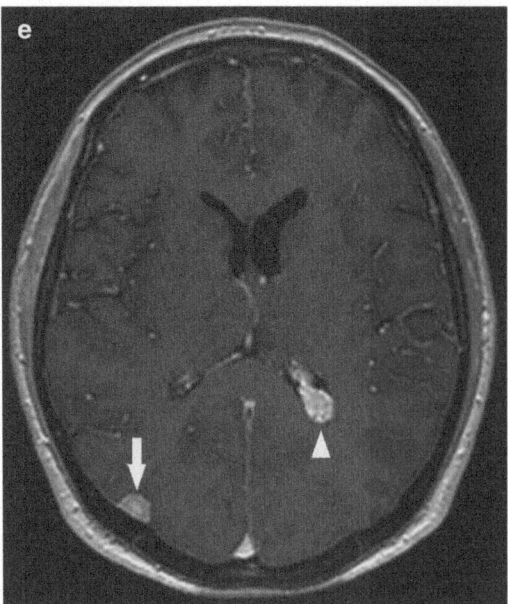

Fig. 14.2 (continued)

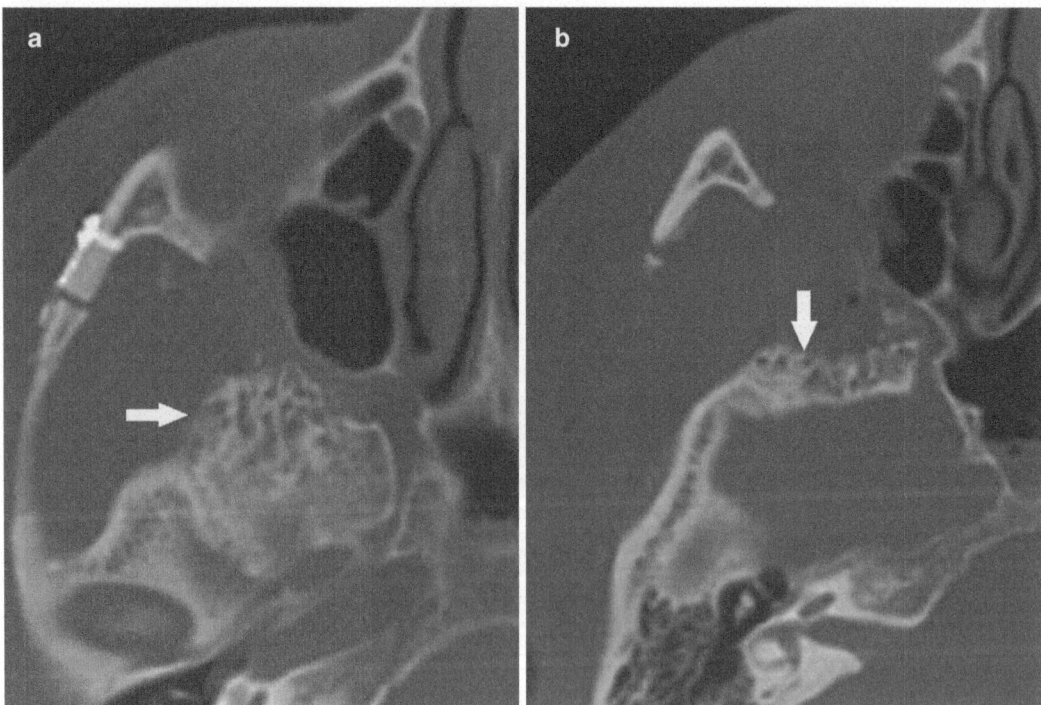

Fig. 14.3 Postoperative CT exam—axial images (**a**, **b**) and coronal reformatted image (**c**) demonstrates osteotomy, with a small residual basal portion of the haemangioma (*arrows*)

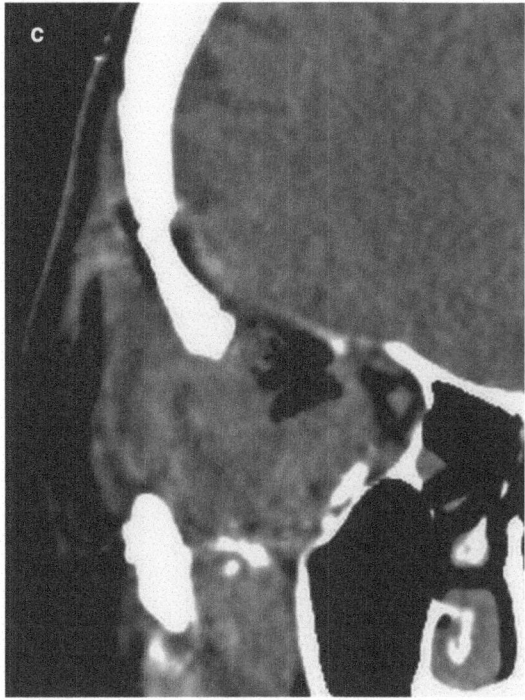

Fig. 14.3 (continued)

expand externally rather than internally. The prevalence is highest among women in the fourth and fifth decade of life. Trauma is considered to be a predisposing factor. If orbit is involved, proptosis and loss of vision are possible; temporal bone involvement may result in hearing loss and facial nerve paralysis, whereas maxillary and mandibular locations are prone to bleeding after tooth extraction and in surgery.

Skull haemangiomas may be venous, cavernous or capillary, according to the predominant vascular network [2]. The cavernous type is composed of large thin-walled vessels and sinusoids lined with a single layer of endothelium; the capillary haemangioma is composed of fine vascular network filled with blood—these two types are frequently seen together, as a mixed-type haemangioma. They may also contain fat, muscle and fibrous tissue and thrombi.

On imaging, intraosseous haemangioma may be misdiagnosed as intraosseous meningioma, as the latter is far more frequent [3]. Confusion with fibrous dysplasia is not uncommon, the main difference being "ground-glass" appearance of the fibrous dysplasia as opposed to "honeycomb" appearance of the haemangioma.

The treatment of choice is en bloc resection with normal bony margin and bone reconstruction. Other treatments include radiation therapy, embolization and curettage. Radiotherapy is generally avoided due to the risk of radiation-induced malignancy; it is the last resort for the unresectable or residual tumours. The drawbacks of curettage are excessive bleeding and high recurrence rate [4].

References

1. Liu JK et al (2003) Primary intraosseous skull base cavernous hemangioma: case report. Skull Base 13(4): 219–228. https://doi.org/10.1055/s-2004-817698
2. Yang Y et al (2016) Primary intraosseous cavernous hemangioma in the skull. Medicine (Baltimore) 95(11):e3069
3. Politti M et al (2005) Intraosseous hemangioma of the skull with dural tail sign: radiologic features with pathologic correlation. Am J Neuroradiol 26(8):2049–2052
4. Park BH et al (2013) Primary intraosseous hemangioma in the frontal bone. Arch Plast Surg 40(3):283–285. https://doi.org/10.5999/aps.2013.40.3.283

Intraosseous Meningioma (of the Greater Wing of the Sphenoid Bone)

15

As an out-hospital patient, a 45-year-old female patient was referred to a head CT due to proptosis of the left eye accompanied with facial asymmetry lasting for several months. Occasionally, she felt sharp pain in the medial angle of the left eye.

Brain CT has revealed a hyperostotic mass of the left greater sphenoid wing with feathered or speculated margins, consistent with intraosseous meningioma (Fig. 15.1).

Due to described CT features, lesion was reported as intraosseous meningioma: MRI of the brain and orbit was recommended and performed several days after the CT examination. MRI confirmed CT finding of intraosseous meningioma causing eye bulb protrusion, while on post-contrast T1WI, it demonstrated adjacent dural thickening and enhancement (Figs. 15.2 and 15.3).

A patient was operated, and part of the hyperostotic intraorbital bone was removed. Pathohistology confirmed intraosseous meningioma. After the operation, left lateral orbital muscle was not compressed, and left bulb did not protrude anymore. Her face did not have asymmetric appearance anymore. Follow-up MRI and CT examinations do not demonstrate enlargement of the rest of the tumour by now.

15.1 Intraosseous Meningioma

Meningiomas are the most frequent benign brain tumours. They arise from meningothelial cells found in the arachnoid membrane and line arachnoid villi associated with intradural venous sinuses and their tributaries. The vast majority are intradural lesions located intracranial in the subdural space, arising along the dural venous sinuses, over the cerebral convexities and in the region of the falx cerebri, although they can develop anywhere in the brain and spine [1]. Extradural meningiomas develop in extracranial sites in the head and neck, but most common are intraosseous meningiomas accounting for about two thirds of all extradural meningiomas [2].

Intraosseous meningiomas (IOMs) are rare, slow-growing tumours, usually involving frontotemporal region of the calvarium and orbits. They are generally benign tumours, but published studies indicate that IOMs are more likely to be malignant than their intradural counterparts. IOMs do not show gender predominance and occur predominantly later in life, with a median patient age at diagnosis in the fifth decade. These tumours have a bimodal incidence peak, one in the second decade, and second peak during the fifth to seventh decades of life [3]. IOM of the greater sphenoid wing clinically presents with pain, proptosis, vision problems, possible swelling and consequently aesthetic problems.

The aetiology is still not clarified: there are several proposed explanations suggesting the origin of intraosseous meningioma. Azar-Kia et al. suggested that IOM arises from ectopic arachnoid cap cells trapped in the cranial sutures during

© Springer International Publishing AG, part of Springer Nature 2018
M. Špero, H. Vavro, *Neuroradiology - Expect the Unexpected*,
https://doi.org/10.1007/978-3-319-73482-8_15

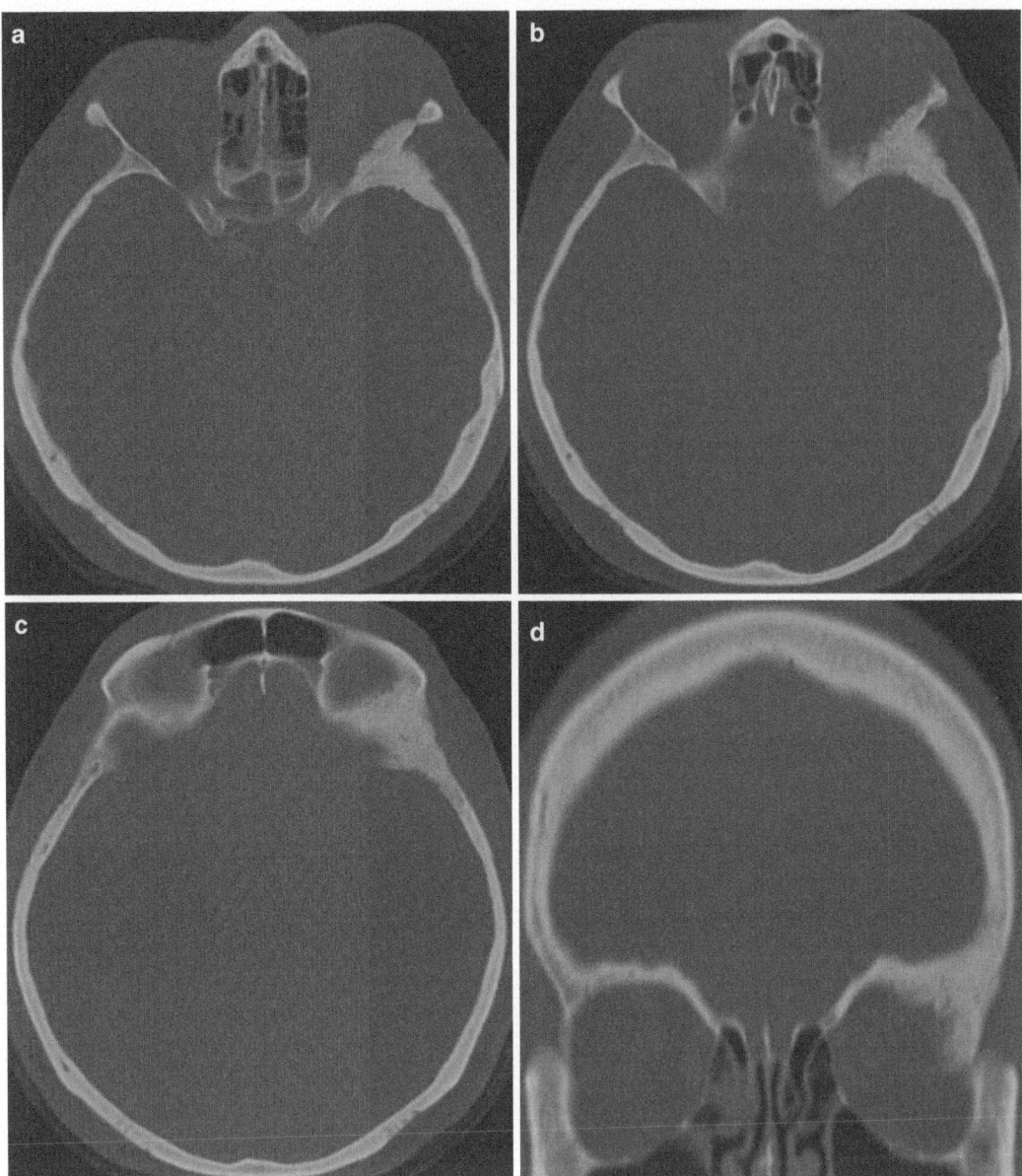

Fig. 15.1 Computed tomography of the brain, axial (**a–c**, **h**), coronal (**d–f**, **i**) sagittal (**g**) planes revealed hyperostotic lesion within the left greater sphenoid wing with extension into the frontal bone and thickening of the lateral orbital wall. The inner and outer tables showed a feathered or speculated appearance, while inner table bowed toward the brain. Left lateral rectus muscle was mildly enlarged and compressed (**e**, **i**), while the left eye bulb protruded (**a**, **b**, **h**)

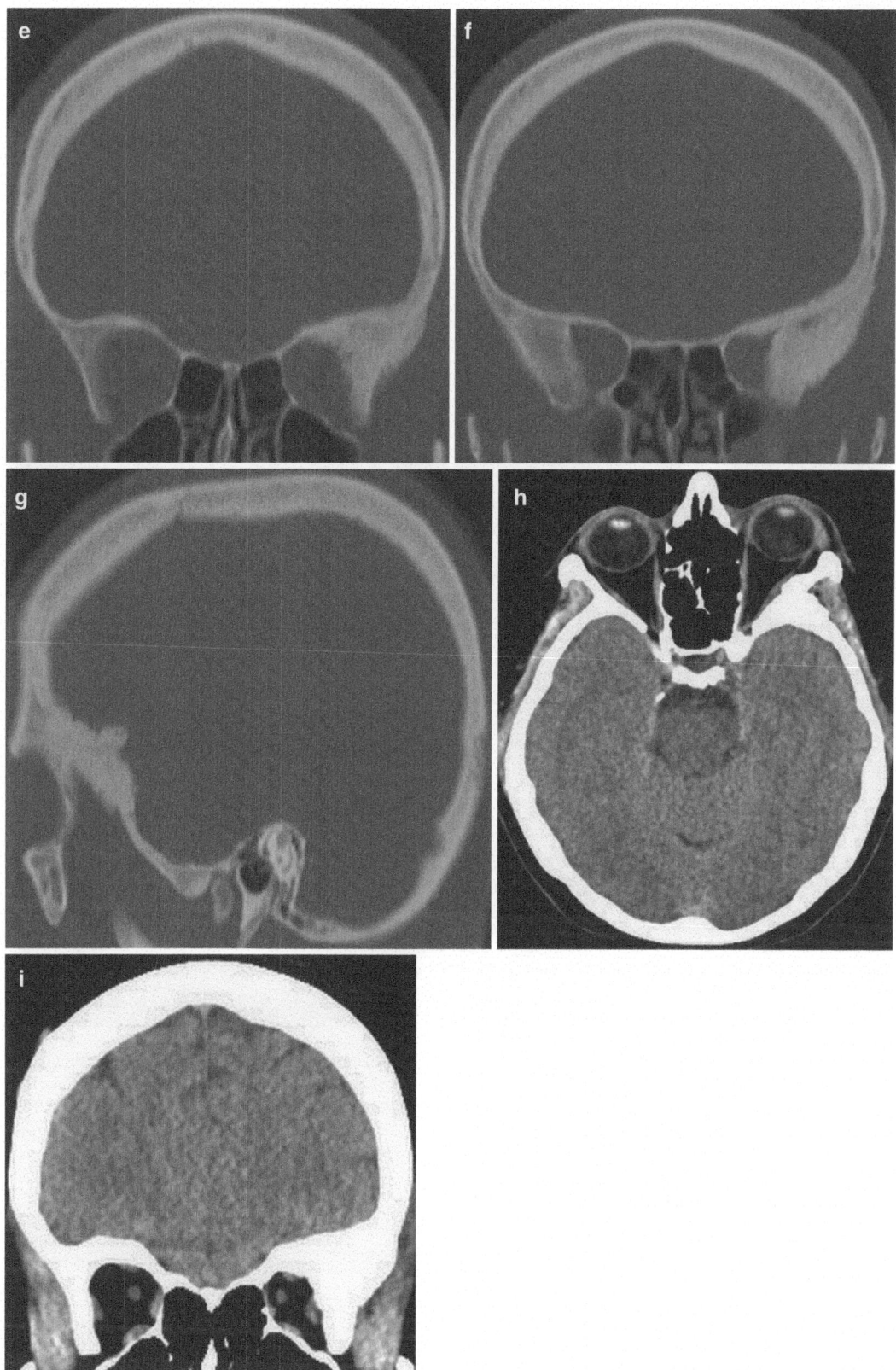

Fig. 15.1 (continued)

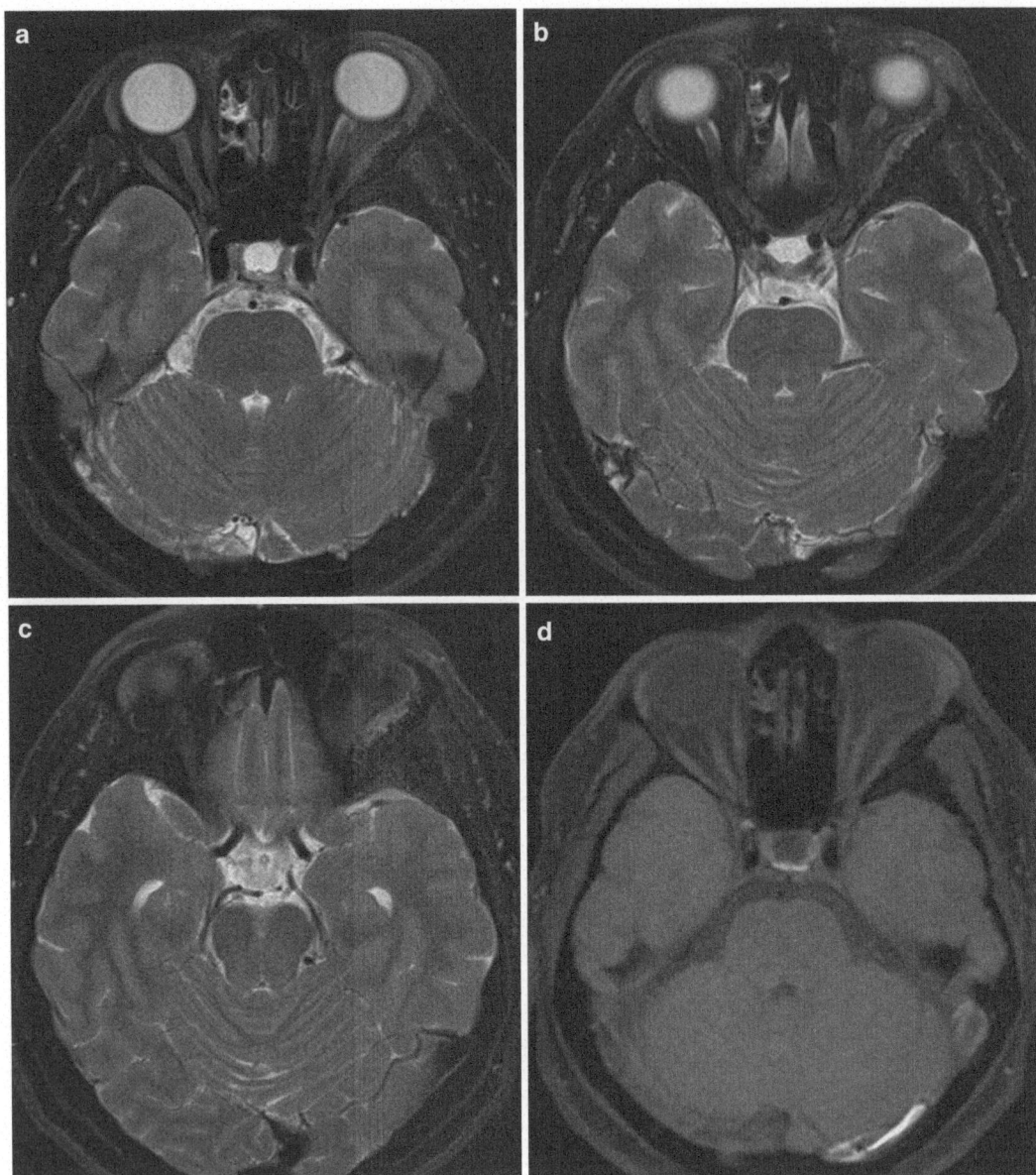

Fig. 15.2 MRI of the orbit, pre-contrast axial T2FSWI (**a–c**) and T1FSWI (**d–f**), post-contrast axial T1FSWI (**g–i**) demonstrated calvarial thickening of the left greater sphenoid wing and left lateral orbital wall, hypointense on pre-contrast T1FSWI and T2FSWI, without contrast enhancement on post-contrast T1FSWI suggesting osteoblastic form of the intraosseous meningioma. Contrast enhancement of the mildly thickened adjacent dura overlying adjacent anterior part of the left temporal lobe, without soft tissue mass. Left eye bulb protruded

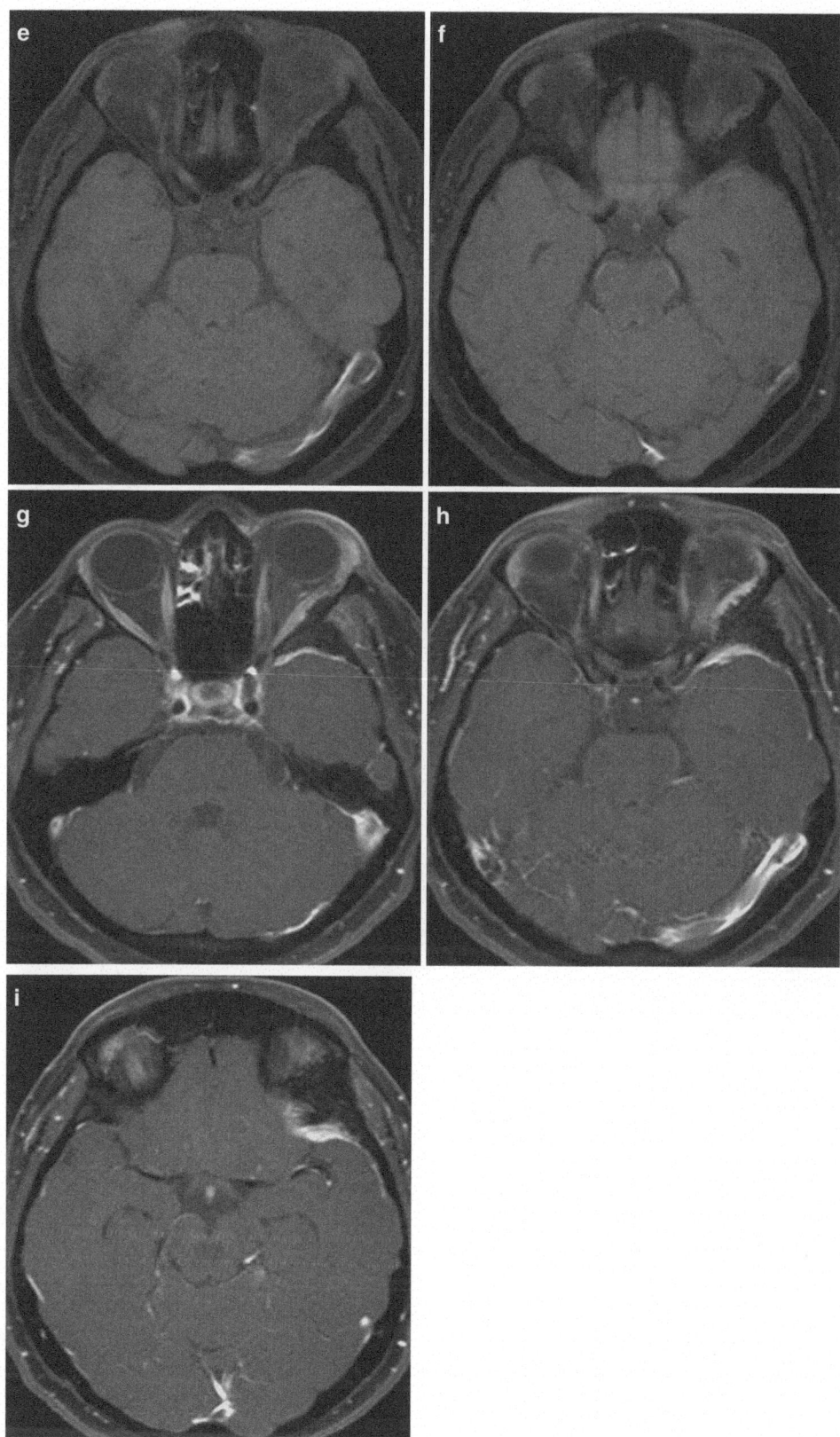

Fig. 15.2 (continued)

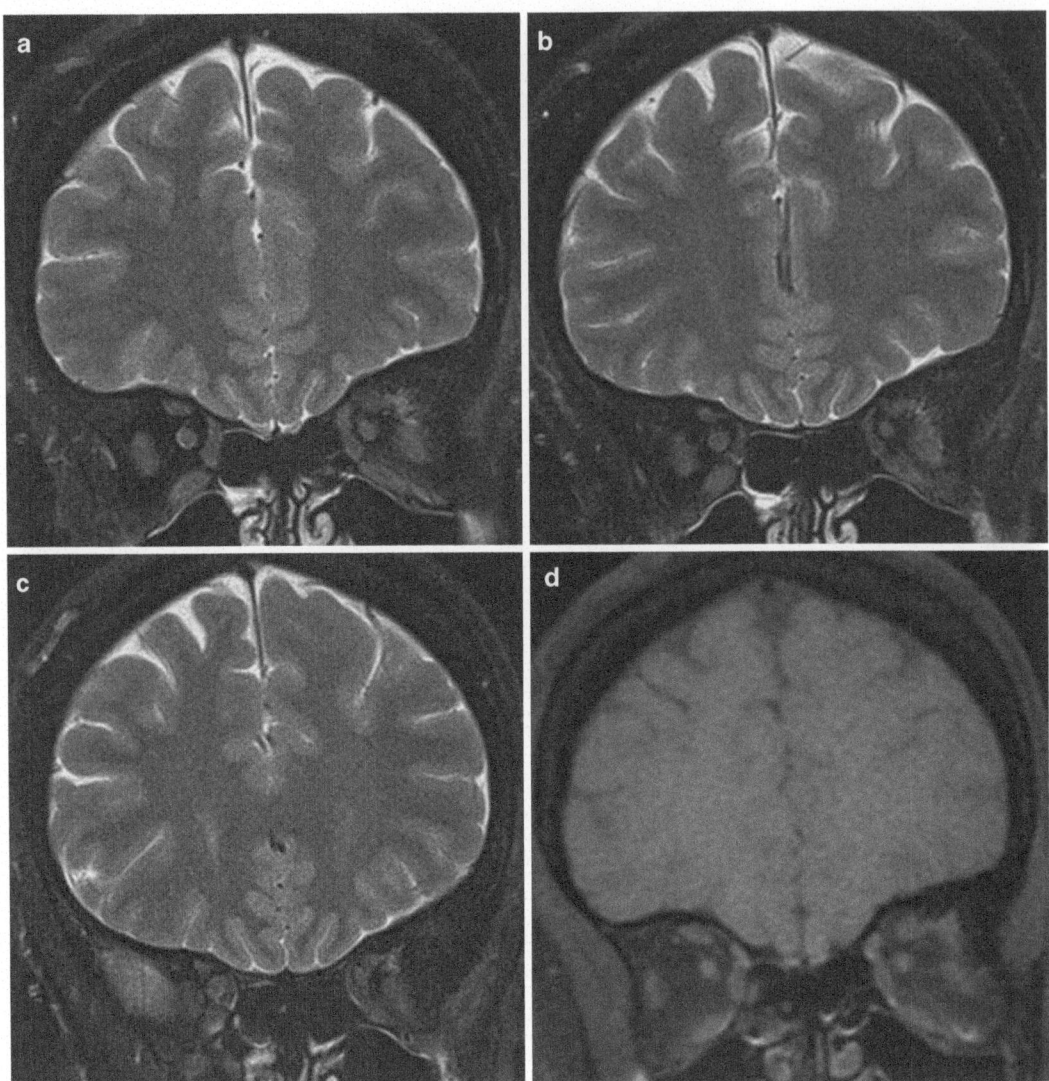

Fig. 15.3 MRI of the orbit, coronal pre-contrast T2FSWI (a–c) and T1FSWI (d–f), post-contrast T1FSWI (g–i). Lateral wall and part of the orbital roof was involved with sclerotic mass. Enhanced dura has encroached planum sphenoidale (h, i). There were mild mass effect on the left lateral rectus muscle and mild intraorbital contrast enhancement of reactive tissue adjacent to the sclerotic bone, between left superior and lateral rectus muscle (g, h)

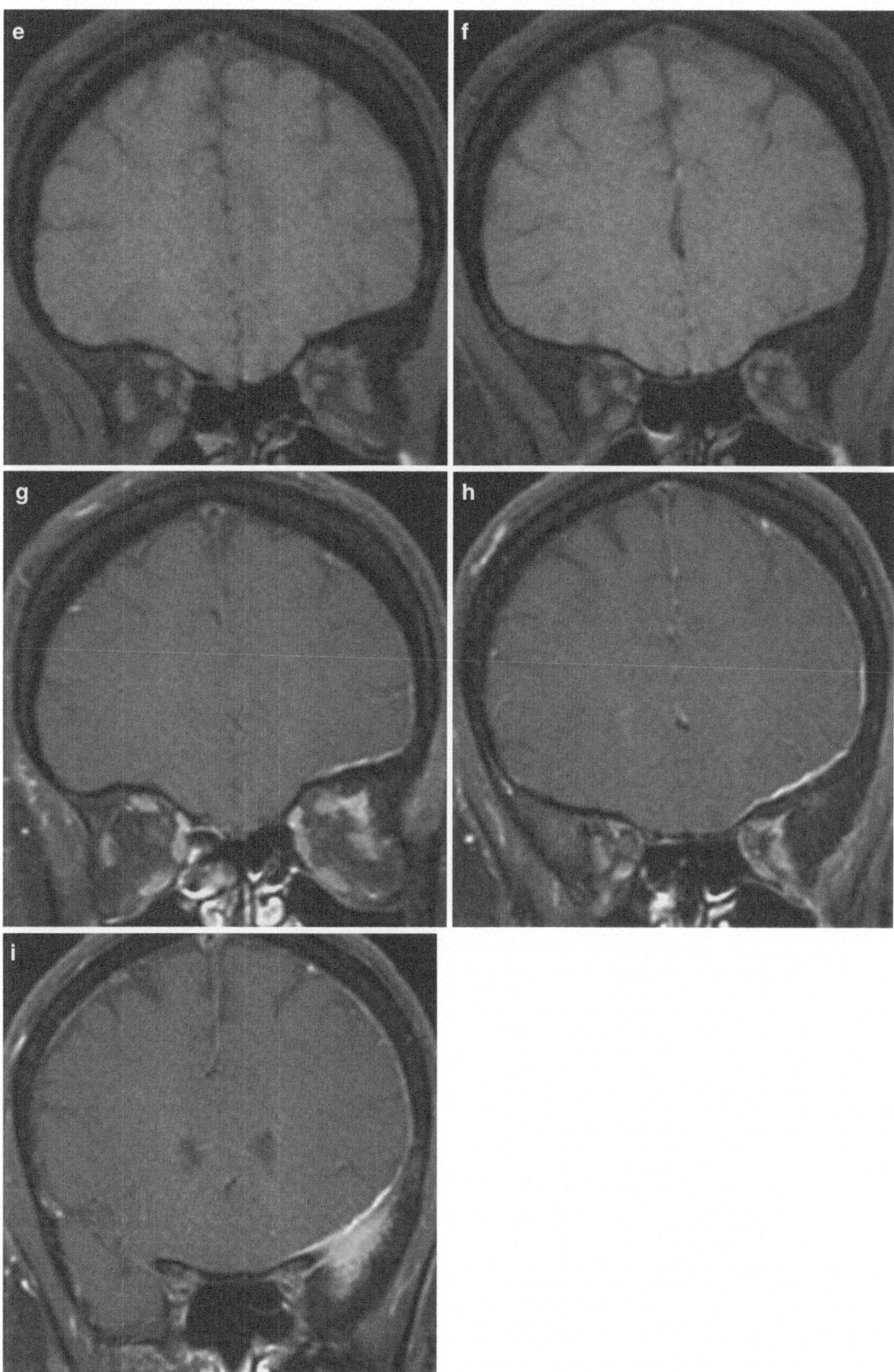

Fig. 15.3 (continued)

moulding of the head at birth: according to the literature, most of IOMs are suture-related masses [4]. Second explanation is that they arise from dura and arachnoid entrapped by previous trauma, while the third suggestion is that extradural meningioma arises from the multipotent mesenchymal cells, explaining mass located far from the head and neck [1, 5].

Lang et al. have suggested to classify primary extradural meningiomas into type I (purely extra-calvarial), type II (purely calvarial) and type III (calvarial lesions extending beyond the calvaria). Each type is further divided into subgroup B (skull base) and C (convexity) [6].

Radiologically, intraosseous meningioma is classified as osteoblastic, osteolytic or mixed osteoblastic-osteolytic type. IOMs are mostly osteoblastic type characterised by intraosseous mass growth leading to significant hyperostosis of an involved bone with, usually, soft tissue growth of a surrounding dura. CT with bone window shows focal hyperostotic bone lesion with feathered appearance of the inner table, which is hypointense on T1WI and T2WI on MRI, while both imaging techniques show contrast enhancement of the adjacent thickened dura and dural soft tissue mass if present [1–3, 5, 7]. MRI allows better delineation in the evaluation of soft tissue component and extradural extension. Thickened and enhanced dura adjacent to the bony tumour is a result of reactive inflammation or tumoural invasion. Pial enhancement, focal dural nodules or dural thickening of more than 5 mm is highly accurate in predicting neoplastic dural invasion [2]. Osteolytic lesions typically cause thinning, expansion and interruption of the inner and outer cortical layers of the skull [3].

In this case, tumour was sphenoid bone lesion extending beyond calvaria, therefore classified as type III B tumour. According to clinical presentation, patient age, typical location of the hyperostotic lesion with lateral orbital wall involvement and other described CT and MRI features (Figs. 15.1, 15.2, and 15.3), diagnosis of the IOM of the greater sphenoid wing was obvious to us and later histologically confirmed. Histological

findings pathognomonic of IOM include uniform spindle-shaped cells arranged in whorls and interconnecting fascicles.

Differential diagnosis includes fibrous dysplasia (FD), meningioma en plaque, osteoma, osteosarcoma and Paget disease. It is important to differentiate IOM from fibrous dysplasia due to different treatment options. FD is a developmental disease that commonly occurs at young age and stops to grow after bone maturation. IOM appears after puberty and continues to grow slowly. IOM and FD expand the bone. In FD the inner table of the skull is typically smooth, while in IOM there is irregularity of the inner table, particularly at the site of origin, almost always with associated dural reaction. Therefore, this irregularity is the key to distinguish IOM and FD on imaging, as well as a soft tissue involvement and contrast enhancement [1, 2, 7].

Total tumour removal with wide surgical resection followed by cranial reconstruction is the treatment of choice. Adjuvant therapy, including gamma knife, chemotherapy and bisphosphonate therapy, is indicated in patients with malignancy and for non-resectable tumours [2, 3].

References

1. Vlychou M et al (2016) Primary intraosseous meningioma: an osteosclerotic bone tumour mimicking malignancy. Clin Sarcoma Res 6:14–19
2. Lee SJ et al (2015) Primary intraosseous meningioma in the orbital bony wall: a case report and review of the literature review. J Korean Soc Radiol 72(1):68–72
3. Elder JB et al (2007) Primary intraosseous meningioma. Neurosurg Focus 23(4):1–9
4. Azar-Kia B et al (1974) Intraosseous meningioma. Neuroradiology 6:246–253
5. Hussaini SM et al (2010) Intraosseous meningioma of the sphenoid bone. Radiol Case Rep 5(1):357–360
6. Lang FF et al (2000) Primary extradural meningiomas: a report on nine cased and review of the literature from the era of computerized tomography scanning. J Neurosurg 93:940–950
7. Shaftel SS et al (2017) Intraosseous meningioma mimicking fibrous dysplasia. Sci Pages Ophthalmol 1(1):25–27

Fibrous Dysplasia: Osteosarcoma

Skull deformity, predominantly frontal, has been something this 62-year-old lady has lived with since childhood. A diagnosis of craniofacial fibrous dysplasia was established by the previous X-ray, CT and MRI exams, as well as by bone biopsy, and the appearances were stable for years. The patient's personal medical history also included surgery and chemotherapy for breast cancer 12 years ago (Fig. 16.1).

Six months before admission to the hospital, the patient noticed a moderate enlargement of the deformity in the left frontal region: at that time, FNA confirmed fibrous dysplasia. Further growth warranted a follow-up CT exam (Fig. 16.2).

A localised resection of the expanded bone in the left frontal region was done. Intraoperative biopsy confirmed fibrous dysplasia. However, postoperative extended histopathology analysis revealed osteosarcoma on grounds of previous fibrous dysplasia. The resection borders could not be determined in the available tissue specimen. Another surgery was done, this time larger in extension (Fig. 16.3).

16.1 Craniofacial Fibrous Dysplasia

Fibrous dysplasia (FD) is a tumour-like, non-neoplastic congenital disease, probably caused by a somatic mutation early in embryonic life, featuring defective osteoblastic differentiation and maturation. Immature bone is intermixed with excessively proliferated fibrous tissue.

It may affect a single bone (monostotic, 70% of cases, most common in ribs) or multiple bones (polyostotic, usually unilateral limb lesions). Any bone may be affected. Craniofacial fibrous dysplasia (CFD) occurring in multiple adjacent craniofacial bones is regarded as monostotic, and it accounts for up to 25% of monostotic form. It may be one of the features in McCune-Albright syndrome [1]. CFD behaves as a chronic, slowly progressive mass lesion, usually self-limiting, rarely progressing after the third decade of life. Complications are usually caused by compression of skull foramina, nerves and vessels—such as visual loss, proptosis, hearing loss and headache.

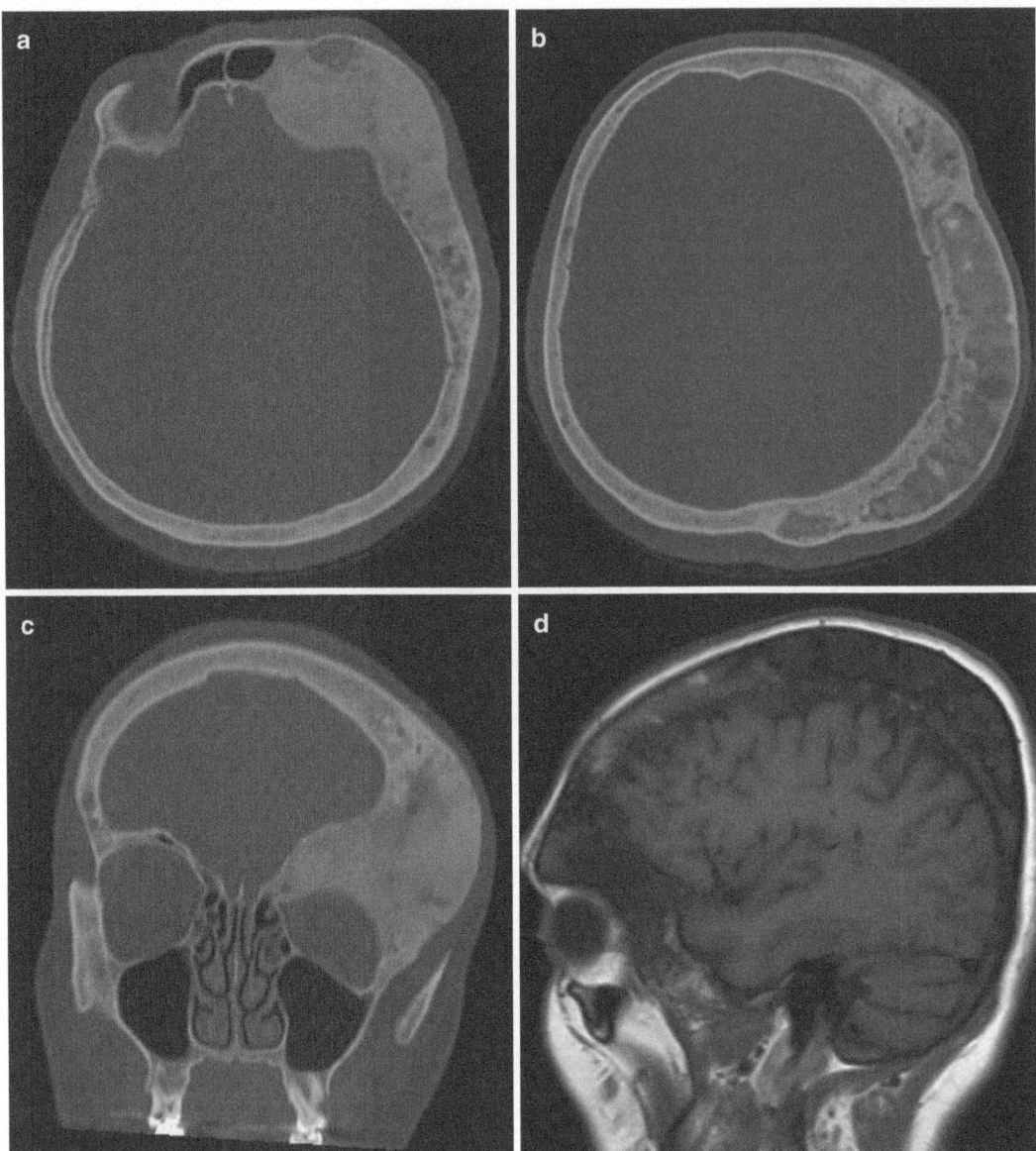

Fig. 16.1 Non-contrast-enhanced axial (**a**, **b**) and coronal (**c**) CT and sagittal T1WI (**d**), axial T2WI (**e**) and coronal T2WI (**f**) MRI images of the (monostotic; see text) fibrous dysplasia involving the left frontal, parietal, sphenoid and temporal bone. Note the facial asymmetry with left orbital deformity (**c**, **f**). CT images demonstrate loss of normal corticomedullary differentiation in the expanded bones, replaced by a ground-glass pattern with focal lucencies and scleroses. MRI images show heterogenous bone signal

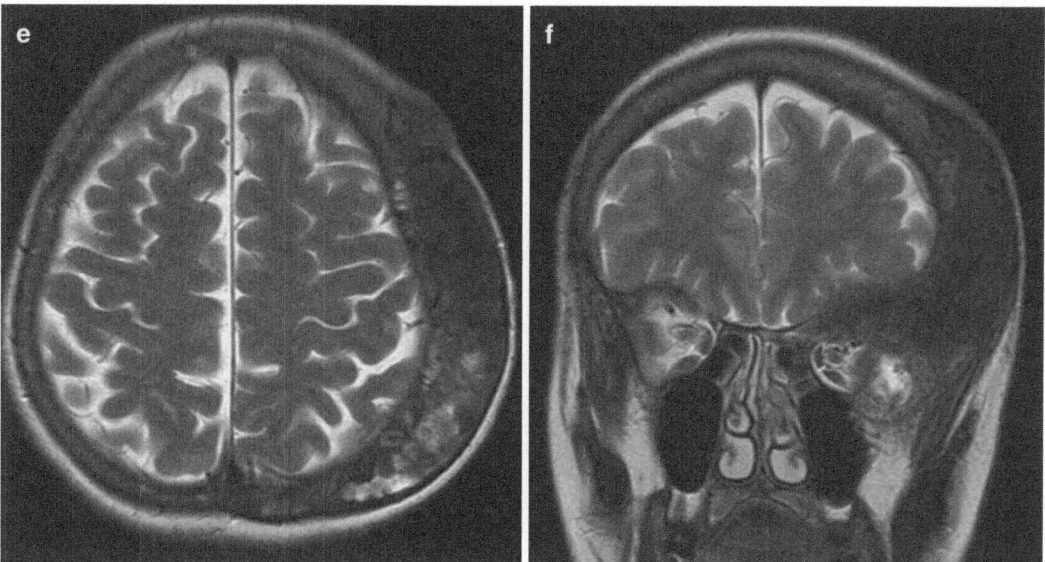

Fig. 16.1 (continued)

CT imaging features ground-glass expansile lesion centred in the medullary bone layer, with inner cortical scalloping and heterogenous sclerosis. There is no periosteal reaction.

MR imaging features consist of heterogenous signal, mostly intermediate in T1WI and low in T2WI and heterogenous contrast enhancement.

The transition to normal bone is often indistinct.

Differential diagnosis includes Paget disease which usually spares facial bones and is more sclerotic; intraosseous meningioma which tends to be sclerotic, does not spare the cortical bone and often abuts the intracranial compartment; sclerotic metastases which are usually smaller in size and focal in distribution; and cemento-ossifying fibroma which is usually distinct from the adjacent normal bone.

The risk for malignant transformation in FD is approximately less than 1% in the monostotic form and up to 4% in the polyostotic form, being the most frequent in McCune-Albright syndrome patients [2]. Prior radiation exposure is also recognized as a risk factor for malignant transformation. The most common sites of malignant transformation in monostotic form of fibrous dysplasia are facial and skull bones. Osteosarcoma accounts for approximately 70% of malignant transformation cases, followed by fibrosarcoma (20%) and chondrosarcoma (10%). The appearance of the benign fibrous dysplasia makes malignant transformation difficult to identify. Sarcomatous transformation may appear in form of cystic osteolytic areas, cortical destruction and heterogeneously enhancing soft tissue mass, such as in this case. The patient should be instructed to bring any change in symptoms to physician's attention. Rapid growth, especially in adults, pain without history of trauma and significant change in radiologic appearance are some of the signs of possible malignant transformation. Yearly X-rays are advocated for screening [3]. The cure for FD or ways to prevent malignant transformation still do not exist.

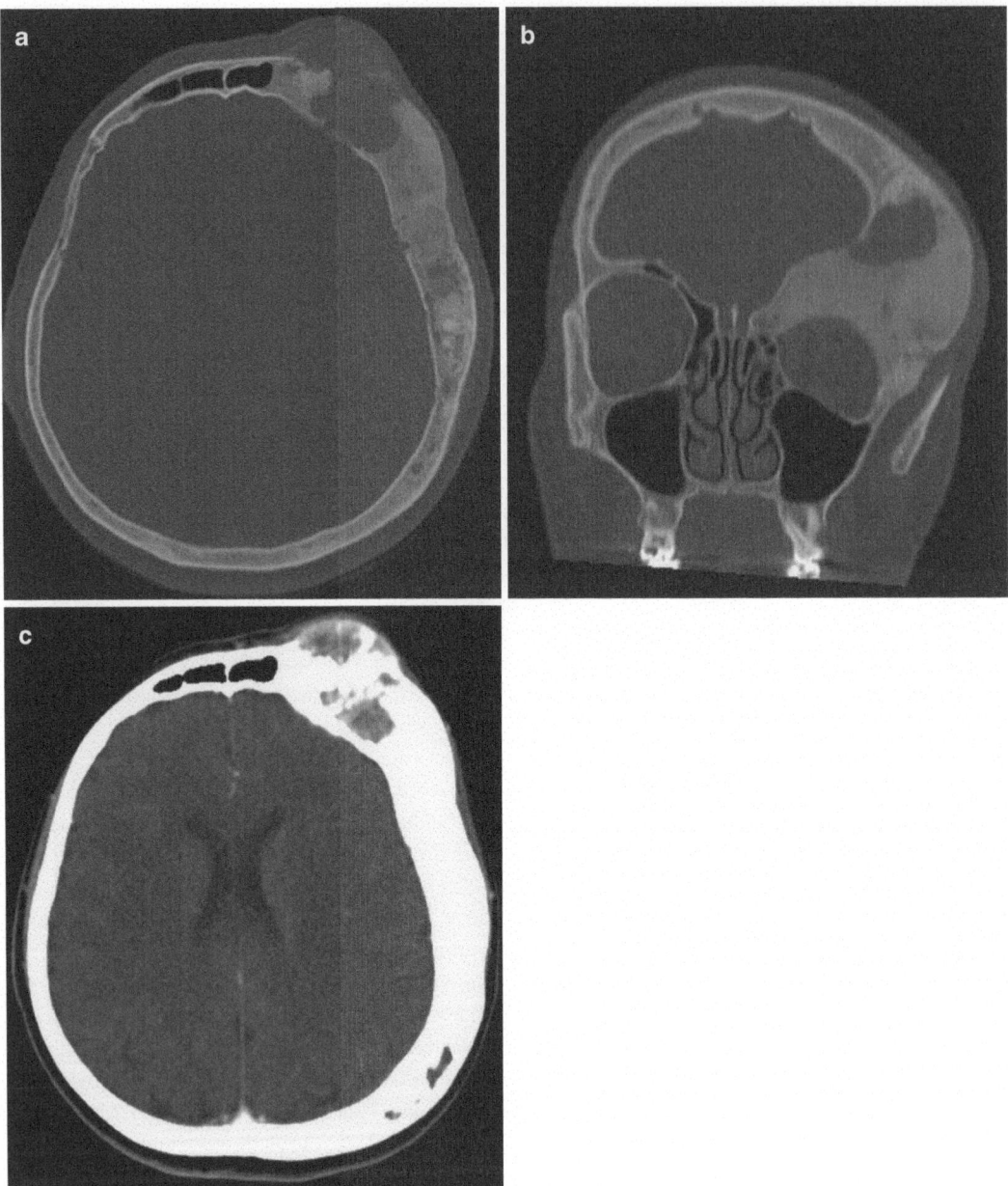

Fig. 16.2 Contrast-enhanced follow-up CT images of the head—note the left frontal bone defect (**a**, **b**) caused by an irregularly enhancing (**c**) osteolytic expansile lesion, not evident in Fig. 16.1

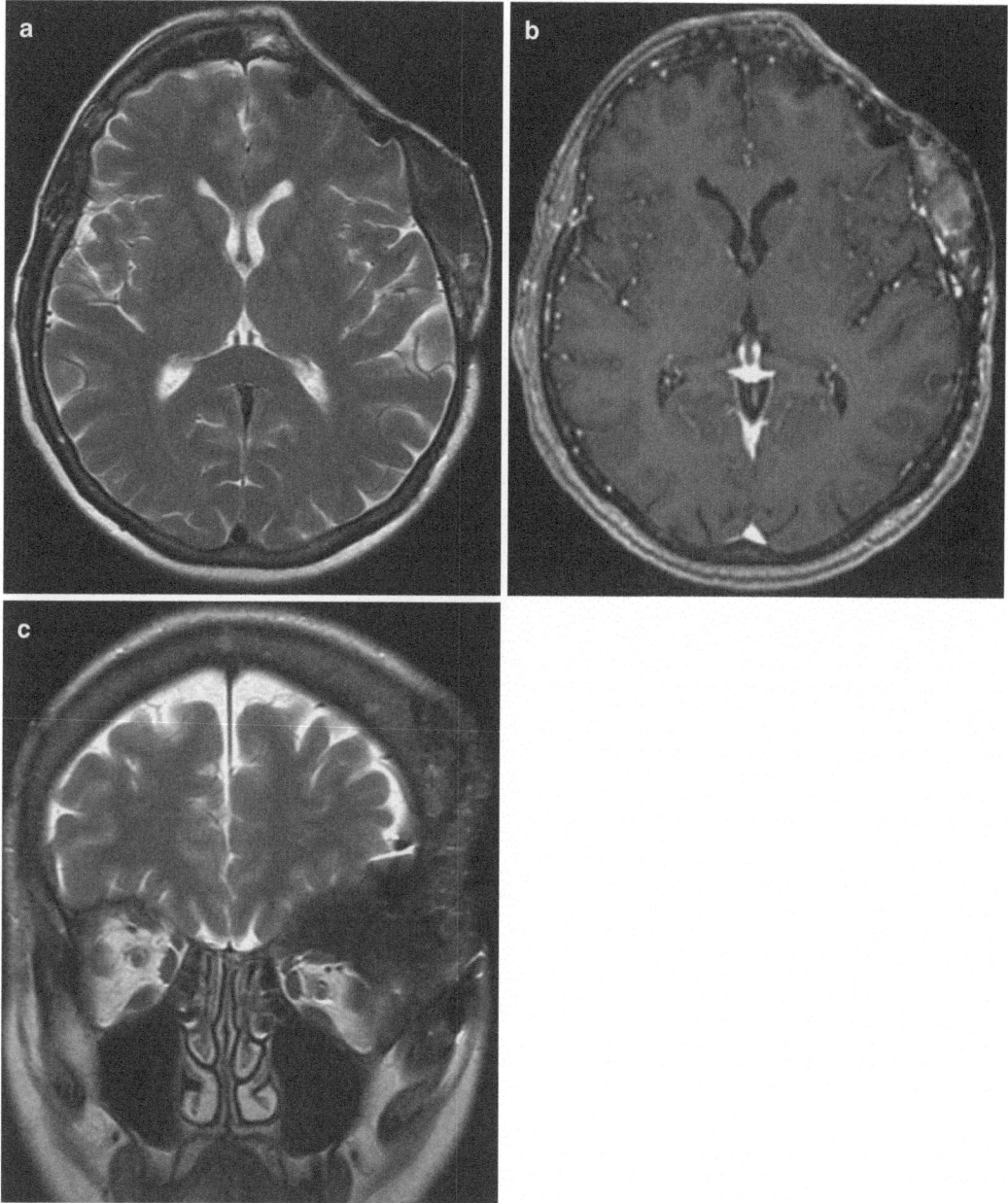

Fig. 16.3 Postoperative MRI of the head—axial T2WI (**a**), axial post-contrast T1WI (**b**), coronal T2WI (**c**). There are postoperative bony defects and characteristic post gadolinium enhancement of the remaining dysplastic bones (**b**)

References

1. Larheim TA, Westesson P-LA (2006) Maxillofacial imaging, vol 81. Springer, Berlin
2. Riddle ND, Bui MM (2013) Fibrous dysplasia. Arch Pathol Lab Med 137(1):134–138
3. Mardekian SK, Tuluc M (2015) Malignant sarcomatous transformation of fibrous dysplasia. Head Neck Pathol 9(1):100–103

Sphenoid Wing Meningocele

At the end of April 2016, a 29-year-old female patient came to our MRI unit, as an out-hospital patient, for a brain MRI (Figs. 17.1 and 17.2). Her only symptom was headache: non-specific diffuse headache during several years, sometimes on daily basis.

About a year ago, she has performed MRI of the brain in a private clinic where radiologist has reported a right temporal arachnoid cyst.

According to the described imaging features (Figs. 17.1 and 17.2), the meningocele of the greater wing of the sphenoid bone was reported spontaneous, because there were no information about other possible aetiologies. Arachnoid cysts represent intra-arachnoid CSF-containing cysts that do not communicate with the ventricular system or adjacent subarachnoid spaces, which are most commonly located supratentorial in the middle cranial fossa. Large anterior temporal arachnoid cyst may thin adjacent greater sphenoid wing but will not cause expansile defect in the bone.

A patient was not a middle-aged obese female; there were no clear information about visual problems, but according to MRI features, there were three imaging characteristics attributable to an idiopathic intracranial hypertension: prominent arachnoid pits, slitlike ventricles and prominent subarachnoid space around the optic nerves showing vertical tortuosity (Fig. 17.2). The lesion

was previously misdiagnosed as temporal arachnoid cyst: in a control interval, it did not change in size. For the time being, follow-up MRI of the brain is recommended, and surgical treatment is a next step in a patient management.

17.1 Sphenoid Wing Meningocele

The term meningocele describes a herniation of meninges and CSF through a bony defect in a skull: CSF egresses from the intracranial cavity through an abnormal communication between the subarachnoid space and a bone. Unless otherwise specified, these lesions are referred as CSF fistulas [1]. Meningocele may be congenital due to a failure of normal skull development with a bone defect, acquired non-traumatic (surgery, tumour, dysplasia, osteoradionecrosis) or posttraumatic, and spontaneous without clear cause [1, 2].

Currently it is widely accepted that spontaneous meningocele in the skull base is a result of a multifactorial process that involves both elevated intracranial pressure and anatomic predisposition involving thinning of the cranial base [1]. Those may occur anywhere in the skull base: in occipital bone, at cribriform plate or temporal bone. Subset of spontaneous meningoceles occur off the midline in the lateral sphenoid bone, known as sphenoid lateral spontaneous cephaloceles (SLSCs).

© Springer International Publishing AG, part of Springer Nature 2018
M. Špero, H. Vavro, *Neuroradiology - Expect the Unexpected*,
https://doi.org/10.1007/978-3-319-73482-8_17

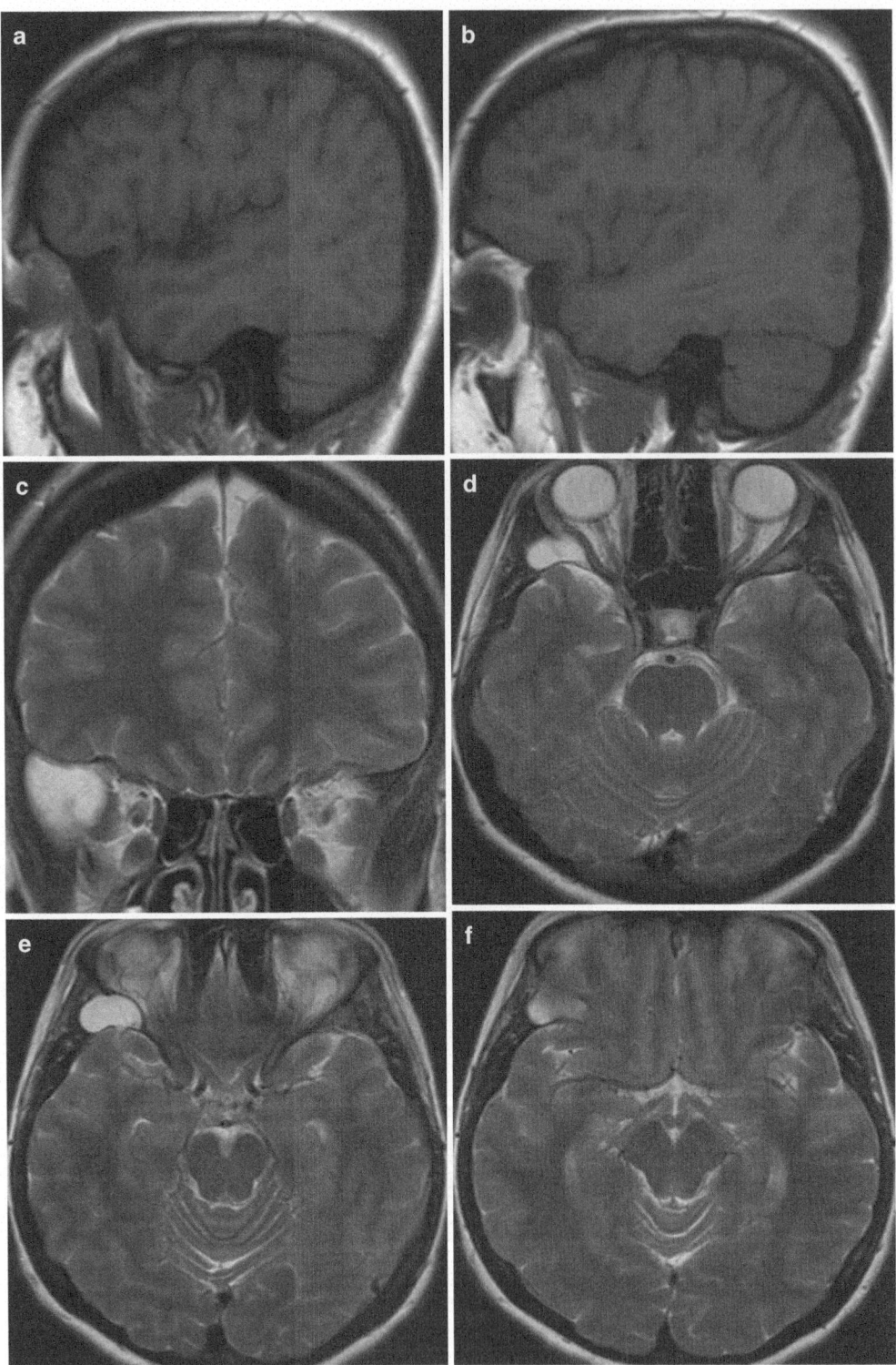

Fig. 17.1 Magnetic resonance imaging of the brain, non-contrast, sagittal T1WI (**a**, **b**), coronal (**c**) and axial (**d**–**f**) T2WI, axial FLAIR (**g**–**i**), axial DWI (**j**), ADC (**k**), SWI (**l**), axial (**m**, **n**) and sagittal (**o**) CISS revealed expansile cystic lesion in the greater wing of the sphenoid bone con- taining only fluid, causing a defect in the bone. Signal intensity of the cyst fluid was similar to CSF on all sequences, while the lesion communicated with adjacent subarachnoid space through a narrow defect

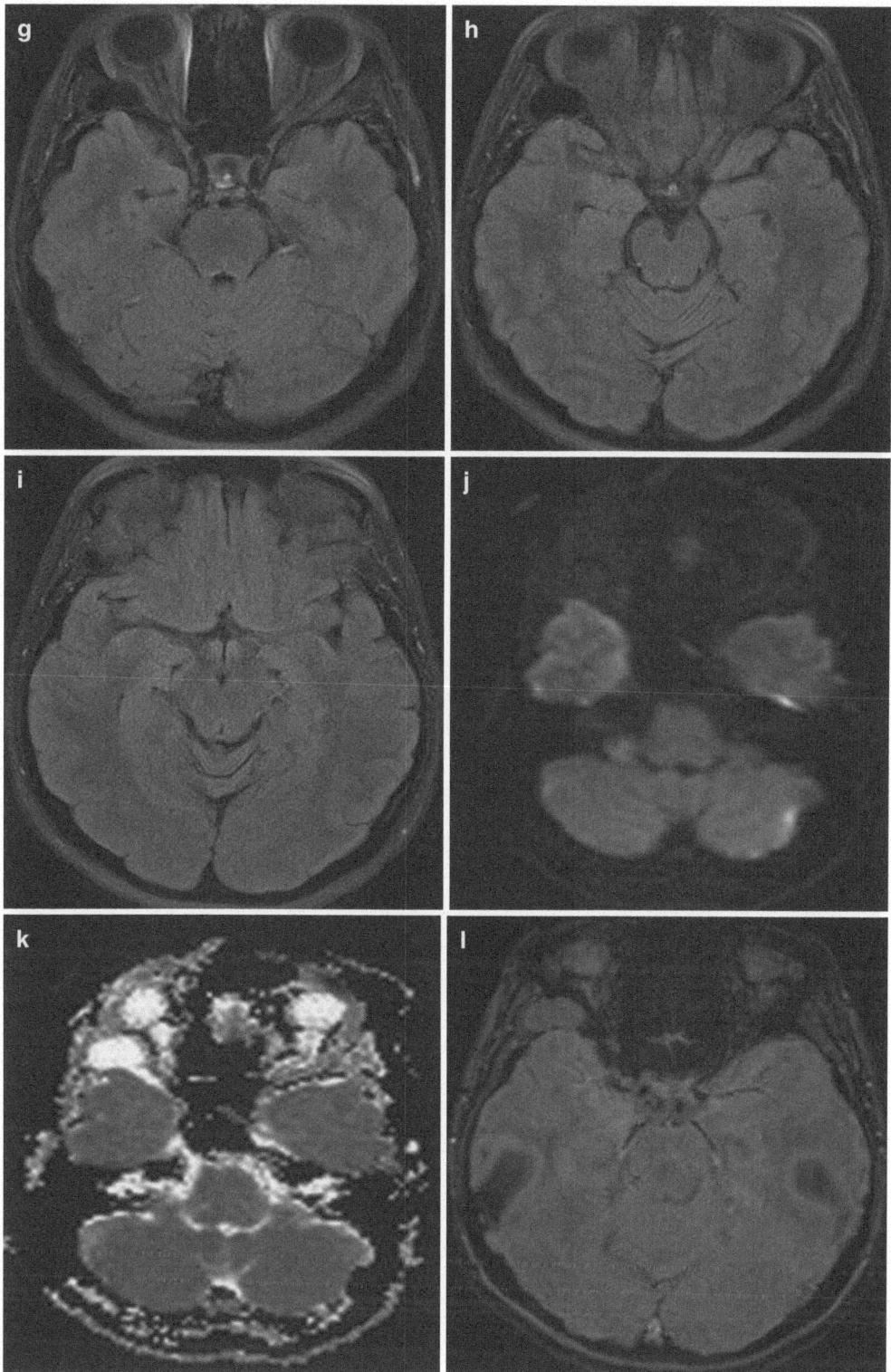

Fig. 17.1 (continued)

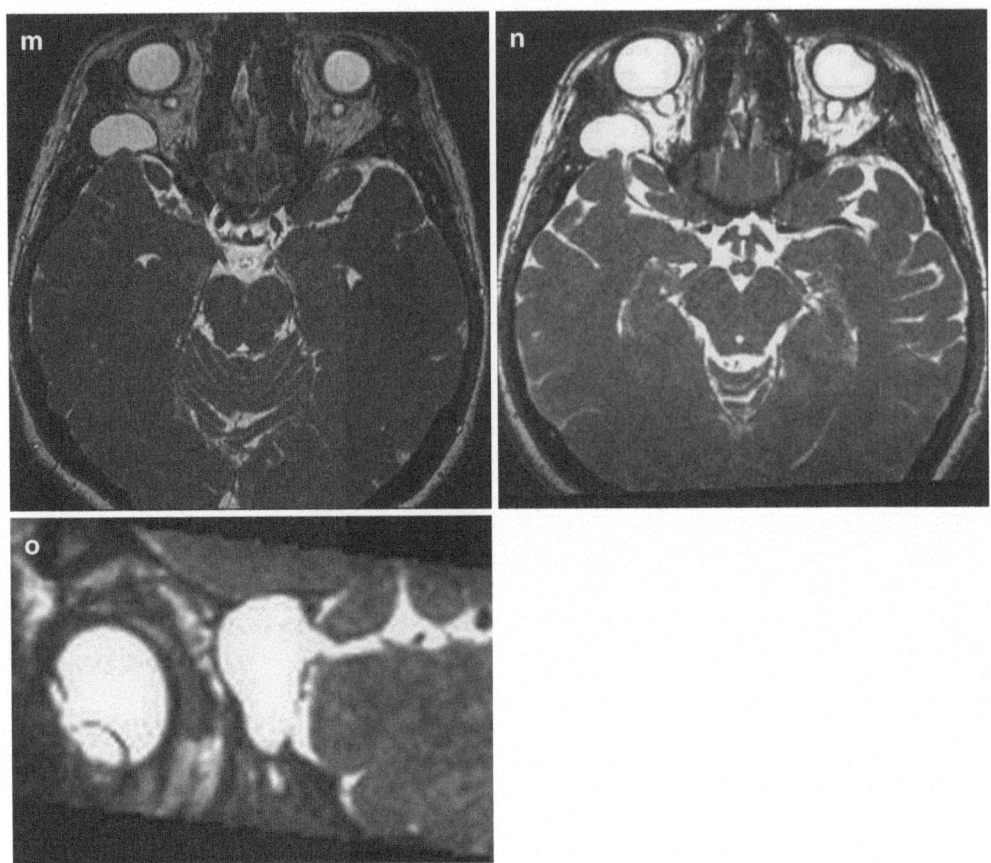

Fig. 17.1 (continued)

There are two types of SLSCs described in the literature: type I herniates into a pneumatised lateral recess of the sphenoid sinus usually presenting with headache and/or CSF leak. Type II herniates into the greater sphenoid wing with scalloping bone defect, may be an incidental finding or may present with headache and/or seizures [2].

The most important mechanism underlying the development of SLSC is likely related to altered CSF dynamics in aberrant arachnoid granulations: those are arachnoid granulations found outside, instead of the inside, dural venous sinuses, resulting in small concave pits in the inner table of the calvaria or the skull base [2–4]. Usually are incidental and asymptomatic, but in the setting of persistently elevated CSF pressure, egress of CSF from the aberrant arachnoid granulations may be impaired leading to granulations'

progressive enlargement and scalloping of the underlying bone [5].

Spontaneous meningoceles most commonly occur in middle-aged obese women with clinical symptoms and imaging features of elevated intracranial pressure.

In the evaluation of SLSC, CT and MRI are complementary imaging techniques: CT demonstrates bone defect and adjacent anatomical structures, and post-contrast CT scans show relation between bone defect and dural sinus, while MRI reveals content of herniated tissue. Three-dimensional CISS sequence provides superior topographic information: therefore I personally use it to investigate a wide range of pathologies when routine MRI sequence does not provide desired anatomic information. In the particular case, I used it to demonstrate more clearly meningocele and

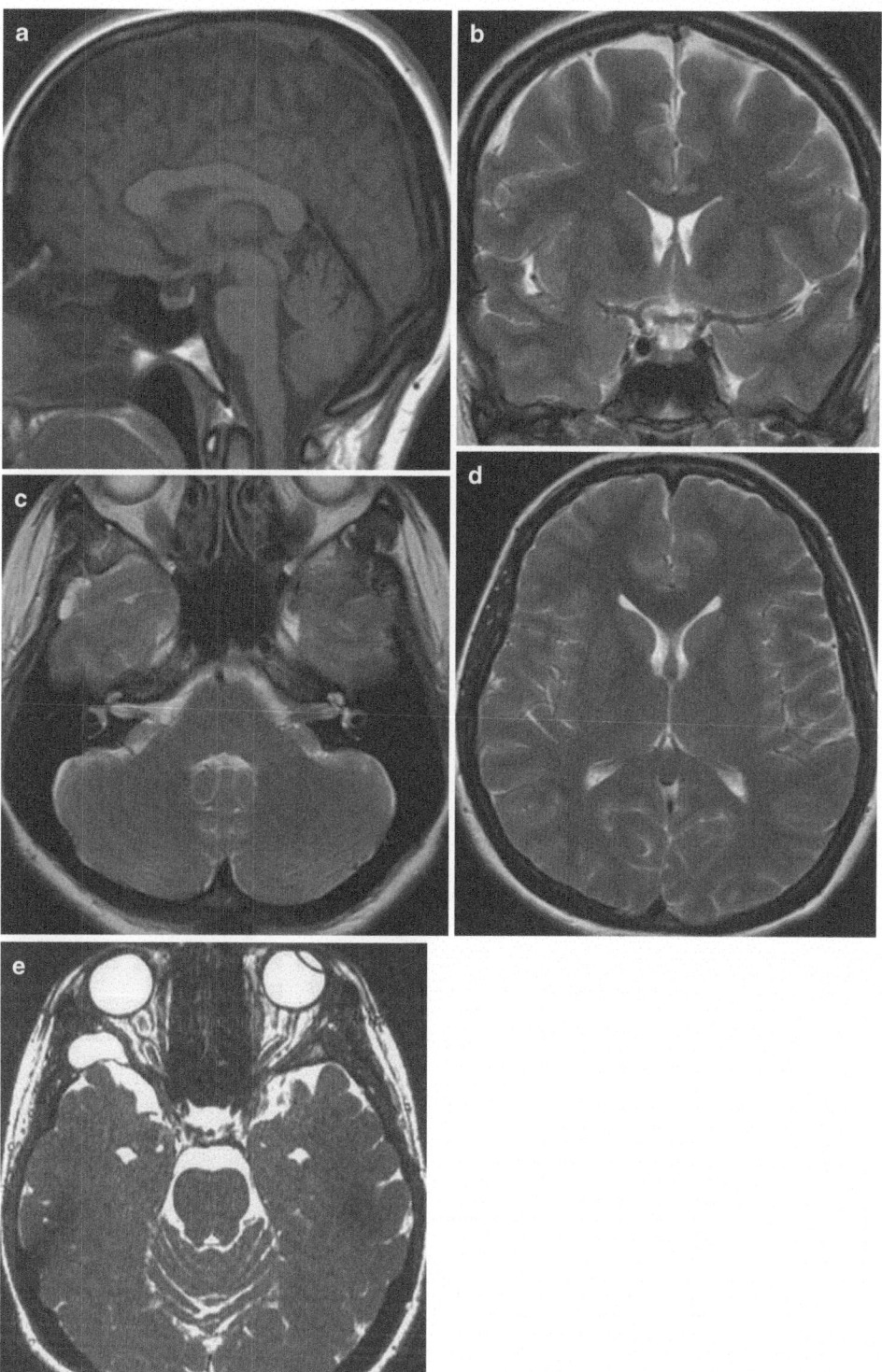

Fig. 17.2 Magnetic resonance imaging of the brain, sagittal T1WI (**a**), coronal (**b**), and axial (**c, d**) T2WI, axial CISS (**e**). Sella and hypophysis were of normal size and shape (**a, b**), there were no tonsillar ectopia (**b**), lateral and third ventricles were narrow and slitlike (**b, d**), and there were prominent arachnoid pits of the sphenoid wing (**c**). CISS sequence more clearly revealed prominent subarachnoid space around the optic nerves and vertical tortuosity of the nerves (**e**)

arachnoid pits, to reveal the exact communication between meningocele and adjacent subarachnoid space and to better visualise optic nerve changes.

Some SLSCs may resolve spontaneously, if are incidental imaging finding and asymptomatic, no treatment is needed. Otherwise, surgical repair is recommended to prevent meningitis or intracranial abscess.

If you see an expansile cystic lesion in the sphenoid bone, do not mistake it for a temporal arachnoid cyst; always ask yourself where the lesion is located, intracranial or extracranial in a bone. If you use 3D CISS sequence, you will be able to report more details regarding anatomical relations and depict communication between a lesion and subarachnoid space at the same time.

References

1. Alonso RC et al (2013) Spontaneous skull base meningoencephaloceles and cerebrospinal fluid fistulas. Radiographics 33:553–570
2. Settecase F et al (2014) Spontaneous lateral sphenoid cephaloceles: anatomic factors contributing to pathogenesis and proposed classification. AJNR Am J Neuroradiol 35(4):784–789
3. Schlosser RJ et al (2006) Spontaneous cerebrospinal fluid leaks: a variant of benign intracranial hypertension. Ann Otol Rhinol Laryngol 115:495–500
4. Almontasheri A et al (2012) Arachnoid pit and extensive sinus pneumatisation as the cause of spontaneous lateral intrasphenoidal encephalocele. J Clin Imaging Sci 2:1–6
5. Connor SEJ (2010) Imaging of skull-base cephaloceles and cerebrospinal fluid leaks. Clin Radiol 65:832–841

Occipital Bone Intradiploic Encephalocele

18

A 77-year-old lady was referred for a routine MRI examination of the brain because of recent intermittent dizziness and unsteadiness. No other neurological abnormalities were noted, and there were no developmental abnormalities nor history of trauma.

MRI did not show any focal cerebellar lesions, but our attention was drawn to an internal table and diploic defect on the right side of the occipital bone, adjacent to the right occipitotemporal suture (Fig. 18.1).

The findings were in keeping with an intradiploic occipital meningoencephalocele.

Additional CT exam was performed (Fig. 18.2).

18.1 Intradiploic Encephalocele

Encephalocele (also, encephalocoele) or meningoencephalocele consists of brain tissue and meninges herniated through a skull defect. They are very rare in adults, and more commonly they are encountered in infants as saclike protrusions of the brain and meninges through openings in the skull, representing incomplete closure of the neural tube during foetal development. Approximately 75% of cases are occipital

Intradiploic encephalocele (IE) is an extremely uncommon entity and usually an incidental finding. In adults it can simulate a lytic lesion, consequently raising suspicion of a number of differential diagnoses, such as eosinophilic granuloma, plasmacytoma, metastasis, osteosarcoma, cavernous haemangioma and epidermoid or dermoid cyst. The presence of CSF within the lytic lesion, lack of outer table bone defect and absence of other malignant features may suggest benign cystic lesions, such as post-traumatic or intradiploic arachnoid cyst and intraosseous leptomeningeal cyst. However, none of them contain herniated brain parenchyma which is a hallmark of an intradiploic encephalocele [1].

So far, there are less than a dozen articles documenting IE [2]. IE aetiology remains unclear, and several possibilities have been considered. The theory proposed by Patil and Etemadrezaie [3] is accepted by most authors—it proposes a blunt trauma as the cause of the internal table rupture, with associated dural tear. The brain tissue subsequently herniates through the dural tear into the diploic defect generated by trauma. Unfortunately, it is difficult to document the trauma which may have caused the defect as minimal trauma is easily forgotten, especially if it

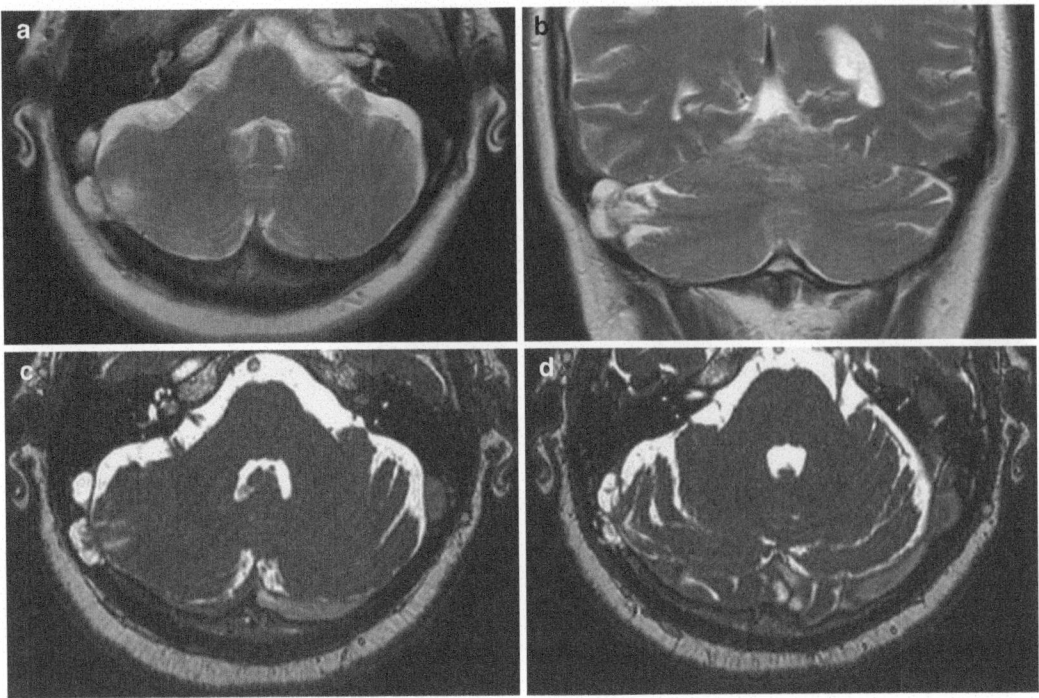

Fig. 18.1 MRI exam of the brain—axial and coronal T2WI (**a**, **b**), axial 3D CISS images (**c**, **d**). There is a 12 mm bony defect in the right side of the occipital bone, adjacent to the occipitotemporal suture and just posterior to the right sigmoid dural venous sinus, involving the inner table and the diploë, reaching the thinned outer table of the bone. The defect is filled with CSF and retracted right cerebellar folia, causing enlargement of the intervening CSF spaces. There is no evidence of gliosis or haemorrhage. The right sigmoid dural venous sinus appears hypoplastic or slightly compressed, with normal flow void. The rest of the appearances is unremarkable

took place many years ago. A congenital anomaly is a less plausible aetiology, given that congenital encephaloceles involve both inner and outer table discontinuity in the midline and are generally accompanied by other malformations, which is not the case with any of the reported IEs. Intracranial hypertension may play a role in IE development, either as idiopathic intracranial hypertension or a short-term increase in intracranial pressure such as in violent cough [4]. Most of the reported IEs were parietal, with exception of a single iatrogenic frontal intradiploic encephalocele. The case reported here seems to be the first case of an occipital IE in an adult reported in literature.

Clinical manifestations are often absent; if there are some symptoms, they affect the functional brain area of the herniated portion of the brain or adjacent parenchyma. While the herniated tissue itself may not be injured, the tension on the adjacent parenchyma may cause symptoms. Another proposed mechanism is vascular constriction with subsequent ischaemic events.

Before deciding on IE treatment, it is necessary to establish a convincing relationship of the parenchymal hernia and the symptoms—functional imaging may be of help. The treatment usually consists of aggressive surgery involving parenchymal amputation, which may be unnecessary in the absence of neurological deficit.

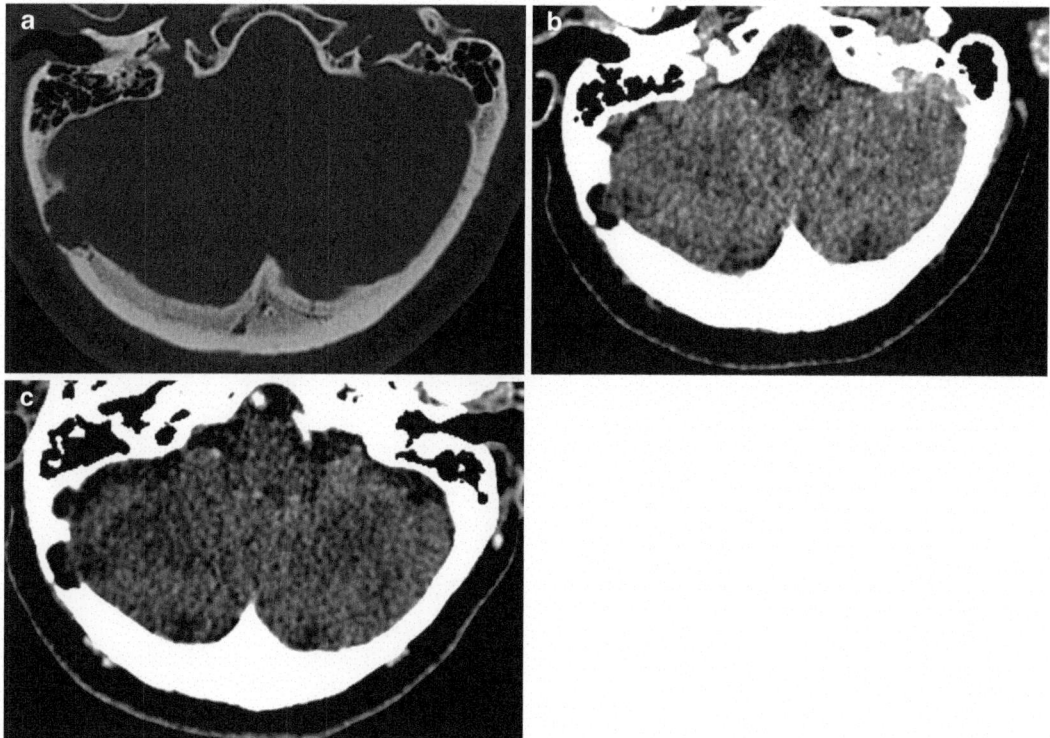

Fig. 18.2 CT exam of the brain, axial images. In the bone window setting (**a**), there is a lytic lesion in the intradiploic space of the right occipital bone, adjacent to the occipitotemporal suture, with a defect of the inner table and marked thinning of the outer table of the bone. In the brain window setting (**b, c**), there is evidence of cerebellar parenchyma protrusion into the bony defect

References

1. Shi C et al (2017) Symptomatic parietal intradiploic encephalocele—a case report and literature review. J Neurol Surg Rep 78(1):e43–e48
2. Arevalo-Perez J, Millán-Juncos JM (2015) Parietal intradiploic encephalocele: report of a case and review of the literature. Neuroradiol J 28(3):264–267
3. Patil AA, Etemadrezaie H (1996) Posttraumatic intradiploic meningoencephalocele. Case report. J Neurosurg 84:284–287
4. Loumiotis I et al (2010) Symptomatic left intradiploic encephalocele. Neurology 75(11):1027

Intraorbital Aspergilloma

Several months after he had undergone heart transplantation and was started on immunosuppressive therapy, this 60-year-old gentleman started feeling retrobulbar pain, redness and swelling of his right eye, with double vision on lateral gaze. On examination, the lateral and downward right eye movement was limited, and there was oedema of the superior and inferior eyelid and proptosis. The left eye was unremarkable.

A CT exam of the orbits was done (Fig. 19.1).

The right-sided intraorbital space occupying lesion was described as inflamed mucocoele. Fine needle aspiration was recommended as the

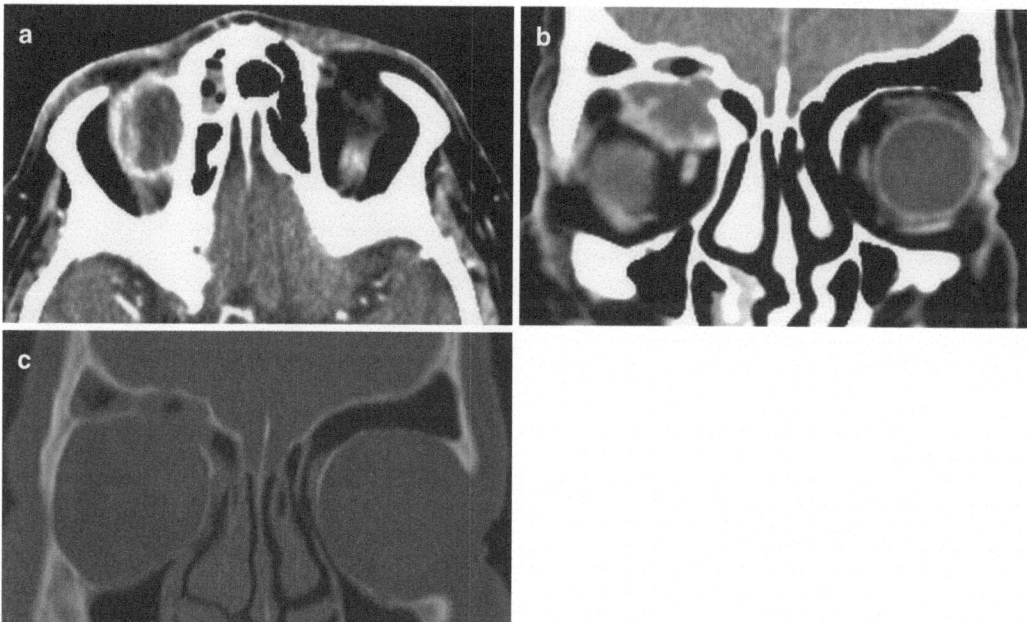

Fig. 19.1 Contrast-enhanced CT exam of both orbits—axial (**a**) and coronal (**b**) soft-tissue imaging and coronal (**c**) bone imaging algorithms show a cystic space occupying lesion with enhancing, irregular, thick margins in the medial superior aspect of the right orbit. Adjacent to it, there is a 7 mm bony defect of the orbital roof/frontal sinus inferior wall (probably due to a previous surgery). The lesion displaces the globe caudally, laterally and anteriorly

© Springer International Publishing AG, part of Springer Nature 2018
M. Špero, H. Vavro, *Neuroradiology - Expect the Unexpected*,
https://doi.org/10.1007/978-3-319-73482-8_19

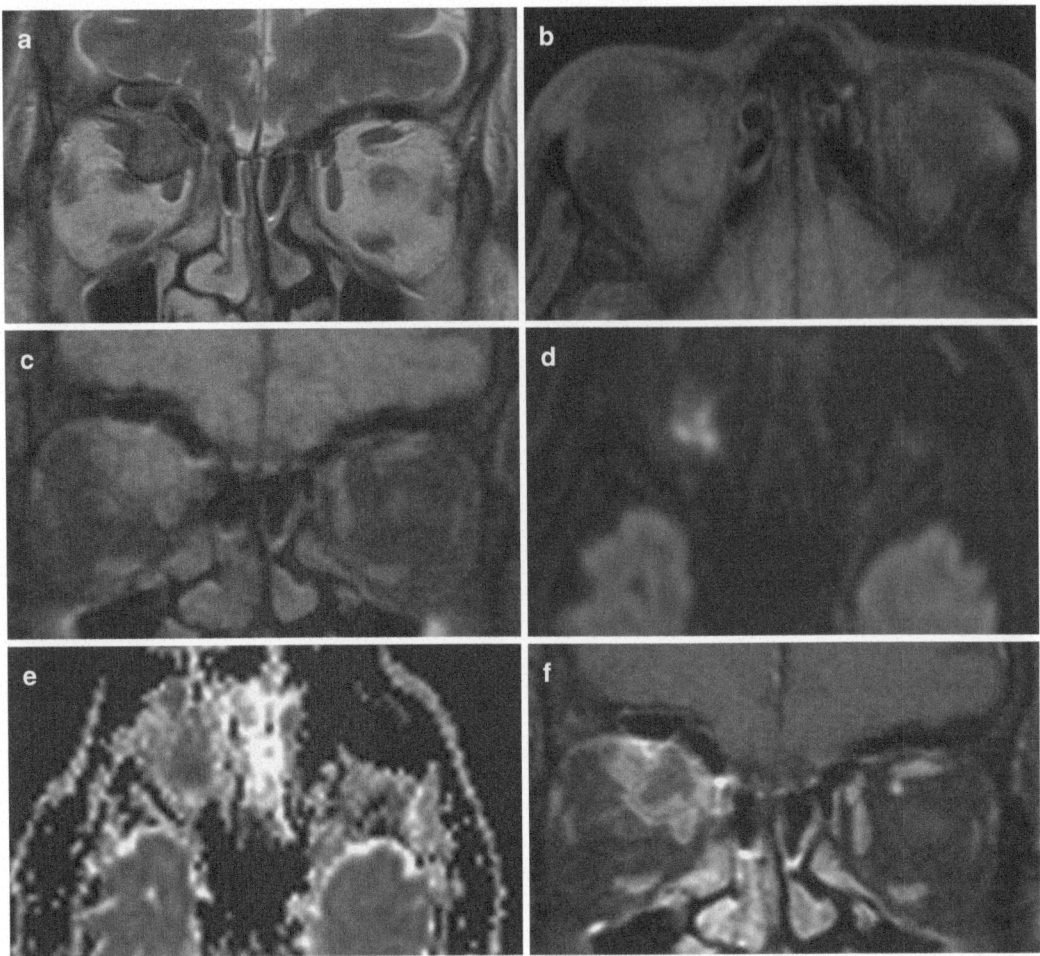

Fig. 19.2 MRI exam of the orbits—coronal T2WI (**a**), axial T2FSWI (**b**), coronal T2FSWI (**c**), axial DWI (**d**), axial ADC map (**e**), post-contrast coronal T1FSWI— shows a space-occupying lesion in the cranial medial aspect of the right orbit, originating in the extraconal compartment, protruding into the intraconal compartment between the upper and medial rectus muscle. There is thick, irregular peripheral enhancement of the lesion. Note the high DWI (**d**) signal coupled with low ADC (**e**) signal in the lesion, indicating thick cyst contents suggestive of an abscess. The right superior oblique muscle is compressed, and it enhances with contrast (**f**) which is probably of reactive inflammatory aetiology

next step, but the cytology report was inconclusive and unremarkable.

Later on, lesion biopsy was performed in a regional hospital, and a diagnosis of intraorbital aspergilloma was established.

A MRI exam of the orbits was recommended (Fig. 19.2).

Three weeks after the MRI exam, the aspergilloma was surgically resected through the upper eyelid (Fig. 19.3).

Four months later, the patient experienced aggravation of the symptoms, and another MRI exam of the orbits was done (Fig. 19.4).

The maxillofacial surgeons performed surgical exploration of the right orbit, with complete resection of the aspergilloma (Fig. 19.5).

The patient has constantly been on immunosuppressive therapy after heart transplantation; regular myocardial biopsies showed no signs of transplant rejection.

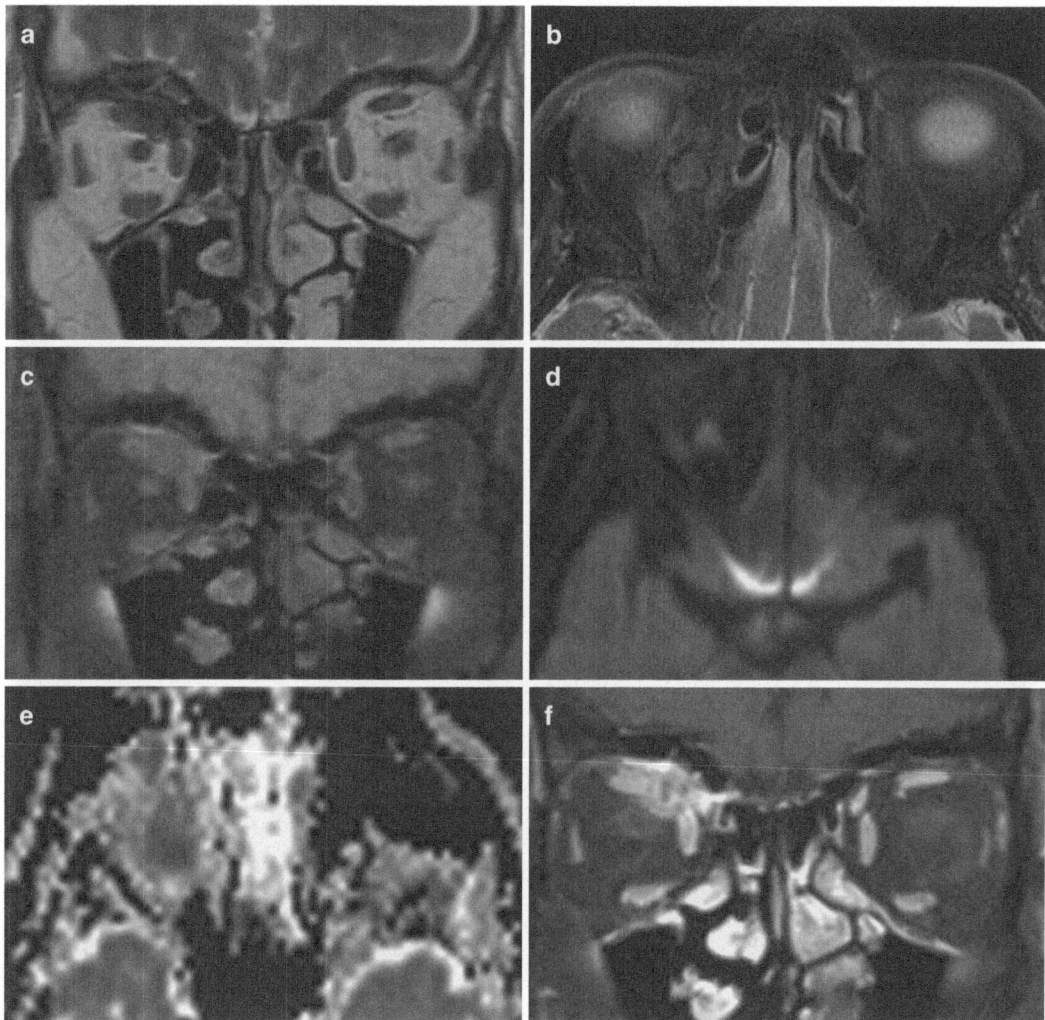

Fig. 19.3 MRI exam of the orbits 2.5 months after evacuation of right orbital aspergilloma. Coronal T2WI (**a**), axial T2FSWI (**b**), coronal T1FSWI (**c**), axial DWI (**d**), axial ADC map (**e**), post-contrast coronal T1FSWI (**f**). There is a residual aspergilloma in the cranial medial aspect of the right orbit, and the mass effect has been partially resolved

19.1   Intraorbital Aspergilloma

Intraorbital aspergilloma is a rare lesion, although aspergillus is a ubiquitous fungus. The spores are found in the soil and decaying organic matter, get airborne and daily get inhaled by most of the people. In the immunocompetent patients, they are usually eliminated by the immune system but can be the cause of a chronic sinusitis, with possible expansion of the sinuses and structural changes of the facial skeleton [1]. An aspergilloma may occur in incompletely aerated sinuses. Generally, no invasion, necrosis or reactive changes of the adjacent tissues are seen in the immunocompetent persons. However, in immunocompromised patients, such as in this case, aspergillus may cause invasive granulomatous inflammation with fibrosis or a fulminant necrotising form with vascular invasion.

Aspergillosis usually spreads to the orbit directly from adjacent paranasal sinuses, rarely haematogenously from the lung. The most

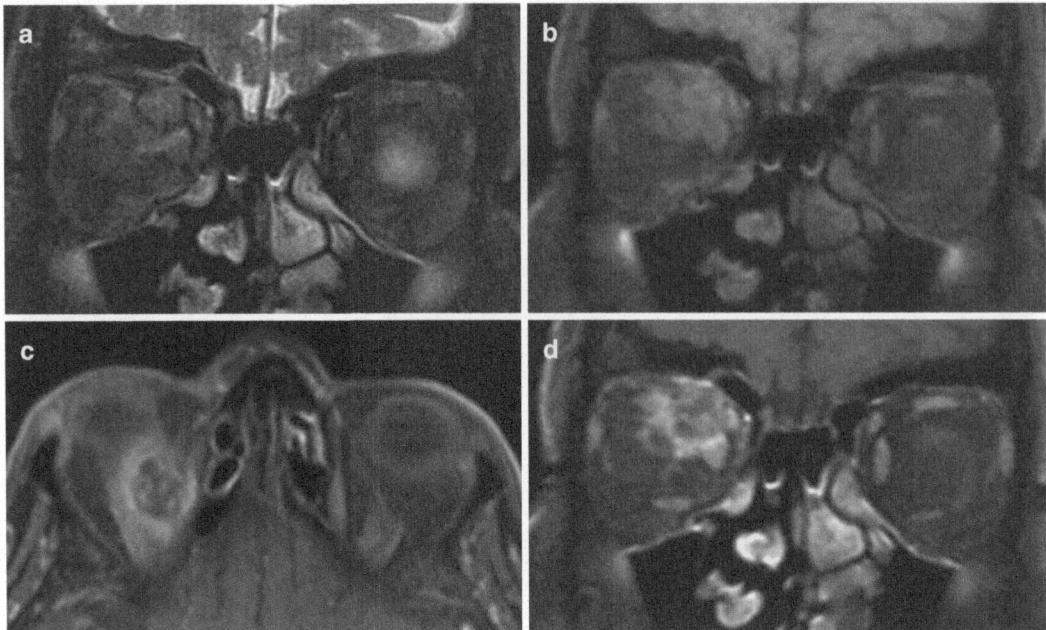

Fig. 19.4 Follow-up MRI exam of the orbits—coronal T2FSWI (**a**), coronal T1FSWI (**b**), post-contrast axial (**c**) and coronal (**d**) T1FSWI—demonstrates progression in size of the irregular aspergilloma residue, with inhomogeneous peripheral enhancement and mild inflammatory reaction of the adjacent soft tissues

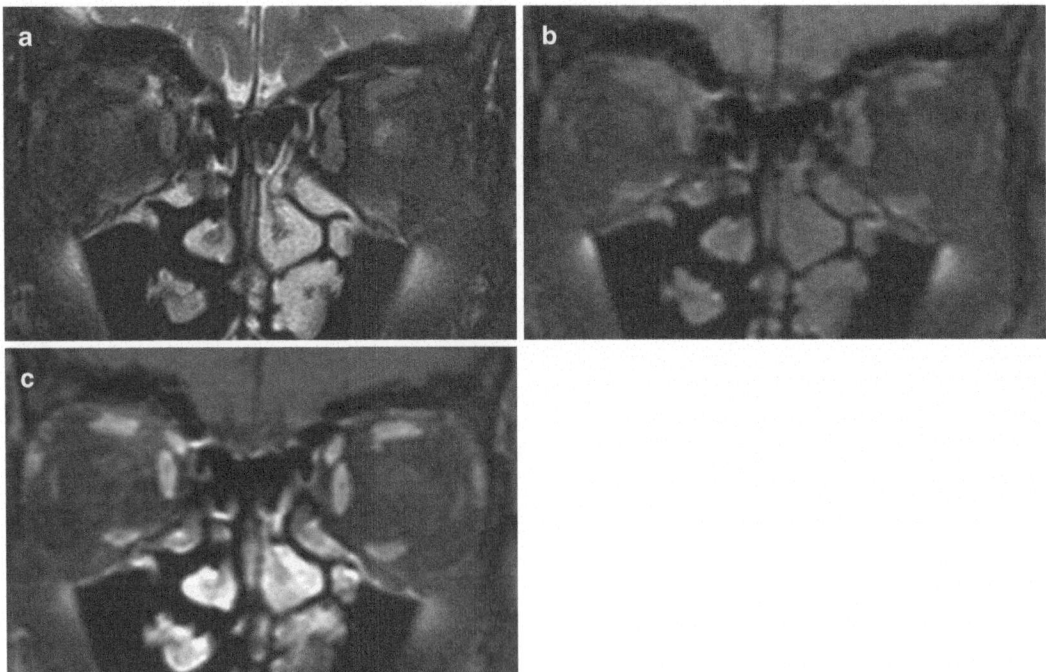

Fig. 19.5 Follow-up MRI exam of the orbits 18 months post surgery—coronal T2FSWI (**a**), coronal T1FSWI (**b**), post-contrast T1FSWI (**c**)—does not show any signs of active inflammation; there are some scarring and a small inactive residual nodal lesion seen in the superior medial aspect of the right orbit. The patient's symptoms have resolved

common site of infection is posterior orbit, presenting as orbital apex syndrome involving ophthalmoplegia, pain, loss of vision, loss of sensation in the infraorbital nerve and proptosis. The cavernous sinus is usually also affected. Invasive form with penetration of bone and blood vessel walls and intracranial spread is not uncommon, presenting a treatment challenge.

CT imaging shows a peripherally or inhomogeneously enhancing intraorbital mass and, usually, opacification of the adjacent paranasal sinuses. In this case the frontal sinus opacification has mostly resolved previously. The characteristic calcification within the mass is only seen in less than 50% of cases. MRI will help differentiate the mass further, showing possible involvement of the optic nerve or adjacent muscles, as well as possible signs of abscess formation with central increased DWI signal and peripheral low T2 signal.

As intraorbital aspergillosis mostly stems from adjacent paranasal sinuses, differential diagnosis includes most of the extraorbital lesions extending into the extraconal space, such as other infections, mucocoele, metastatic tumours and sinonasal tumours (squamous cell carcinoma, adenocarcinoma, adenoid cystic carcinoma, lymphoma). Differential diagnosis may be narrowed if there are MRI features of abscess, such as in this case.

For definitive diagnosis of invasive aspergillosis, a tissue sample is needed, obtained either by FNA or biopsy.

Systemic and local antifungal therapy remains the mainstay of treatment, but surgical debridement is often performed [2]. Reversal of immunosuppression is important, if at all possible.

References

1. Karcioglu ZA (ed) (2015) Orbital tumors diagnosis and treatment. Springer, New York
2. Sivak-Callcott JA et al (2004) Localised invasive sino-orbital aspergillosis: characteristic features. Br J Ophthalmol 88:681–687

Van Buchem Disease, Sclerosteosis or Something Else?

20

Due to dull headaches and enlarged hands, feet and mandible, endocrinologist referred a 39-year-old female patient to MRI of the brain (Fig. 20.1).

In 2009, during preoperative preparation due to collateral ligament injury, knee X-rays have been performed and have demonstrated bone thickening: bone biopsy and histomorphometry have been proposed, but never performed, because a patient has been avoiding diagnostic workup until the autumn 2016.

According to anamnestic data, she had "drumstick"-shaped fingers since birth, during childhood she has been a little bit higher compared to other children, childhood photos have showed mildly pronounced mandible. Family photos have showed her father and grandfather had mild mandibular prognathism. Menstrual cycle has always been normal.

In the age of 30, she has noticed hand, feet and mandible enlargement—now without further enlargement. Diffuse dull headaches occur periodically once a month and resolve completely on analgesic drugs. During the last 6 years, she noticed mild hearing loss in the left ear and vague mild balance disorder. For several years, she has suffered from sleep apnea symptoms.

In late autumn 2016, an extensive diagnostic workup was commenced and revealed normal hormone levels, no abnormalities in routine blood tests (alkaline phosphatase level was normal), bilateral mixed hearing loss and small hard palate exostosis. Officially, serum sclerostin levels are not possible to measure in any of biochemical laboratories in our country, only abroad.

MRI Imaging features suggested sclerosteosis (Fig. 20.1). Due to generalised thickening of the skull, cranial CT was recommended to assess degree of the bone thickening as well as the possible narrowing of the neural exit foramina and canals (Fig. 20.2).

Differential diagnosis included sclerosteosis and Van Buchem disease. Regarding patient phenotype, as an adult, she is not much taller than female coevals and does not have finger abnormality characteristic for patients with sclerosteosis like radial deviation, syndactyly or both; Van Buchem disease was a more obvious diagnosis. To confirm or exclude possible differential diagnosis, a genetic testing has been conducted at Department of Medical Genetics, University of Antwerp in Belgium. By the time we concluded this manuscript, we have got the information that mutation in the SOST gene seemed to be excluded, and testing of a few other candidate genes was in progress. Such information was expected because a patient does not have a Duch ancestry, and "de novo" mutation was presumed.

© Springer International Publishing AG, part of Springer Nature 2018
M. Špero, H. Vavro, *Neuroradiology - Expect the Unexpected*,
https://doi.org/10.1007/978-3-319-73482-8_20

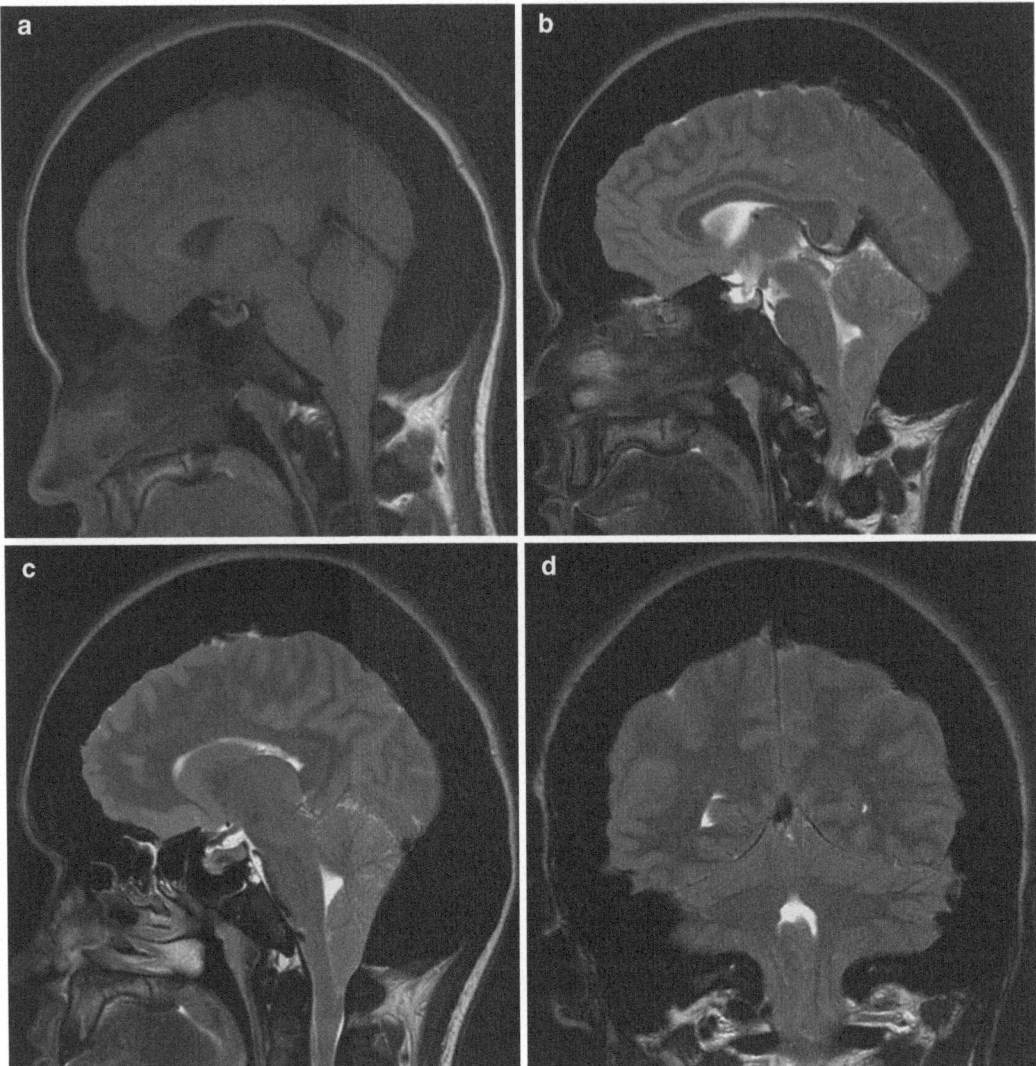

Fig. 20.1 Magnetic resonance of the brain, sagittal T1WI (**a**) and T2WI (**b**, **c**), coronal T2WI (**d–f**) and axial T2WI (**g–i**), revealed generalised thickening of the skull with irregularities of the brain surface due to bony elevations of the inner table: occipital bone was thick as 3.5 cm, sphenoid bone as 10 mm, rest of the skull bones up to 2.5 cm. Sella turcica was shallow, but widened, pituitary gland had concave cranial surface, and stalk was narrow as well as the infundibular recess of the third ventricle. Cerebellar tonsils were elongated, beak-like in shape, and descended below the level of foramen magnum. Subarachnoid space over the convexity was reduced; sulci over the convexity were narrow. Hypoglossal canals were not compressed (**g**), and cisternal space surrounding the brainstem was reduced and narrow as well as pontocerebellar angles (**g**, **h**). Lateral ventricles appeared normal (**i**)

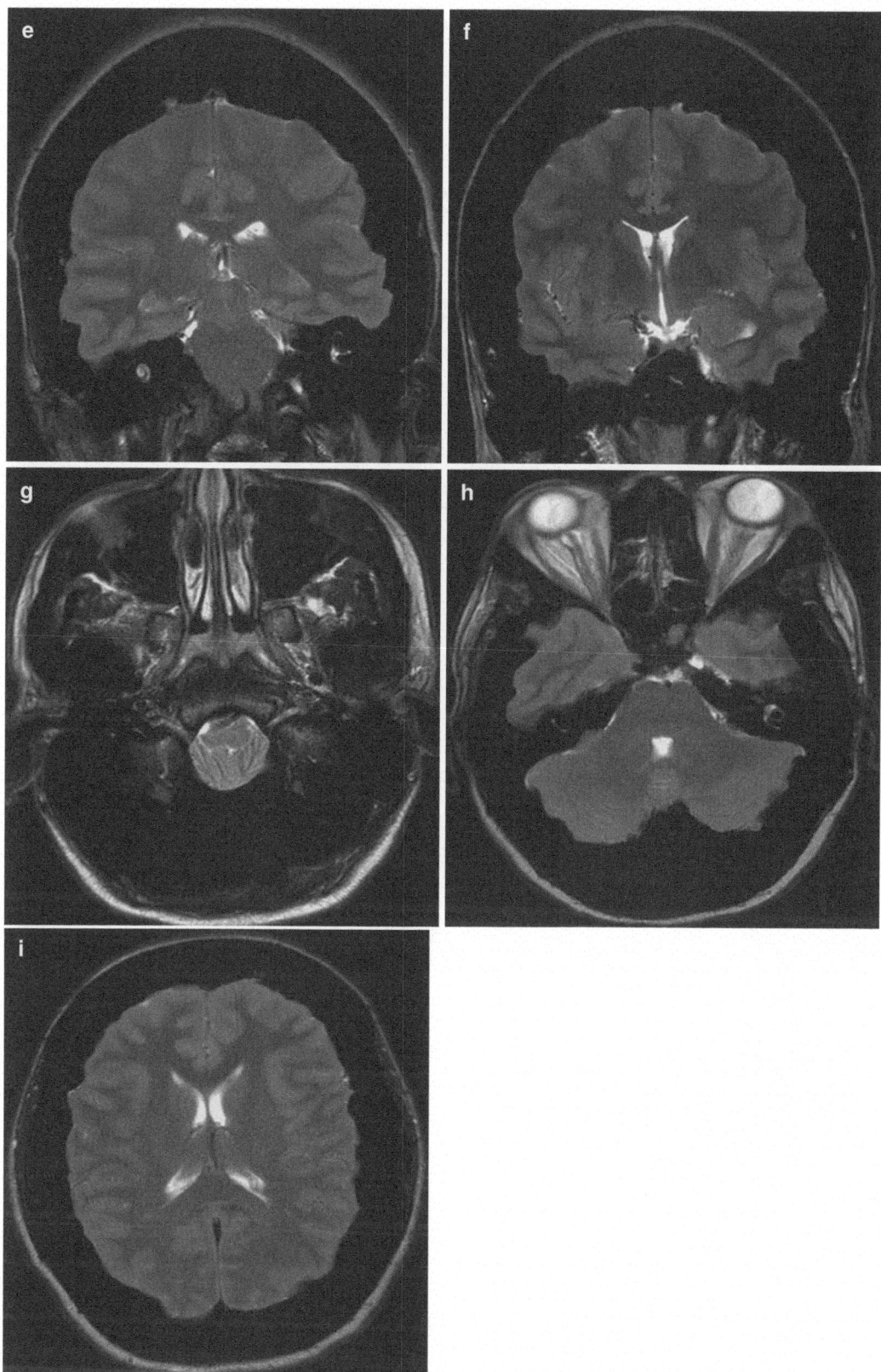

Fig. 20.1 (continued)

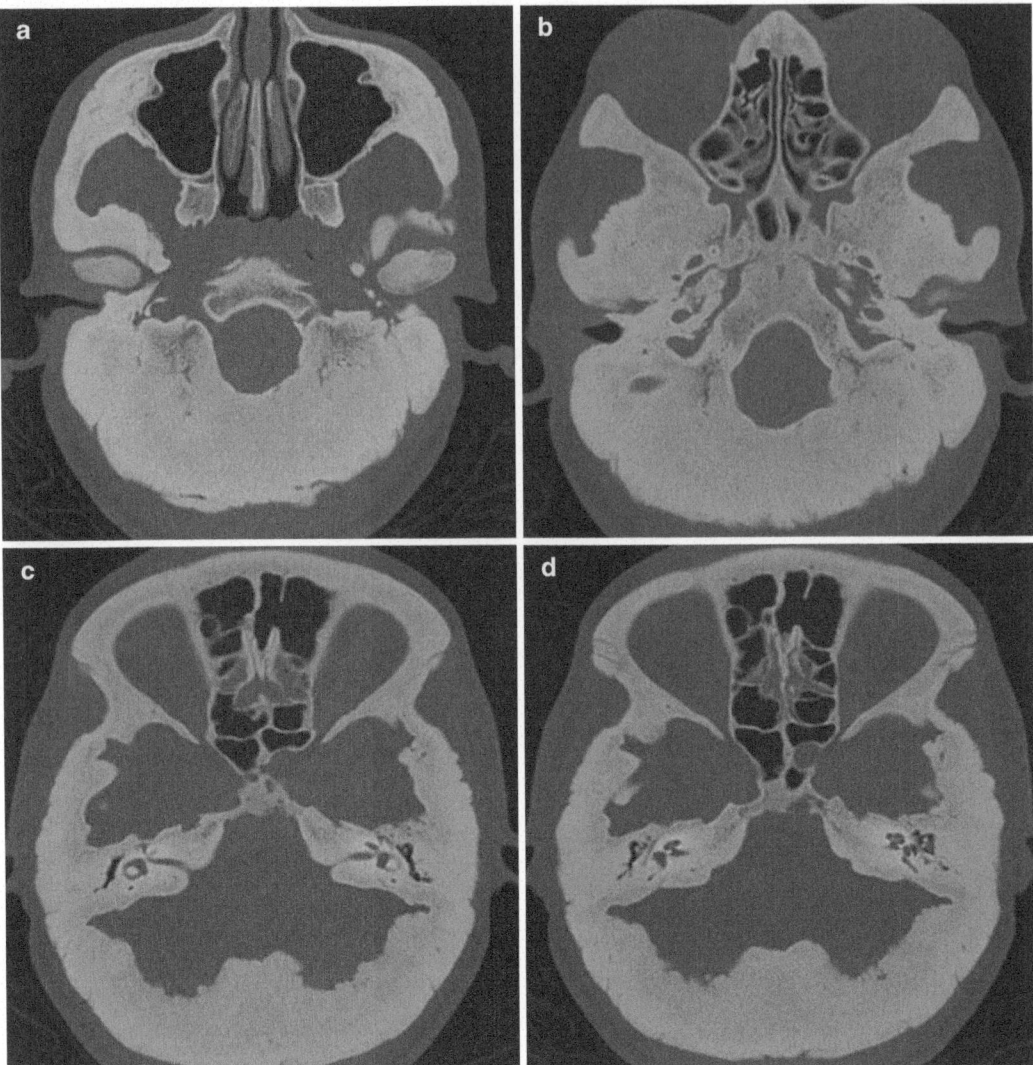

Fig. 20.2 Computed tomography of skull bones (high-spatial-resolution bone algorithm), axial scans (**a–f**) and sagittal scan (**g**) of the skull base and the rest of the cranium (**a–f**) and coronal (**h**) and oblique (**i**) VRT. Massive hyperostosis of the skull base and vault, as well as the mandible (**h, i**) and petrous bones: bones were dense and thick with loss of diploe due to cortical thickening. Mandible was particularly enlarged, assuming a square form, prognathic. Hypoglossal canals (**a**) and foramen ovale (**b**) were not compressed, while foramen rotundum (**b**) was narrowed. Internal auditory canals were extremely narrow, while external auditory canals were not occludes. Mastoid cells were not developed; dense abnormal bone was encroaching upon otherwise normal inner ear structures in the narrow tympanic cavities (**c, d**). Facial canals were compressed (**d**). Upper orbital fissures and optic canals were mildly narrow due to involvement of lateral orbital walls (**e, f**). Small exostosis in the posterior part of hard palate (**g**)

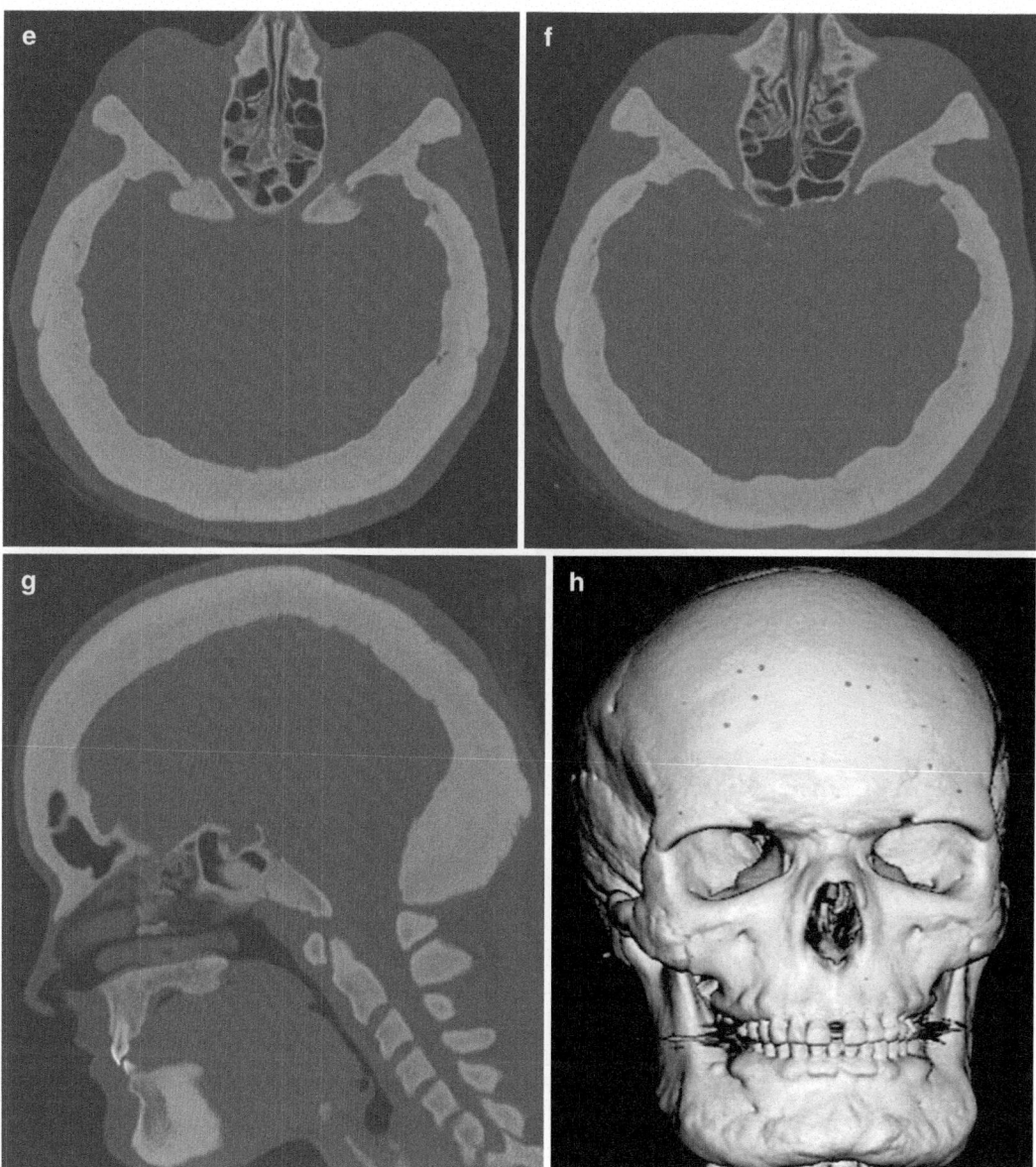

Fig. 20.2 (continued)

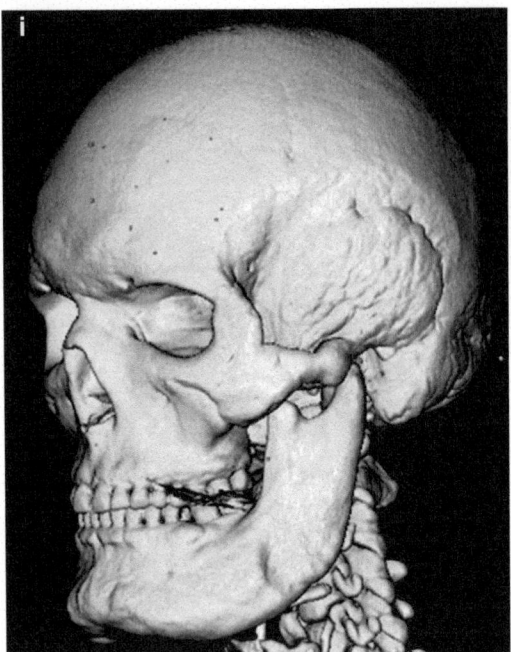

Fig. 20.2   (continued)

20.1   Van Buchem Disease or Sclerosteosis

Van Buchem disease (VBD) and sclerosteosis are very rare diseases that belong to the group of craniotubular hyperostoses or osteopetroses that involve bony overgrowths that alter contour and increase skeletal density, mainly involving the skull and long, tubular bones. Sclerosteosis was first described in 1958 and is most common among Afrikaners, mainly white, of Dutch origin in South Africa, although small number of individuals and families have been reported in other parts of the world, including Brazil, United States, Germany, Senegal and Turkey. Van Buchem disease was first described in 1955 by Van Buchem as "hyperostosis corticalis generalisata familiaris", in a fishing village in the Netherlands among descendants from 151 inhabitants who survived the plague in 1637 and appears more frequently in persons of Dutch ancestry [1–3].

Both are autosomal recessive disorders: sclerosteosis is caused by mutation in the SOST gene encoding sclerostin on chromosome 17q12-q21 which leads to osteoblast hyperactivity, while VBD is caused by a 52 kb deletion downstream of the SOST gene on chromosome 17q12-q21, which results in lack of a SOST-specific regulatory element in osteoblasts leading to impaired inhibition of osteoblastic bone formation [3, 4]. Sclerostin is a protein produced almost exclusively from osteocytes that inhibits bone formation by both osteoblasts and osteocytes. It acts as a negative regulator of bone formation inhibiting the Wnt signalling pathway on molecular level, which plays a critical role in osteoblast development and function [4, 5]. Undetectable levels in sclerosteosis and very low levels of sclerostin in VBD result in excessive bone growth and increased bone strength: mainly affected are cranial bones and diaphysis of long, tubular bones.

Described neuroimaging features are similar in sclerosteosis and VBD: you will not be able to distinguish it only on cranial CT and MRI. Associated clinical features, age of onset, molecular genetic test results and disease progression must be taken into account when establishing a differential diagnosis.

Sclerosteosis is characterised by a progressive bone thickening, tall stature, finger abnormalities—syndactyly and/or radial deviation—and enlargement of the skull. Patients usually appear normal at birth, with possible exception of syndactyly, while other manifestations appear early in life during the first decade of life [4, 6].

Patients with VBD have phenotype similar to patients with sclerosteosis but less severe including increased bone mass with enlargement of the mandible and macrocephaly, normal stature and no finger abnormalities [4, 6].

In both conditions, in the third decade of life, clinical features and complications usually stabilise, with no new clinical findings or progression, but are less severe in VBD because of slower progression of the bone overgrowth after the first years, in comparison to sclerosteosis [4].

Hyperostotic skull and facial bones distort the shape of a patient's face who usually has massive square prognathic chin, in sclerosteosis also frontal bossing, and cause foraminal stenosis resulting in cranial nerve compression with facial palsy, hearing loss and increased intracranial pressure that may result in sudden death from impaction of the brainstem into the foramen magnum in sclerosteosis, while in VBD is not so frequent and usually craniotomy is not necessary.

Mixed hearing loss, in those patients, could be explained by marked narrowing of the external and internal auditory canals and impediment of the bony middle and inner ear structures. Neuroradiologist should look for signs of increased intracranial pressure like herniation of cerebellar tonsils, depletion of subarachnoid space and distension of the subarachnoid space along the optic nerves which can alternatively be caused by narrowing of the optic nerve canals preventing fluid drainage. Low position of cerebellar tonsils could also be a result of occipital bone hypertrophy. On imaging methods, ventricles appear normal in size and shape because elevated intracranial pressure is not a result of obstructed CSF flow and/or absorption [6].

Van Buchem disease is clinically similar to sclerosteosis; however, the main clinical differences between two diseases are gigantism and hand abnormalities present in sclerosteosis but never in VBD. Therefore if you have a patient with imaging features described above, look for clinical signs which can help you in reporting more obvious diagnosis, and always recommend genetic test to confirm or exclude possible diagnosis.

References

1. Fayez A et al (2015) A novel loss-of-sclerostin function mutation in a first Egyptian family with sclerosteosis. Biomed Res Int 2015:517815, 8 pages. https://doi.org/10.1155/2015/517815
2. Bhadada SK et al (2013) Novel SOST gene mutation in a sclerosteosis patient and her parents. Bone 52(2):707–710
3. Van Hul W et al (1998) Van Buchem disease (hyperostosis corticalis generalisata) maps to chromosome 17q12-q21. Am J Hum Genet 62:391–399
4. Yavropoulou MP et al (2014) The sclerostin story: from human genetics to the development of novel anabolic treatment for osteoporosis. Hormones 13(4):476–487
5. Lewiecki EM (2014) Role of sclerostin in bone and cartilage and its potential as therapeutic target in bone disease. Ther Adv Musculoskelet Dis 6(2):48–57
6. Wengenroth M et al (2009) Case 150: Van Buchem disease (hyperostosis corticalis generalisata). Radiology 253:272–276

Neurinoma: Chondrosarcoma of the Thoracic Spine

A 29-year-old female patient suffered from sideropenic anaemia due to a menorrhagia: in October 2013, during preoperative workup of uterine myoma, chest X-ray was performed and revealed large left-sided paravertebral expansile mass at a level of left upper lobe of a lung. Anamnestic data disclosed that in 2007 she occasionally felt thoracic back pain but recommended chest X-ray was not performed. Due to anaemia, she was feeling fatigue in physical activity: she did not have other symptoms.

In November 2013, she was admitted to a hospital, and diagnostic workup has been commenced. CT of the thorax (Fig. 21.1) and MRI of the thoracic spine (FIg. 21.2) were performed and revealed large, oval expansile left paravertebral lesion at the level of T4–T5 segment involving and widening left neural foramina.

According to described CT and MRI features (Figs. 21.1 and 21.2), paraspinal thoracic tumour of possible neural origin was reported, although calcifications in extradural schwannoma are rare. Chondrosarcoma, due to "benign" imaging features, was not our first choice. A patient was operated in November 2013: total resection was performed, while pathohistology revealed chondrosarcoma grade II. There was no tumour recurrence on regular MRI follow-ups (previous MRI examination was in January 2017).

21.1 Spinal Chondrosarcoma

Chondrosarcoma is a malignant tumour of connective tissue, characterised by formation of cartilage matrix by tumour cells. It is the second most common primary malignant tumour of the spine in adults. Males are affected two to four times more frequently than female, with a peak prevalence between 30 and 70 years. Most spinal chondrosarcomas are low-grade tumour; hence clinical course is usually long. Clinically they are presented with pain, palpable mass and neurological deficit [1–3].

Thoracic and lumbar spine are more frequently affected, while sacrum is affected rarely. Primary chondrosarcoma originates "de novo" in the vertebral body, posterior element or both, while secondary chondrosarcoma occurs mostly as a result of malignant transformation within the cartilage cap of a pre-existing benign tumour such as osteochondroma.

Primary and secondary chondrosarcoma are histologically similar: three different grades are recognized for both, representing the most reliable predictors of clinical behaviour. Grade I chondrosarcoma grows relatively slow; histological appearance is similar to cells of normal cartilage, and is less aggressive, and rarely metastasize. Grade III chondrosarcoma is faster-growing

M. Špero, H. Vavro, *Neuroradiology - Expect the Unexpected*,
https://doi.org/10.1007/978-3-319-73482-8_21

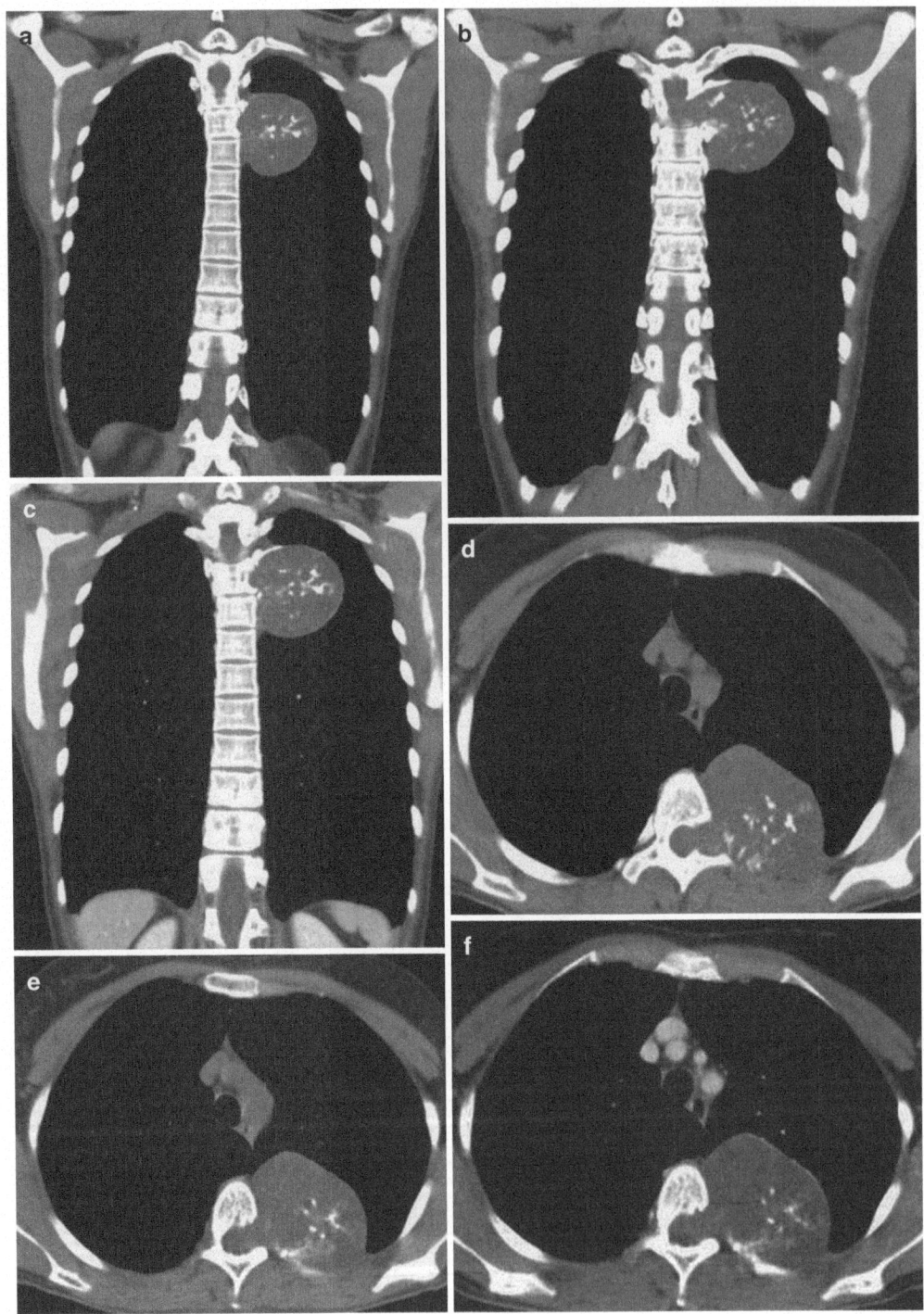

Fig. 21.1 CT of the thorax, pre-contrast coronal (**a**, **b**) and axial (**d**, **e**) plane and post-contrast coronal (**c**) and axial (**f**) scans demonstrated large (44 × 72 × 64 mm) soft tissue left paravertebral mass at the level of T4–T5 segment. Tumour was oval and well-circumscribed, hypodense with amorphous calcifications and did not reveal contrast enhancement on post-contrast scans. Tumour has widened left neural foramina of the T4–T5 segment and did not destruct adjacent third, fourth and fifth left rib or left transverse process of the fourth and fifth thoracic vertebra. Left transverse process of the T4 vertebra and left fourth rib were scalloped, while left lamina of the fourth vertebra was thinned and scalloped. There was no pulmonary metastases or mediastinal lymphadenopathy

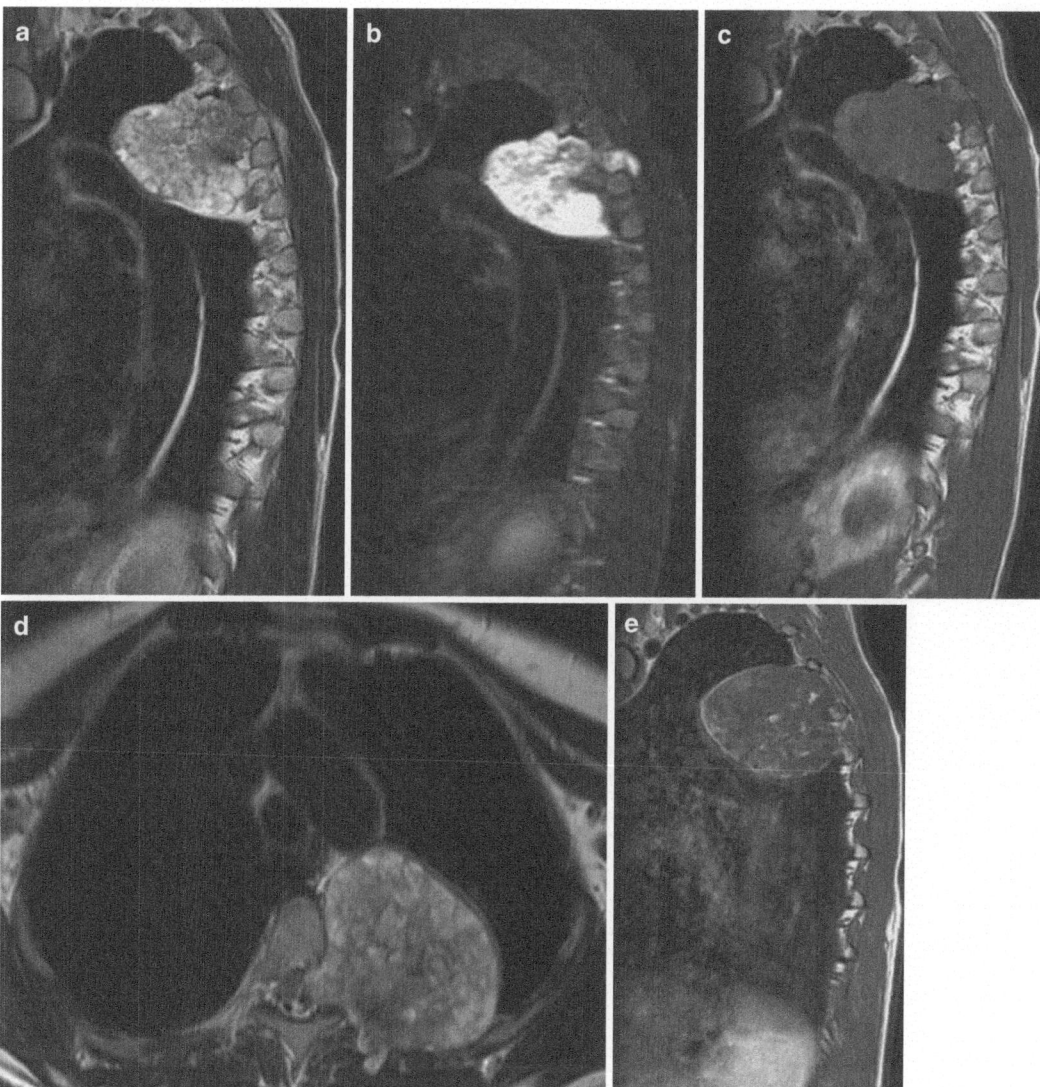

Fig. 21.2 Magnetic resonance of the thoracic spine, pre-contrast sagittal T2WI (**a**), TIRM (**b**) and T1WI (**c**), axial T2WI (**d**) and T1WI (**g**), post-contrast sagittal (**e**), coronal (**f**) and axial (**h**) T1WI showed oval, well-circumscribed tumour, heterogenous, but predominantly hyperintense on T2WI and hypointense on T1WI, which on post-contrast T1WI demonstrates peripheral and heterogeneous contrast enhancement. Tumour widened left neural foramina of the T4–T5 segment, entered left lateral epidural space and mildly compressed thoracic medulla, without signal intensity changes in terms of compressive myelopathy. There was no bone oedema of the adjacent part of the fourth and fifth vertebral body, left lamina and transverse process

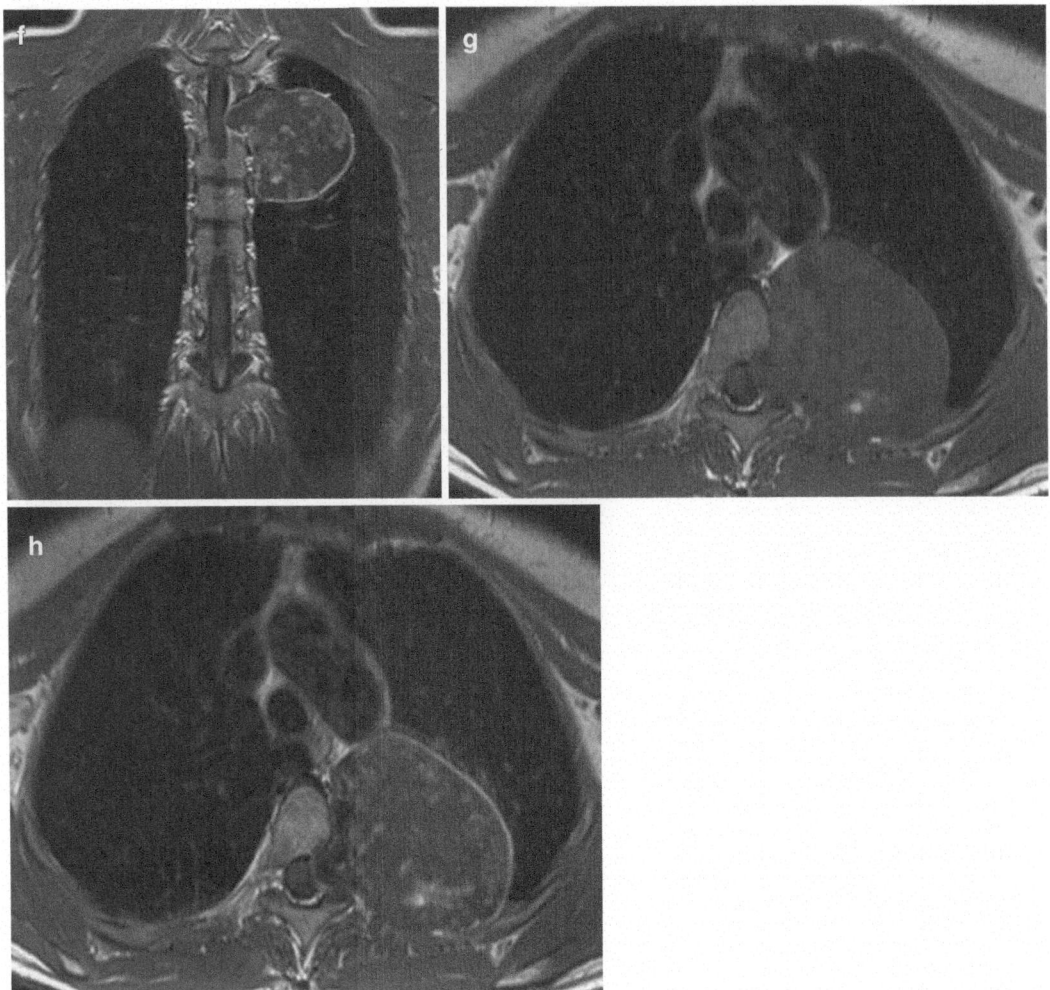

Fig. 21.2 (continued)

tumour, more anaplastic and invasive to surrounding tissues, lymph nodes and organs:
metastases occurs in 70% of patients. Grade II
chondrosarcoma holds some of the characteristics of grade I and grade II [3].

Imaging features of chondrosarcoma include
large mass with bone destruction and mineralised
chondroid matrix in the form of amorphous calcification seen as rings and arcs on CT, while non-
mineralised part of a tumour is hypodense. On
MRI, non-mineralised part of chondrosarcoma
has low to intermediate signal intensity on T1WI

and is heterogeneously hyperintense on T2WI
due to a high water content of hyaline cartilage,
while calcifications are seen as signal void.
Contrast enhancement may be lobular, septal,
nodular or diffuse. Surrounding bone oedema,
soft tissue and spinal canal involvement is best
evaluated by MRI [1–4].

Spinal chondrosarcoma may present diagnostic difficulties [5]. Differential diagnosis includes
chondroblastic osteosarcoma, chondromatosis,
chordoma, ganglioneuroblastoma and schwannoma. Neuroblastic tumours are rare after the age

of 10, while schwannomas rarely have calcifications. Location, no evidence of surrounding bone destruction, widening of neural foramina, propagation into spinal canal and signal intensities lead us to think maybe it could be an atypical or degenerated tumour originating from a nerve sheath. Malignant tumour was not our top differential diagnosis. But if you have a patient with a paraspinal mass which imaging features refer to "benign" type of tumour, think about possible malignant diagnosis, especially if one imaging feature of a lesion does not fit into differential diagnosis you consider.

Chondrosarcomas are not considered sensitive to radiotherapy or chemotherapy. The most successful treatment for spinal chondrosarcoma is complete en bloc resection: it provides the best chance of survival and the lowest rate of local recurrence. When en bloc resection is not possible, partial removal followed by radiotherapy is an optional treatment [2, 3, 5].

References

1. Razek A, Castillo M (2010) Imaging appearance of primary bony tumors and pseudo-tumors of the spine. J Neuroradiol 37:37–50
2. Lloret I et al (2006) Primary spinal chondrosarcoma: radiologic findings with pathological correlation. Acta Radiol 47(1):77–84
3. Katonis P et al (2011) Spinal chondrosarcoma: a review. Sarcoma 2011:378957, 10 pages
4. Rodallec MH et al (2008) Diagnostic imaging of solitary tumors of the spine: what to do and say. Radiographics 28:1019–1041
5. Strike SA, McCarthy EF (2011) Chondrosarcoma of the spine: a series of 16 cases and a review of the literature. Iowa Orthop J 31:154–159

Sacral Aneurysmal Bone Cyst

An 18-year-old female was referred to the MRI unit due to the pain in the left coxofemoral region with slightly increased urge to urinate which she developed after falling from a train stairs on iced ground about 2 years before the symptom onset. After the fall, bone X-ray was not performed, and, for a short period of time after the fall, she was treated with non-steroidal anti-inflammatory drugs.

Magnetic resonance imaging of the lumbosacral spine was performed using gadolinium contrast media (Fig. 22.1).

Computed tomography of the sacrum was performed after the MRI to demonstrate bone changes, cortical changes and possible periosteal reaction (Fig. 22.2).

Due to the anamnesis of previous trauma, patient age, location as well as lesion imaging features, main differential diagnosis was sacral aneurysmal bone cyst (ABS). Due to patient age and imaging features of the lesion, differential diagnosis also included a GCT of the bone (GCTOB) without solid component and a telangiectatic osteosarcoma. Bone biopsy is the only method to confirm the exact pathological process. In this case, bone biopsy confirmed ABC without elements of possible underlying process.

Due to the size and location of the sacral ABC, denosumab treatment was conducted during 12 months: 120 mg subcutaneous per week during the first month of treatment and 120 mg subcuta-

neous per month during the following 11 months, with vitamin D2 and calcium carbonate supplementation to prevent hypocalcaemia, a rare but serious toxicity of denosumab.

After 1-year denosumab treatment (April 2017), pain in the left coxofemoral region regressed and by now is rarely present, but during the second 6 months of the treatment, she still had increased urge to urinate, especially during at night. After completing 1-year denosumab treatment, physical examination is unremarkable, while CT and MRI revealed evidence of bone formation without further tumour progression in size (Figs. 22.3 and 22.4).

22.1 Sacral Aneurysmal Bone Cyst

Going through the literature, you can find resembling definitions of ABC, defining it as rare benign expansile and osteolytic bone lesion consisting of blood-filled spaces, separated by fibrous septa containing osteoclast giant cells and trabeculae of the bone or osteoid, not lined by endothelium. It may affect all age groups; most common are in the first two decades of life with slightly higher prevalence in females [1, 2]. ABCs most commonly occur in the metaphyseal region of long bones, especially distal femur or proximal tibia; pelvis and posterior elements of the spine are also commonly involved, while sacrum is rarely involved (3%) [2, 3].

© Springer International Publishing AG, part of Springer Nature 2018
M. Špero, H. Vavro, *Neuroradiology - Expect the Unexpected*,
https://doi.org/10.1007/978-3-319-73482-8_22

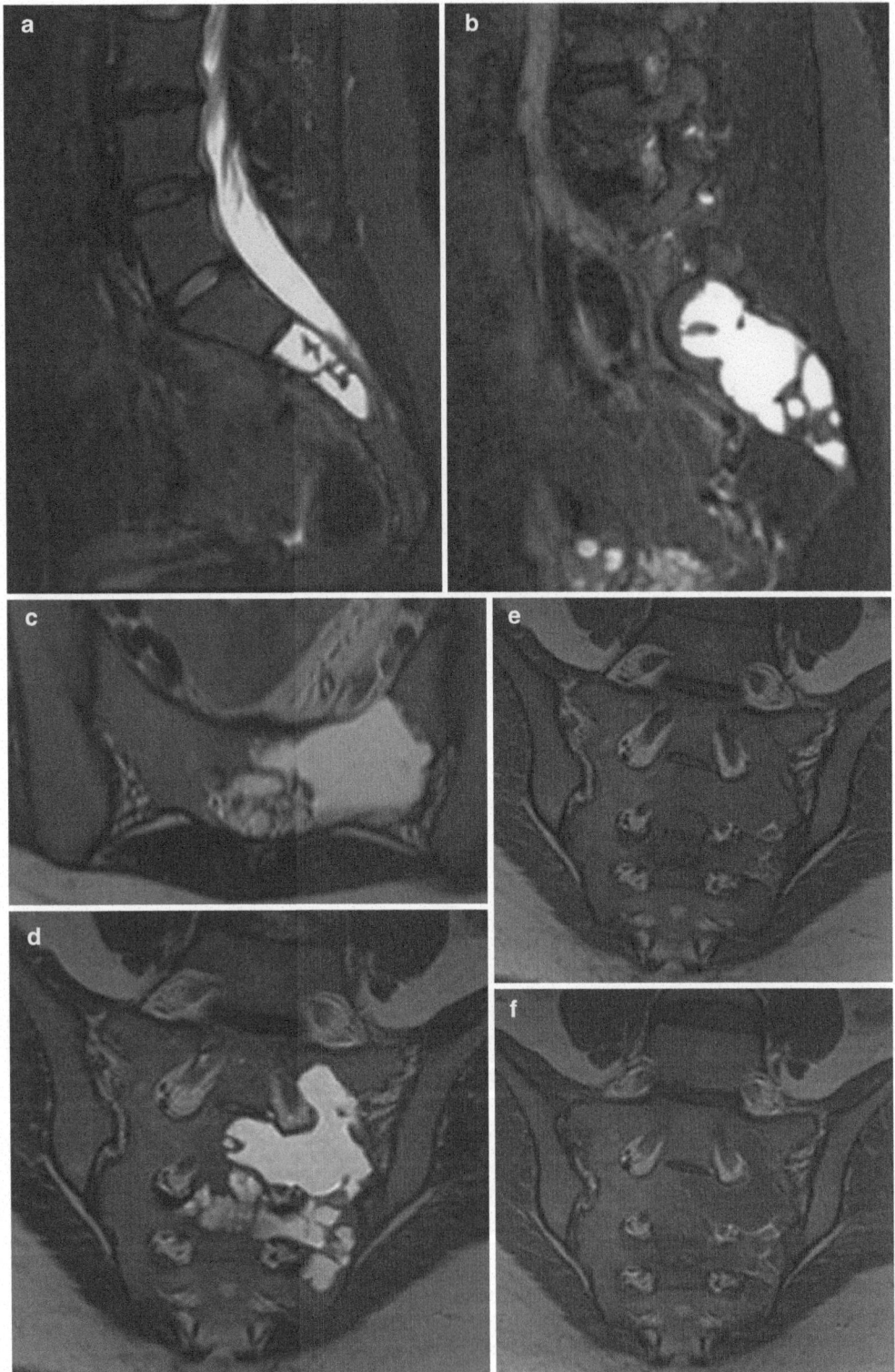

Fig. 22.1 Pretreatment magnetic resonance imaging, sagittal STIR (**a**, **b**), axial T2WI (**c**), coronal T2WI (**d**) and pre-contrast (**e**) and post-contrast (**f**) T1WI revealed expansile, lobulated, multiseptated lytic, cystic lesion in the left sacrum: hypointense on T1WI and hyperintense T2WI with several discreet dark fluid-fluid levels. Septa and cyst walls were enhanced. After intravenous administration of gadolinium contrast media, the septa and the cyst walls enhanced

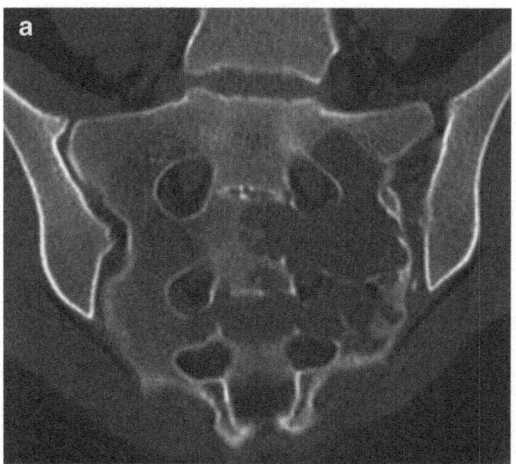

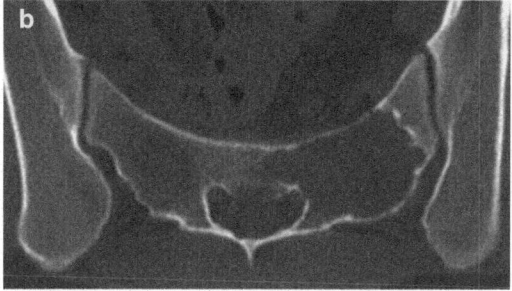

Fig. 22.2 Pre-treatment computed tomography of the sacrum, coronal (**a**) and axial (**b**) scan, demonstrated expansile, lobulated lytic lesion in the left sacrum: S1 to S4 vertebra, mainly involving S2 and S3 vertebra at which level lesion crossed the midline and reached right neural foramina – there was no clear solid component or periosteal reaction, cortical bone was slightly to moderately thinned, while lateral margin of the lesion was slightly sclerotic

Although the condition was first described in 1942 by Jaffe and Lichtenstein [4], its etiopathogenesis is still uncertain: lesions may be primary (70%) or secondary (30%). For primary ABC it is now proven that those can be real benign primary tumour associated with a specific pattern of genetic alterations that result in the activation of the gene USP6 located on chromosome 17p13 [5, 6]. Vascular factors and trauma are considered an initiating factor in their pathogenesis as well. Secondary ABC can arise within pre existing bone tumours such as GCT of the bone, chondroblastoma, chondromyxoid fibroma, osteoblastoma and fibrous dysplasia or malignant tumours such as osteosarcoma, chondrosarcoma and hemangioendothelioma [7].

Clinical presentation in sacral ABC includes pain, bowel or urinary bladder symptoms and possible neurological symptoms.

CT and MRI are imaging methods of choice in assessment of the ABCs revealing expansive and lytic, well-circumscribed lesions. Overlying cortex is thinned and generally intact, lacking any periosteal reaction [8]. CT allows the exact three-dimensional location and measuring of an ABC, which usually has density of about 20 Hounsfield units, and may show the cavitary septa structure and fluid-fluid (serum/blood) levels as well [7, 8]. MRI shows fluid content in multilobulated cystic lesion with intracavitary fluid-fluid levels detected on T2WI, which are not specific but are highly suggestive for ABC. High-to-low T1- and T2-weighted signal intensity in the fluid-fluid levels is due to blood product of baring age. Oedema of a surrounding bone may be present on MRI [8–10]. After gadolinium injection, post-contrast T1WI shows enhancement of the cyst walls and internal septa. Solid tissue component in an ABC may suggest osteosarcoma or secondary ABC [1]. CT and MRI should be carefully studied in order to identify any concomitant tumour.

Biopsy is essential for diagnosing ABC and differentiating it from GCT of bone and telangiectatic osteosarcoma, as well as from other tumours in spinal location [1, 8]. The fluid-fluid levels on MRI and CT are not sufficient to elucidate the differential diagnose of primary ABC because telangiectatic osteosarcoma as well as GCT of the bone may contain those levels. Osteoblastoma, eosinophilic granuloma or malignant tumour can be mistaken for ABC in spinal locations, and only biopsy enables diagnosis. Histopathologically, there are two varieties of ABC: classic cavitary (95%) and solid (5%) form [8].

It is recommended to wait 4–6 weeks after the biopsy, if possible, before initiating treatment, to allow the trepanation orifice to fill and, in some cases, the cyst to begin involution, which is rare, but not surprising in case of ABC [1, 11].

Treatment of pelvic and sacral ABC is difficult due to the relative inaccessibility of the lesions, associated intraoperative bleeding, proximity of a lesion to neurovascular structures

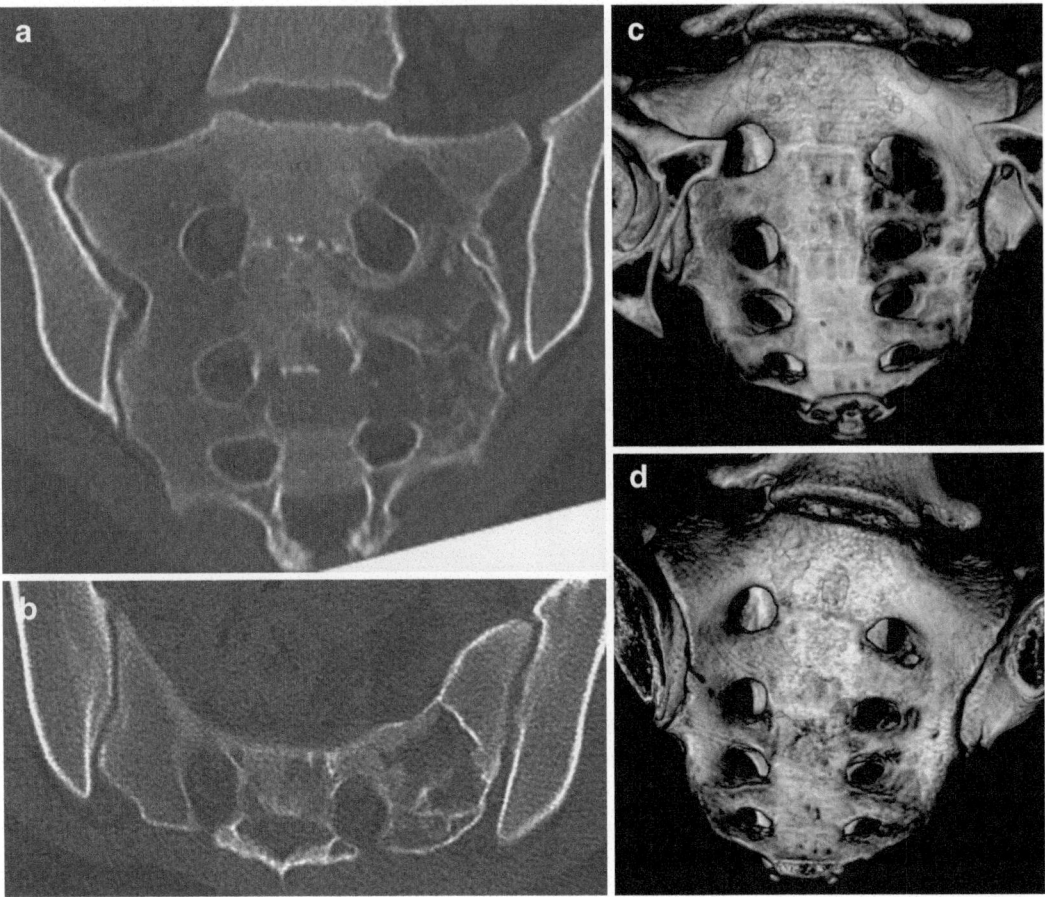

Fig. 22.3 Computed tomography of the sacrum, coronal (**a**) and axial (**b**) scan, 12 months after denosumab treatment, coronal pretreatment (**c**) and post-treatment (**d**) volume rendering technique (VRT). CT revealed regression of the cystic formation in the lesion and partial replacement of the cystic formation with solid, bone marrow-like tissue in peripheral parts of the lesion in S1, S2 and S4 vertebra, while the cystic lesion persisted in the S3 vertebra

and vulnerability of the acetabulum or sacroiliac joint. Therefore, the method of treatment (wide resection, intralesional curettage and filling by graft, cement or bone substitute, selective embolisation, radiotherapy) of sacral and pelvic ABCs must be individualized based on location, extent and aggressiveness of the lesion [12].

In a GCT of the bone, tumour cells secrete the cytokine receptor activator of nuclear factor κ-B ligand (RANKL), which initiates bone turnover upon binding to its cognate receptor, receptor-activator of nuclear κ-B (RANK). Therefore, RANKL is an essential factor in the development and progression of the bone GCT [13]. Denosumab is a human monoclonal antibody that binds RANKL, thus preventing its binding to RANK,

reducing osteoclasts and decreasing bone destruction [13, 14]. By altering tumour environment, it may lead to bone formation as well. Therefore, denosumab has been used with excellent results in the treatment of osteoporosis, skeletal metastases and GCTs of the bone [14, 15]. Recent studies have suggested clear immunohistochemical similarity and relationship between GCTs of the bone and ABCs justifying the hypothesis that denosumab may also have positive effects on ABCs. From 2013 to 2016, seven cases of ABCs (one forearm, three spinal, three sacral) treated with denosumab were published in the literature: all revealed resolution or recovery from initial symptoms, no progression in size of the lesion and evidence of bone formation on CT or MRI, while one

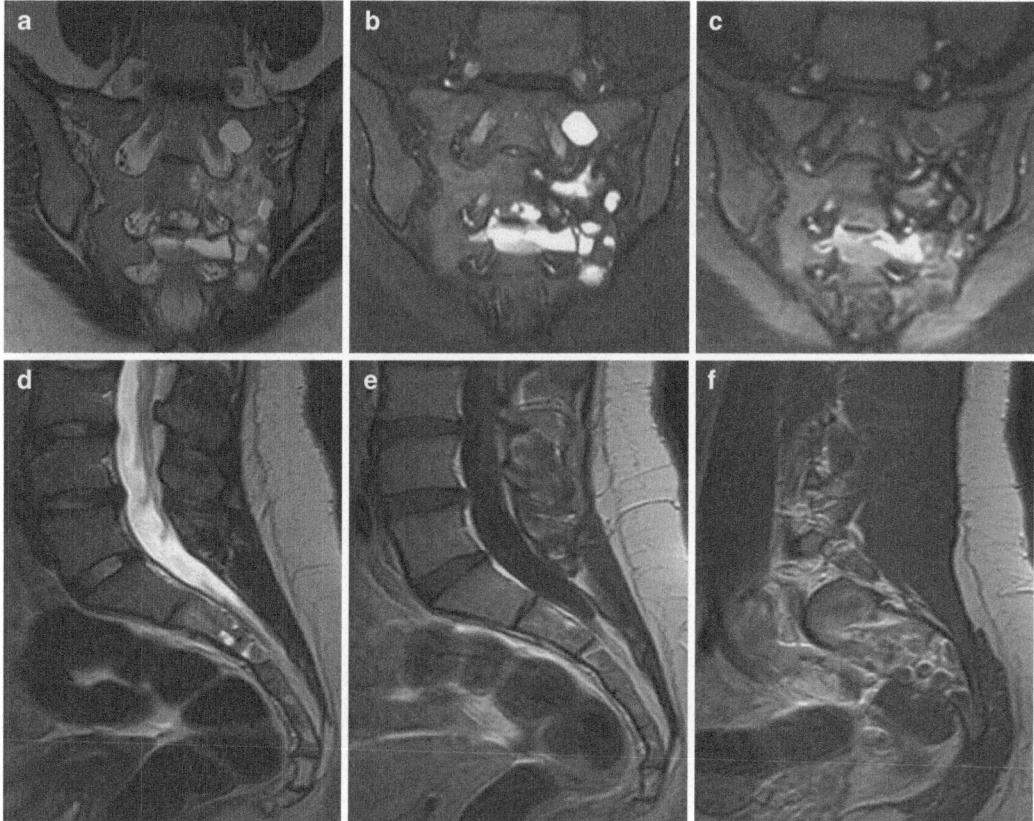

Fig. 22.4 Magnetic resonance imaging coronal T2WI (**a**), coronal T2FS (**b**), post-contrast coronal T1FSWI (**c**), sagittal T2WI (**d**) and sagittal post-contrast T1WI (**e, f**), after 12 months of denosumab treatment: there was no further progression in ABC size, with clear signal alterations; fluid-fluid levels in S3 vertebra and peripheral contrast enhancement were more pronounced

revealed almost complete ossification of the lesion [5, 14–16]. These data support the idea of a prospective study to confirm the effectiveness of denosumab as a treatment option in ABCs.

References

1. Mascard E et al (2015) Bone cysts: unicameral and aneurysmal bone cyst. Orthop Traumatol Surg Res 101:S119–S127
2. Yalcinkaya M et al (2016) Surface aneurysmal bone cyst: clinical and imaging features in 10 new cases. Orthopedics 39(5):897–903
3. Brastianos P et al (2009) Aneurysmal bone cysts of the sacrum: a report of ten cases and review of the literature. Iowa Orthop J 29:74–78
4. Jaffe HL, Lichtenstein L (1942) Solitary unicameral bone cyst with emphasis on roentgen picture, the pathologic appearance and the pathogenesis. Arch Surg 44(6):1004–1025
5. Pauli C et al (2014) Response of an aggressive periosteal aneurysmal bone cyst (ABC) of the radius to denosumab therapy. World J Surgl Oncol 12:17
6. Oliveira AM et al (2004) USP6 and CDH11 oncogenes identify the neoplastic cell in primary aneurysmal bone cysts and are absent in so-called secondary aneurysmal bone cysts. Am J Pathol 165(5):1773–1780
7. Bajracharya G et al (2007) Aneurysmal bone cyst of the pelvis: a challenge in treatment: review of the literature. Int J Orthop Surg 8(1):1–6
8. Radulescu R et al (2014) Aneurysmal bone cyst–clinical and morphological aspects. Romanian J Morphol Embryol 55(3):977–981
9. Girish G et al (2012) Imaging review of skeletal tumours of the pelvis – part i: benign tumours of the pelvis. Sci World J 2012:290930. https://doi.org/10.1100/2012/290930
10. Diel J et al (2001) The sacrum: pathologic spectrum, multi-modality imaging, and subspecialty approach. Radiographics 21:83–104

11. Cottalorda J, Bourelles S (2007) Aneurysmal bone
    cyst in 2006. Rev Chir Orthop Reparatrice Appar Mot
    93(1):5–16
12. Yildirim E et al (2007) Treatment of pelvic aneu-
    rysmal bone cysts in two children: selective arterial
    embolization as an adjunct to curettage and bone
    grafting. Diagn Interv Radiol 13:49–52
13. Pelle DW et al (2014) Targeting RANKL in aneurys-
    mal bone cysts: verification of target and therapeutic
    response. Transl Res 164(2):139–148

14. Lange T et al (2013) Denosumab: a potential new
    and innovative treatment option for aneurysmal bone
    cysts. Eur Spine J 22:1417–1422
15. Skubitz KM et al (2015) Response of aneurysmal
    bone cyst to denosumab. Spine (Phila Pa 1976)
    40(22):E1201–E1204
16. Ghermandi R et al (2016) Denosumab: non-surgical
    treatment option for selective arterial embolization
    resistant aneurysmal bone cyst of the spine and sacrum.
    Case report. Eur Rev Med Pharmacol Sci 20:3692–3695

Postductal Coarctation of the Aorta with Neurovascular Conflict

23

A 54-year-old lady working as a kindergarten teacher has been complaining of several years' history of left-sided cervical brachial syndrome recently in progression, not reacting to medication or physical therapy. She had bilateral tinnitus and occasional dizziness, not dependent on head movements. There was no history of headache, no hand weakness and no trunk or leg neurological abnormalities.

Duplex Doppler ultrasound demonstrated normal carotid and vertebral artery haemodynamics within the neck but slower blood flow within the intracranial segments of both vertebral arteries. A physiatrist recommended MRI exam of the cervical spine (Fig. 23.1).

The multiple aberrant arteries raised suspicion of a structural arterial abnormality, so a CT angiography of the aortic arch and supra-aortic arteries was recommended for further analysis (Fig. 23.2).

The patient was not prone to any surgical or interventional treatment.

23.1 Coarctation of the Aorta

Coarctation of the aorta is a congenital malformation which may only be presented by subtle and non-specific clinical signs and thus overlooked until older age. It ranges from discrete narrowing at the insertion of the ductus arteriosus (which may be patent) to severe tubular hypoplasia. The common feature to all grades of coarctation is flow disturbance in the thoracic aorta, increased afterload on the left ventricle, hypertension in the upper body and hypoperfusion of the lower body. The incidence is approximately 4 in 10,000 live births and accounts for 5–8% of all congenital heart defect. If untreated, mean life expectancy of patients is 35 years, with 90% of patients not reaching the age of 50 [1] due to complications such as congestive heart failure, aortic dissection, systemic hypertension, coronary heart disease and stroke.

Native coarctation is caused by either a ridge-like protrusion of the thickened aortic wall media into the aortic lumen or, less frequently, by tubular hypoplasia. Recoarctation refers to restenosis after initially successful surgical or endovascular treatment (up to 10% of treated cases, mostly in children) [2].

Chronic aortic lumen stenosis in coarctation of the aorta provokes enlargement of collateral vessels, including spinal cord arteries which may dilate enough to produce compressive myelopathy [3]. Compression by enlarged arteries may affect not only the spinal cord but the spinal nerves as well, such as in this case. The spinal and intracranial arteries in patients with aortic coarctation are prone to developing aneurysms—in case of rupture, subarachnoid haemorrhage will develop.

Treatment of aortic coarctation in adults consists of surgical approach or percutaneous balloon angioplasty, usually with subsequent stent placement and medical therapy.

M. Špero, H. Vavro, *Neuroradiology - Expect the Unexpected*,
https://doi.org/10.1007/978-3-319-73482-8_23

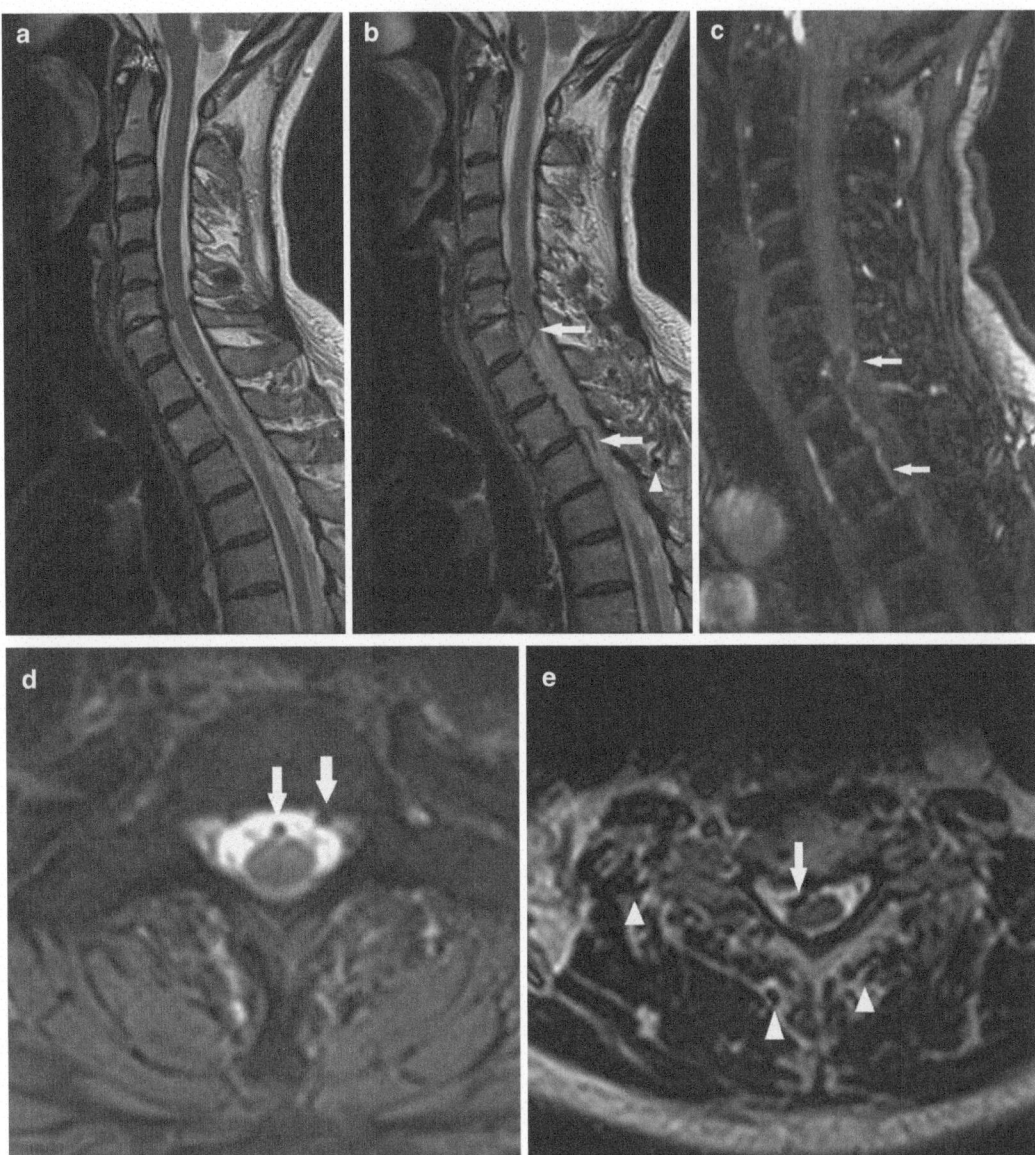

Fig. 23.1 MRI exam of the cervical and proximal thoracic spine. Sagittal T2WI (**a**, **b**), sagittal MIP 3D-TOF MRA reformatted image (**c**), axial T2WI (**d**, **e**), axial 3D-TOF MRA reformatted image (**e**). There is multilevel mild to moderate intervertebral disc degeneration (**a**, **b**) but without evidence of spinal nerve or spinal cord compression by the discs. However, in the lower cervical and upper thoracic spinal canal, several abnormal flow voids are visible, both intradural and extradural (arrows in (**b**, **d**, **e**)). There are also numerous serpiginous flow voids (arrowheads in (**b**, **e**)) in the paravertebral soft tissues of the cervical-thoracic junction. 3D-TOF MRA (**c**, **f**) sequence shows high-flow vessels consistent with hypertrophic arteries in the paravertebral space; there are also enlarged arteries in the extradural space and subdural space within the spinal canal (arrows in (**c**, **f**)). Bilateral intradural and extradural arteries cross the spinal neural foramina at the C7–T1 level bilaterally, especially on the left (**f**) with compression of the left-sided C8 spinal nerve

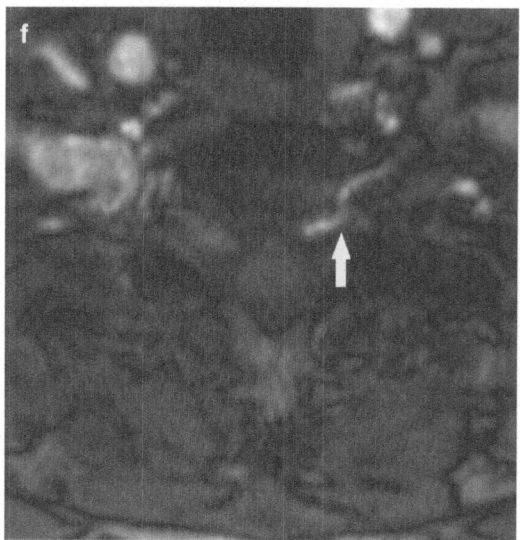

Fig. 23.1 (continued)

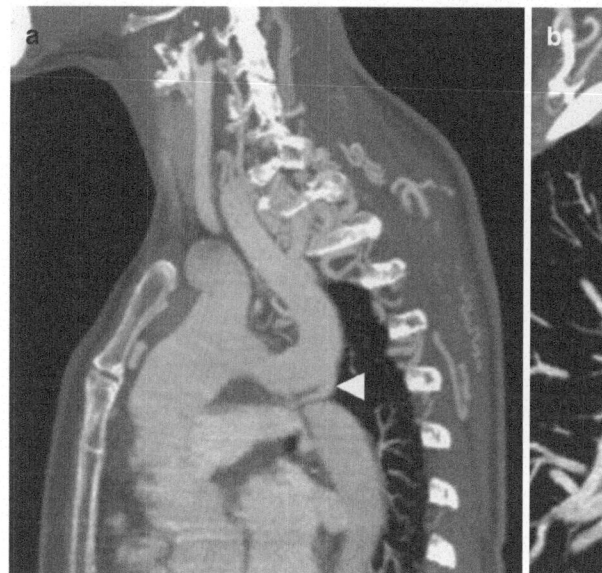

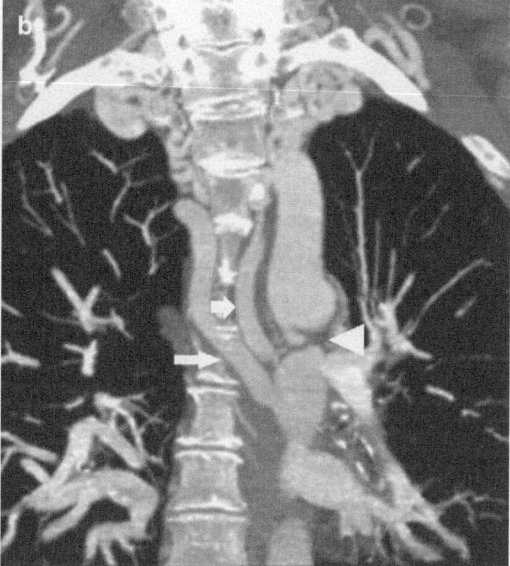

Fig. 23.2 CTA of the aortic arch and supra-aortic arteries demonstrates a high-grade aortic coarctation distal to the origin of the left subclavian artery (arrowhead in (**a**, **b**)), with extensive collateral arterial network consisting of enlarged internal thoracic, intercostal (**c**), thoracoacromial and subscapular arteries, thyrocervical trunks and vertebral arteries with their respective branches. VRT image (**d**) shows hypertrophic posterior rami of the posterior intercostal arteries. Hypertrophic radicular arteries are clearly visible in neural foramina at C7–Th1 level (**e**). Collateral arteries (**f**) are supplied from the moderately hypertrophic brachiocephalic trunk, left common carotid and left subclavian artery. Note the two hypertrophic paravertebral arteries supplying the aorta immediately distal to the coarctation (arrows in (**b**)). The pulmonary arteries are normal. The descending thoracic aorta distal to the coarctation is mildly hypoplastic

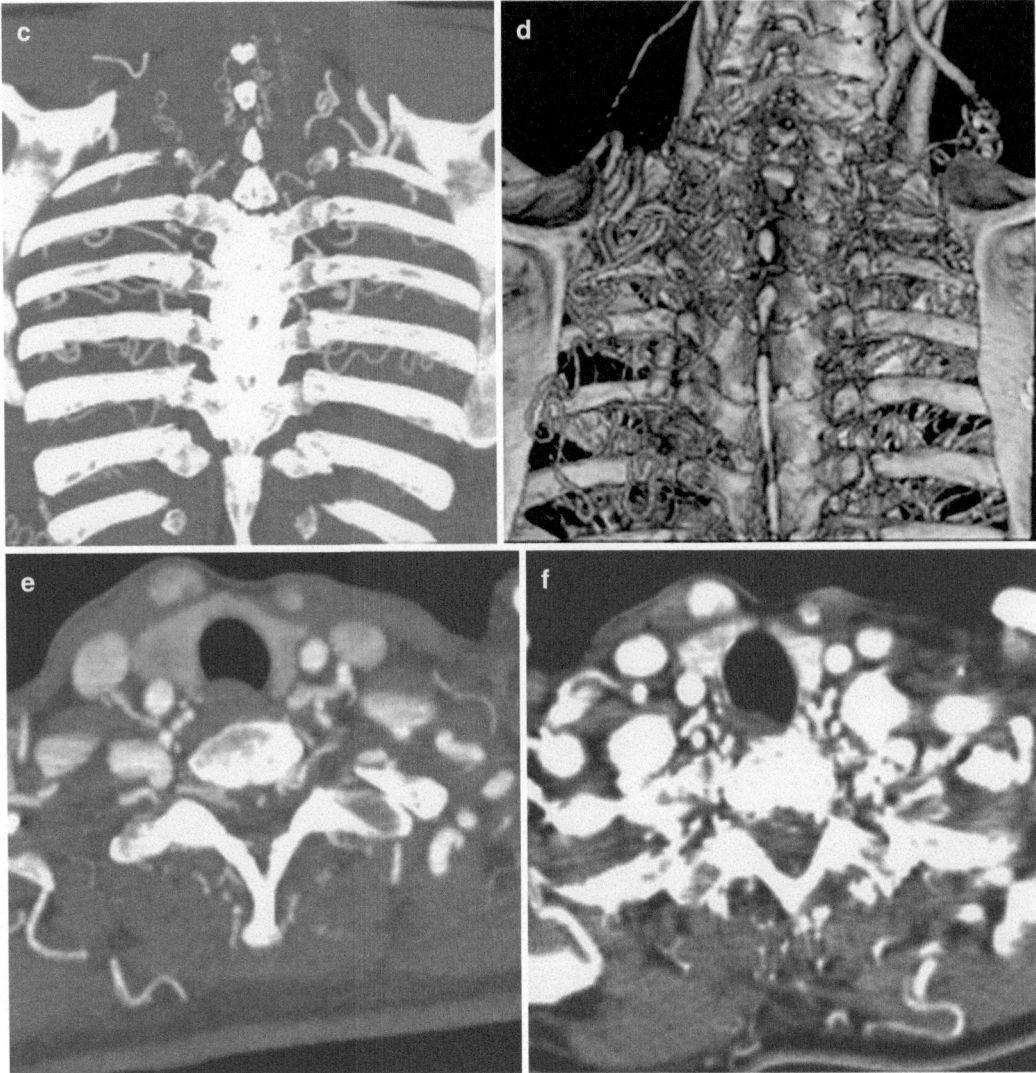

Fig. 23.2 (continued)

References

1. Jurcut R et al (2011) Coarctation of the aorta in adults: what is the best treatment? Case report and literature review. J Med Life 4(2):189–195
2. Suradi H, Hijazi ZM (2015) Current management of coarctation of the aorta. Glob Cardiol Sci Pract 2015:44. https://doi.org/10.5339/gcsp.2015.44
3. Mourya C et al (2016) Myelopathy in adult aortic coarctation: causes and caveats of an atypical presentation. Indian J Radiol Imaging 26(4):451–454. https://doi.org/10.4103/0971-3026.195775

Acute Transverse Myelitis: Primary Spinal Cord Lymphoma

24

Three weeks prior to admission, this 66-year-old lady complained of paraesthesiae in her feet, with cranial progression to the umbilical level and bilateral leg weakness. She also lost the urge to urinate and defecate. In the following 2 weeks, she developed paraplegia and incontinence. Personal medical history was unremarkable, with no evidence of trauma, fever or tick bite and no pain at all.

EMG study results of both upper and lower extremities were unremarkable. Brain CT was normal.

A MRI exam of the spine was done (Fig. 24.1).

Methylprednisolone therapy had been started, and the patient was transferred to a larger clinical hospital for further workup where samples of serum and CSF were taken for analysis and a follow-up MRI exam was performed (Fig. 24.2).

The serum and CSF were negative for oligoclonal bands (for demyelination) and AQP4 antibodies (for NMO). However, there was a large number of cells within the CSF, predominantly blasts. The immunophenotype analysis revealed a B-cell non-Hodgkin lymphoma. The peripheral blood analysis and bone marrow analysis did not show evidence of lymphoma infiltration.

It was concluded that this was a case of a primary spinal cord lymphoma.

24.1 Primary Spinal Cord Lymphoma

Primary spinal cord lymphoma is extremely rare, accounting for approximately 3.3% of all primary CNS lymphomas (PCNSL), and only 1% of or lymphoma is in the body. Eighty-five percent are non-Hodgkin lymphomas [1]. Most of them are B-cell type tumours. The classification as "primary" implicates there is no evidence of systemic lymphoma at the time of diagnosis. Somewhat more commonly lymphoma involves the vertebral bodies or epidural compartment. Secondary intramedullary invasion of the spinal cord by leptomeningeal disease is also possible [2].

Common presentation is focal neurologic deficit, including pain, paraesthesias and paresis. On MRI imaging, there is typically an intramedullary T2 hyperintense lesion, as opposed to the brain lymphoma where T2 signal tends to be hypointense. The gadolinium enhancement is often avid. There may be some surrounding oedema. They usually do not feature cysts, and secondary syringomyelia is rare. CSF analysis is often non-specific, requiring additional histopathological evaluation [3].

M. Špero, H. Vavro, *Neuroradiology - Expect the Unexpected*, https://doi.org/10.1007/978-3-319-73482-8_24

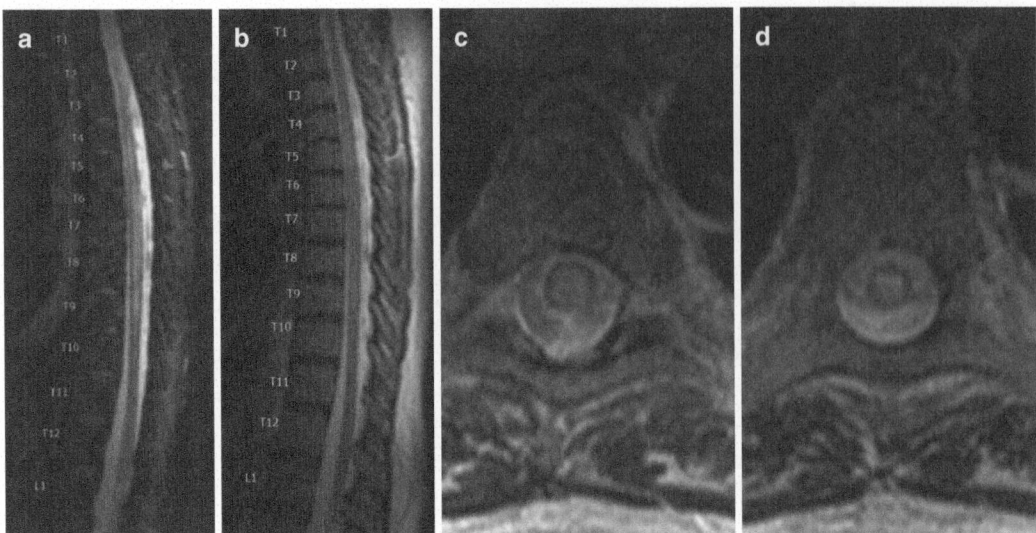

Fig. 24.1 Initial MRI of the thoracic spine—sagittal STIR sequence (**a**), sagittal T2WI (**b**), axial T2WI at the T6 level (**c**), axial T2WI at the T8 level (**d**)—reported as "prominent central cord canal in segments T4–T10 in keeping with hydromyelia"

The differential imaging considerations include glioma, metastasis and inflammatory processes such as multiple sclerosis or acute transverse myelitis. In series of cases analysed by Guzey et al. [4], out of 46 cases diagnosed with MRI, there was an initial misdiagnosis in 24 cases—10 of them were diagnosed as transverse myelitis or multiple sclerosis.

Transverse myelitis features extension through at least 3–4 spinal segments and involvement of more than two thirds of the cross-sectional area of the cord. It does not involve diffusion abnormalities. The enhancement pattern varies from no enhancement to homogenous enhancement (Fig. 24.3). Symptoms and signs are bilateral, evolve over hours or days and include paraparesis, tetraparesis, sphincter dysfunction and a clearly defined level of sensory impairment.

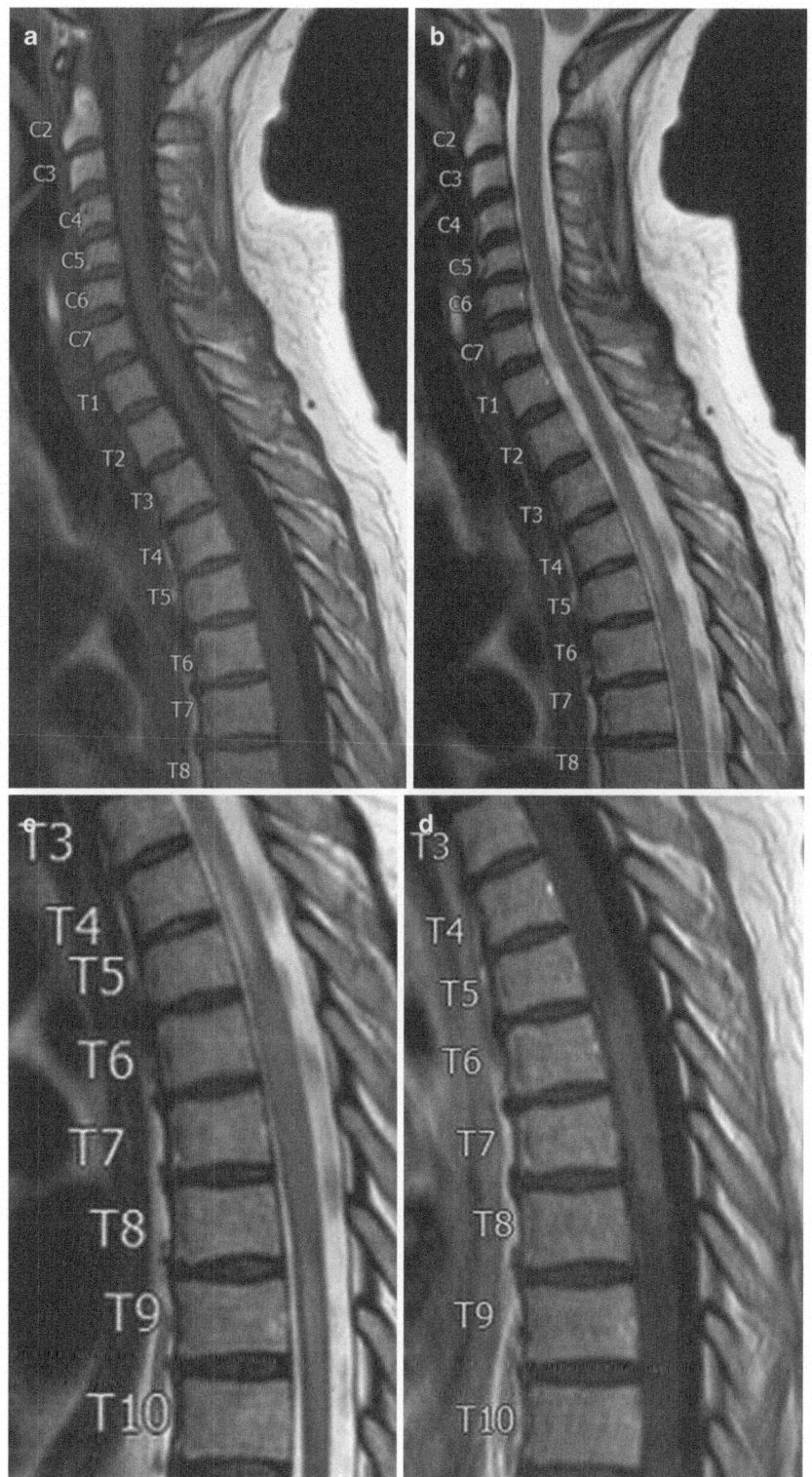

Fig. 24.2 MRI exam of the cervical and thoracic spinal cord. Sagittal T1WI (**a**), T2WI (**b,c**), post-contrast T1WI (**d**), axial T2WI (**e–g**). There is a structural spinal cord lesion at levels T5–T8, enhancing with contrast. At the proximal and distal end of the lesion, there are T2 hyper-intense areas which do not enhance, consistent with oedema rather than syrinx or hydromyelia. There is minimal cord expansion. The features were thought to be compatible with transverse myelitis; the differential diagnosis included neuromyelitis optica (NMO)

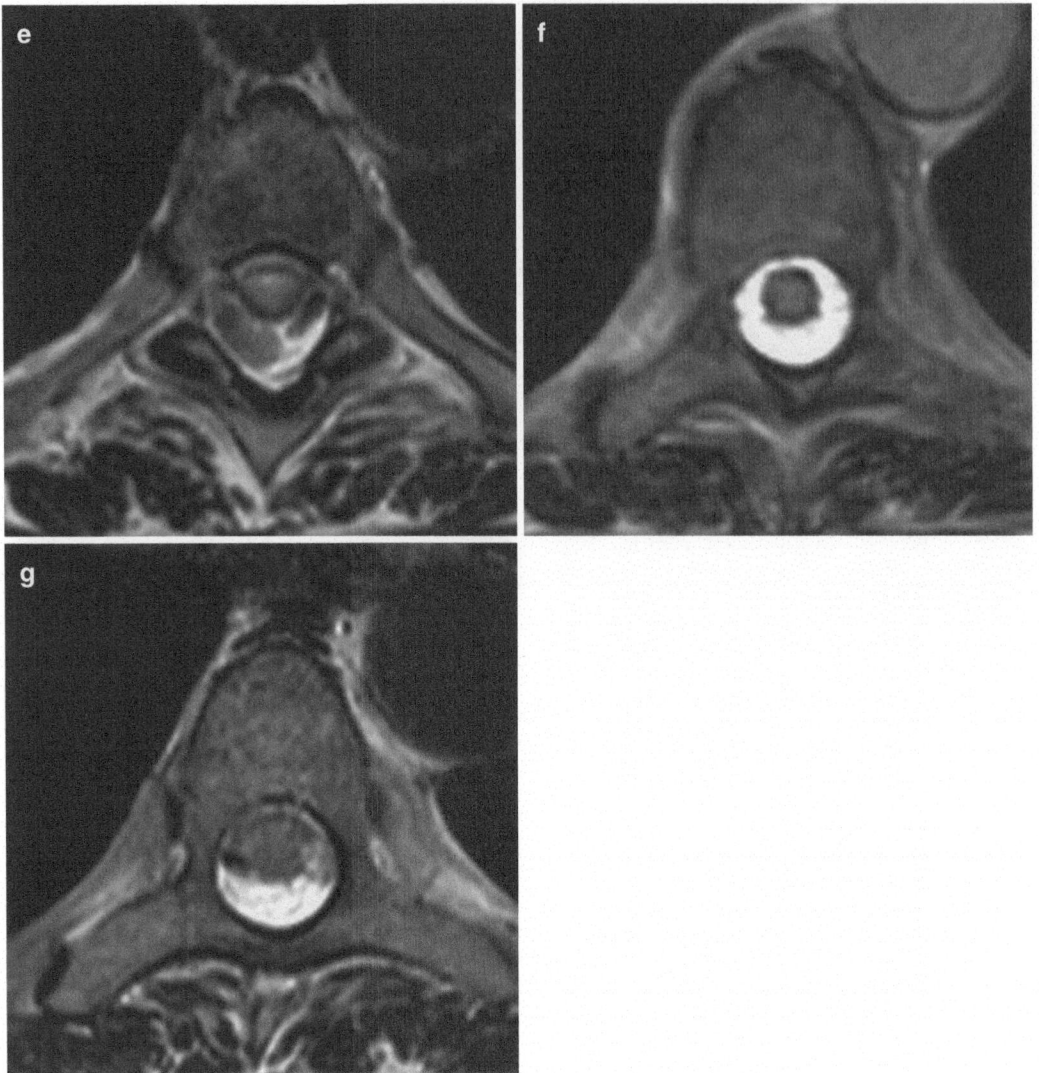

Fig. 24.2 (continued)

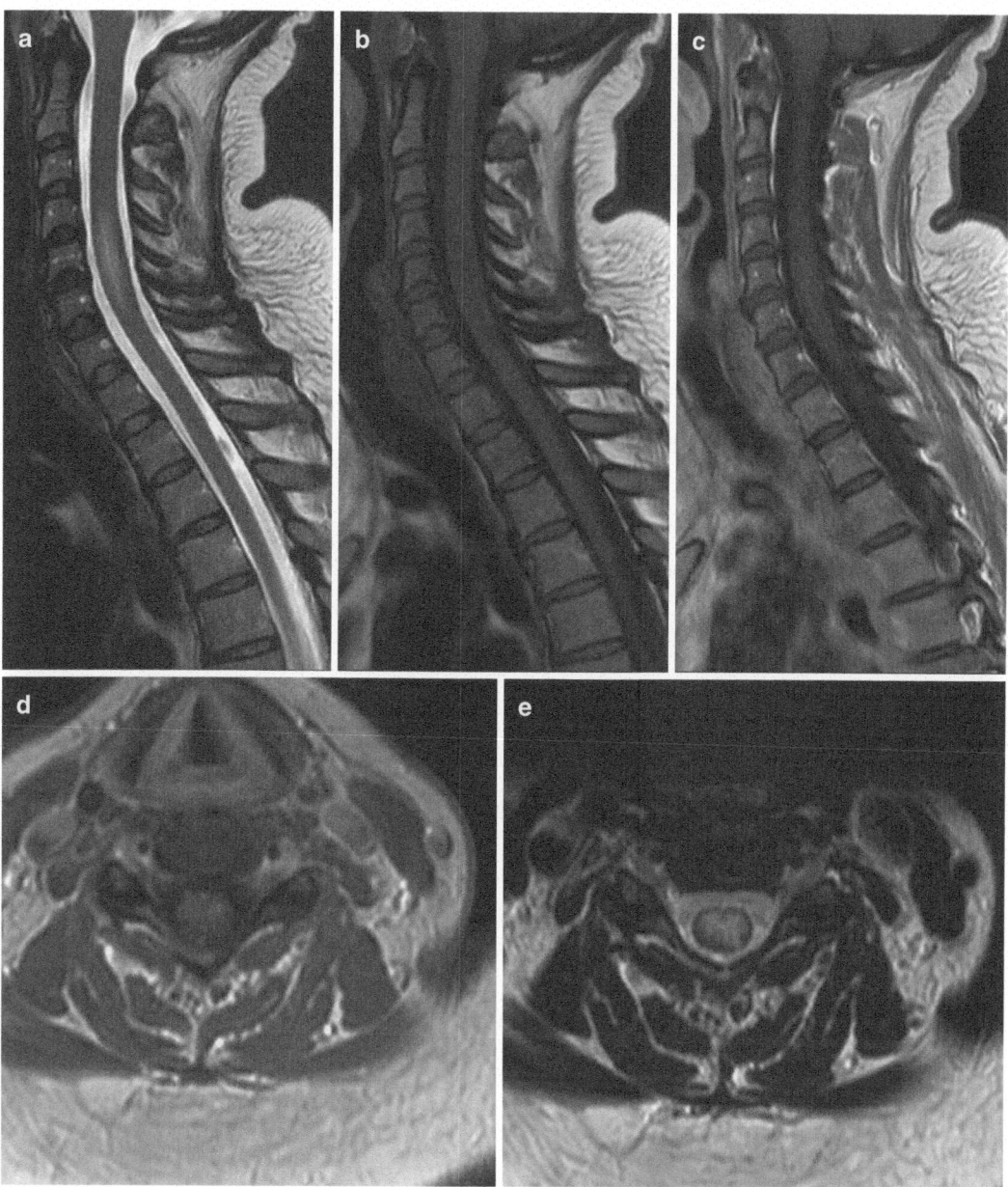

Fig. 24.3 MR images of transverse myelitis. Compare with Fig. 24.1. Sagittal T2WI (**a**) and T1WI (**b**), post-contrast sagittal (**c**) and axial (**d**) T1WI, axial T2WI (**e**). There is a faintly and inhomogeneously enhancing central spinal cord lesion in segments C4–C6, mildly expanding the cord

References

1. Abul-kasim K et al (2008) Intradural spinal tumors: current classification and MRI features. Neuroradiology 50(4):301–314. https://doi.org/10.1007/s00234-007-0345-7
2. Haque S et al (2008) Imaging of lymphoma of the central nervous system, spine, and orbit. Radiol Clin North Am 46(2):339–361. https://doi.org/10.1016/j.rcl.2008.04.003
3. Newton HB, Jolesz FA (2008) Handbook of neuro-oncology neuroimaging. Academic Press, Amsterdam, p 479
4. Guzey FK et al (2015) Primary spinal intramedullary lymphoma: a case report and review of the literature. JSM Neurosurg Spine 3(1):1049

Part VI

Something Different

Garfish Sting

This is a bit bizarre case about a 36-year-old woman who was spending summer vacation on an island on the Adriatic Coast. One morning at the beginning of August 2016, she was swimming in shallow waters along a beach when, quite bizarre, a garfish or sea needle jumped out from the sea and plunged its sharp beak into patient's right eye. Garfish has elongated jaws presenting as a long, narrow beak.

Patient was transported to a hospital on a mainland from where she was transported to one of the several hospitals in the capital city where ophthalmologists tried to remove the beak. When she arrived at a university hospital, computed tomography of the orbit was performed (Fig. 25.1).

Due to a near vicinity of the inferior rectus muscle and the optic nerve, precise procedure of the beak removal was required. Therefore, a patient was transferred to our hospital where maxillofacial surgeon was able to remove the rest of the beak without any damage to the adjacent orbital structures, especially the optic nerve and inferior rectus muscle; thus the vision and eye movements were preserved. There was no eye infection afterwards (Fig. 25.2).

25.1 Garfish Sting

The garfish or needlefish (family Belonidae) is a pelagic fish primarily inhabiting close to a water surface, in very shallow marine waters, or at the surface of the open sea of the Atlantic, the Mediterranean Sea, the Caribbean Sea and the Baltic Sea. The needlefish is a long and slender fish with a laterally compressed body and elongated jaws with sharp teeth forming a beak, which can grow to about 50–75 cm in length [1–3].

All needlefish feed primarily on smaller fishes, which they catch with an upward sweep of the head. When undisturbed, needlefishes move along with an undulating motion of the body. Needlefish is capable of making short jumps out of the water: this jumping activity is greatly excited by artificial light from fishing boats at night. In a case of "human-needlefish" encounter, a fish is usually excited or chased by larger fishes and on rare occasion inflicts injuries and deep puncture wounds to the chest, abdomen, arms, legs or neck, often breaking off inside the victim in the process [4].

This is a really bizarre case because a needlefish inflicted an injury by plunging a beak into a patient's eye. At the time, most of the daily newspapers reported about the case and medical procedures resulting in successful removal of the beak from the eye. In this particular case, ichthyologist has explained that, while swimming in the sea, our patient probably found herself in a way of a moving needlefish flock; this particular garfish was probably catching a prey when jumped out of the sea and "stumbled upon" our patient's eye. Probably a fish body broke off in the process

© Springer International Publishing AG, part of Springer Nature 2018
M. Špero, H. Vavro, *Neuroradiology - Expect the Unexpected*,
https://doi.org/10.1007/978-3-319-73482-8_25

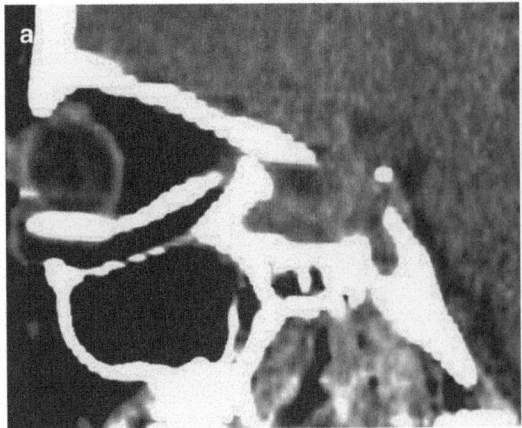 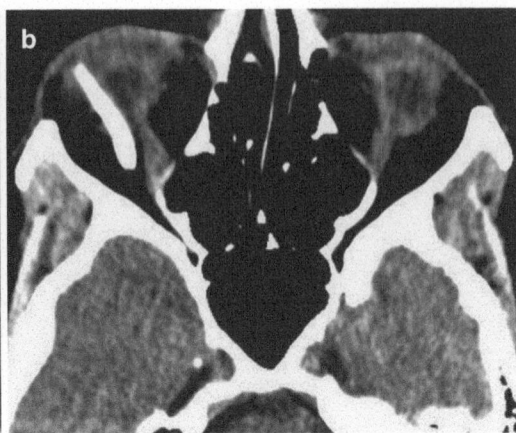

Fig. 25.1 Computed tomography of the orbit, sagittal (**a**) and coronal (**b**) scan, demonstrated the beak extending just below the inferior part of the eye bulb, right next to the inferior rectus muscle, few millimetres away from the optic nerve, through the orbital fat tissue, ending in the posterior part of the inferior rectus muscle. Tissue around the beak, just below the eye bulb, was oedematous; orbital fat tissue did not reveal density changes. Ophthalmologists tried to remove the beak but were able to remove the small part of the beak placed just below the eye bulb; they were not able to remove the rest of the beak

while the beak remained deep in a patient eye. Our patient was lucky because the beak did not damaged the inferior rectus muscle and because it did not hit the optic nerve. At the end, joint forces and knowledge of ophthalmologist and maxillofacial surgeon resulted in a successful removal of the beak from the eye, while vision and eye movements remained intact. This is one of the many injuries inflicted by a garfish and published in daily newspapers or even published in scientific literature. Those injuries could have a serious sequel, like a case of a traumatic carotid-cavernous sinus fistula in a boy due to a penetrating injury caused by a needlefish while he was fishing with his father on Hawaii [4], or even a death outcome [5]. This is a really bizarre case of a garfish sting with a positive outcome for a patient with a preserved eyesight after medical intervention.

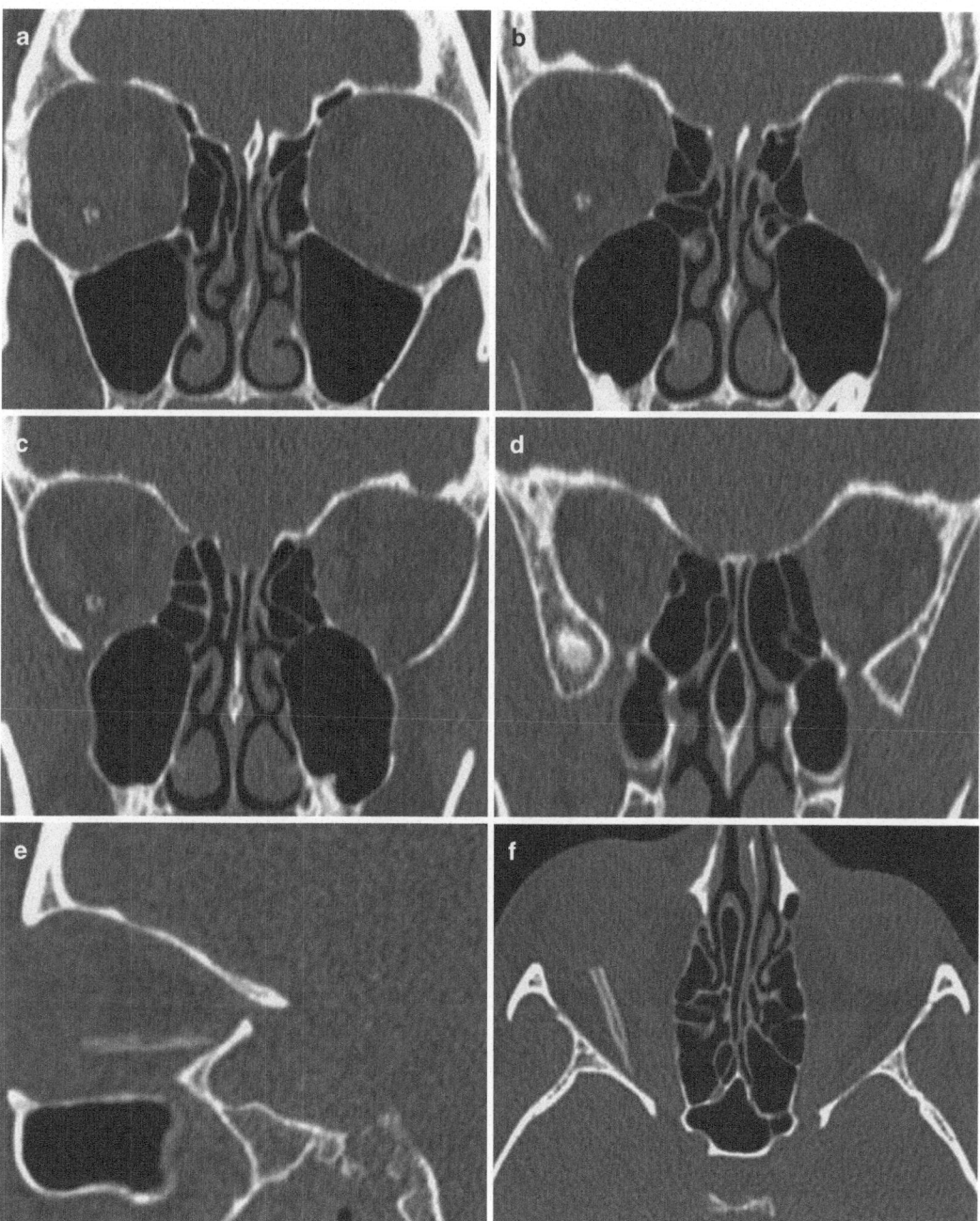

Fig. 25.2 Computed tomography of the orbit, coronal (**a**–**d**, **g**–**j**), sagittal (**e**, **k**) and axial (**f**, **l**) scans, performed just before maxillofacial surgeon removed the rest of the beak. Ophthalmologist managed to remove a part of the beak just below the eye bulb. The rest of the beak remained in the orbit, extending through the orbital fat tissue, just next to the inferior rectus muscle, few millimetres away from the optic nerve, and ended in the posterior part of the inferior rectus muscle

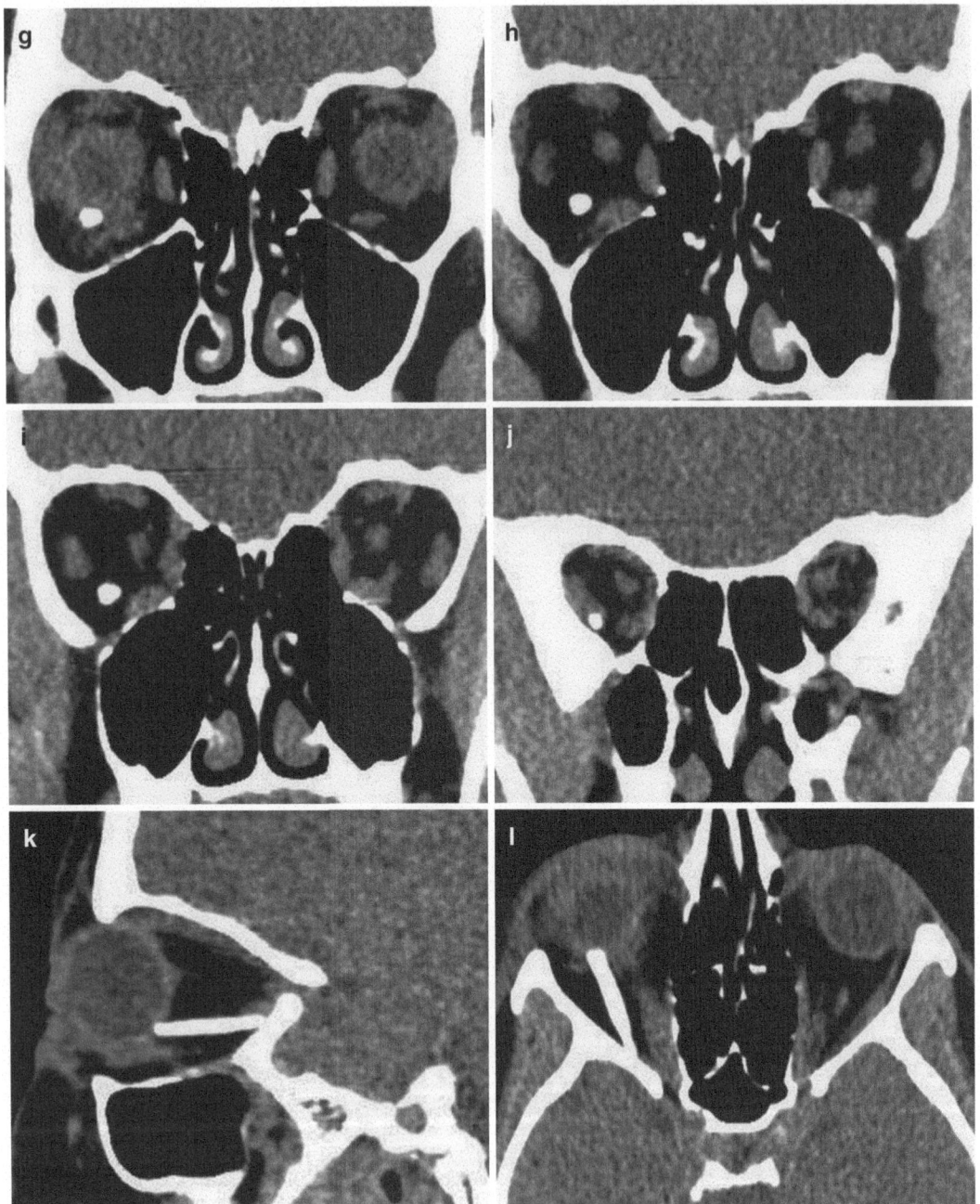

Fig. 25.2 (continued)

References

1. Collette BB et al (1998) Encyclopedia of fishes. Academic Press, San Diego. pp 144–145. isbn: 0-12-547665-5
2. Colette BB, Parin NV (1986) Belonidae. In: Whitehead PJP (ed) Fishes of the north-eastern Atlantic and the Mediterranean. UNESCO, Paris, pp 604–609
3. Zorica B, Čikeš Keč V (2013) Age, growth and mortality of the garfish, belone belone (L. 1761) in the Adriatic Sea. J Mar Biol Assoc U K 93(2):365–372
4. McCabe MJ et al (1978) A fatal brain injury caused by a needlefish. J Neuroradiol 5(3):137–139
5. Needlefish stabs diver to death in Vietnam (2007) Deutsche Press Agenteur. http://www.digitaljournal.com/article/226080/Needlefish_stabs_diver_to_death_in_Vietnam. Accessed 02 Sept 2017

A Dural Surprise

26

In April 2017 this previously healthy young gentleman (34) started suffering from occasional headaches in the right frontal region. MRI imaging he was referred to in May showed somewhat unexpected pathology (Fig. 26.1).

The patient was scheduled for surgery; a contrast-enhanced CT scan of the head was performed as part of preoperative neuronavigation workup(Fig. 26.2).

The surgery was uneventful, the involved dura and bone were resected, and intraoperative histopathology report was compatible with a meningioma.

However, after detailed histopathology analysis of all resected tissue samples, the histopathological diagnosis was changed to non-Hodgkin lymphoma—diffuse large B-cell lymphoma (DLBCL).

Subsequently, CT screening of the thorax, abdomen and pelvis was requested, as well as follow-up MRI of the whole neural axis. The body CT was negative, as well as whole neural axis MRI. The bone marrow biopsy was unremarkable.

There were no other foci of lymphoma (Fig. 26.3).

It was concluded that the lesion was a primary dural aggressive non-Hodgkin lymphoma-diffuse large B-cell lymphoma. Immunochemotherapy (R-CHOP protocol) was started.

26.1 Intracranial Primary Dural Diffuse Large B-Cell Lymphoma

Primary dural lymphoma (PDL), without leptomeningeal, parenchymal or systemic involvement, is very rare, making less than 1% of all brain lymphomas. Most of the cases are low-grade B-cell lymphomas [1]. High-grade primary diffuse large B-cell lymphoma (DLBCL) of the dura, such as in this case, is an extremely rare entity.

PDL differs from the primary central nervous system lymphoma (PCNSL; see Chap. 2) by the clinical presentation, prognosis and tumour biology. It originates outside of the central nervous system, in immunocompetent patients. The dura normally does not contain any lymphoid tissue; it is presumed that a chronic inflammatory meningeal process may precede the occurrence of PDL [2].

The rarity of the PDL and the imaging characteristics which include en plaque dural infiltration, enhancement (with dural tail signs), increased DWI signal and intraosseous propagation are the reasons why this lesion is commonly mistaken for an aggressive meningioma. If there is vasogenic oedema of the underlying brain parenchyma and/or osteolysis rather than hyperostosis of the adjacent bone, it is more likely that the lesion represents a lymphoma than a meningioma [1, 2]. The clinical appearances are also similar to meningioma. Symptoms depend on the

M. Špero, H. Vavro, *Neuroradiology - Expect the Unexpected*,
https://doi.org/10.1007/978-3-319-73482-8_26

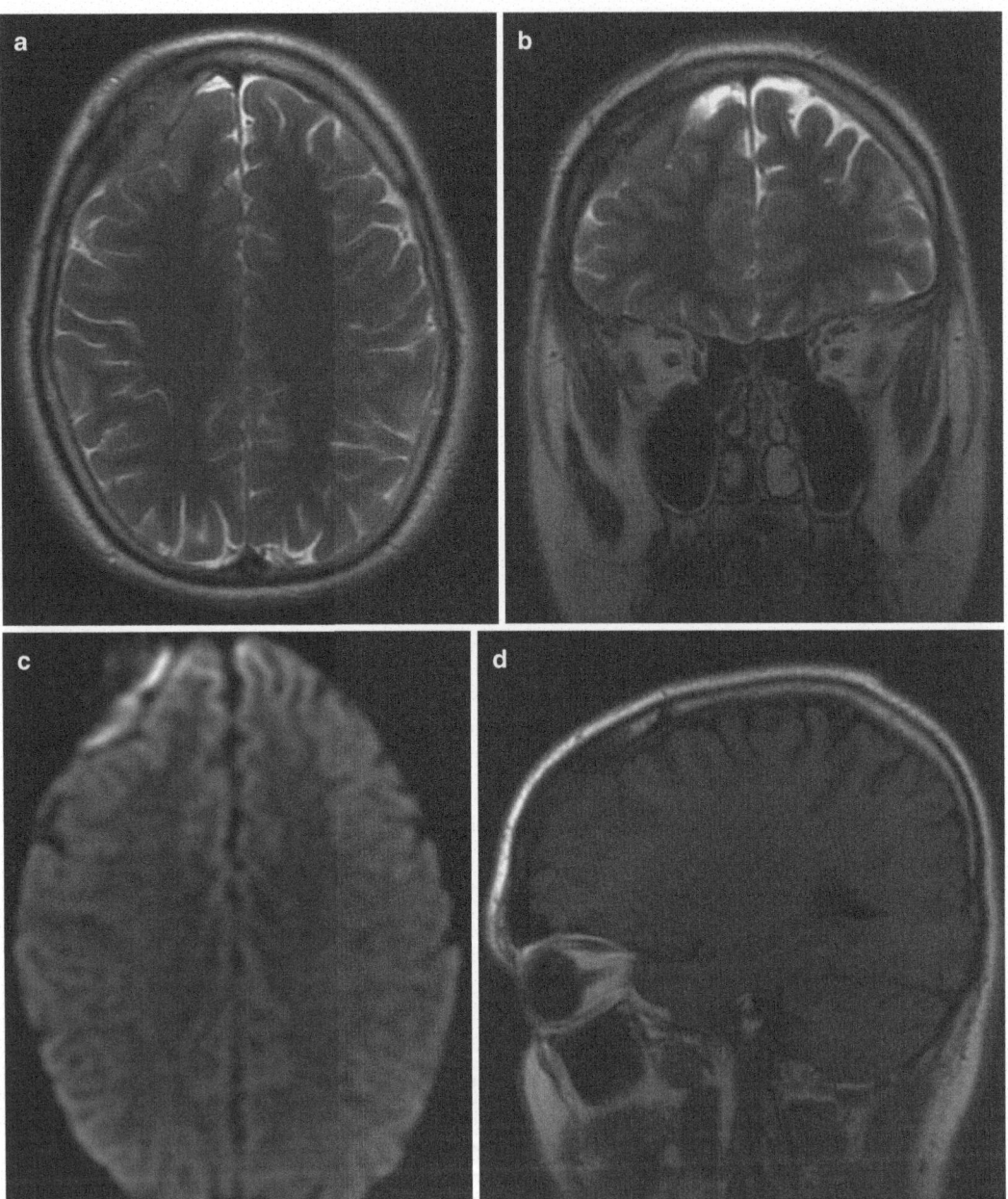

Fig. 26.1 Initial MRI exam of the head. Axial (**a**) and coronal (**b**) T2WI, axial DWI (**c**), sagittal non-contrast (**d**) and contrast-enhanced (**e**) T1WI, axial contrast-enhanced T1WI (**f**). There is a right-sided frontal extra-axial space-occupying lesion, isointense in T1WI (**d**), hypointense in T2WI (**a–c**), avidly enhancing with gadolinium contrast (**e, f**), with evidence of intradiploic propagation. Note the increased DWI signal of the lesion (**c**) which indicates compact cellularity. The lesion abuts the brain parenchyma, without evidence of brain infiltration. Most probable diagnosis stated in the report was meningioma with intraosseous invasion

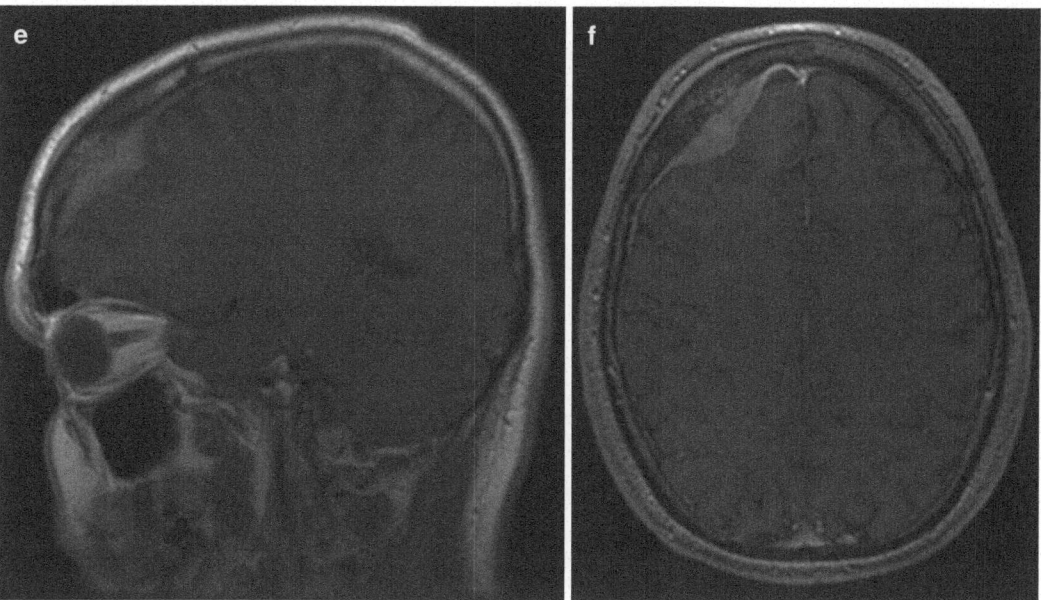

Fig. 26.1 (continued)

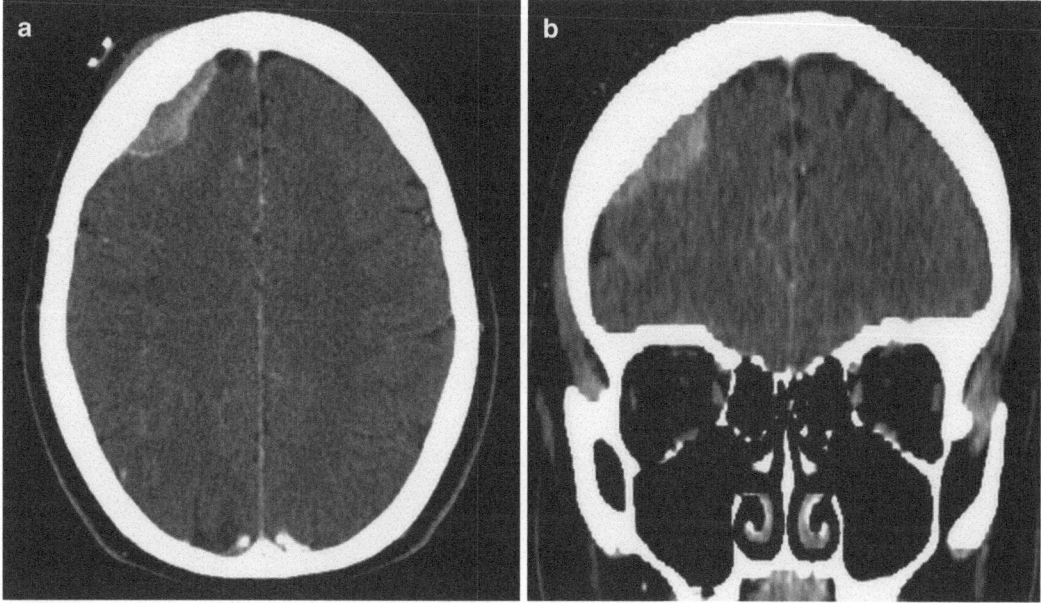

Fig. 26.2 Initial CT exam of the head (for neuronavigation purposes). As on previous MRI exam, there is a right frontal extra-axial enhancing space-occupying lesion (**a, b**) with evidence of bone infiltration (**c**)

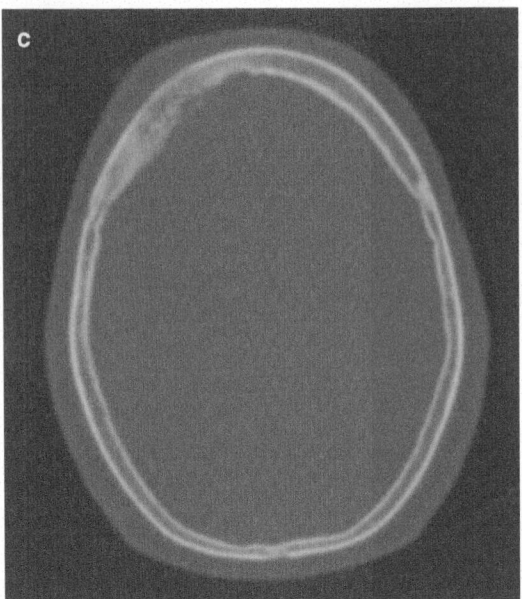

Fig. 26.2 (continued)

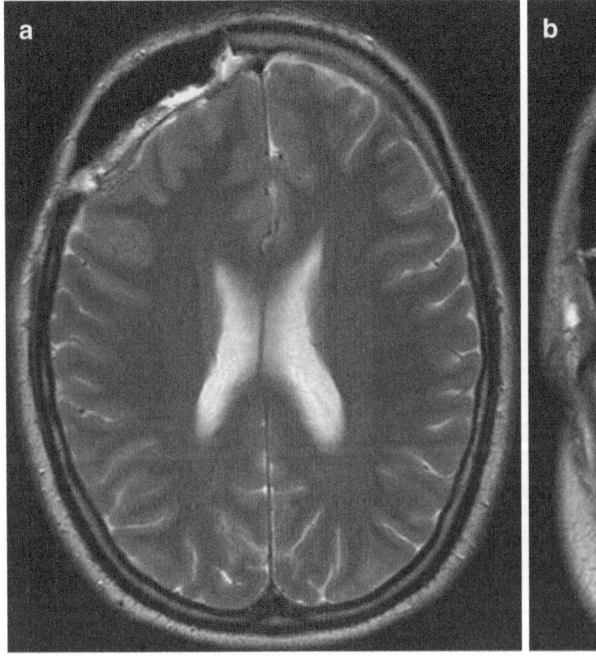

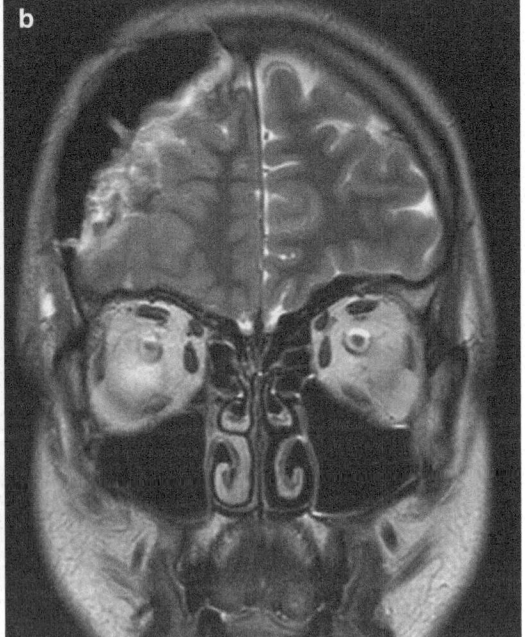

Fig. 26.3 Follow-up MRI of the brain with MRI of the whole spine. Axial (**a**) and coronal (**b**) T2WI and post-contrast axial T1WI (**c**) show evidence of right-sided frontal craniectomy with a small extradural postsurgical collection, without significant compression of the brain parenchyma. There is no evidence of residual tumour. In sagittal T2WI (**d–f**) and post-contrast T1WI (**g, h**), there is no evidence of space-occupying lesions or abnormal enhancement in the spinal canal. The spinal cord is unremarkable

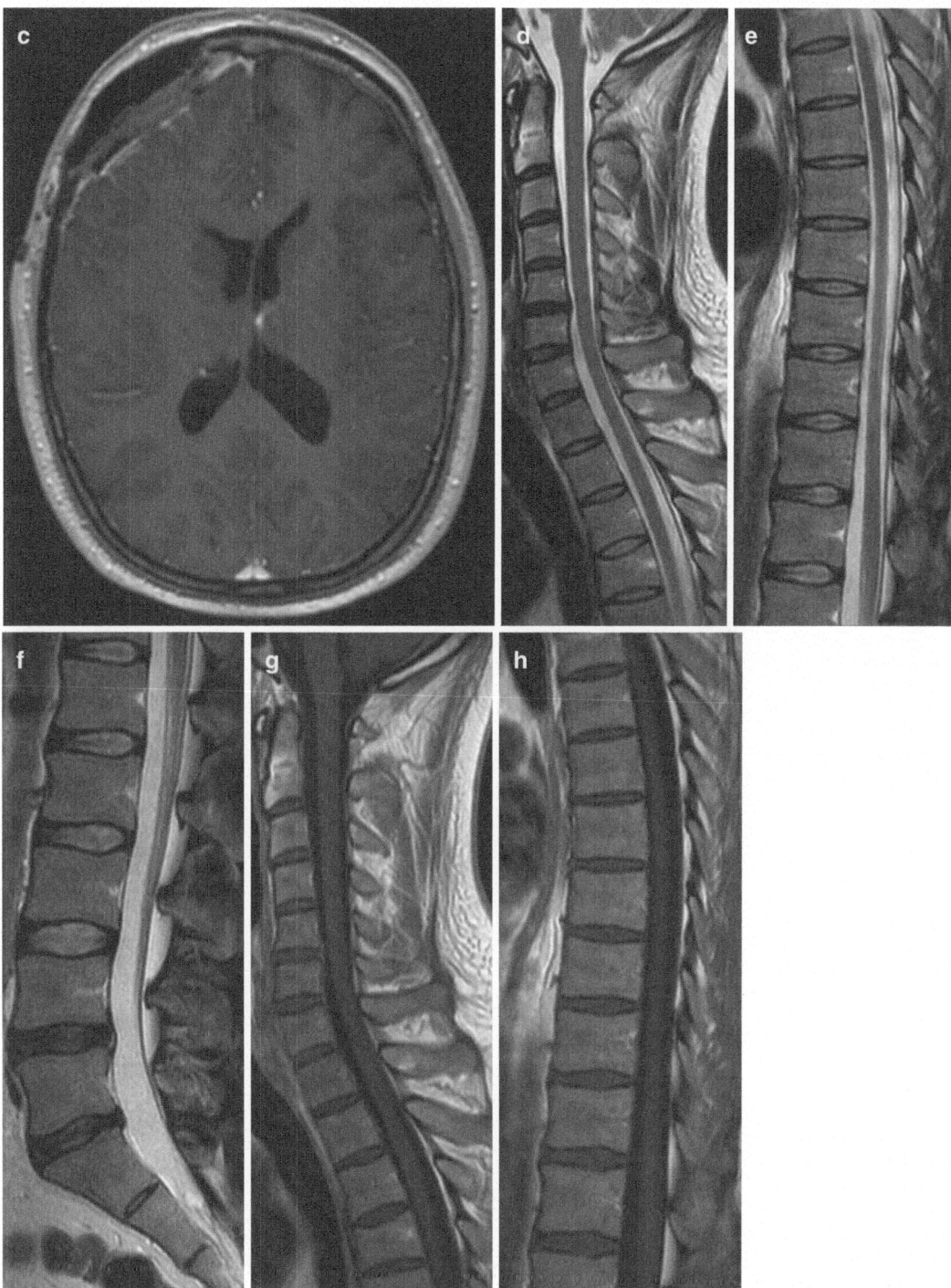

Fig. 26.3 (continued)

tumour location and may include headaches, nausea, ataxia, seizures, focal sensory or motor deficits and loss of hearing and vision in case of progressive dural involvement. Spinal PDL often presents with radicular pain and paraparesis [3].

Apart for meningioma, differential diagnoses include dural metastasis, gliosarcomas, leiomyosarcomas, haemangiopericytomas, plasmacytomas, solitary fibrous tumours, neurosarcoidosis and tuberculomas.

References

1. Brito ABC et al (2014) Intracranial primary diffuse large B-cell lymphoma successfully treated with chemotherapy. Int J Clin Exp Med 7(2):456–460
2. Iwamoto FM, Abrey LE (2006) Primary dural lymphomas: a review. Neurosurg Focus 21(5):E5
3. Said R et al (2011) Clinical challenges of primary diffuse large B-cell lymphoma of the dura: case report and literature review. ISRN Hematol:945212. https://doi.org/10.5402/2011/945212

Leptomeningeal Surprise

At the beginning of February 2017, a 59-year-old male patient was admitted to the EHD of our hospital due to ataxia, headache with nausea and vomiting, lasting for 7 days. He was not febrile; he did not have any other symptoms like abdominal pain, loss of weight or problems with swallowing. According to anamnestic data, he was taking medications for arterial hypertension. CT of the brain was performed at the admittance: radiologist who was on call reported small oval, mildly hyperdense lesion in the roof of the fourth ventricle surrounded with mild vasogenic oedema, possible expansile, neoplastic process (Fig. 27.1).

MRI of the brain was the next diagnostic procedure that was performed (Figs. 27.2 and 27.3).

MRI of the brain demonstrated T2 and FLAIR slightly hyperintense content diffusely distributed along the folia of both cerebellar hemispheres and vermis, showing nodular and linear contrast enhancement due to leptomeningeal spread of malignant cells or leptomeningeal carcinomatosis. Both vestibulocochlear and left trigeminal cranial nerves demonstrated contrast enhancement consisted with perineural spread of malignant cells.

Lumbar puncture and CSF analysis were recommended: CSF analysis confirmed malignant cells of epithelial origin. Laboratory data revealed slightly enlarged serum levels of urea, bilirubin and gamma-glutamyltransferase, as well as high levels of tumour markers, carcinoembryonic antigen, alpha-fetoprotein and cancer antigens 19-9 and 125.

CT of the chest and abdomen was performed revealing only several celiac lymph nodes measuring up to 10 mm: there were no metastasis in the lung parenchyma or liver and no enlarged mediastinal or hilar lymph nodes. There were no signs of oesophageal process on CT scans as well. Finally, esophagogastroduodenoscopy revealed small (10 mm) polypoid lesion above the oesophageal Z line involving one third of the oesophageal circumference: biopsy was performed, and oesophageal adenocarcinoma was confirmed.

Patient died 14 days after the admittance, before there was a chance to start with oncological treatment.

27.1 Leptomeningeal Carcinomatosis

Leptomeningeal carcinomatosis (LMC) is one of the most serious complications that can occur in cancer patients representing metastatic tumour cells involving leptomeninges and circulating CSF. It usually occurs in case of a breast or lung cancer and melanoma or in case of lymphoma and leukaemia [1]. It is very rare in case of gastrointestinal malignancy. Gastrointestinal solid tumours usually give metastasis in liver, lung, peritoneal cavity or abdominal lymph nodes.

M. Špero, H. Vavro, *Neuroradiology - Expect the Unexpected*,
https://doi.org/10.1007/978-3-319-73482-8_27

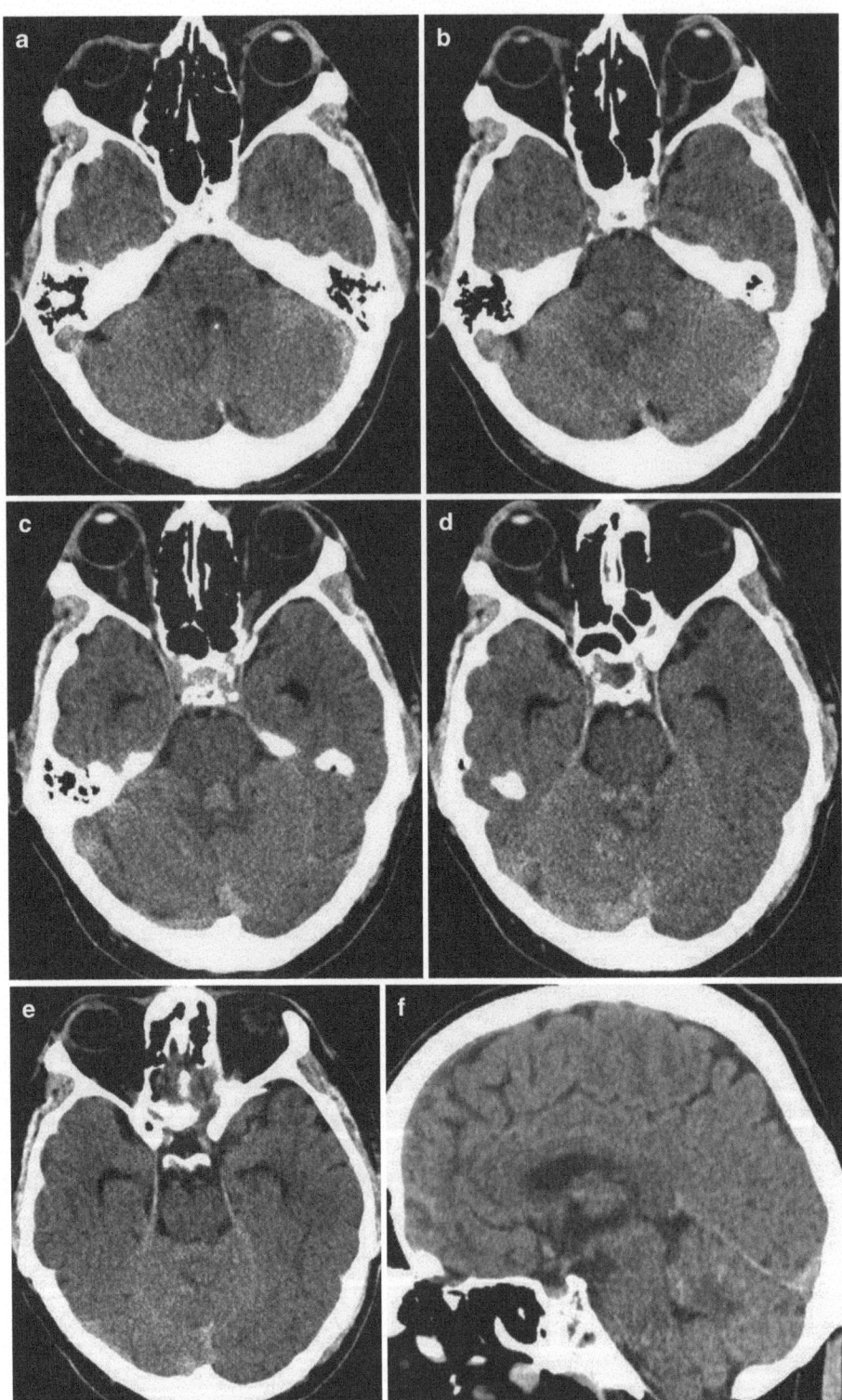

Fig. 27.1 Pre-contrast CT of the brain revealed oval, expansile slightly hyperdense lesion in the vermis, surrounded with mild vasogenic oedema (**a–c**). If you look closely, there was also slightly hyperdense content in the folia of the right cerebellar hemisphere (**d–f**)

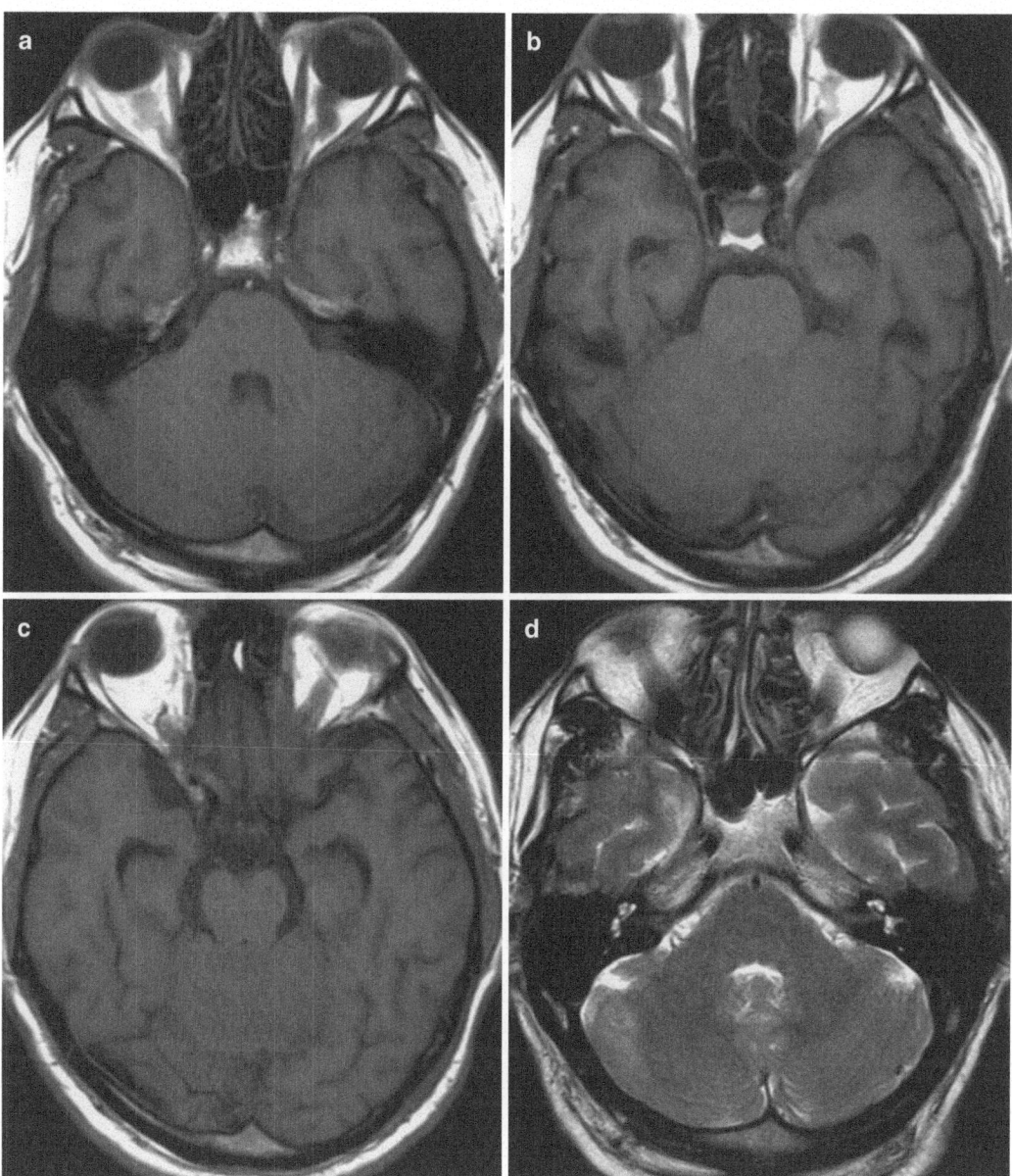

Fig. 27.2 Non-contrast MRI of the brain, axial T1WI (**a–c**), axial T2WI (**d–f**) and axial FLAIR (**g–i**), revealed slightly hyperintense content on T2WI and FLAIR in the folia of both cerebellar hemispheres and vermis that was hypointense on T1WI. Both vestibulocochlear nerves were hypointense on T2 and FLAIR sequences, slightly enlarged. CSF flow was not obstructed

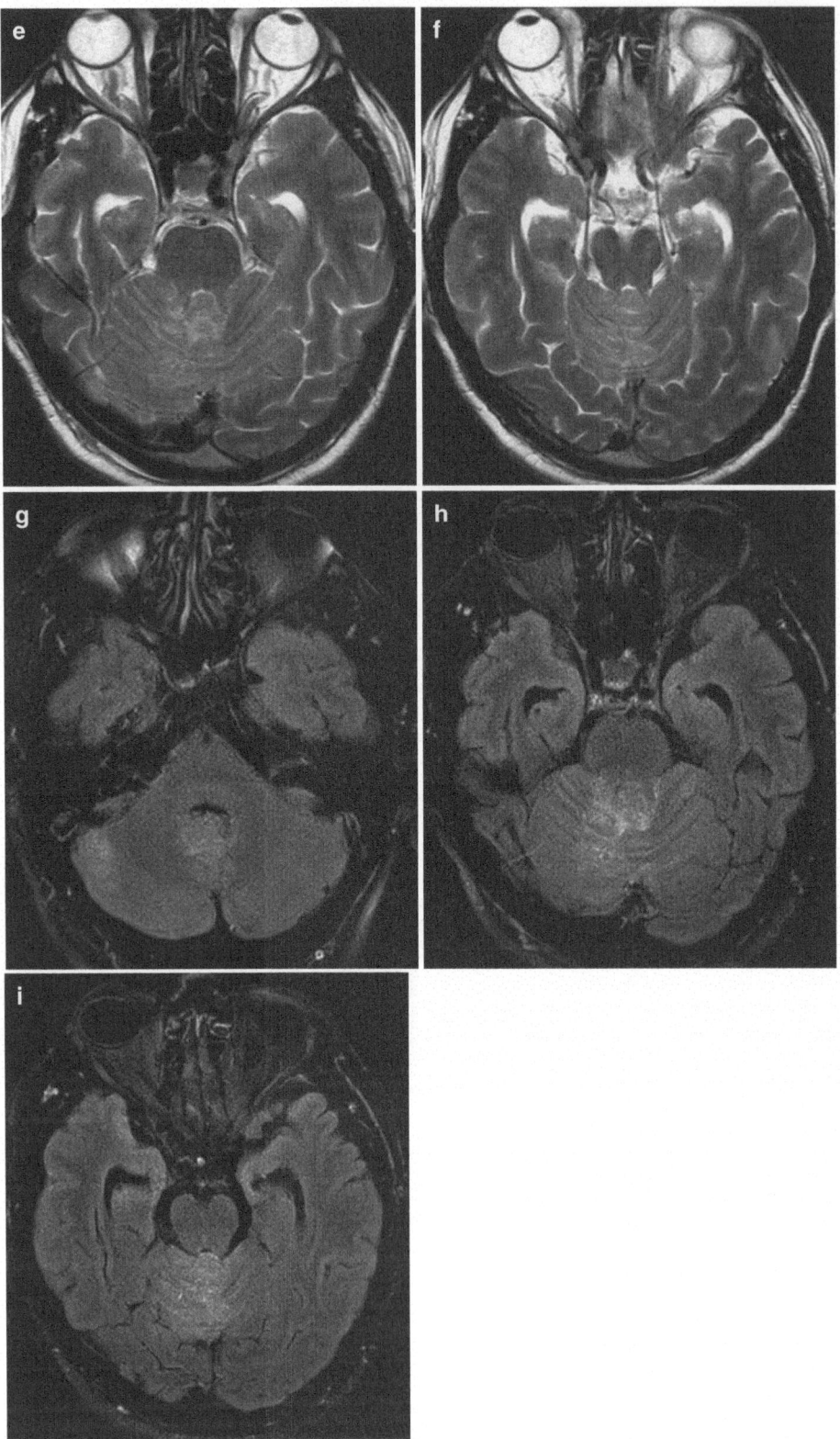

Fig. 27.2 (continued)

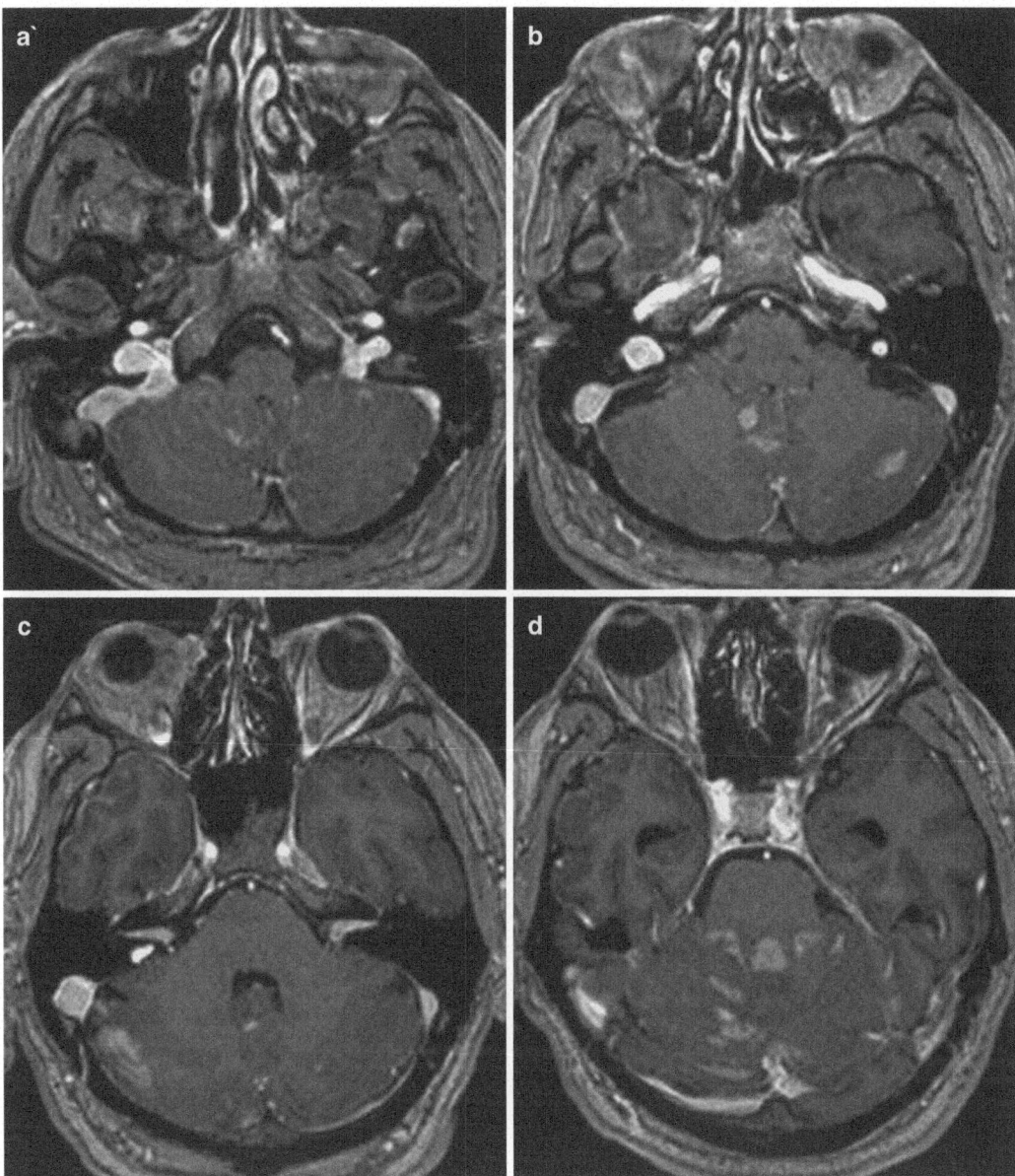

Fig. 27.3 Post-contrast MRI of the brain, axial (**a–f**), sagittal (**g–i**) and coronal (**j–l**) T1WI, demonstrated linear and nodular contrast enhancement of the content distributed diffusely along the folia of both cerebellar hemi- spheres and vermis, protruding towards the roof of the forth ventricle. Both vestibulocochlear nerves were enhanced; left fifth cranial nerve was not enlarged but mildly enhanced

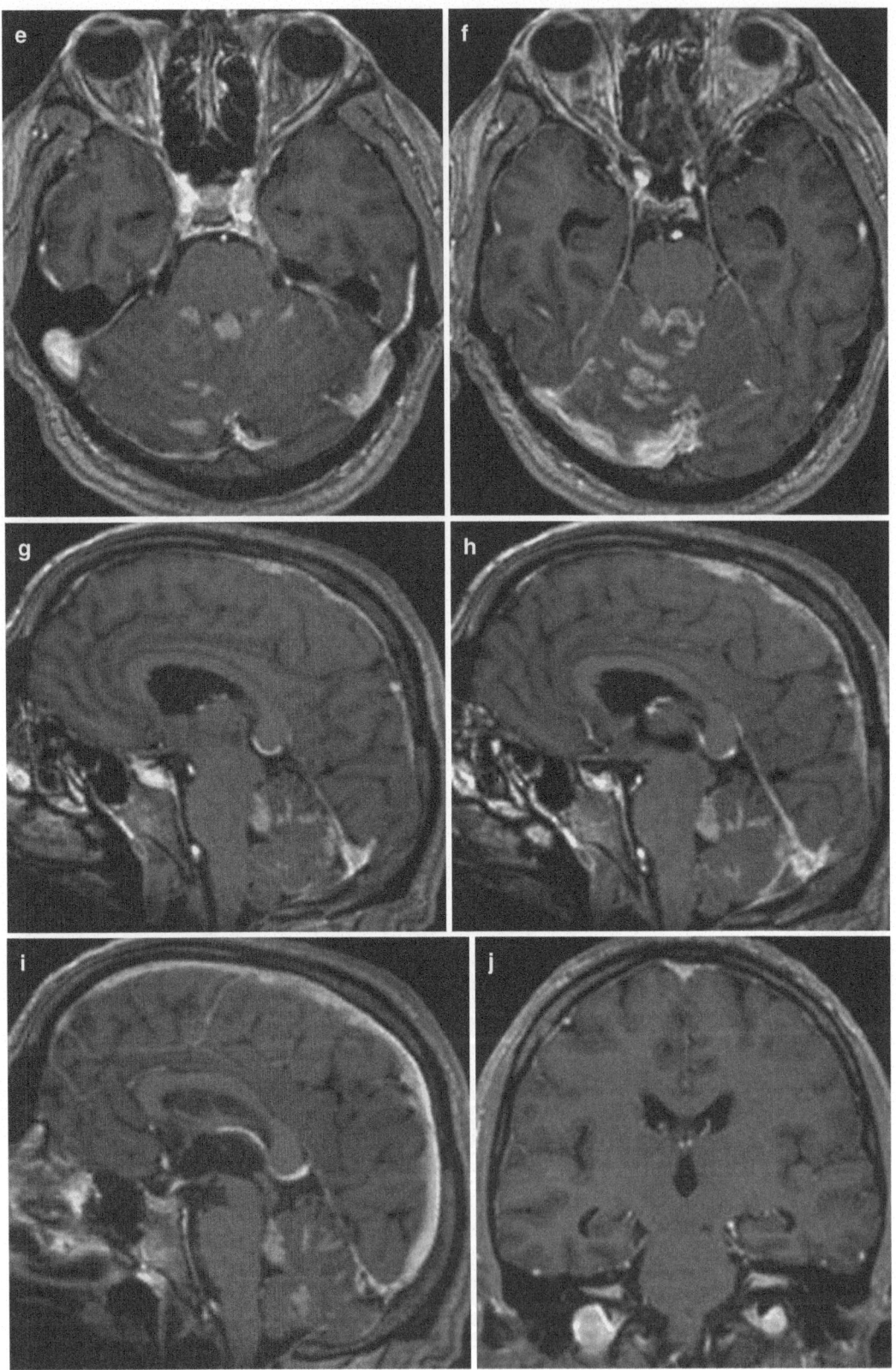

Fig. 27.3 (continued)

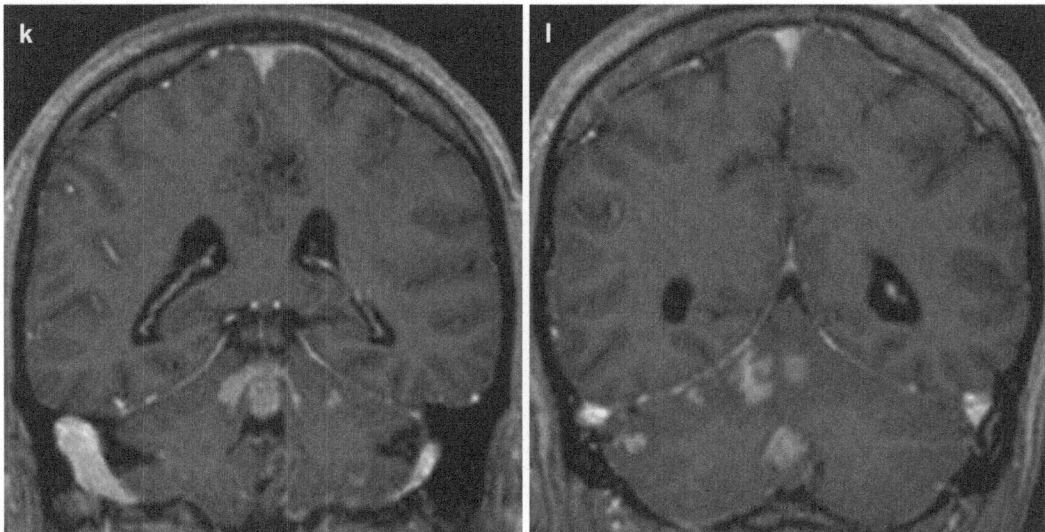

Fig. 27.3 (continued)

CNS metastasis of solid gastrointestinal tumours is usually in a form of parenchymal metastasis, sometimes dural metastasis, but leptomeningeal involvement is extremely rare.

Leptomeningeal carcinomatosis is very rare in oesophageal cancer. Cancer cells may invade the meninges through different pathways including haematogenous spread and endoneural or perineural spread and through perivascular lymphatic routes, or it may be a case of a direct spread from the CNS. The most common presenting features of leptomeningeal metastasis are headache, changes in mental status, cranial nerve palsies and neck stiffness [2].

The diagnosis of LMC is a combination of cytological examination and neuroimaging methods, CT and MRI [3].

It is not easy to detect LMC on non-contrast brain CT: if it is not suspected and contrast media applied, it could be misdiagnosed.

FLAIR imaging has been known to be sensitive for parenchymal lesions but also have shown sensitivity for leptomeningeal processes [4]. Hyperintense signal in sulci, folia or cisternal spaces on FLAIR images should warn radiologist of possible pathological content, like blood, pus in infectious inflammation, granulomatous inflammation due to a systemic disease or malignant cells in case of a malignant process. In case

of a haemorrhage, signal intensity of blood on other standard sequences depends on the age of haemoglobin degradation products, but CT is usually helpful, as well as clinical presentation. In case of granulomatous or infectious inflammation, patient data, clinical presentation, laboratory data and CSF analysis help us in decision-making. When primary malignant process is known, it is not a problem to make a diagnosis. When it is unknown, neuroradiologist should recommend further workup, possibly in right direction regarding expected malignancies as well as unexpected one like oesophageal or gastric tumour.

LMC gives linear and/or nodular pattern of leptomeningeal contrast enhancement. Contrast-enhanced T1W imaging is the most sensitive single sequence for depicting leptomeningeal metastases. Therefore, FLAIR imaging gives us information of a leptomeningeal content, while contrast-enhanced T1W imaging confirms LMC.

If you have a patient without signs of haemorrhage or infectious inflammatory disease, systemic disease is unknown, as well as primary malignant process, think about a possible metastatic leptomeningeal involvement from an unknown oesophageal or gastric malignancy. Therefore, recommend further diagnostic workup of gastrointestinal tract. In recent times, there are more and more reports of LMC due to oesophageal carcinoma spread, maybe because now those patients live longer than before and have a time to develop LMC.

Despite oncological treatment like intrathecal chemotherapy or radiation therapy, survival of patients with LMC due to oesophageal carcinoma is poor: median survival is 3–6 months [3, 5].

References

1. Oh SY et al (2009) Gastric leptomeningeal carcinomatosis: multi-center retrospective analysis of 54 cases. World J Gastroenterol 15(40):5086–5090

2. Akhavan A, Navabii H (2012) Leptomeningeal metastasis from squamous cell carcinoma of oesophagus with unusual presentation. BMJ Case Rep 2012:bcr0220125846

3. Aulakh AS et al (2012) Leptomeningeal carcinomatosis in esophageal cancer: case report and review of literature. J Gastrointest Cancer 43(Suppl 1):S84–S88

4. Singh SK et al (2002) MR imaging of leptomeningeal metastases: comparison of three sequences. AJNR Am J Neuroradiol 23:817–821

5. Dam T et al (2013) Meningeal carcinomatosis: a metastasis from gastroesophageal junction adenocarcinoma. Case Rep Med 2013:245654, 4 pages. https://doi.org/10.1155/2013/245654

The manufacturer's authorised representative in the EU is Springer
Nature Customer Service Centre GmbH, Europaplatz 3, 69115 Heidelberg,
Germany. If you have any concerns regarding our products, please
contact ProductSafety@springernature.com

Printed and bound by CPI Group (UK) Ltd, Croydon, CR0 4YY

29/04/2026

02099517-0001

Emergency Imaging of Pregnant Patients

Michael N. Patlas · Douglas S. Katz
Mariano Scaglione

Editors

Emergency Imaging of Pregnant Patients

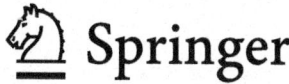 Springer

Editors
Michael N. Patlas
Hamilton General Hospital
McMaster University
Hamilton
ON
Canada

Douglas S. Katz
Department of Radiology
NYU Winthrop Hospital
Mineola
NY
USA

Mariano Scaglione
Department of Radiology
Pineta Grande Hospital
Castel Volturno
Italy

James Cook University Hospital
Middlesbrough
YSN
UK

Teeside University, School of health
and Life Sciences
Middlesbrough
YSN
UK

ISBN 978-3-030-42721-4   ISBN 978-3-030-42722-1   (eBook)
https://doi.org/10.1007/978-3-030-42722-1

This Springer imprint is published by the registered company Springer Nature Switzerland AG
The registered company address is: Gewerbestrasse 11, 6330 Cham, Switzerland

Foreword

It is broadly understood that optimal patient care is rarely one-size-fits-all, but must rather be tailored to the unique needs of the patient. This is a daily truth to practitioners of emergency imaging, a field in which diagnostic decisions and exam performance must be optimized to the specific patient's presentation and physical characteristics.

Pregnant patients pose unique challenges to those participating in their emergent care needs. Care teams must consider the diagnostic and therapeutic needs not only of the mother, but of her unborn child as well. Presenting signs and symptoms may be modified, masked, or accentuated. Differential diagnostic considerations fluctuate in their likelihoods over the course of the pregnancy. Risk–benefit considerations of imaging may be altered by unique concerns about ionizing radiation exposure or intravenous contrast agents. Physiologic changes of pregnancy introduce specific challenges to optimal image acquisition and may impose diagnostic limitations unique to this population. All of these factors impact decisions about how best to image and to diagnose these women and their unborn children.

Our imaging technologies and understanding of how best to personalize imaging decisions have evolved tremendously in the past decade. For example, following heightened concerns about ionizing radiation exposure in the mid-2000s, the CT manufacturers responded by developing many new tools to enable high-quality imaging at progressively lower radiation doses. Many physician-scientists have studied methods to best implement these and preexisting dose reduction techniques into routine clinical practice. As a result, optimally planned examinations can now be performed at substantially lower radiation doses than was previously possible, potentially reducing concerns about clinically indicated modest levels of ionizing radiation during pregnancy.

In *Emergency Imaging of Pregnant Patients,* Drs. Patlas, Katz, Scaglione, and colleagues explore these and other key considerations in this unique patient population. They highlight the relevant merits and limitations of CT, ultrasound, and MRI and delineate special clinical considerations organized by body region and the nature of the emergency. Ultimately, the first priority of imaging pregnant patients must be to optimally care for the mother. This book provides a roadmap to do so and will help practitioners make thoughtful, patient-centered care decisions for expectant mothers and their unborn children.

Aaron Sodickson
American Society of Emergency Radiology
East Dundee, IL, USA

Brigham and Women's Hospital
Boston, MA, USA

Contents

Emergency Imaging of the Pregnant Patient: General Principles

Nanxi Zha, Michael N. Patlas, and Douglas S. Katz

Contents

1.1 Epidemiology

In the United States, 6.2 million women become pregnant each year [1]. The pregnant woman typically makes an average of 5.3 unscheduled health care visits, 10% of which are secondary to non-obstetrical medical or surgical issues [2]. Altered physiology associated with a pregnancy can complicate emergency presentations. For example, the gravid uterus can lead to atypical presentations for acute appendicitis, the hypercoagulable state associated with pregnancy predisposes an otherwise healthy woman to deep vein thrombosis and pulmonary embolism, and adverse complications to the fetus should not limit workup or management in the setting of trauma [3]. Complications secondary to trauma are observed in 6–7% of pregnancies, and are the leading cause of non-obstetrical maternal death [4]. Common mechanisms of injury in pregnant trauma patients include domestic violence (an estimated 8,307 per 100,000 live births), motor vehicle collisions (207 per 100,000 live births), and falls (49 per 100,000 live births) [3]. Specific obstetrical-related traumatic complications include placental abruption, which occurs in 20–50% of major traumatic injuries [4], uterine rupture, which is observed in approximately 1% of obstetrical trauma and carries a poor prognosis for both the mother and the fetus [5], and preterm labor, which affects 11.4% of traumas in pregnancy [6]. Overall, fetal demise is estimated to occur in 42–71% of pregnant

N. Zha · M. N. Patlas (✉)
Department of Radiology, McMaster University, Hamilton, ON, Canada
e-mail: patlas@HHSC.CA

D. S. Katz
NYU Winthrop Hospital, Mineola, New York, USA

© Springer Nature Switzerland AG 2020
M. N. Patlas et al. (eds.), *Emergency Imaging of Pregnant Patients*,
https://doi.org/10.1007/978-3-030-42722-1_1

women with penetrating trauma [7]. Non-traumatic emergent conditions, particularly an acute surgical abdomen, are experienced by 1 in 500–635 pregnant patients [8]. Due to the pregnancy-associated hypercoagulable state, venous thrombosis is experienced by 100 per 100,000 pregnant patients, with an incidence of deep vein thrombosis estimated at 152 per 100,000 pregnancies, and with the pulmonary embolism incidence at 48 per 100,000 pregnancies [9]. Otherwise normal physiologic changes, especially later in gestation, predispose the pregnant patient to an increased risk of serious complications from a variety of conditions when presenting to the emergency department. In this chapter, we will examine the normal physiologic changes in pregnancy, which will help to understand how to optimize management of the pregnant patient from the radiologist and the clinical perspectives, as well as introduce the specific roles of various imaging modalities and their applications in the emergency setting in pregnancy.

1.2   Physiologic Changes in Pregnancy

There are multi-organ physiologic changes that occur during pregnancy. These changes predispose the pregnant patient to unique challenges in accurate clinical diagnosis of emergency presentations, and also have implications for imaging and image interpretation.

Otherwise normal and expected hemodynamic changes can complicate the analysis of pregnant trauma patients, and require careful consideration in correctly managing such patients. In preparation for the expected blood loss at the time of delivery, increased osmoregulation and the renin–angiotensin system lead to fluid retention in pregnancy [10]. This is facilitated primarily by high levels of estrogen produced by the placenta, which increases angiotensin, and results in elevated aldosterone levels [11, 12]. The aldosterone increase leads to the retention of sodium by 500–900 mEq [13], and subsequently fluid retention. This hemodynamic change begins at 12 weeks gestational age, and volume retention of 6–8 L is noted by the third trimester [11]. The

volume expansion predominantly correlates to plasma volume, which increases by 1300 mL [14]. Despite ramped-up erythropoiesis in pregnancy, there is only a 40% increase in red blood cell production, which translates to a red blood cell volume increase by 400 mL [14, 15]. The constellation of findings results in a physiologic anemia in pregnancy. Hemoglobin levels at 11 g/dL are still considered to be within the physiological normal limits for a pregnant patient in later stages of gestation [15]. The increased blood volume in pregnancy is necessary to perfuse the growing fetus, and to prepare for the impending blood loss during delivery [16]. When assessing the pregnant patient in the trauma setting, the patient can remain asymptomatic until approximately a 35% blood loss has been reached because of physiologic anemia [11]. In the non-traumatic setting, emergencies including pre-eclampsia are observed more frequently in patients who fail to increase their blood volume [17], while patients with pre-existing poor cardiac function can experience cardiogenic pulmonary edema due to increased blood volume [15].

During pregnancy, cardiac output is increased primarily due to stroke volume in the first two trimesters, and heart rate elevation in the third trimester [18]. To meet this demand, the heart undergoes ventricular dilatation to allow higher end diastolic volume and increased myocardial contractility [15]. Normal physiologic changes, including a bounding pulse and an ejection murmur, are commonly found on physical examination [15]. In the latter stages of pregnancy, the heart rotates upwards and leftwards secondary to diaphragm elevation by the gravid uterus, which results in cardiomegaly on chest radiography [18]. The gravid uterus can exert substantial compression on the inferior vena cava in the supine position, leading to reduced venous return and potentially compromise of uteroplacental blood flow [15]. Venous stasis caused by this phenomenon combined with increased blood volume and decreased anticoagulant response results in a hypercoagulable state during pregnancy [19]. Acute myocardial infarction, while rare in pregnancy, can lead to devastating outcomes, which is in part due to lack of consensus on treatment [20]. An increased risk of acute myocardial infarction in pregnancy is observed because of elevated progesterone, leading to intimal and medial coronary wall degeneration, increased blood volume, and pregnancy-related hypertension [20]. A rare entity is spontaneous coronary arterial dissection associated with pregnancy, which can result in serious myocardial infarction and other sequelae [21]. Accurate and urgent diagnosis is best performed on coronary angiography (although the diagnosis can be suggested on emergency coronary CT angiography), and is associated with high mortality [21].

The main changes in the respiratory system of a pregnant woman are due to increased uterine size. The diaphragm is elevated by approximately 4 cm, and the chest diameter is elevated by about 2 cm [22]. Bibasilar atelectasis is commonly observed due to the diaphragmatic elevation [23]. The diaphragm morphology change also leads to a barrel-chest appearance of the thoracic cavity on chest radiography (and on other imaging) [24]. This physiologic change should also be taken into consideration in the setting of interventional procedures, including chest tube insertion [11]. Chest wall compliance is lowered which in combination with diaphragm elevation leads to a decrease in total lung capacity by 5%, but without changes to the vital capacity [25]. Minute ventilation increases by 20–40% in pregnancy, commonly resulting in feelings of hypoxia or breathlessness [24]. The hypercoagulable state in pregnancy can predispose the patient to pulmonary embolism, as noted, which requires special consideration for radiation reduction. This will be further discussed in the next section of this chapter [26]. Elevated progesterone during pregnancy can cause delayed gastric emptying and decreased tone of the lower esophageal sphincter, which increases the risk of aspiration [11, 27]. In the peripartum and delivery stages, acute shortness of breath can be the sequela of amniotic fluid embolism. The patient can rapidly develop shock, fulminant pulmonary edema, and cardiovascular collapse. Urgent chest radiography can play a role in identifying pulmonary edema. Further workup with chest computed tomography (CT), while non-specific as the

emboli are not directly visualized, can help exclude other etiologies, including venous thromboembolism, pneumonia, or aspiration [26].

During pregnancy, an estimated 1 in 500–635 patients experience an abdominal emergency [8]. The gravid uterus during pregnancy causes stretching and desensitization of the peritoneum, which can confound the abdominal examination [27]. Such atypical presentations and possible associated resultant delays in management can substantially increase morbidity for the pregnant patient [28]. Therefore, imaging investigations play a crucial role in arriving at an accurate diagnosis. Aside from pregnancy-related abdominal pain without a specific identifiable underlying pathologic diagnosis, the most common etiologies include acute appendicitis, urinary tract stasis, urinary tract infection, urolithiasis (or a combination of these three), cholecystitis, and bowel obstruction [28]. Appendicitis in pregnancy has an estimated incidence of 1 per 500–1000 patients. During the second and third trimesters, the appendix frequently migrates to the level of the iliac crests due to mass effect from the uterus/fetus and other adnexal structures, and then can present with right flank or even right upper quadrant pain [28]. A mild physiologic leukocytosis is commonly observed in pregnancy, and can further obscure diagnosis. Ultrasound is useful for the assessment of right lower quadrant pain in early pregnancy, while magnetic resonance imaging (MRI) is the primary modality of choice in later trimesters, following non-diagnostic ultrasound [28].

Cholestasis develops in 3.5–10% of pregnant patients, and subsequent acute cholecystitis occurs in 1 in 1600–10,000 pregnancies [28]. The expected cholestatic symptoms, including nausea, biliary colic, and intolerance to fat-containing foods, are commonly observed in the pregnant patient; however, the reliability of a clinical Murphy's sign is poor, especially in advanced pregnancy [28]. Ultrasound is the initial imaging modality of choice in suspected cholelithiasis and/or cholecystitis in pregnancy [28].

Bowel obstruction has an incidence rate of 1 in 1500–16,000 pregnancies. The most common etiologies are post-surgical adhesions and volvulus. An increased rate of cecal volvulus is observed in the later stages of pregnancy [28]. The precipitating factors are intra-abdominal migration of the uterus in the second trimester, and pelvic descent of the fetus in the third trimester [28]. Typical symptoms of bowel obstruction, including nausea, vomiting, and obstipation, can be masked by similar physiologic symptoms related to pregnancy, which can potentially confound the diagnosis [27].

Anatomical and physiological changes in the genitourinary system of the pregnant patient are more prevalent later in gestation [29]. The glomerular filtration rate increases by 50% [30]. Fluid retention secondary to activation of the renin–aldosterone–angiotensin system results in enlargement of the kidneys by 1–1.5 cm lengthwise [31]. Physiological hydronephrosis is extremely common in pregnancy, especially on the right side, affecting 43–100% of the patient population [29]. This puts the pregnant patient at relatively substantially increased risk for urinary stasis and subsequent urinary tract infection compared to a non-pregnant population, and there is an associated increased incidence of urolithiasis in pregnancy [32].

Physiologic changes in pregnancy predispose the otherwise healthy woman to acute intracranial abnormalities such as infarct and hemorrhage. Hypercoagulability in pregnancy occurs due altered coagulation factors secondary to estrogen, vasodilation due to elevated progesterone levels, and mechanical compression of the inferior vena cava by uterine enlargement [33]. This physiologic change predisposes the pregnant patient to ischemic brain infarcts (frequency of 25–34 in 100,000 pregnancies), as well as cerebral venous thrombosis (frequency of 12 in 100,000 pregnancies) [33]. Additionally, the elevated progesterone changes the collagen and elastin of vessel walls, leading them to become more friable, thereby increasing the risk of hemorrhage transformation for ischemic strokes. CT and MRI remain the first steps for investigation. Pre-eclampsia and eclampsia are the most common etiology for ischemic and hemorrhagic strokes. While the pathophysiology of pre-eclampsia and eclampsia is not completely understood, it is likely due to poor placentation,

and decreased trophoblastic activity, resulting in poor blood flow through the uterine arteries, which leads to an excessive inflammatory response, which eventually leads to systemic autoregulation failure. During this process, the blood brain barrier is compromised and the patient is predisposed to developing intracranial hemorrhage, which is the most common cause of death in a patient with eclampsia [33].

The pregnant state leads to multi-systemic physiologic changes that not only predisposes to atypical presentations of acute conditions, but also require considerations to alternative diagnoses unique to the pregnant patient. Accurate diagnosis and prompt management of acute presentations lowers morbidity and mortality. Urgent imaging plays a vital role in patient care, as will be emphasized throughout this book. Imaging safety considerations for the fetus are discussed in the following sections.

1.3 Radiation Considerations in Pregnancy

In the pregnant patient, diagnostic imaging is an integral part in the workup of a patient. Radiographs and computed tomographic examinations are vital in emergency medicine because of their relative low costs, accessibility, and fast acquisition times. However, limiting radiation exposure to the fetus must be balanced with the necessity for urgent imaging.

The average fetal radiation due to background radiation during pregnancy is estimated to be 1 mGy [34]. According to the American College of Obstetricians and Gynecologists, the risk of total fetal radiation exposure is thought to be negligible below 50 mGy [35]. Radiation exposure and associated risks during the first 2 weeks after fertilization and before implantation are thought to be an "all or none" phenomenon, resulting in either death or in insignificant consequence to the embryo. During the organogenesis period (2–8 weeks after fertilization), the fetal tube can be affected when radiation dose exceeds 200 mGy, and can leads to congenital anomalies of the eyes, skeleton, and genitals. Growth restrictions are potential complications at radiation levels above 200–250 mGy [34]. At 8–15 weeks, radiation exposure leads to a high risk of intellectual disability (threshold beyond 60–310 mGy) or microcephaly (radiation beyond 200 mGy). Gestational ages beyond 15 weeks carry a low risk of severe intellectual disability at radiation levels of 250–280 mGy [36]. The risk of carcinogenesis from *in utero* radiation exposure is uncertain, to our knowledge. The theoretical risk of prenatal radiation exposure based on atomic bomb survivors suggest the risk of developing childhood leukemia is doubled, compared to a baseline risk of 1 in 3000 [34, 37]. A more recent population-based study, however, suggested that prenatal fetal radiation exposure from medical imaging did not lead to a statistically significant increase in relative risk for childhood cancers [38].

In the acute trauma setting, the stability of the mother is prioritized. Radiation dosage to the fetus from commonly performed imaging examinations are listed in Table 1.1 [39]. It is important to note that not one single diagnostic imaging examination exceeds the recommended radiation dose. Examinations where the fetus is outside the field of view, such as the head, cervical spine, or extremities, can be performed safely in the emergent setting without further consideration [36]. A computed tomography (CT) of the chest has low radiation

Table 1.1 Radiation dosage to the fetus from commonly performed imaging examinations

Type of imaging examination	Estimated range of fetal dose[a] (mGy)
Head or neck CT	0.001–0.01
Chest CT or CT pulmonary angiography	0.01–0.66
Low-dose perfusion scintigraphy	0.1–0.5
Abdominal CT	1.3–35
Pelvic CT	10–50

Annual average background radiation: 1.1–2.5 mGy
Estimated fetal exposure to background radiation during pregnancy: 1 mGy
Modified from Tremblay E, Thérasse E, Thomassin Naggara I, Trop I (2012) Quality initiatives: guidelines for use of medical imaging during pregnancy and lactation. Radiographics 32:897–911
CT computed tomography
[a]Fetal exposure varies with gestational age, maternal body habitus, and exact acquisition parameters

exposure if the fetus is excluded from the primary beam [36]. Low-exposure techniques should be employed, in particular, if there is fetal exposure from the primary beam. For example, a "routine" CT of the pelvis can result in a radiation dose of 50 mGy, but can be reduced to as low as 2.5 mGy [34]. Techniques for dose reduction include dynamic adaptive section collimation, automatic tube current modulation, and adaptive statistical iterative reconstruction [40, 41]. Dynamic adaptive section collimation involves collimator movement during scanning to the attenuate X-ray beam in the z-axis, thereby limiting radiation to tissue outside the field of view [41]. Automatic tube current modulation adjusts the mA based on the patient's body habitus to reduce radiation dose [42]. Noise reduction can be achieved by using adaptive statistical iterative reconstruction, allowing a lower tube current to be utilized [41].

1.4 Introduction to Imaging Modalities in Pregnancy

1.4.1 Ultrasonography

Ultrasound employs sound waves for image acquisitions and does not emit ionizing radiation. The spatial peak-temporal average intensity threshold is limited to 720 mW/cm^2 in pregnancy, which translates to a theoretical temperature elevation to the fetus of 2 °C [34]. M mode has the lowest temperature increase (intensity of 34 mW/cm^2), whereas color Doppler and spectral Doppler have the highest temperature increase (potential to reach intensity of 1180 mW/cm^2) [34]. Exposure time and intensity should be minimized to comply with the acceptable intensity threshold. The fetus is particularly susceptible to thermal damage before 10–12 weeks gestational age, which can potentially result in congenital anomalies [43, 44]. Currently, there are no reported definitive cases of adverse fetal outcomes from diagnostic ultrasound, to our knowledge, even using Doppler imaging, when the intensity threshold is observed [34].

While ultrasound is often the modality of choice for non-obstetrical emergencies due to its safety profile and ease of access, several limitations exist. They include patient body habitus, intraluminal air, and intra-operator variability [45]. For example, in the workup of acute appendicitis, graded compression of the appendix on ultrasound is difficult to attain after 35 weeks of gestational age due to the gravid uterus, and can also be challenging in many patients earlier in pregnancy [45]. Baruch et al. observed a statistically significantly higher rate of inconclusive or negative US results for appendicitis in the pregnant population compared to a non-pregnant control group—39 pregnant patients (or 43% of the pregnant patient group) compared to ten non-pregnant patients (or 11% of the non-pregnant patient group) [46]. Due to the potential increased morbidity from a delay in the diagnosis of appendicitis in pregnancy when present, or in a delay in other potential diagnoses presenting with an acute abdomen or pelvis in pregnancy if not identified on sonography, the negative or equivocal ultrasound examination should prompt further assessment with a second-line imaging modality, particularly MRI, as noted [45, 46].

1.4.2 Computed Tomography

Computed tomography (CT) is generally avoided in the pregnant patient, whenever possible, particularly when the fetus is in or near the field of view, due to the potential risk of ionizing radiation, as we have noted above. However, due to high diagnostic accuracy and ease of access, CT remains a mainstay modality in the acute trauma setting, in suspected pulmonary embolism, and in other selected scenarios such as rapid neurological deterioration, where fast acquisition of a CT examination outweighs benefits of MRI.

In the setting of trauma, patients with a positive focused assessment with sonography in trauma (FAST) examination should be evaluated emergently with an IV contrast-enhanced CT [47]. While multi-phasic CT of the torso is usually performed for trauma evaluation of the non-pregnant adult patient, a single-phase CT may be performed to reduce radiation [47]. If CT cystography is

required, radiation can be reduced by increasing the noise index [48].

For the evaluation of suspected pulmonary embolism in the pregnant patient, bilateral leg ultrasound should be initially performed for the evaluation of possible associated deep vein thrombosis, as per the American Thoracic Society, the Society of Thoracic Radiology, and the American College of Radiology guidelines [47, 49]. CT pulmonary angiography (CTPA) generally should be performed only if the ultrasound is negative. Further assessment with CTPA may not be necessary if the ultrasound is positive for deep vein thrombosis, as it may not change management. However, a dose-adjusted CTPA which results in a low fetal radiation dose, may be useful in confirming the diagnosis of PE, or can provide an alternative diagnosis in patients without PE. When compared to ventilation–perfusion (V/Q) scintigraphy, pulmonary CT angiography generally results in a lower radiation dose to the fetus, particularly early in the pregnancy [47]. Radiation dosages from the two imaging modalities are similar in late pregnancy, because the enlarged uterus rises to the level of the diaphragm. Additionally, techniques can be used to decrease the radiation dose from V/Q scintigraphy, by reducing the radiation dose of the perfusion portion, or by eliminating the ventilation portion if the perfusion component of the examination is already strongly suggestive of pulmonary embolism [47].

Scattered fetal radiation absorbed when the fetus is outside the field of view is considered negligible from current CT units. Radiation exposure should take the ALARA (as low as reasonably achievable) principle into consideration. Standardized protocols should not be used, but rather techniques to minimize radiation exposure, including lowering tube potential based on the patient's weight, decreasing the tube-time product, increasing pitch, and decreasing the z-axis to decrease image length, should all be considered [47]. Dose adjustment in pregnancy needs to be carefully balanced, especially in late gestational age where increased abdomen circumference would require higher radiation dosage to maintain image quality. This requires teamwork amongst technologists, radiologists, and medical physicists.

Contrast is used for CT in the pregnant patient when clinically necessary. Oral contrast does not get absorbed by the patient, and theoretically does not cause harm [34]. Intravenous iodinated contrast agents can cross the placenta. There are no definitive teratogenic effects in animal-based studies to date, but no formal published studies have been performed in pregnant women, to our knowledge. The American College of Obstetricians and Gynecologists' recommendation is to limit use of intravenous contrast to only when necessary [34].

1.4.3 Magnetic Resonance Imaging

Aside from emergent traumatic scenarios, MRI is the preferred imaging modality when the fetus in the field of view, and generally following initial non-diagnostic sonography. While ultrasound remains a cheaper and more accessible option, substantial shortcomings with ultrasound in pregnancy, particularly later in gestation, including intra-operator variability and patient size, leading to usually poor diagnostic accuracy in several common scenarios [45]. For intra-abdominal pathologies, MRI is usually the second choice for imaging after ultrasound, as noted. For example, the diagnosis of appendicitis in pregnancy can be made with upwards of 100% sensitivity and 94% specificity, based on multiple small-to-medium-sized published studies. The high diagnostic accuracy of MRI extends to inflammatory bowel disease (sensitivity of 91% and specificity of 71%) and diverticulitis (sensitivity of 86–94% and specificity of 88–92%), although the latter diagnosis is rather uncommon in pregnancy [50]. In addition, the high soft-tissue resolution provided by MRI can reveal alternative diagnoses if the initial leading clinical diagnosis has been excluded.

There are theoretical concerns with MRI usage in the pregnant patient. Specifically, concerns exist regarding tissue heating and subsequent teratogenesis, as well as acoustic damage; however, there is no definite evidence supporting these claims [34]. Tissue heating is the result of multiple factors, including the strength of the static magnetic field, the radiofrequency (RF) pulse used, the repetition time, the RF coil used, and the volume of tissue within the field of view [51]. Increase in body temperature should be limited to be below 0.5 °C [51]. It is worthwhile to note that although the spin-echo sequences utilized for fast fetal imaging do have higher RF energy than standard gradient-echo sequences, the heat deposited is below the teratogenic threshold. A review of health care databases by Ray et al. demonstrated no increased risk of harm to the fetus or in subsequent early childhood due to first trimester MRI [38]. In the second and third trimesters, excessive levels of noise generated by an MRI system may theoretically lead to acoustic damage. While the American College of Radiology approves of the use of MRI in all stages of pregnancy, careful consideration must be given to the necessity of the MRI and whether imaging can be delayed until post-partum [50].

If IV contrast agents are required for MR imaging, gadolinium is the preferred choice. In animal studies, there are reports of teratogenic effects at high or repeated doses [34]. This is thought to be due to the conversion of chelated gadolinium to toxic-free gadolinium over time. Injected gadolinium is water soluble, and does cross the placenta and can dissolve into the amniotic fluid, and thus is swallowed by the fetus. It is uncertain how long gadolinium remains in the fetal system (and whether it persists into infancy and beyond). The longer gadolinium stays in the body, the more likely it is to be converted to the free form. There is currently no study, either retrospective or prospective, to our knowledge, which has indicated any definite harm to the human fetus due to IV gadolinium use at current clinical dosages similar to those used in non-pregnant patients. Gadolinium, however, should only be used when there is a perceived potential benefit [34].

1.5 Conclusion

Non-obstetric emergencies affecting various parts of the mother's body are experienced by a non-trivial minority of pregnant patients.

Complex physiologic changes in pregnancy, from expected elevated normal ranges in blood work, to the gravid uterus confounding physical examination findings, complicate accurate diagnosis. Physiologic changes experienced by the pregnant patient places her at increased risk for potential complications. Since these factors can confound clinical findings and assessment, the use of imaging is crucial to assist in accurate diagnosis and management of emergencies in the pregnant patient. Due to the risk of radiation exposure to the fetus, the use of CT for intra-abdominal pathology is generally limited to assessment of acute traumatic injuries and in the workup for suspected pulmonary embolism. Scattered radiation to the fetus when the imaging is performed away from the abdomen (i.e., imaging the head, cervical spine, or extremities) can be considered if clinically indicated. MRI plays a vital role in the workup of intra-abdominal pathology in the pregnant patient, because it does not use ionizing radiation, and due to its ability to display soft tissues in high contrast resolution. Imaging the pregnant patient can be challenging for all the before mentioned reasons. The purpose of this book is, therefore, to examine in depth the complexities of imaging the acutely ill pregnant patient, to assist in accurate clinical diagnosis in the setting of emergency medicine.

References

1. CDC. NVSS - birth data. 2019. http://www.cdc.gov/nchs/nvss/births.htm. Accessed 23 Feb 2019.
2. Magriples U, Kershaw TS, Rising SS, et al. Prenatal health care beyond the obstetrics service: utilization and predictors of unscheduled care. Am J Obstet Gynecol. 2008;198:75.e1–7.
3. Mendez-Figueroa H, Dahlke JD, Vrees RA, Rouse DJ. Trauma in pregnancy: an updated systematic review. Am J Obstet Gynecol. 2013;209:1–10.
4. Hill CC, Pickinpaugh J. Trauma and surgical emergencies in the obstetric patient. Surg Clin North Am. 2008;88:421–40. viii.
5. El-Kady D, Gilbert WM, Anderson J, et al. Trauma during pregnancy: an analysis of maternal and fetal outcomes in a large population. Am J Obstet Gynecol. 2004;190:1661–8.
6. Connolly AM, Katz VL, Bash KL, et al. Trauma and pregnancy. Am J Perinatol. 1997;14:331–6.
7. Brown HL. Trauma in pregnancy. Obstet Gynecol. 2009;114:147–60.
8. Augustin G, Majerovic M. Non-obstetrical acute abdomen during pregnancy. Eur J Obstet Gynecol Reprod Biol. 2007;131:4–12.
9. Heit JA, Kobbervig CE, James AH, et al. Trends in the incidence of venous thromboembolism during pregnancy or postpartum: a 30-year population-based study. Ann Intern Med. 2005;143:697–706.
10. Hill CC, Pickinpaugh J. Physiologic changes in pregnancy. Surg Clin North Am. 2008;88:391–401. vii.
11. Petrone P, Marini CP. Trauma in pregnant patients. Curr Probl Surg. 2015;52:330–51.
12. Oelkers WK. Effects of estrogens and progestogens on the renin-aldosterone system and blood pressure. Steroids. 1996;61:166–71.
13. Koller O. The clinical significance of hemodilution during pregnancy. Obstet Gynecol Surv. 1982;37:649–52.
14. Troiano NH. Physiologic and hemodynamic changes during pregnancy. AACN Adv Crit Care. 2018;29:273–83.
15. Sanghavi M, Rutherford JD. Cardiovascular physiology of pregnancy. Circulation. 2014;130:1003–8.
16. West CA, Sasser JM, Baylis C. The enigma of continual plasma volume expansion in pregnancy: critical role of the renin-angiotensin-aldosterone system. Am J Physiol Renal Physiol. 2016;311:F1125–34.
17. de Haas S, Ghossein-Doha C, van Kuijk SMJ, et al. Physiological adaptation of maternal plasma volume during pregnancy: a systematic review and meta-analysis. Ultrasound Obstet Gynecol. 2017;49:177–87.
18. Fujitani S, Baldisseri MR. Hemodynamic assessment in a pregnant and peripartum patient. Crit Care Med. 2005;33:S354–61.
19. Elliott CG. Evaluation of suspected pulmonary embolism in pregnancy. J Thorac Imaging. 2012;27:3–4.
20. Ismail S, Wong C, Rajan P, Vidovich MI. ST-elevation acute myocardial infarction in pregnancy: 2016 update. Clin Cardiol. 2017;40:399–406.
21. Appleby CE, Barolet A, Ing D, et al. Contemporary management of pregnancy-related coronary artery dissection: a single-centre experience and literature review. Exp Clin Cardiol. 2009;14:e8–e16.
22. Elkus R, Popovich J. Respiratory physiology in pregnancy. Clin Chest Med. 1992;13:555–65.
23. Costantine MM. Physiologic and pharmacokinetic changes in pregnancy. Front Pharmacol. 2014;5:65.
24. Lee S-Y, Chien D-K, Huang C-H, et al. Dyspnea in pregnancy. Taiwan J Obstet Gynecol. 2017;56:432–6.
25. Farman JV, Thorpe ME. Static compliance before and after vaginal delivery. Br J Anaesth. 1971;43:418.
26. Plowman RS, Javidan-Nejad C, Raptis CA, et al. Imaging of pregnancy-related vascular complications. Radiographics. 2017;37:1270–89.
27. Tan EK, Tan EL. Alterations in physiology and anatomy during pregnancy. Best Pract Res Clin Obstet Gynaecol. 2013;27:791–802.

28. Bouyou J, Gaujoux S, Marcellin L, et al. Abdominal emergencies during pregnancy. J Visc Surg. 2015;152:S105–15.

29. Faúndes A, Brícola-Filho M, Pinto e Silva JL. Dilatation of the urinary tract during pregnancy: proposal of a curve of maximal caliceal diameter by gestational age. Am J Obstet Gynecol. 1998;178:1082–6.

30. Cheung KL, Lafayette RA. Renal physiology of pregnancy. Adv Chronic Kidney Dis. 2013;20:209–14.

31. Bailey RR, Rolleston GL. Kidney length and ureteric dilatation in the puerperium. J Obstet Gynaecol Br Commonw. 1971;78:55–61.

32. Rasmussen PE, Nielsen FR. Hydronephrosis during pregnancy: a literature survey. Eur J Obstet Gynecol Reprod Biol. 1988;27:249–59.

33. Haber MA, Nunez D. Imaging neurological emergencies in pregnancy and puerperium. Emerg Radiol. 2018;25:673–84.

34. Jain C. ACOG committee opinion no. 723: guidelines for diagnostic imaging during pregnancy and lactation. Obstet Gynecol. 2019;133:186.

35. Brent RL, Mettler FA. Pregnancy policy. AJR Am J Roentgenol. 2004;182:819–22. author reply 822.

36. Patel SJ, Reede DL, Katz DS, et al. Imaging the pregnant patient for nonobstetric conditions: algorithms and radiation dose considerations. Radiographics. 2007;27:1705–22.

37. Gjelsteen AC, Ching BH, Meyermann MW, et al. CT, MRI, PET, PET/CT, and ultrasound in the evaluation of obstetric and gynecologic patients. Surg Clin North Am. 2008;88:361–90. vii.

38. Ray JG, Schull MJ, Urquia ML, et al. Major radiodiagnostic imaging in pregnancy and the risk of childhood malignancy: a population-based cohort study in Ontario. PLoS Med. 2010;7:e1000337.

39. Tremblay E, Thérasse E, Thomassin-Naggara I, Trop I. Quality initiatives: guidelines for use of medical imaging during pregnancy and lactation. Radiographics. 2012;32:897–911.

40. Solomou G, Papadakis AE, Damilakis J. Abdominal CT during pregnancy: a phantom study on the effect of patient centring on conceptus radiation dose and image quality. Eur Radiol. 2015;25:911–21.

41. Chatterson LC, Leswick DA, Fladeland DA, et al. Fetal shielding combined with state of the art CT dose reduction strategies during maternal chest CT. Eur J Radiol. 2014;83:1199–204.

42. Kalra MK, Maher MM, Toth TL, et al. Comparison of Z-axis automatic tube current modulation technique with fixed tube current CT scanning of abdomen and pelvis. Radiology. 2004;232:347–53.

43. Abramowicz JS. Benefits and risks of ultrasound in pregnancy. Semin Perinatol. 2013;37:295–300.

44. Abramowicz JS, Barnett SB, Duck FA, et al. Fetal thermal effects of diagnostic ultrasound. J Ultrasound Med. 2008;27:541–59. quiz 560–563.

45. Diegelmann L. Nonobstetric abdominal pain and surgical emergencies in pregnancy. Emerg Med Clin North Am. 2012;30:885–901.

46. Baruch Y, Canetti M, Blecher Y, et al. The diagnostic accuracy of ultrasound in the diagnosis of acute appendicitis in pregnancy. J Matern Fetal Neonatal Med. 2019:1–6.

47. Tirada N, Dreizin D, Khati NJ, et al. Imaging pregnant and lactating patients. Radiographics. 2015;35:1751–65.

48. Sadro C, Bernstein MP, Kanal KM. Imaging of trauma: part 2, abdominal trauma and pregnancy — a radiologist's guide to doing what is best for the mother and baby. Am J Roentgenol. 2012;199:1207–19.

49. Leung AN, Bull TM, Jaeschke R, et al. An official American Thoracic Society/Society of Thoracic Radiology clinical practice guideline: evaluation of suspected pulmonary embolism in pregnancy. Am J Respir Crit Care Med. 2011;184:1200–8.

50. Spalluto LB, Woodfield CA, DeBenedectis CM, Lazarus E. MR imaging evaluation of abdominal pain during pregnancy: appendicitis and other nonobstetric causes. Radiographics. 2012;32:317–34.

51. Patenaude Y, Pugash D, Lim K, et al. The use of magnetic resonance imaging in the obstetric patient. J Obstet Gynaecol Can. 2014;36:349–63.

Imaging of Neurological Emergencies During Pregnancy and the Puerperium

2

Carlos Torres, Nader Zakhari, Diego B. Nunez, Angela Guarnizo-Capera, Paulo Puac, and Francisco Rivas-Rodriguez

Contents

C. Torres (✉)
Department of Radiology, University of Ottawa, Ottawa, ON, Canada

Department of Diagnostic Imaging, The Ottawa Hospital, Ottawa, ON, Canada

Ottawa Hospital Research Institute OHRI, Ottawa, ON, Canada
e-mail: catorres@toh.ca

N. Zakhari
Department of Radiology, University of Ottawa, Ottawa, ON, Canada

Department of Diagnostic Imaging, The Ottawa Hospital, Ottawa, ON, Canada
e-mail: nzakhari@toh.ca

D. B. Nunez
Brigham and Women's Hospital, Harvard Medical School, Boston, MA, USA
e-mail: dnunez@bwh.harvard.edu

A. Guarnizo-Capera · P. Puac
Department of Radiology, University of Ottawa, Ottawa, ON, Canada
e-mail: aguarnizocapera@toh.ca; ppuacpolanco@toh.ca

F. Rivas-Rodriguez
Department of Radiology, University of Michigan, Ann Arbor, MI, USA
e-mail: frivasro@med.umich.edu

© Springer Nature Switzerland AG 2020
M. N. Patlas et al. (eds.), *Emergency Imaging of Pregnant Patients*,
https://doi.org/10.1007/978-3-030-42722-1_2

The physiologic changes which occur during pregnancy and the peripartum period place female patients at risk for several acute neurological conditions that can have deleterious effects to both the mother and the fetus. These obstetric emergencies may be unique to pregnancy and the puerperium, including the pre-eclampsia/eclampsia syndrome, or may rather be related to the effect of predisposing factors associated with pregnancy, including ischemic and hemorrhagic stroke, cerebral venous thrombosis, reversible vasoconstriction syndrome, and posterior reversible encephalopathy. Among the risk factors commonly associated with the development of peripartum and puerperium "stroke" are cesarean section, fluid overload, electrolyte disturbance, and hypertension. Pregnant women are also at risk for hypophyseal diseases including pituitary apoplexy and lymphocytic hypophysitis.

Overall, acute neurological symptoms in pregnant and post-partum patients can be the result of exacerbation of a pre-existing condition or the initial presentation of a pregnancy or non-pregnancy-related problem [1]. Regardless of the individual underlying condition, throbbing headaches, acute neurological deficit, and/or seizures are among the most common clinical presentations. Pregnant and post-partum patients complaining of headache and neurological deficits are frequently diagnosed with pre-eclampsia/eclampsia, but a wider range of etiologies must be considered. Understanding the pathogenesis and physiopathology of these disorders allows for prompt and accurate diagnosis, which is key to establish subsequent adequate treatment [1]. The radiologist plays therefore a fundamental role, not only in guiding appropriate management, but also contributing as a consultant regarding the risk of imaging to the fetus, and helping to balance those risks with those of the mother.

This chapter reviews the scope of computed tomography (CT) and magnetic resonance imaging (MRI) features of the various entities responsible for acute neurological syndromes in pregnant and post-partum women, and highlights the role of the radiologist as an important consultant of the managing team.

2.1 Neurovascular Complications of Pregnancy

Pregnancy and the puerperium have unique pathophysiological states, including increased levels of estrogen and progesterone, as well as elevated plasma and total blood volumes. Elevated estrogen levels increase the production of clotting factors with a higher resultant risk of thromboembolic events. Vasodilation effect of progesterone during late pregnancy increases venous capacity and facilitates capillary leakage. Higher blood and plasma volumes during pregnancy render an elevated risk of hypertension. The combination of these hormonal and hemodynamic changes may result in leaky capillaries and vasogenic edema, which contribute to the genesis of neurological complications of pregnancy [2].

2.2 Pre-eclampsia and Eclampsia, Including HELLP Syndrome

Pre-eclampsia is a multi-system disorder defined as the new onset of hypertension and proteinuria later than 20 weeks of gestation in a previously normotensive woman. Mild pre-eclampsia criteria include blood pressure higher than 140/90 mmHg, and proteinuria greater than 0.3 g in a 24-h urine sample. Severe pre-eclampsia is diagnosed with two blood pressures of or greater than 160/110 mmHg, proteinuria greater than 5 g per 24 h, and signs of end-organ injury. Eclampsia is defined as pre-eclampsia and grand mal seizures in the absence of other conditions that may account for the genesis of seizures [3]. At advanced disease stages, the combination of endothelial injury, systemic vasoconstriction, reduced intravascular volume, hemoconcentration, and systemic edema leads to hepatic ischemia with liver dysfunction, hemolysis, elevated liver enzymes, and low platelets (HELLP) syndrome, which is a part of the spectrum of pre-eclampsia/eclampsia disease [4].

Pre-eclampsia occurs in 2–8% of pregnancies. Eclampsia develops in up to 0.6% of mildly pre-eclamptic and 2–3% of severely pre-eclamptic pregnant women. Eclampsia is diagnosed before term in 50% of patients, intrapartum in 25%, and within 48 h of delivery in 25%. Eclampsia may occur in normotensive patients without proteinuria in up to one-quarter of patients [5]. Patients with post-partum eclampsia have a higher incidence of cerebral venous thrombosis (CVT), intracranial hemorrhage (ICH), and acute ischemic stroke (AIS) than in those diagnosed prepartum [6].

Neurological events in eclampsia may be acute and transient, with long-term deficits being rare when prompt diagnosis and proper management are stabilized. Poor blood pressure control in pre-eclamptic pregnancies may result in severe vasoconstriction of the intracranial vasculature, with increased risk of ischemic brain injury and ICH, the most common causes of maternal eclampsia-related death. Eclampsia mortality varies between 0% and 14%, being higher in less developed countries [6, 7].

Pregnant women with new-onset headaches should be screened for pre-eclampsia. Pre-eclamptic women may complain of bilateral throbbing headache, blurred vision, scintillating scotomata, epigastric/right upper quadrant pain, edema, agitation, and restlessness. On physical examination, hypertension and hyperreflexia may be found. Proteinuria, thrombocytopenia, hemoconcentration, and elevated transaminases and creatinine levels may be also documented [8]. In pre-eclamptic pregnancies, prophylaxis with magnesium sulfate reduces the incidence of eclampsia. Although delivery is the definitive treatment for pre-eclampsia and eclampsia, post-partum seizures may still occur in the first 48 h after termination of pregnancy [9].

2.3 Imaging in Pre-eclampsia and Eclampsia

Neuroimaging in the setting of uncomplicated well-defined pre-eclampsia may not be necessary, but in the setting of neurological deficits, including seizures, and/or clinical deterioration, imaging should be performed [10].

The target for imaging evaluation is the documentation of brain edema, ischemic brain injury, and intracranial hemorrhage. MRI demonstrates increased symmetric signal on T2-weighted and FLAIR sequences in the deep and subcortical white matter, often widespread, but with predominance for the posterior circulation, with involvement of the parietal and occipital lobes. MR signal abnormalities correspond to areas of low attenuation on CT [11]. Imaging abnormalities may also occur in the basal ganglia, pons, and brainstem. Preferential involvement of the posterior circulation and watershed zones is believed to be related to a decrease in vasomotor sympathetic innervation, in comparison with the anterior circulation [12] (Fig. 2.1).

Signal intensity changes may be reversible (Fig. 2.2) or can evolve into infarction and/or ICH. T2-weighted signal abnormalities with increased diffusivity represent reversible vasogenic edema; while increased DWI signal and low ADC values represent infarction or tissue

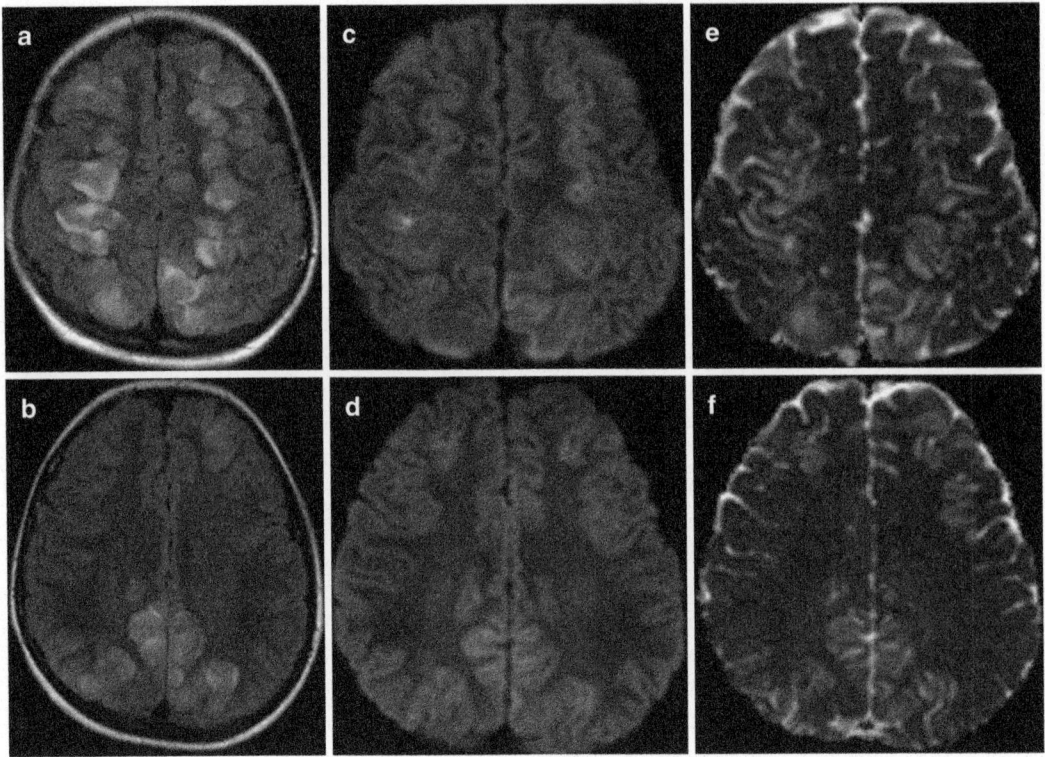

Fig. 2.1 Thirty-eight-year-old woman at 39 weeks' gestational age and pre-eclampsia presents with worsening headaches, vertigo, and confusion. Axial FLAIR images (**a**, **b**) demonstrate symmetric parenchymal edema, with increased cortical subcortical signal intensity in the medial aspect of the frontal and parietal lobes. Axial DWI and ADC map images (**c–f**) demonstrate T2-shine-through consistent with vasogenic edema

injury from cytotoxic edema, the latter of which is associated with an adverse outcome [11] (Fig. 2.3). Brain edema in pre-eclampsia and eclampsia is associated with laboratory-based evidence of endothelial damage, including abnormal red cell morphology and elevated levels of lactic dehydrogenase [13].

In patients with severe pre-eclampsia and eclampsia, vasospasm may be documented with CT angiography (CTA) and/or MR angiography (MRA), as well as with conventional cerebral angiography. Diffuse or focal vasoconstriction with a "string-of-beads" appearance can be identified [14] (Fig. 2.4). Corresponding elevated MCA velocities can be found on intracranial Doppler examinations [15]. Cerebral vasospasm is uncommon in mild or moderate pre-eclampsia.

Cerebral hemorrhage is identified in approximately one-third of eclampsia-related fatalities. Hemorrhagic patterns range from petechial hemorrhage and convexal subarachnoid hemorrhage (SAH), to parenchymal hematomas (Fig. 2.5). Coexisting coagulopathies, including thrombocytopenia and disseminated intravascular coagulation, commonly seen in the setting of severe pre-eclampsia and eclampsia, exacerbate intracranial hemorrhage in these patients [10].

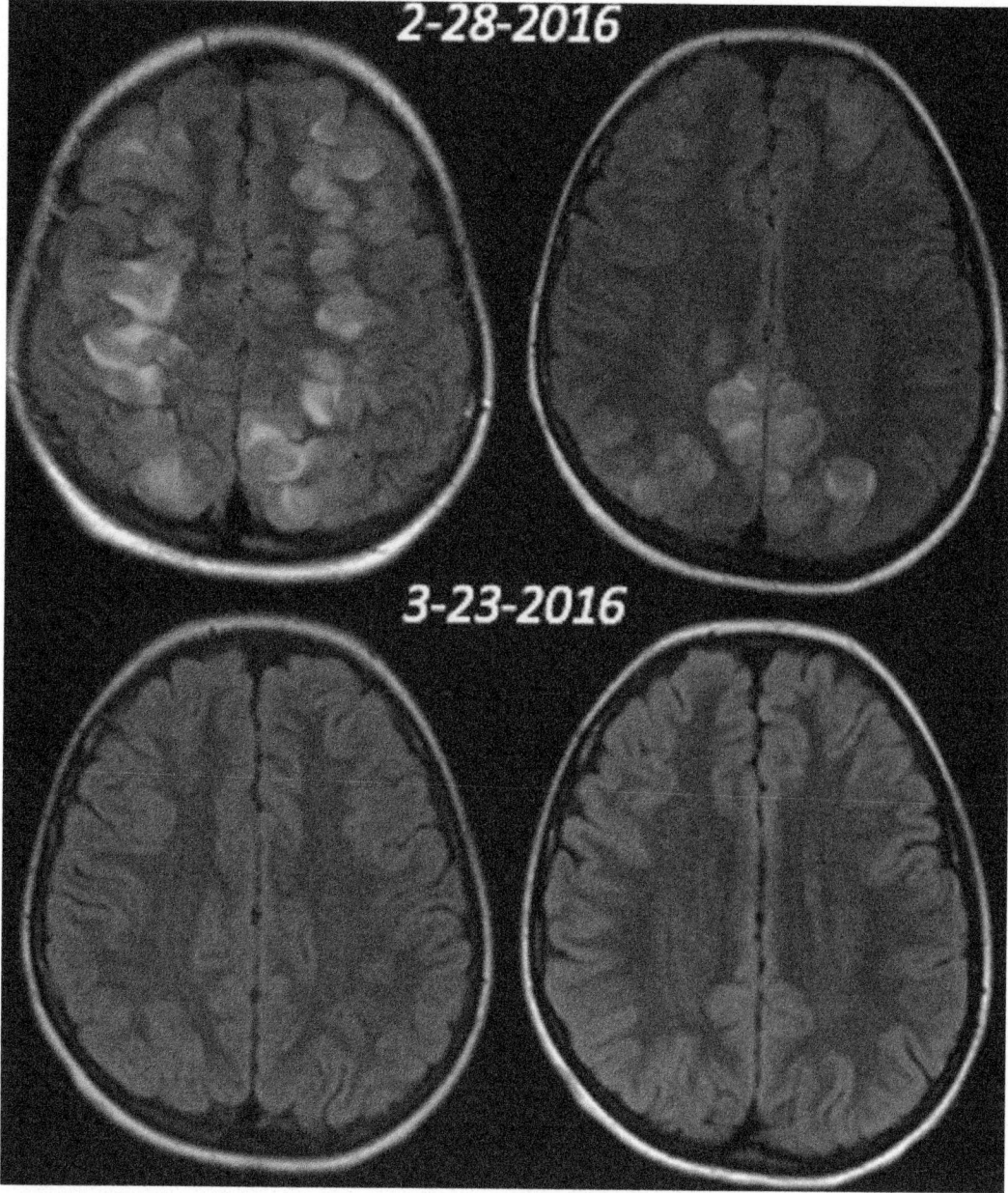

Fig. 2.2 Follow-up MR imaging 3 weeks after C-section demonstrate complete interval resolution of the signal abnormalities in the axial FLAIR sequences (same patient as in Fig. 2.1)

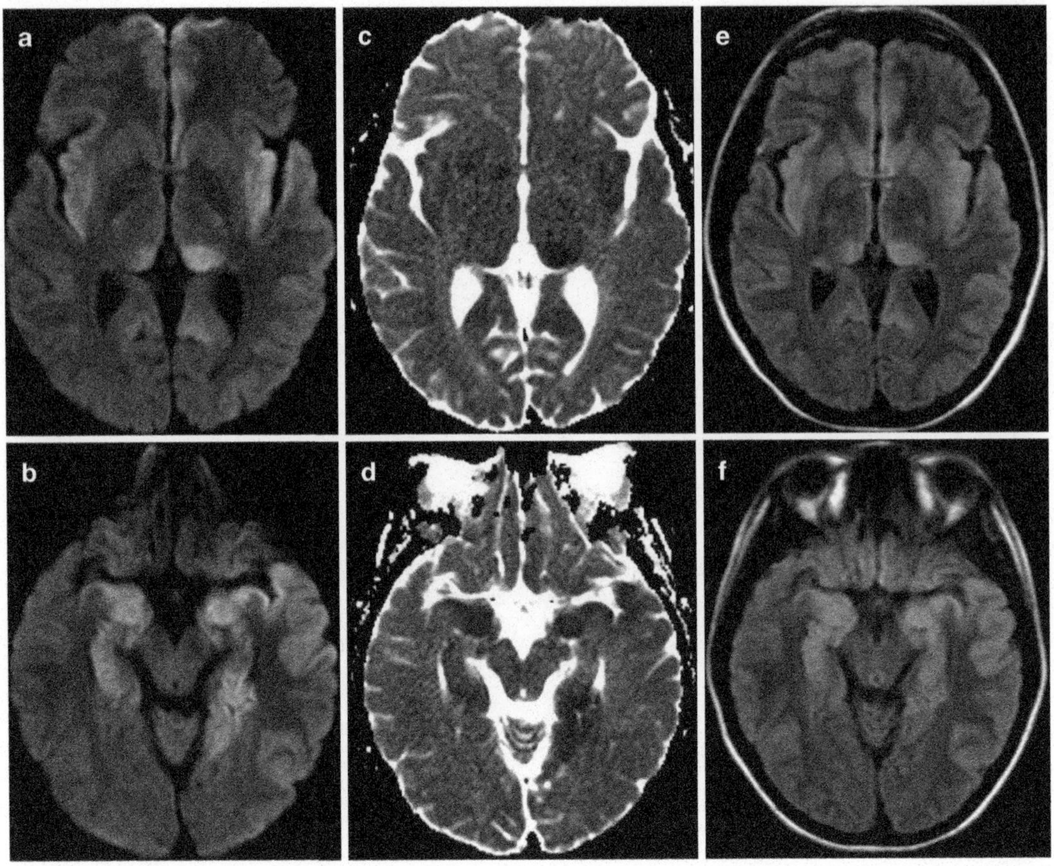

Fig. 2.3 Twenty-five-year-old woman at 33 weeks' gestational age following c-section, with eclampsia. Axial DWI and ADC map images (**a–d**) demonstrate restricted diffusion with corresponding FLAIR hypersignal (**e, f**) consistent with subacute infarcts in the left insula, left thalamus, and bilateral mesial temporal regions. Vasogenic edema is also identified in the right insula and right thalamus

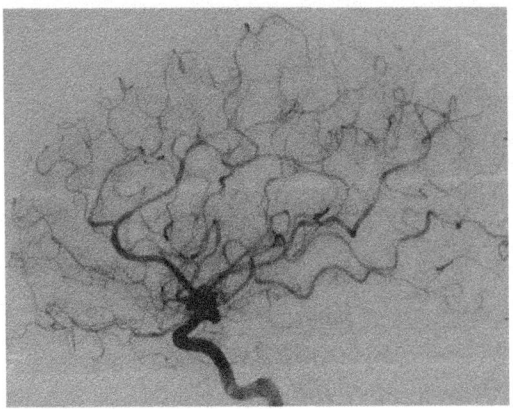

Fig. 2.4 Post-partum cerebral catheter angiogram in the same patient as in Fig. 2.3 demonstrates a vasculopathy pattern with multiple areas of vasospasm with segmental luminal narrowing and alternating luminal dilatation

2.4 Acute Ischemic Stroke (AIS) and Intracranial Hemorrhage (ICH)

Approximately 60% of strokes during pregnancy are ischemic, either embolic or watershed. The remaining 40% strokes are hemorrhagic in nature [16, 17].

Pregnancy and the puerperium are considered hypercoagulable states due to increased fibrinogen levels, platelet aggregability, and factors VIII, IX, X; additionally, fibrinolytic activity is decreased with reduced levels of protein S and antithrombin III, as well as the suboptimal therapeutic effect of heparin [16, 17].

While rare in pregnancy, there is an increased risk for stroke during late pregnancy and in the early puerperium [16, 17]. A large Swedish population study found a significant increase in neurovascular complications during the puerperium, including cerebral infarction, venous sinus thrombosis, intracerebral hemorrhage, and subarach- noid hemorrhage [18]. Risk factors for stroke in pregnancy include pre-eclampsia/eclampsia, age older than 35 years, African-American race, hypertension, cesarean delivery, migraine, thrombophilia, systemic lupus erythematosus, sickle cell disease, post-partum cardiomyopathy, and thrombocytopenia [19]. Complications of pregnancy, including post-partum hemorrhage, pre-eclampsia/eclampsia, gestational hypertension, transfusion, and post-partum infection, all have a substantially associated increased stroke risk [20].

Pregnant and post-partum women with thunderclap headache need prompt CT evaluation to exclude or diagnose SAH, ICH, and CVT. Underlying structural abnormalities including aneurysms, vascular malformations, and CVT should be promptly investigated.

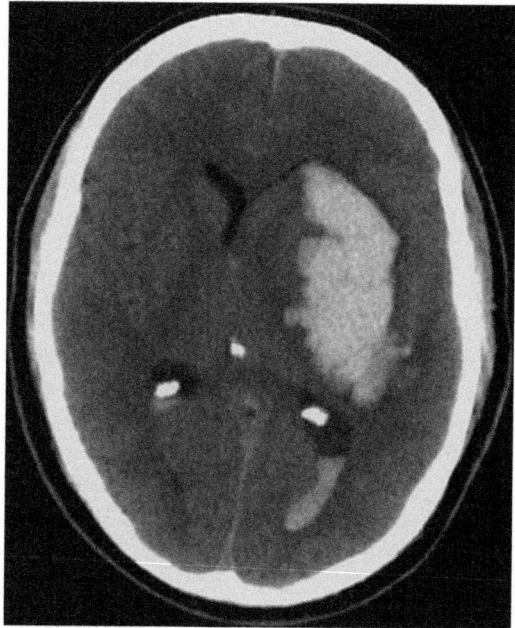

Fig. 2.5 Axial image of a non-contrast head CT in a 40-year-old post-partum woman with severe headache and eclampsia shows an acute intraparenchymal hemorrhage in the left basal ganglia region with extension into the ventricular system. There is associated mass effect causing partial effacement of the left lateral ventricle, and midline shift to the right

2.5   Acute Ischemic Stroke

Acute ischemic brain injury during pregnancy may result from arterial thrombotic/embolic occlusions, or from watershed infarctions.

Thrombotic arterial occlusions result from thrombus formation on pre-existing atherosclerotic plaques or in thrombophilic conditions (Fig. 2.6). Pre-existing atherosclerotic plaques are associated with underlying hypertension, diabetes, hyperlipidemia, or premature atherosclerosis. Thrombophilic conditions include antiphospholipid syndrome, factor V Leiden

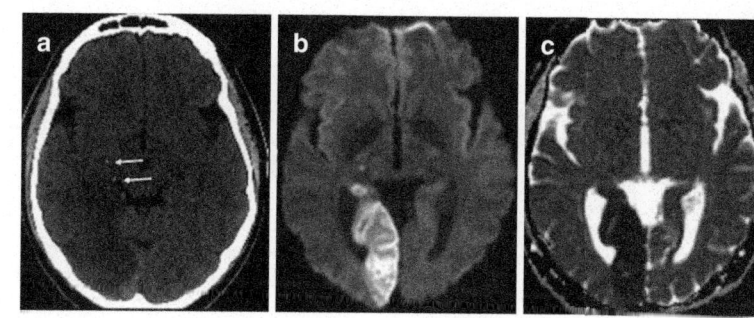
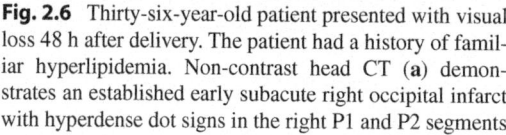
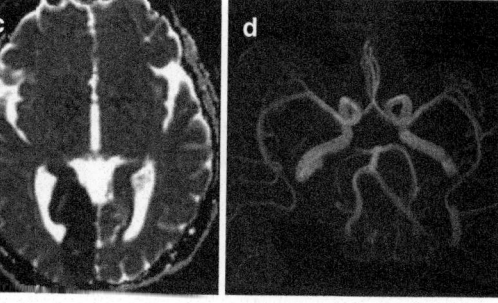

Fig. 2.6 Thirty-six-year-old patient presented with visual loss 48 h after delivery. The patient had a history of familiar hyperlipidemia. Non-contrast head CT (**a**) demonstrates an established early subacute right occipital infarct with hyperdense dot signs in the right P1 and P2 segments topography (arrows). Axial DWI and ADC map images (**b**, **c**) show corresponding diffusion restriction in the right occipital lobe, and the time-of-flight MR angiogram (TOF-MRA) of the circle of Willis (**d**) shows an occlusion at the distal P1 segment of the right posterior cerebral artery

mutation, and deficiency of protein C, S, and antithrombin III [20].

Cardio-embolic cerebral arterial occlusions may result from underlying valvular disease or from peripartum cardiomyopathy [10]. The strain of pushing during labor increases the right atrial pressure, which may facilitate paradoxical embolization through a patent foramen ovale in patients with lower extremity venous thrombosis [21]. While cervico-cranial arterial dissection (CCAD) has been described as an unusual cause of stroke in post-partum women, related to valsalva maneuvers during labor or neck hyperextension during anesthesia, no strong epidemiological evidence of an increased incidence of CCAD in pregnancy has been documented, to our knowledge [22].

Watershed infarcts result from parenchymal ischemic brain injury in the deep white matter between two major vascular territories secondary to hypotension from massive obstetric hemorrhage, sepsis, or pulmonary embolus [10].

2.6 Subarachnoid Hemorrhage (SAH)

While subarachnoid hemorrhage is a rare occurrence during pregnancy, there is a five times higher prevalence of SAH during pregnancy than that in non-pregnant women. Ruptured saccular aneurysm remains the leading cause of SAH during pregnancy. The risk of aneurysm rupture during pregnancy is increased due to hemodynamic and hormonal alterations. It commonly occurs in primigravida during the third trimester. A ruptured aneurysm is a serious condition associated with high rates of fetal (~17%) and maternal (~35%) mortality [23].

Non-contrast CT of the head demonstrates subarachnoid space hyperdensity in the suprasellar and perimesencephalic cisterns, as well as in the interhemispheric or sylvian fissures (Fig. 2.7a). Intraventricular hemorrhage may also be present. CT additionally permits evaluation of complications of SAH, including ventriculomegaly and ischemic brain injury from SAH-induced

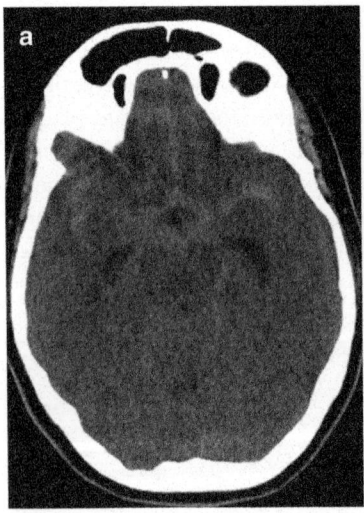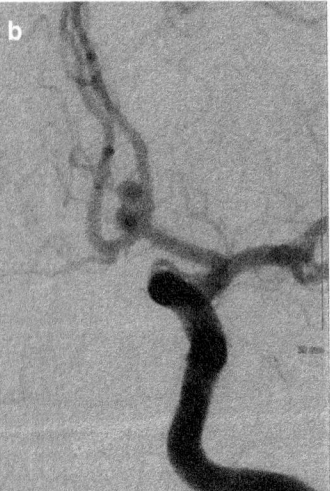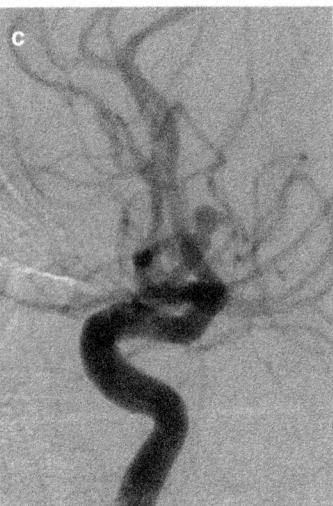

Fig. 2.7 Thirty-three-year-old primigravida, with 35 weeks' gestational age and family history of aneurysmal subarachnoid hemorrhage (SAH), presents with the worst headache of her life. Non-contrast CT scan of the head (**a**) demonstrates extensive subarachnoid hemorrhage in the suprasellar and perimesencephalic cisterns, as well as in the interhemispheric and bilateral sylvian fissures. Cerebral angiography (**b**, **c**) demonstrates a large, irregular, multi-lobulated saccular aneurysm at the junction of the A1-A2 segments of the left ACA with the anterior communicating artery

vasospasm. SAH in the perimesencephalic and/or suprasellar cisterns supports the diagnosis of a ruptured saccular aneurysm, while convexal SAH suggests RCVS of CVT. Cross-sectional vascular imaging with CTA and/or MRA are excellent ways to reveal an underlying saccular aneurysm. Aneurysms are more likely to be identified at the bifurcation of the vessels of the circle of Willis (COW) or at the origin of their main branches, for example, at the anterior communicating artery complex, middle cerebral artery bifurcation, basilar tip, or at the origins of the ophthalmic, posterior communicating, or posterior–inferior cerebellar arteries. Conventional cerebral angiography, although invasive, remains the reference standard imaging examination for the characterization of aneurysms (Fig. 2.7b, c), vascular malformations, and vasculopathy.

Ruptured intracranial aneurysms during pregnancy should be treated as they would be in non-pregnant patients. Unruptured aneurysms should be treated only if symptomatic or enlarging.

Few clinical cases of primary non-aneurysmal SAH have been reported in patients with pregnancy-induced hypertension, to our knowledge. Presenting symptoms included sharp headaches, and seizures within 2 days after delivery. CT demonstrates a small amount of unilateral SAH confined to the frontal or parietal convexities. No aneurysm is documented on cerebral angiograms performed within 2 days following the initial head CT in such patients [24].

2.7 Intracranial Hemorrhage (ICH)

ICH can occur in pregnancy as a complication of venous or arterial infarctions, or from ruptured saccular intracranial aneurysms or arteriovenous malformations (AVM). No increase in relative risk for AVM rupture has been described during pregnancy, to our knowledge [25]. Pregnancy-specific causes of ICH include eclampsia, bleeding cerebral metastases from disseminated choriocarcinoma, and pituitary apoplexy. Nonetheless, ICH in an eclamptic patient may result from a ruptured AVM (Fig. 2.8), and therefore, further imaging investigation with catheter angiography or with a dedicated MRA/CTA is indicated (Fig. 2.9).

2.8 Cerebral Venous Sinus Thrombosis (CVT)

While rare in the general population, CVT is an important and potentially fatal diagnostic consideration in pregnant women presenting with neurologic symptoms. More than 75% of CVT cases present in the post-partum period. Risk factors include caesarean section, dehydration, traumatic delivery, anemia, intracranial hypotension, puerperal infection, and poor nutrition. Presenting symptoms may mimic those of postdural puncture headache in parturient women who underwent regional anesthesia. Differential clinical diagnosis includes SAH and migraine headache [26].

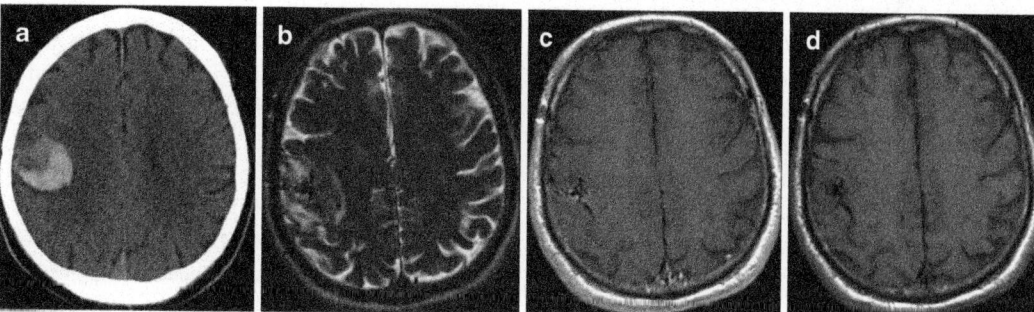

Fig. 2.8 Post-partum woman with thunderclap headache. CT head without contrast (**a**) demonstrates a right frontal ICH. An underlying structural abnormality was investigated with MRI, which demonstrated abnormal flow voids on the T2-weighted sequence (**b**) as well as on the T1-weighted sequences pre- and postintravenous contrast injection (**c**, **d**), demonstrating a vascular malformation

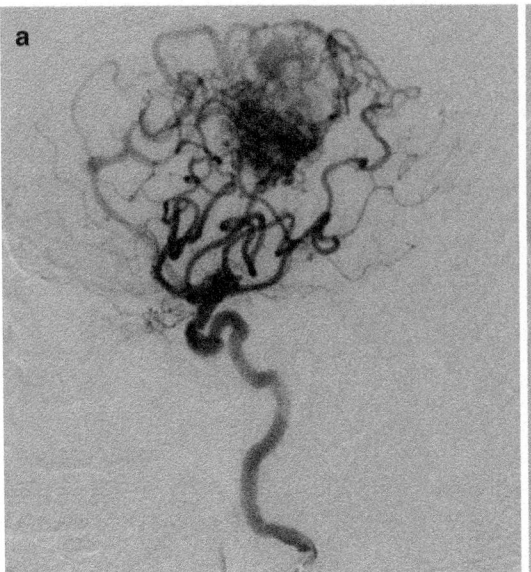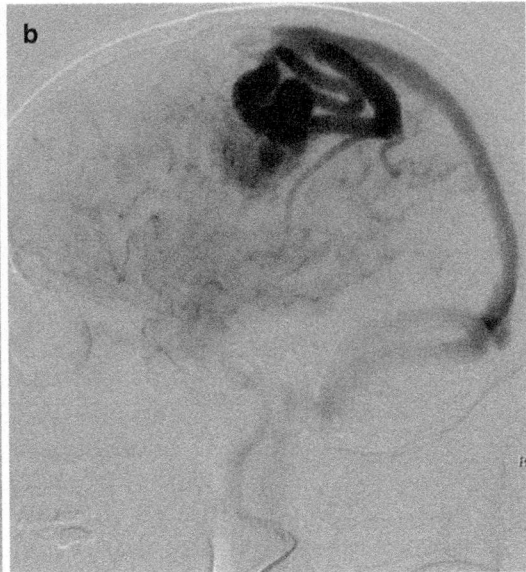

Fig. 2.9 Cerebral catheter angiogram confirms the presence of a large arteriovenous malformation (AVM) in the right fronto-parietal region. The lateral view in the arterial phase (**a**) shows multiple feeders arising from the right middle cerebral artery, a large nidus, and early drainage into a parietal cortical vein. The venous phase (**b**) shows tortuous dilated draining veins, as well as venous pouches in the region of the AVM

Intracranial venous thrombosis presents with a wide range of non-specific symptoms. The majority of patients experience progressively severe, constant, and diffuse headache which may result in focal neurological deficits and seizures. The specific clinical presentation varies according to the location and extent of thrombosis, the degree of venous collateral circulation, and associated cortical abnormalities. The intensity of symptoms fluctuates as thrombosis and fibrinolysis occur simultaneously during the course of the disease. The severity of symptoms is related to the effects of increased intracranial pressure and the presence of ICH [27]. The clinical course of CVT is unpredictable, and the clinical picture may worsen after the diagnosis. Predictors for poor outcome include alteration in consciousness and intracranial hemorrhage [28].

Treatment of CVT is supportive; while anticoagulation seems to be the treatment of choice, its use remains somewhat controversial, as approximately 50% of patients have hemorrhagic cerebral infarcts. Endovascular thrombolysis and surgical thrombectomy may be considered in severe cases [29–32].

Neuroimaging is required to confirm the diagnosis of intracranial venous thrombosis. A CT of the head is diagnostic in only one-third of patients. For stable cooperative patients, MRI of the brain and MR venography (MRV) have become the standard for diagnosis of CVT [26].

Early in the course of the disease, non-contrast head CT is likely to be unrevealing; however, hyperattenuation associated with a thrombosed venous sinus can be seen. Venous ischemic brain injury results in low attenuation of the parenchyma and loss of gray-white matter differentiation which does not conform to an arterial vascular territory (Fig. 2.10a–d) and is often associated with hemorrhagic transformation. CT venography (CTV) demonstrates filling defects representing the thrombus within the involved venous sinus (Fig. 2.10e, f).

MRI of the brain with MRV has the advantage of greater spatial and soft-tissue contrast resolution, which allows for better characterization of parenchymal edema, ischemic changes, and parenchymal hemorrhage (Fig. 2.10). MR has greater sensitivity than CT for the detection of early venous infarction, and is able to show sub-

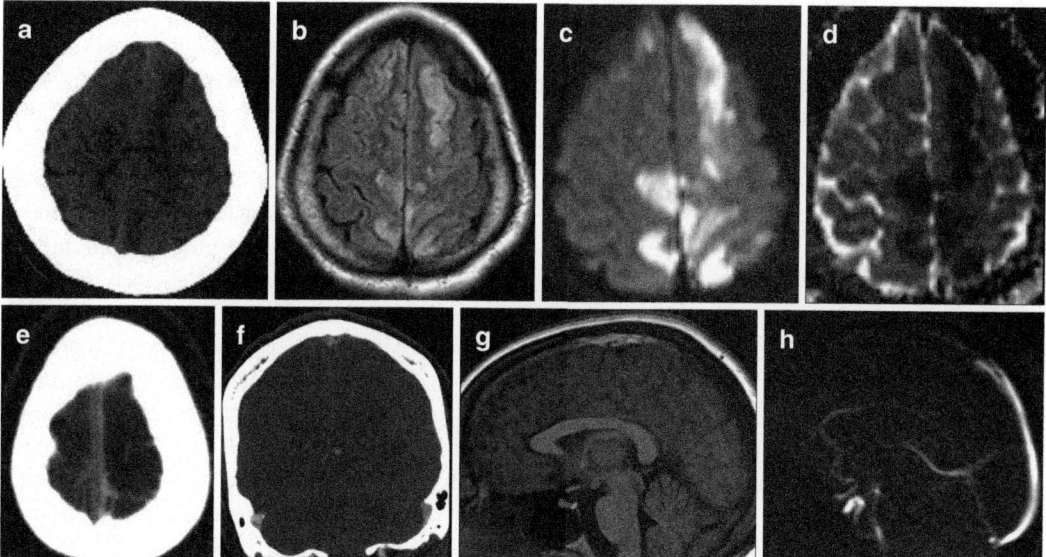

Fig. 2.10 Thirty-three-year-old woman following C-section complains of low abdominal pain, fever, and vaginal discharge as well as progressive and worsening headache 48 h after delivery. The patient was brought to the ER due to seizures. Non-contrast head CT (**a**) demonstrates abnormal low attenuation in the cortical and subcortical parenchyma of the bilateral parasagittal frontal lobes. Axial FLAIR sequence (**b**) shows corresponding signal abnormality. Axial DWI and ADC maps (**c, d**) demonstrate restricted diffusion consisting with acute/early subacute ischemic brain injury on a non-vascular territorial distribution, which in this clinical setting confirm the presence of nonhemorrhagic venous infarcts. Post-contrast CT venography of the head in the axial and coronal planes (**e, f**) demonstrates an extensive tubular filling defect along the superior sagittal sinus, which represents venous thrombosis. The sagittal T1-weighted sequence of a follow-up MRI (**g**) performed the same day, shows the hyperintense thrombus along the anterior two-thirds of the superior sagittal sinus, and a corresponding filling defect on the TOF MR venogram (**h**)

stantial differences between arterial and venous infarcts [33–35]. In venous infarcts, unlike in arterial infarcts, diffusion-weighted imaging does not exactly match the FLAIR signal abnormality, and therefore, the venous infarct will appear larger on FLAIR [35, 36]. In addition, vasogenic edema is more evident on MRI. MRI may demonstrate a lack of a normal flow void within a cerebral venous sinus as well as marked hypointensity/magnetic susceptibility within the thrombosed sinus on T2*-weighted imaging [35, 36]. An acute thrombus within a vein is isointense on T1-weighted imaging, and is hypointense on T2-weighted imaging due to the T2-shortening effect of deoxyhemoglobin, which may mimic the normal flow void within a normal sinus, and thus can potentially prevent an accurate diagnosis on conventional imaging [33–35]. A subacute thrombus, on the other hand, shows hyperintensity on both T1- and T2-weighted sequences, and is easier to identify [33–35].

MR venography adds diagnostic certainty by confirming the presence of a filling defect within a suspected thrombosed venous sinus (Fig. 2.10g, h). Time-of-flight (TOF) MRV does not require contrast, and is the preferred imaging examination when venous sinus thrombosis is suspected during pregnancy, when gadolinium should be avoided [35, 37, 38].

Both MRI/MRV and CT/CTV offer advantages and disadvantages for the diagnosis of CVT. Imaging acquisition is much faster with CT than MRI, which makes CT an extremely valuable examination for those unstable patients not able to hold still long enough for MRI acquisition. MRV prevents unnecessary ionizing radiation, but also has two potential pitfalls: difficulty in revealing the presence of clots within small cortical veins, and in revealing the difference between true thrombosis versus venous hypoplasia [35, 36]. In addition, T1 hyperintense venous clot in the subacute phase may mimic normal flow-related enhancement, and therefore, during the puerperium, gadolinium should be given as it will show lack of enhancement within the thrombosed sinus [1, 35].

2.9 Post-partum Angiopathy

Post-partum angiopathy (PPA) is one of the entities now encompassed under reversible cerebral vasoconstriction syndrome (RCVS). The common features of this syndrome are its presentation with acute severe headache and the presence of segmental constriction of the intracranial arteries, which is reversible within 3 months [39, 40].

PPA occurs usually between 1 and 3 weeks after pregnancy. Later presentations can occur but are uncommon [1]. PPA commonly follows an uncomplicated pregnancy, although some studies reported increased incidence of PPA in pregnancies complicated by proteinuria, suggesting an overlap between eclampsia and PPA [41].

RCVS occurs secondary to derangement of the cerebral autoregulation needed to maintain the cerebral blood flow [42]. PPA is thought to be related to rapid drop of progesterone levels with loss of its vasodilator effects as well as the increased levels of both pro- and antiangiogenic

factors, e.g., placental growth factor [34, 39]. Bromocriptine and ergot alkaloids sometimes used in the post-partum period can be additional triggers for PPA [34].

PPA presents with recurring thunderclap headache, which can be associated with nausea, vomiting, and photosensitivity. Other clinical manifestations include seizure, altered mental status, and focal neurological deficits if infarction or intracranial hemorrhage develops [34, 39]. While RCVS usually carries a very good prognosis with symptoms resolution in 3 weeks, it has been reported that PPA is more likely to follow a more fulminant course [39, 41, 42]. Treatment is usually supportive with administration of calcium channel blockers and discontinuation of trigger medication [34, 39, 42].

On imaging, the hallmark of PPA is the presence of multifocal stenosis giving a beaded appearance to the small and medium intracranial arteries. The changes in PPA predominantly involve the anterior circulation, as opposed to vascular changes in eclampsia predominantly affecting the posterior circulation [34]. Conventional cerebral angiography is the most sensitive modality for revealing arterial narrowing (Fig. 2.11). CT and MR angiography can also be used, with a reported sensitivity of approximately 80% of that of conventional angiography [43, 44].

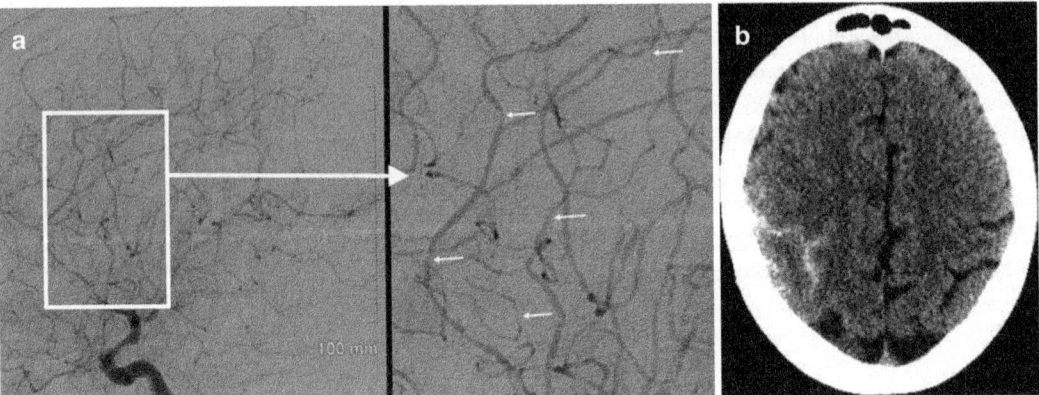

Fig. 2.11 Cerebral angiogram in a 38-year-old woman with severe headache 1 week post-partum. Injection of the right ICA reveals in the catheter angiogram (**a**) innumerable stenoses of multiple small arterial vessels (white arrows), which is highly consistent with post-partum angiopathy. The CT scan of the head (**b**) of the same patient demonstrates subarachnoid hemorrhage in the right cerebral convexity at presentation. This finding triggered the catheter angiogram in this patient

These vascular findings can be absent early after the presentation, and may only become conspicuous after the third day [42, 43, 45]. On follow-up imaging, a mixed evolution can be seen with improved stenosis in some arteries, and worsening in other arteries [43]. The vasoconstriction resolves by 3 months [39].

Other imaging findings that can be seen on non-enhanced CT and MRI include convexal subarachnoid hemorrhage (SAH) (Fig. 2.11b), which is confined to cerebral convexity sulci as opposed to the basal aneurysmal SAH, and parenchymal hemorrhage and small infarcts, usually in a watershed distribution [34, 41, 42]. Parenchymal findings of posterior reversible encephalopathy syndrome (PRES) can also be encountered in up to 38% of patients with RCVS [43].

2.10 Posterior Reversible Encephalopathy Syndrome

Posterior reversible encephalopathy syndrome (PRES) occurs with failure of cerebral autoregulation due to rapid increase in arterial blood pressure or due to endothelial dysfunction from circulating endogenous or exogenous toxins, resulting in cerebral hyperperfusion with vascular leakage and vasogenic edema [46].

Typically, PRES presents clinically with headache, altered mental status, visual symptoms, and seizures. Headache in PRES is dull in character, not thunderclap. Visual disturbances are common (40%). A seizure occurs in 90% of the patients, and usually precedes headache and visual changes. It can be focal or progress to tonic-clonic seizures [1]. The symptoms can occur in the absence of hypertension [1, 46]. It has been reported that PRES in pregnancy more commonly presents with headache, and less frequently with confusion compared to PRES secondary to other causes [47].

On imaging, PRES presents with cortical/subcortical vasogenic edema, which can be seen on CT, but which is better appreciated on MRI as symmetric T2/FLAIR hyperintensity with no diffusion restriction that resolves on follow-up

(Fig. 2.12). The parieto-occipital regions are the most common areas of involvement; however, other commonly involved areas include the superior frontal gyrus posteriorly, the precentral gyrus, the inferior temporo-occipital region, and the cerebellum [14, 48, 49].

The involvement of the brain stem and basal ganglia is less common, and can be challenging when it presents as an isolated "central variant." In these instances, alternate differential diagnoses, e.g., osmotic demyelination and encephalitis, need to be excluded [50]. While PRES is commonly symmetric, asymmetric or unilateral presentations occur and may pose diagnostic difficulty [49]. In cases of cerebellum and brainstem PRES, patients should be monitored for hydrocephalus [14]. In a few rare patients, the initial MR of the brain may be negative [51].

True diffusion restriction is atypical and occurs in a minority of patients as punctate foci within larger areas of vasogenic edema, and usually resolves with no sequelae, although larger gyral areas of diffusion restriction may occur and can progress to encephalomalacia [42, 49].

Another atypical PRES manifestation is hemorrhage, which can be subarachnoid or parenchymal. While this was thought not to be common (up to 17% of cases), some studies using susceptibility-weighted imaging (SWI) have reported a higher frequency of microhemorrhage (>50%); however, this does not correlate with the imaging or clinical severity of PRES [52].

Catheter angiography, if performed, can show reversible segmental narrowing of large and medium-sized cerebral arteries, similar to RCVS, in >85% of patients, highlighting the overlap between the two syndromes [39, 51].

2.11 Pituitary Apoplexy

Pituitary apoplexy is an uncommon condition which refers to hemorrhage or infarction of an enlarged pituitary which outgrows its blood supply in the setting of a pituitary adenoma or less likely in a physiologically enlarged pituitary

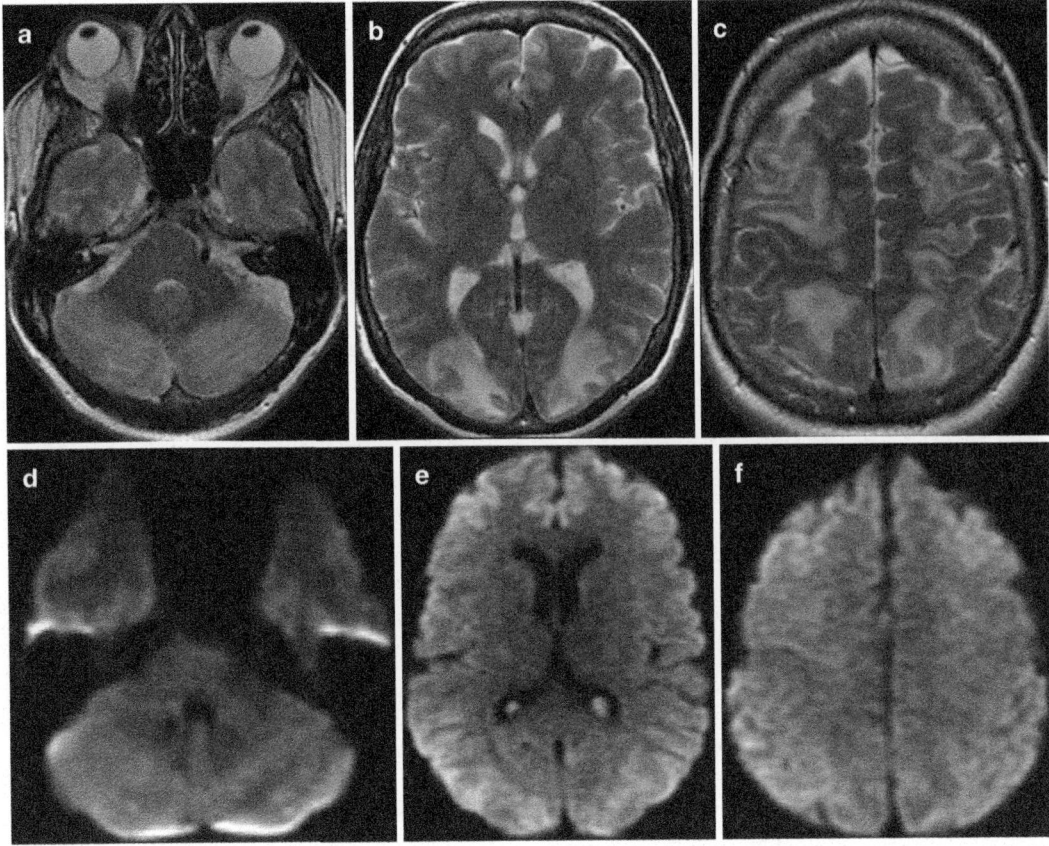

Fig. 2.12 Twenty-eight-year-old pregnant woman in her third trimester presents to the emergency department with a 2-day history of dull headache and visual disturbance. Axial T2-weighted sequences (**a–c**) show symmetric cortical/subcortical T2/FLAIR hyperintensity in the frontal, parietal, and occipital lobes, as well as in both cerebellar hemispheres without diffusion restriction (**d–f**), which is highly consistent with posterior reversible encephalopathy syndrome PRES. These findings completely resolved on follow-up imaging (not shown)

gland without an underlying focal abnormality [53–55]. The enlarged pituitary gland in pregnancy is at risk for apoplexy, although the overall incidence remains low [55, 56]. Pituitary apoplexy is often the first manifestation of a previously unknown adenoma [53, 57].

Pituitary apoplexy is a medical emergency, and a potentially fatal condition which can be diagnosed only when it presents with an acute clinical syndrome, including sudden severe headache, nausea, vomiting, decreased visual acuity, visual field deficits, ophthalmoplegia, deteriorated level of consciousness, and panhypopituitarism [54, 55].

On imaging, a sellar/suprasellar mass can be seen with possible mass effect on the optic apparatus and the hypothalamus. Patchy hyperdensity can be identified on CT, while on MRI the abnormality appears iso to hypointense on T1WI and hypointense on T2WI initially, then T1 and T2 hyperintense in the subacute phase (Fig. 2.13). T1 hyperintensity is more commonly seen along the periphery of the mass [34, 54, 57]. Pituitary apoplexy is associated with blooming on gradient echo/T2∗ imaging, and shows diffusion restriction on DWI. Non-hemorrhagic pituitary infarction is T2 hyperintense, and demonstrates diffusion restriction without blooming [54, 57].

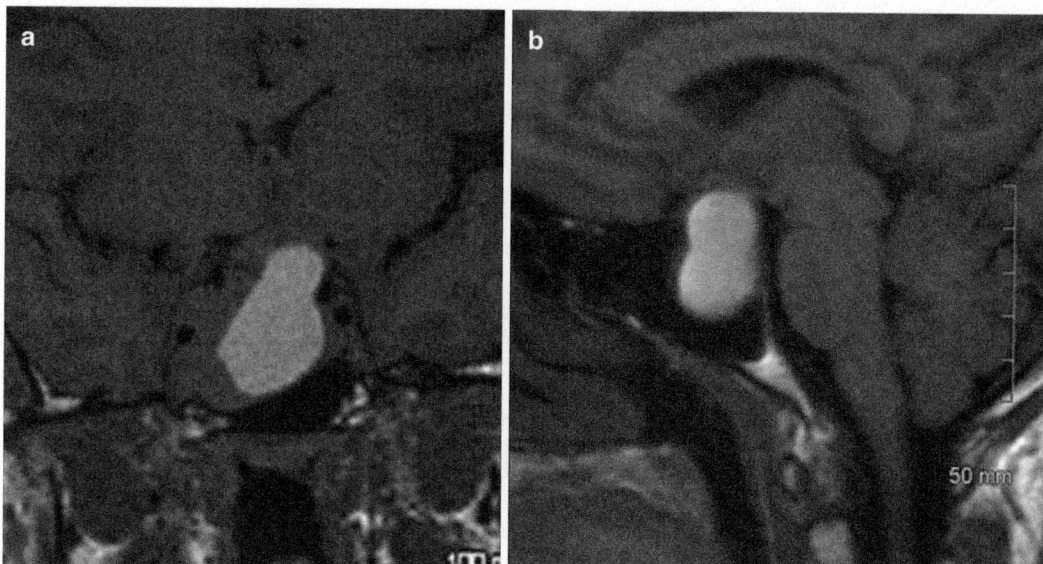

Fig. 2.13 Pituitary apoplexy. A pregnant patient presented with sudden severe headache and visual disturbance. Coronal (**a**) and sagittal (**b**) T1-weighted MR sequences show a large hyperintense sellar/suprasellar mass with a fluid level consistent with hemorrhage within an underlying adenoma, causing superior displacement and mild compression of the optic chiasm

After contrast administration, heterogenous enhancement can be seen with internal necrotic nonenhancing areas. Rim enhancement is suggestive but not pathognomonic for apoplexy. Fluid-debris level(s) are considered a specific sign for apoplexy. Sphenoid sinus mucosal thickening is also a highly indicative sign of pituitary apoplexy. Other imaging findings in pituitary apoplexy include mild adjacent dural thickening and enhancement, and rarely subarachnoid hemorrhage [54, 57].

MRI is superior to CT for the diagnosis of pituitary apoplexy, as the imaging findings can be subtle or missed on CT [54, 57]. Other differential diagnoses associated with various combinations of CT hyperdensity, T1 hyperintensity, and T2 hypointensity need to be carefully excluded, including sellar aneurysm (relation to parent artery, flow void, or opacification on angiography, and onion-skin pattern of internal signal intensity in a thrombosed aneurysm), Rathke's cleft cyst (T2 hypointense intracystic nodule and lack of enhancement or a fluid level), and craniopharyngioma (predominantly suprasellar, mixed solid and cystic with calcifications and solid enhancement) [54, 57].

2.12 Lymphocytic Hypophysitis

Lymphocytic hypophysitis (LH) is a rare inflammatory condition characterized by lymphocyte and plasma cell infiltration of the pituitary, which is idiopathic autoimmune in origin in most of the affected patients, and is due to antibodies targeting the pituitary antigens [58, 59]. LH occurs more commonly in women, and up to 70% of cases occur during pregnancy or during the post-partum period [58].

It is classified based on the site of involvement into adenohypophysitis when the anterior pituitary is involved, infundibuloneurohypophysitis when the pituitary stalk and neurohypophysis are infiltrated, and panhypophysitis when the whole pituitary is affected [34]. LH presents clinically with symptoms of endocrine dysfunction (hypopituitarism, amenorrhea, failure to lactate, and diabetes insipidus), and symptoms related to

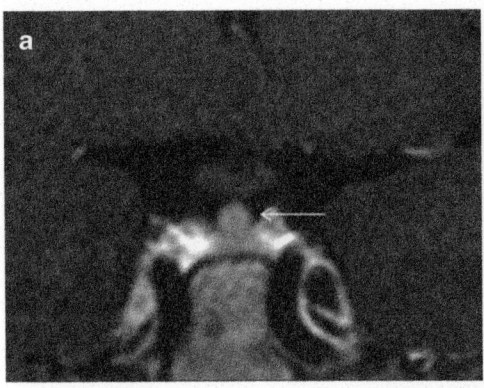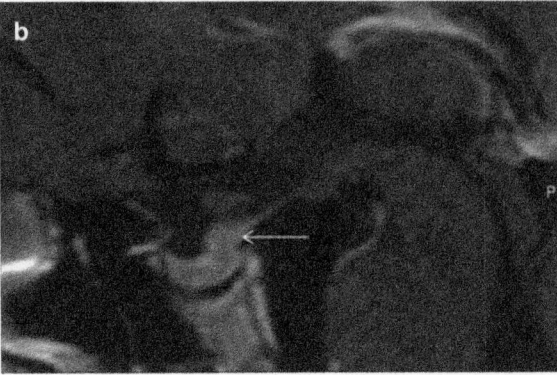

Fig. 2.14 Lymphocytic hypophysitis. Thirty-year-old post-partum woman presents with symptoms of endocrine dysfunction and diabetes insipidus. The coronal T1 (**a**) and sagittal T1-weighted (**b**) MR sequences post-contrast show substantial thickening and enhancement of the pituitary stalk (arrows). Of note, the bright spot of the neurohypophysis is not visualized

mass effect from the enlarged pituitary, including headache and visual changes [34, 59, 60].

MRI is the main imaging modality for the assessment of LH. There is usually enlargement of the gland, thickening of the pituitary stalk (>3 mm), with loss of its normal superior–inferior tapering with homogeneous enhancement (Fig. 2.14). On pre-contrast T1WI, there is loss of the posterior pituitary bright spot. The MR findings can still be confused with the more common pituitary adenoma, with 37.5% of LH cases misdiagnosed as pituitary adenoma in one report [60, 61]. Helpful MR signs favoring LH over pituitary adenoma include the loss of pituitary bright spot, intact sellar floor, thickened stalk without deviation, and homogeneous enhancement [34, 60]. On follow-up imaging, a partially empty sella can be seen as sequelae of destruction and fibrosis of the pituitary tissue [34, 60]. Conservative management with steroids and hormone replacement is the mainstay of treatment [60].

2.13 Intracranial Hypotension Syndrome Associated with Epidural Anesthesia

Intracranial hypotension syndrome is an important differential diagnosis consideration for post-partum headache in patients who were given spinal anesthesia. The onset of positional and predominantly occipital/nuchal headache occurs between 1 and 7 days post-partum. Additional symptoms include tinnitus, diplopia, and hyperacusia. Low-pressure headaches have been reported to occur in 0.5–1.5% of patients who have had spinal anesthesia. This clinical scenario has also been described during the puerperium of women without previous spinal anesthesia, presumably secondary to dural tears from labor-related pushing [62, 63].

Symptoms are likely to resolve within 48 h of a blood patch. Reported complications of intracranial hypotension, although rare, include subdural hematoma and CVT. Subdural hematomas may be either intracranial or spinal in location [62, 63].

Imaging examinations demonstrate sagging of supratentorial and infratentorial structures, pseudoenlargement of the pituitary, effacement of the suprasellar cistern, tectal beaking, flattening of the anterior pontine curvature, ectopic cerebellar tonsils (Fig. 2.15a, b), linear diffuse pachymeningeal enhancement, and decreased size of transverse and sigmoid venous sinuses. Complications of intracranial hypotension, including subdural hematomas and fluid collections, can also be identified with CT or MRI (Fig. 2.15c–f).

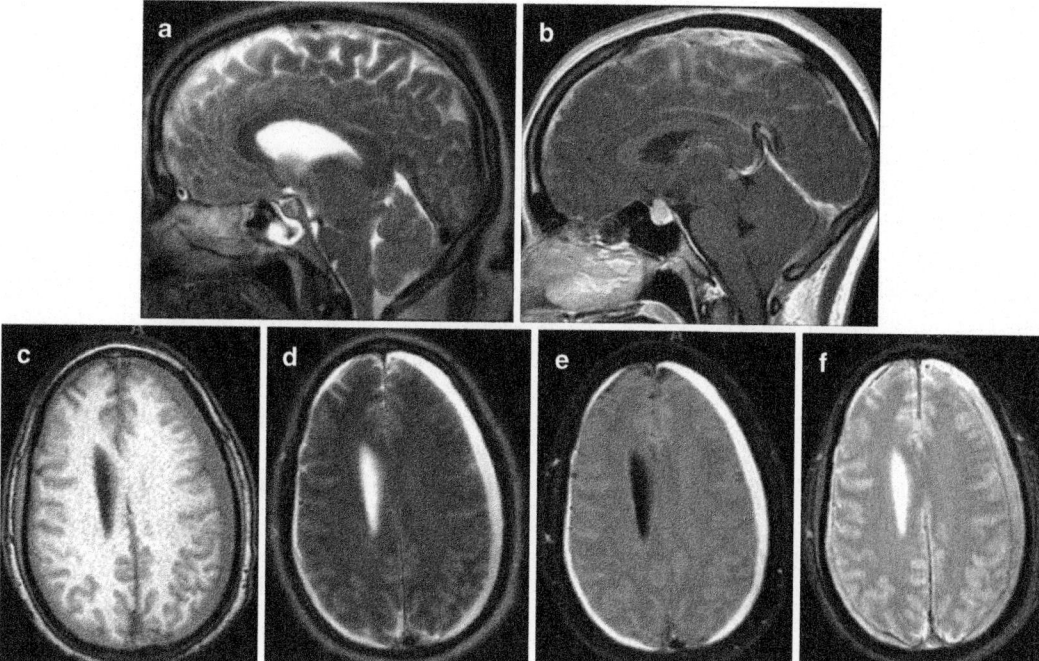

Fig. 2.15 Intracranial hypotension syndrome in a 35-year-old woman with a 10-day history of positional headaches. Symptoms developed in the immediate post-partum period. She had had spinal epidural anesthesia with accidental dural puncture. Sagittal T2 (**a**) and sagittal T1-weighted MR sequences post-contrast (**b**) demonstrate pseudo-enlargement of the pituitary, tectal beaking, ecto- pic cerebellar tonsils, flattening of the anterior curvature of the pons, and abnormal pachymeningeal enhancement, reflecting intracranial hypotension. Axial T1 (**c**), T2 (**d**), FLAIR (**e**) and gradient-echo (**f**) MR sequences demonstrate bilateral subacute subdural hematomas which predominantly contain extracellular methemoglobin with a thin peripheral rim of hemosiderin

2.14 Safety of Contrast Material Use During Pregnancy and Lactation

The movement of iodinated contrast media and gadolinium-based contrast agents (GBCAs) between the maternal and fetal circulation is partially restricted by the single-layer chorionic epithelium of the placenta [35, 64]. Therefore, studies have demonstrated measurable quantities of these agents in the fetus after intravenous administration to the mother [64, 65].

After entering the fetal bloodstream, iodinated and GBCAs could enter a vicious cycle in which they will be cleared by the kidneys into the amniotic fluid, being subsequently swallowed by the fetus and eliminated back into the amniotic fluid. It is also possible that some swallowed-contrast agent will be reabsorbed from the gut to the fetal bloodstream [35, 65, 66]. Because of this cycle, the half-life of iodinated and GBCAs in the fetal circulation is unknown, to our knowledge.

2.15 Iodinated Contrast Agents

Pregnant patients have the same risk factors as the general population for adverse reactions to iodinated contrast media [66]. Diagnostic low-osmolality contrast media (LOCM) crosses the human placenta and enters the fetus when given in usual clinical doses [65, 67, 68].

No mutagenic nor teratogenic effects have been demonstrated in in vivo tests in animals; however, no well-controlled studies of the teratogenic effects of these agents have been tested in pregnant women, to our knowledge [65, 69, 70]. As a result, LOCM is considered a U.S. FDA category-B drug (no risk demonstrated in animal studies, but no controlled studies in pregnant women) [35, 65, 66].

There has been concern regarding the use of iodinated contrast agents during pregnancy and secondary induced hypothyroidism in the fetus related to excess iodine exposure [66, 70, 71]. To date, there has been no documented case of neonatal hypothyroidism from intravascular administration of iodinated contrast agents during pregnancy, to our knowledge [70, 71]. If iodinated contrast agent has to be given during a gestation, the infant should be screened for hypothyroidism, which is a standard practice anyway in many countries; however, an extra recommendation is not worthless, since approximately 70% of babies worldwide are born in a location without established newborn screening programs for hypothyroidism [65, 72, 73].

No other adverse effects have been reported in the fetus or neonate following administration of LOCM [65]. Given there are still no available data to suggest any potential harm to the fetus from exposure to iodinated contrast media to the mother, the current recommendations are to not routinely screen for pregnancy prior to contrast media use and not to withhold its use in pregnant patients. A recommendation also supported by the FDA, as mentioned before, classifying most iodinated contrast agents as category B medications [65, 66].

2.16 Iodinated Contrast Agents During Breastfeeding

Concerns remain regarding potential toxicity to the infant from contrast media which is excreted into the breast milk. Studies have shown that limited amounts at a low rate (<1% in 24 h) of contrast media are transferred into the breast milk, and thus, the expected dose of contrast medium swallowed by an infant is extremely low [65, 74]. Also, less than 1% of the contrast media ingested is absorbed from its gastrointestinal tract. Overall, the total expected systemic dose from breast milk is 0.01%, which is far below the threshold of 10% of the therapeutic dose considered safe when

contrast media is prescribed related to an imaging examination [64, 65]. The likelihood of either directly toxic or allergic-like manifestations resulting from ingested iodinated contrast material in the infant is very low.

These findings led to the conclusion that it is safe for the mother and infant to continue breastfeeding after receiving iodinated contrast agents [35, 65, 66, 75]. If any concern remains, the mother may abstain from breastfeeding 12–24 h from the time of contrast administration, during which time breast milk should be discarded from both breasts. There is no value to stop breastfeeding for more than 24 h since contrast agents are undetectable beyond this point [65, 75].

2.17 Gadolinium-Based Contrast Agents

MR imaging is an excellent imaging modality when evaluating pregnant patients for diagnostic purposes due to its ability to image deep soft tissues without the use of ionizing radiation. In some instances, the use of intravenous GBCAs is utilized in order to add diagnostic value to MR, and thus knowing its utility and safety in this group of patients is imperative [65, 66, 76].

In animal models, GBCAs have demonstrated teratogenicity when high doses are administrated during the first trimester [35, 65]. There is a potential risk for the development of nephrogenic systemic fibrosis (NSF) in the child or mother secondary to GBCAs administration due to accumulation of gadolinium chelates in the amniotic fluid with the potential dissociations of the toxic-free gadolinium ion [76]. In a large retrospective study of over one million deliveries in Ontario, Canada, the occurrence of NSF was extremely rare, yet the use of gadolinium had a statistically significantly greater risk to the fetus of developing any rheumatological, inflammatory, or infiltrative skin condition, as well as stillbirth or neonatal death [77].

The FDA classified GBCAs as category-C drugs given the adverse effects in animal models at repeated supraclinical doses; however, they have not been thoroughly tested in humans [64, 66, 78]. The current guidelines of the FDA require labeling to indicate that the safety of GBCAs with regard to the fetus "has not been established."

The ACR Committee on Drugs and Contrast Media recommends that GBCAs should only be used if their usage is considered critical, and the potential benefits justify the potential unknown risk to the fetus. Each case should be reviewed carefully by clinicians and radiologists. When GBCAs cannot be avoided, macrocyclic agents (gadobutrol, gadoteridol, and gadoterate meglumine) should be used as they possess the highest stability with the lowest risk of gadolinium ions being released into tissues [65, 66, 76]. The lowest possible dose to achieve diagnostic results should be administered.

After an adequate explanation is given to the patient, informed consent should be obtained before the administration of any gadolinium-based contrast agent during breastfeeding.

The water solubility of GBCAs limits their excretion into breast milk. Similar to iodinated contrast media, GBCAs are nearly entirely cleared from the bloodstream in patients with normal renal function within 24 h. During this time, less than 0.04% of the intravascular dose given to the mother is excreted into the breast milk. Moreover, also similar to iodinated contrast media, less than 1% of the contrast medium ingested by the infant is absorbed from its gastrointestinal tract [71, 79]. It is likely that the minute fraction of gadolinium excreted in the breast milk is in its stable form, and thus, the likelihood of an adverse effect is remote [65].

The last ACR guidelines on this topic state that it is safe for the mother and infant to continue breastfeeding after receiving GBCAs [65]. If the mother remains concerned after facts are communicated, she may stop breastfeeding for 12–24 h after the administration of GBCAs. She may use a breast pump to obtain milk before contrast administration in order to feed the infant during the 24 h following the examination [65, 71, 79].

2.18   Conclusion

Pregnant patients have an increased risk of developing potentially life-threatening neurological disorders during and immediately after pregnancy, due to substantial physiological changes associated with the pregnant state [65]. Both CT and MRI are fundamental imaging modalities for the diagnosis of acute neurological emergencies that can compromise the life of the mother and the fetus, and therefore, the radiologist plays a key role, not only in guiding appropriate management but also contributing as a consultant regarding the risk of imaging to the fetus, helping to balance those risks with those of the mother.

References

1. Edlow JA, Caplan LR, O'Brien K, Tibbles CD. Diagnosis of acute neurological emergencies in pregnant and post-partum women. Lancet Neurol. 2013;12(2):175–85.
2. Cipolla MJ. Cerebrovascular function in pregnancy and eclampsia. Hypertension. 2007;50(1):14–24.
3. Kaplan PW, Repke JT. Eclampsia. Neurol Clin. 1994;12(3):565–82.
4. Cunningham F, Leveno K, Bloom S, Spong CY, Dashe J. Williams obstetrics. 24th ed. New York, NY: McGraw-Hill; 2014.
5. Dekker GA, Sibai BM. Etiology and pathogenesis of preeclampsia: current concepts. Obstet Gynecol. 1998;179(5):1359–75.
6. Sibai BM. Diagnosis, prevention, and management of eclampsia. Obstet Gynecol. 2005;105(2):402–10.
7. Sibai BM, Spinnato JA, Watson DL, Lewis JA, Anderson GD. Eclampsia: IV. Neurological findings and future outcome. Obstet Gynecol. 1985;152(2):184–92.
8. Steegers EA, Von Dadelszen P, Duvekot JJ, Pijnenborg R. Pre-eclampsia. Lancet. 2010;376(9741):631–44.
9. Altman D, Carroli G, Duley L, et al. Magpie Trial Collaboration Group. Do women with pre-eclampsia, and their babies, benefit from magnesium sulphate? The Magpie Trial: a randomised placebo-controlled trial. Lancet. 2002;359(9321):1877–90.
10. Dineen R, Banks A, Lenthall R. Imaging of acute neurological conditions in pregnancy and the puerperium. Clin Radiol. 2005;60(11):1156–70.
11. Watanabe Y, Mitomo M, Tokuda Y, et al. Eclamptic encephalopathy: MRI, including diffusion-weighted images. Neuroradiology. 2002;44(12):981–5.
12. Sheth RD, Riggs JE, Bodenstenier JB, Gutierrez AR, Ketonen LM, Ortiz OA. Parietal occipital edema in

hypertensive encephalopathy: a pathogenic mechanism. Eur Neurol. 1996;36(1):25–8.

13. Schwartz RB, Feske SK, Polak JF, et al. Preeclampsia-eclampsia: clinical and neuroradiographic correlates and insights into the pathogenesis of hypertensive encephalopathy. Radiology. 2000;217(2):371–6.

14. Bartynski WS. Posterior reversible encephalopathy syndrome, part 1: fundamental imaging and clinical features. Am J Neuroradiol. 2008;29(6):1036–42.

15. Lewis LK, Hinshaw DB, Will AD, Hasso AN, Thompson JR. CT and angiographic correlation of severe neurological disease in toxemia of pregnancy. Neuroradiology. 1988;30(1):59–64.

16. Kittner SJ, Stern BJ, Feeser BR, et al. Pregnancy and the risk of stroke. N Engl J Med. 1996;335(11):768–74.

17. Tiel Groenestege AT, Rinkel GJ, van der Bom JG, Algra A, Klijn CJ. The risk of aneurysmal subarachnoid hemorrhage during pregnancy, delivery, and the puerperium in the Utrecht population: case-crossover study and standardized incidence ratio estimation. Stroke. 2009;40(4):1148–51.

18. Ros HS, Lichtenstein P, Bellocco R, Petersson G, Cnattingius S. Increased risks of circulatory diseases in late pregnancy and puerperium. Epidemiology. 2001;12(4):456–60.

19. Kuklina EV, Tong X, Bansil P, George MG, Callaghan WM. Trends in pregnancy hospitalizations that included a stroke in the United States from 1994 to 2007: reasons for concern? Stroke. 2011;42(9):2564–70.

20. James AH, Bushnell CD, Jamison MG, Myers ER. Incidence and risk factors for stroke in pregnancy and the puerperium. Obstet Gynecol. 2005;106(3):509–16.

21. Daehnert I, Ewert P, Berger F, Lange PE. Echocardiographically guided closure of a patent foramen ovale during pregnancy after recurrent strokes. J Interv Cardiol. 2001;14(2):191–2.

22. Tettenborn B. Stroke and pregnancy. Neurol Clin. 2012;30(3):913–24.

23. Dias MS, Sekhar LN. Intracranial hemorrhage from aneurysms and arteriovenous malformations during pregnancy and the puerperium. Neurosurgery. 1990;27(6):855–66.

24. Shah AK. Non-aneurysmal primary subarachnoid hemorrhage in pregnancy-induced hypertension and eclampsia. Neurology. 2003;61(1):117–20.

25. Horton JC, Chambers WA, Lyons SL, Adams RD, Kjellberg RN. Pregnancy and the risk of hemorrhage from cerebral arteriovenous malformations. Neurosurgery. 1990;27(6):867–72.

26. Bousser M. Cerebral venous thrombosis: diagnosis and management. J Neurol. 2000;247(4):252–8.

27. Cantu C, Barinagarrementeria F. Cerebral venous thrombosis associated with pregnancy and puerperium. Review of 67 cases. Stroke. 1993;24(12):1880–4.

28. Masuhr F, Mehraein S, Einhäupl K. Cerebral venous and sinus thrombosis. J Neurol. 2004;251(1):11–23.

29. De Bruijn S, Stam J. Randomized, placebo-controlled trial of anticoagulant treatment with low-molecular-weight heparin for cerebral sinus thrombosis. Stroke. 1999;30(3):484–8.

30. Mas J, Lamy C. Stroke in pregnancy and the puerperium. J Neurol. 1998;245(6-7):305–13.

31. Philips MF, Bagley LJ, Sinson GP, et al. Endovascular thrombolysis for symptomatic cerebral venous thrombosis. J Neurosurg. 1999;90(1):65–71.

32. Weatherby S, Edwards NC, West R, Heafield M. Good outcome in early pregnancy following direct thrombolysis for cerebral venous sinus thrombosis. J Neurol. 2003;250(11):1372–3.

33. Alvis JS, Hicks RJ. Pregnancy-induced acute neurologic emergencies and neurologic conditions encountered in pregnancy. Semin Ultrasound CT MR. 2012;33(1):46–54.

34. Kanekar S, Bennett S. Imaging of neurologic conditions in pregnant patients. Radiographics. 2016;36(7):2102–22.

35. Haber MA, Nunez D. Imaging neurological emergencies in pregnancy and puerperium. Emerg Radiol. 2018;25(6):673–84.

36. Ferro JM, Canhão P. Cerebral venous sinus thrombosis: update on diagnosis and management. Curr Cardiol Rep. 2014;16(9):523.

37. Klein JP, Hsu L. Neuroimaging during pregnancy. Semin Neurol. 2011;31(04):361–73.

38. Razmara A, Bakhadirov K, Batra A, Feske SK. Cerebrovascular complications of pregnancy and the postpartum period. Curr Cardiol Rep. 2014;16(10):532.

39. Miller TR, Shivashankar R, Mossa-Basha M, Gandhi D. Reversible cerebral vasoconstriction syndrome, part 1: epidemiology, pathogenesis, and clinical course. Am J Neuroradiol. 2015;36(8):1392–9.

40. Singhal AB, Bernstein RA. Postpartum angiopathy and other cerebral vasoconstriction syndromes. Neurocrit Care. 2005;3(1):91–7.

41. Fugate JE, Ameriso SF, Ortiz G, et al. Variable presentations of postpartum angiopathy. Stroke. 2012;43(3):670–6.

42. Hacein-Bey L, Varelas PN, Ulmer JL, Mark LP, Raghavan K, Provenzale JM. Imaging of cerebrovascular disease in pregnancy and the puerperium. Am J Roentgenol. 2016;206(1):26–38.

43. Miller TR, Shivashankar R, Mossa-Basha M, Gandhi D. Reversible cerebral vasoconstriction syndrome, part 2: diagnostic work-up, imaging evaluation, and differential diagnosis. Am J Neuroradiol. 2015;36(9):1580–8.

44. Ducros A. Reversible cerebral vasoconstriction syndrome. Lancet Neurol. 2012;11(10):906–17.

45. Lemmens R, Smet S, Wilms G, Demaerel P, Thijs V. Postpartum RCVS and PRES with normal initial imaging findings. Acta Neurol Belg. 2012;112(2):189–92.

46. Fischer M, Schmutzhard E. Posterior reversible encephalopathy syndrome. J Neurol. 2017;264(8):1608–16.

47. Liman TG, Bohner G, Heuschmann PU, Scheel M, Endres M, Siebert E. Clinical and radiological

differences in posterior reversible encephalopathy syndrome between patients with preeclampsia-eclampsia and other predisposing diseases. Eur J Neurol. 2012;19(7):935–43.

48. Pereira PR, Pinho J, Rodrigues M, et al. Clinical, imagiological and etiological spectrum of posterior reversible encephalopathy syndrome. Arq Neuropsiquiatr. 2015;73(1):36–40.

49. McKinney AM, Short J, Truwit CL, et al. Posterior reversible encephalopathy syndrome: incidence of atypical regions of involvement and imaging findings. Am J Roentgenol. 2007;189(4):904–12.

50. McKinney AM, Jagadeesan BD, Truwit CL. Central-variant posterior reversible encephalopathy syndrome: brainstem or basal ganglia involvement lacking cortical or subcortical cerebral edema. Am J Roentgenol. 2013;201(3):631–8.

51. Junewar V, Verma R, Sankhwar PL, et al. Neuroimaging features and predictors of outcome in eclamptic encephalopathy: a prospective observational study. Am J Neuroradiol. 2014;35(9): 1728–34.

52. McKinney AM, Sarikaya B, Gustafson C, Truwit CL. Detection of microhemorrhage in posterior reversible encephalopathy syndrome using susceptibility-weighted imaging. Am J Neuroradiol. 2012;33(5):896–903.

53. Abraham RR, Pollitzer RE, Gokden M, Goulden PA. Spontaneous pituitary apoplexy during the second trimester of pregnancy, with sensory loss. BMJ Case Rep. 2016;2016:bcr2015212405.

54. Boellis A, di Napoli A, Romano A, Bozzao A. Pituitary apoplexy: an update on clinical and imaging features. Insights Image. 2014;5(6):753–62.

55. Schoen JC, Campbell RL, Sadosty AT. Headache in pregnancy: an approach to emergency department evaluation and management. West J Emerg Med. 2015;16(2):291.

56. De Heide LJ, Van Tol KM, Doorenbos B. Pituitary apoplexy presenting during pregnancy. Neth J Med. 2004;62(10):393–6.

57. Goyal P, Utz M, Gupta N, et al. Clinical and imaging features of pituitary apoplexy and role of imaging in differentiation of clinical mimics. Quant Imag Med Surg. 2018;8(2):219.

58. Imber BS, Lee HS, Kunwar S, Blevins LS, Aghi MK. Hypophysitis: a single-center case series. Pituitary. 2015;18(5):630–41.

59. Tirosh A, Hirsch D, Robenshtok E, et al. Variations in clinical and imaging findings by time of diagnosis in females with hypopituitarism attributed to lymphocytic hypophysitis. Endocr Pract. 2015;22(4): 447–53.

60. Gubbi S, Hannah-Shmouni F, Stratakis CA, Koch CA. Primary hypophysitis and other autoimmune disorders of the sellar and suprasellar regions. Rev Endocr Metab Disord. 2018;19(4):335–47.

61. Leung GK, Lopes MS, Thorner MO, Vance ML, Laws ER. Primary hypophysitis: a single-center experience in 16 cases. J Neurosurg. 2004;101(2):262–71.

62. Oliver CD, White SA. Unexplained fitting in three parturients suffering from postdural puncture headache. Br J Anaesth. 2002;89(5):782–5.

63. Vaughan DJ, Stirrup CA, Robinson PN. Cranial subdural haematoma associated with dural puncture in labour. Br J Anaesth. 2000;84(4):518–20.

64. Tirada N, Dreizin D, Khati NJ, Akin EA, Zeman RK. Imaging pregnant and lactating patients. Radiographics. 2015;35(6):1751–65.

65. ACR Committee on Drugs and Contrast Media. ACR manual on contrast media, version 10.3. 2018.

66. Puac P, Rodríguez A, Vallejo C, Zamora CA, Castillo M. Safety of contrast material use during pregnancy and lactation. Magn Res Imag Clin. 2017;25(4):787–97.

67. Moon AJ, Katzberg RW, Sherman MP. Transplacental passage of iohexol. J Pediatr. 2000;136(4):548–9.

68. Vanhaesebrouck P, Verstraete AG, De Praeter C, Smets K, Zecic A, Craen M. Transplacental passage of a nonionic contrast agent. Eur J Pediatr. 2005;164(7):408–10.

69. Morisetti A, Tirone P, Luzzani F, de Haën C. Toxicological safety assessment of iomeprol, a new X-ray contrast agent. Eur J Radiol. 1994;18:S31.

70. Tremblay E, Thérasse E, Thomassin-Naggara I, Trop I. Quality initiatives: guidelines for use of medical imaging during pregnancy and lactation. Radiographics. 2012;32(3):897–911.

71. Bourjeily G, Chalhoub M, Phornphutkul C, Alleyne TC, Woodfield CA, Chen KK. Neonatal thyroid function: effect of a single exposure to iodinated contrast medium in utero. Radiology. 2010;256(3):744–50.

72. Dayal D, Prasad R. Congenital hypothyroidism: current perspectives. Res Rep Endocr Disord. 2015;5(5):91–102.

73. LaFranchi SH. Worldwide coverage of newborn screening for congenital hypothyroidism-a public health challenge. US Endocrinol. 2014;10(2):115–6.

74. Nielsen ST, Matheson I, Rasmussen JN, Skinnemoen K, Andrew E, Hafsahl G. Excretion of iohexol and metrizoate in human breast milk. Acta Radiol. 1987;28(5):523–6.

75. Parkash V, Fadare O, Tornos C, McCluggage WG. Committee Opinion No. 631: endometrial intraepithelial neoplasia. Obstet Gynecol. 2015;126(4):897.

76. Czeyda-Pommersheim F, Martin DR, Costello JR, Kalb B. Contrast agents for MR imaging. Magn Reson Imag Clin. 2017;25(4):705–11.

77. Ray JG, Vermeulen MJ, Bharatha A, Montanera WJ, Park AL. Association between MRI exposure during pregnancy and fetal and childhood outcomes. JAMA. 2016;316(9):952–61.

78. De Santis M, Straface G, Cavaliere AF, Carducci B, Caruso A. Gadolinium periconceptional exposure: pregnancy and neonatal outcome. Acta Obstet Gynecol Scand. 2007;86(1):99–101.

79. Sachs HC. The transfer of drugs and therapeutics into human breast milk: an update on selected topics. Pediatrics. 2013;132(3):e809.

Imaging of Thoracic and Cadiovascular Emergencies During Pregnancy

3

Pratik Mukherjee, Shobhit Mathur,
Omar Metwally, Saman Fouladirad,
Ana-Maria Bilawich, and Savvas Nicolaou

Contents

P. Mukherjee (✉)
Woodlands Health Campus, Singapore, Singapore

S. Mathur
University of British Columbia,
Vancouver, BC, Canada

University of Toronto, Toronto, ON, Canada

O. Metwally · S. Fouladirad · A.-M. Bilawich
S. Nicolaou
University of British Columbia,
Vancouver, BC, Canada
e-mail: saman.fouladirad@alumni.ubc.ca;
savvas.nicolaou@vch.ca

© Springer Nature Switzerland AG 2020
M. N. Patlas et al. (eds.), *Emergency Imaging of Pregnant Patients*,
https://doi.org/10.1007/978-3-030-42722-1_3

3.1   Introduction

Imaging has become a mainstay of evaluation of patients presenting with thoracic emergencies in the emergency department (ED). Of all the patients presenting to an ED, pregnant patients are a unique cohort. Pregnancy is a special condition in a woman's life and warrants a particularly specialized approach to imaging. The reason for this is twofold. First, a pregnant patient cannot be considered as only one patient, as the life of the fetus is directly related to the mother and, secondly, radiation concerns in this cohort of patients are of paramount importance, especially the dose to the fetus. Ionizing radiation from medical imaging should be avoided as much as possible in principle, especially during the first trimester, when organogenesis takes place [1, 2].

Most of the thoracic emergencies arising in pregnant women are not much different from those arising in the general population, except for a few conditions which warrant special mention, including pulmonary embolism, amniotic fluid embolism (AFE), peripartum cardiomyopathy, and pregnancy-associated spontaneous coronary artery disease (P-SCAD). Maternal cardiovascular collapse arising in the third trimester is now rare, with the overall reported risk of maternal death estimated at 6.5 in 100,000 deliveries. The most common etiologies are pre-eclampsia (16%), AFE (14%), hemorrhage (12%), cardiac disease (11%), and pulmonary thromboembolism (9%) [3, 4].

For this chapter, we have broadly divided the thoracic emergencies as follows:

Classification of Thoracic Emergencies
- Lung:
  – Pulmonary embolism.
  – Infection/pneumonia.
  – Pulmonary arteriovenous malformation (PAVM).
  – Amniotic fluid embolism.
- Cardiac:
  – Pregnancy-associated spontaneous coronary artery disease (P-SCAD).
  – Peri-partum cardiomyopathy (PCM).
  – Mitral stenosis.
  – Myocardial infarction.
- Others:
  – Chest trauma: rib fractures, aortic injury, etc.

3.2   Physiological Changes in Pregnancy

During pregnancy, the mother undergoes remarkable changes, both anatomical and physiological [5]. Table 3.1 lists the major cardiovascular and respiratory changes which routinely occur in pregnancy. For this chapter, we will only consider the changes in coagulation system, as the female body goes into a physiological hypercoagulable state with increasing concentration of certain clotting factors, particularly VIII, IX, and X, and fibrinogen levels, which rise up to 50% [7, 8]. Thus, pregnancy alters the balance within the coagulation system in favor of clotting, predisposing the pregnant and the post-partum woman to venous thrombosis. This state persists from the first trimester until at least 12 weeks following

Table 3.1 Normal physiological changes in pregnancy

Cardiovascular		Respiratory	
Increased	Cardiac output	Increased	Tidal volume
	Total blood volume (35–50%)		Minute ventilations
	Plasma volume (up to 1.5 L)		Central respiratory drive
Decreased	Systolic and diastolic BP	Decreased	Total respiratory compliance
	Pulmonary vascular resistance		DLCO
	Serum proteins (increased hypercoagulability)		
Others	Dilutional anemia	Others	Mild compensatory alkalosis
			Hyperemia and edema of airway mucosa

Reference: Adapted from [6]

delivery. The mother is predisposed to deep venous thrombosis and an increased risk of pulmonary embolism, which can be aggravated by other factors, including prolonged periods of bed rest in the third trimester, reduced exercise, and long-haul airline flights [9].

3.3 First-Line Conventional Imaging Modalities

3.3.1 Radiographs

Chest radiographs are the first-line imaging modality which should be used in mos patients presenting with thoracic emergencies. Chest radiography is routinely used in the emergency setting and is a low radiation dose examination for screening and, in many patients, obviates the need for further imaging involving higher radiation dose, particularly CT. In the example below, a pregnant patient presented with shortness of breath, and the initial diagnosis was pulmonary embolism. However, the chest radiograph revealed a pneumothorax, thereby revealing the correct diagnosis quickly without requiring CT (Fig. 3.1).

Further discussion of the role of chest radiographs will be covered in specific conditions in the later sections.

3.3.2 Ultrasound

Ultrasound has a relatively limited role in thoracic emergencies, including in pregnancy. It can occasionally be used for pneumothorax evalua-

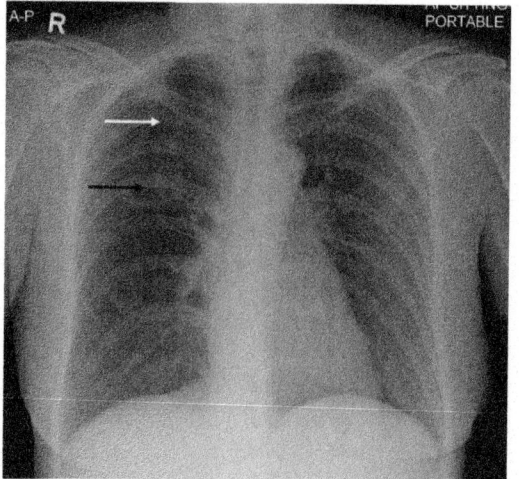

Fig. 3.1 Frontal chest radiograph of a pregnant woman shows a moderately sized right pneumothorax (white arrow). Note the increased density (black arrow) in the upper zone of the collapsed right lung which was described as a cavitating mass. This turned out to be a primary malignancy (adenocarcinoma) on histopathology

tion while also performing a bedside ultrasound of the abdomen in trauma patients. The diagnostic value is, however, operator dependent, as with any sonographic examination, and radiography is still the preferred imaging modality to diagnose or exclude a pneumothorax.

Transesophageal ultrasound is a very useful imaging examination in very selected circumstances in pregnant and non-pregnant patients, to look for valvular infection, blood clots, or other cardiac disorders which cannot be detected on routine echocardiography or on other less invasive cross-sectional imaging examinations [4].

3.4 Second-Line Imaging Modalities

We will discuss the role of advanced imaging modalities in the relevant sections.

3.5 Lung Emergencies

3.5.1 Pulmonary Embolism

Pulmonary embolism (PE) is partial or complete obstruction of a pulmonary artery or usually one or more of its branches unilaterally or bilaterally, which is usually produced by a blood clot which has originated in a deep vein of the leg or pelvis, and which has travelled to the lungs. When the clot burden is acute and substantial, signs and symptoms in both pregnant and non-pregnant patients can include labored breathing, chest pain, fainting, rapid heart rate, cyanosis, shock, and sometimes death. Pregnancy is associated with an up to fivefold increased prevalence of venous thromboembolism due to the factors discussed in earlier sections [10]. It is the leading preventable cause of maternal death during pregnancy. It is of paramount importance to diagnose PE in pregnant patients as it has important implications in terms of delivery planning, prolonged anticoagulation therapy, and possible prophylaxis for future pregnancies [11].

Due to variable institutional practices worldwide depending on resource availability and individual practices of clinicians and radiologists, the clinical pathway for evaluating this subset of patients is highly variable. In this chapter, we will familiarize radiologists with the current available guidelines, the advantages, and disadvantages of different tests available, and introduce our own institutional algorithm [12–14]. We will briefly discuss the current estimates of radiation exposure to mother and fetus from the relevant imaging examinations for suspected pulmonary embolism in pregnancy.

3.5.1.1 Diagnostic Dilemma
While the diagnosis of pulmonary embolism based on the clinical features is challenging in the non-pregnant patient population, the clinical diagnosis of pulmonary embolism in pregnant patients is further complicated by the overlap of usual signs and symptoms of PE (and deep venous thrombosis) with the usual physiological changes of pregnancy, including leg swelling, pain, tachycardia, tachypnea, and dyspnea [15]. For the treating physician or other health care practitioner, it is a clinical dilemma to triage these patients based on established parameters, including the Wells and Geneva criteria, which have not been validated for pregnant patients [13, 16]. Dyspnea in pregnancy has a broad differential diagnosis, which includes physiological changes, PCM, pulmonary edema, AFE, spontaneous pneumothorax, and complications of rare conditions including gestational trophoblastic disease [17].

3.5.1.2 D-dimer Assay
A relatively reliable laboratory examination in the non-pregnant adult population, D-dimer assays are generally elevated in pregnancy and progressively increase as the pregnancy advances, thereby increasing false-positive results [18]. Table 3.2 summarizes the gestation-specific D-dimer values in a longitudinal cohort

Table 3.2 Gestational age-specific D-dimer reference intervals

	2.5th percentile (90% CI)	97.5th percentile (90% CI)	Samples	Outliers
First trimester Gestational weeks <15	0.2 (0.2–0.2)	0.9 (0.8–0.9)	222	13
Second trimester Gestational weeks 15–27	0.2 (0.2–0.2)	1.5 (1.4–1.6)	1412	12
Third trimester Gestational weeks >27	0.4 (0.4–0.5)	2.8 (2.6–3.1)	971	20

The 2.5th and 97.5th percentiles with 90% confidence intervals (in brackets) are given
Reference: Adapted from [19]

study performed between June 2006 and October 2007 on 801 healthy Danish women with expected normal pregnancies. D-dimer values were repeatedly measured during pregnancy, at active labor, and on the first and second post-partum days and gestation-specific percentiles were calculated and were subsequently transformed to percentiles for the relevant gestational age or delivery group.

The authors concluded that the conventional negative predictive threshold of 0.5 mg/L for D-dimer is of limited use during pregnancy due to a high number of false positives and, hence, a particularly elevated D-dimer threshold throughout pregnancy cannot be provided. A gestational age-specific reference interval is required and, even then, due to the presence of many outliers, D-dimer values should be interpreted with caution [19].

3.5.1.3 Chest Radiography

Chest radiography is the first-line imaging modality in a pregnant patient presenting with dyspnea and other signs or symptoms of suspected PE. It is a baseline low radiation dose examination and is used to screen and to diagnose or exclude other causes of thoracic signs and symptoms, including pneumothorax and pneumonia. A definitive alternate diagnosis generally obviates the need for further imaging, particularly computed tomography (CT). A normal radiograph does not exclude pulmonary embolism [10], but helps to determine the need to perform lung scintigraphy (Fig. 3.2) [20].

3.5.1.4 Lower Extremity Ultrasound (US)

Lower extremity sonography is a non-invasive imaging examination with no known contraindications in pregnancy. As in non-pregnant individuals, it allows for direct evaluation of deep venous thrombosis with gray-scale imaging, compression technique, and color and spectral flow Doppler. Failure of a vein or veins to compress completely indicates the presence of a DVT. This method has limitations, particularly a large body habitus and/or overlying edema. In

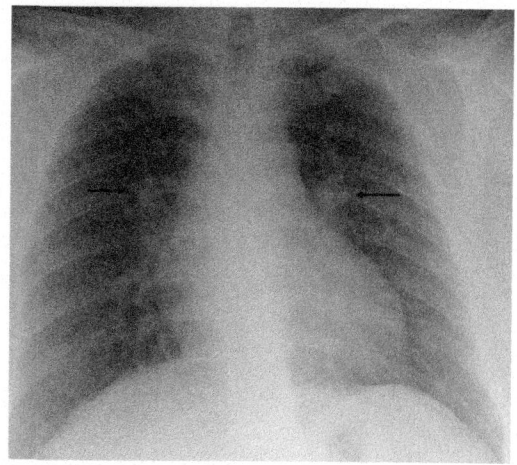

Fig. 3.2 Frontal chest radiograph of a 26-year-old pregnant woman presenting with chest pain and shortness of breath. Note perihilar vascular prominence (black arrows). No focal consolidation or pleural effusion was detected. The patient had a history of pulmonary embolism

obese patients, the use of color Doppler is helpful to adequately localize and evaluate the vessels. In a recently published article by Cascio et al., the authors recommended the use of low frequency (2 MHz) transducers and tissue harmonic imaging in obese patients as beneficial. The technique is based on the concept that sound intensity increases with depth to a point proportional to the non-linearity coefficient of a tissue, fat in this context [21]. Augmentation of the veins by compressing the calf and/or performing plantar flexion complements the analysis [22]. Graded-compression sonography has a sensitivity of 97% and a specificity of 94% for the diagnosis of symptomatic femoral-popliteal DVT in the general population [23].

The main advantage of US is that a positive result excludes the need to do any further imaging in most patients, especially involving ionizing radiation, and anticoagulation therapy can be started if there are no contraindications (Fig. 3.3).

Overall, the estimated prevalence of venous thrombosis in pregnant patients ranges between 0.06% and 8%, although the actual prevalence among clinically suspected PE cases is uncertain to our knowledge [24, 25]. Of note is a unique

Fig. 3.3 Ultrasound of the left lower limb reveals a thrombus in the mid-segment of the left femoral vein

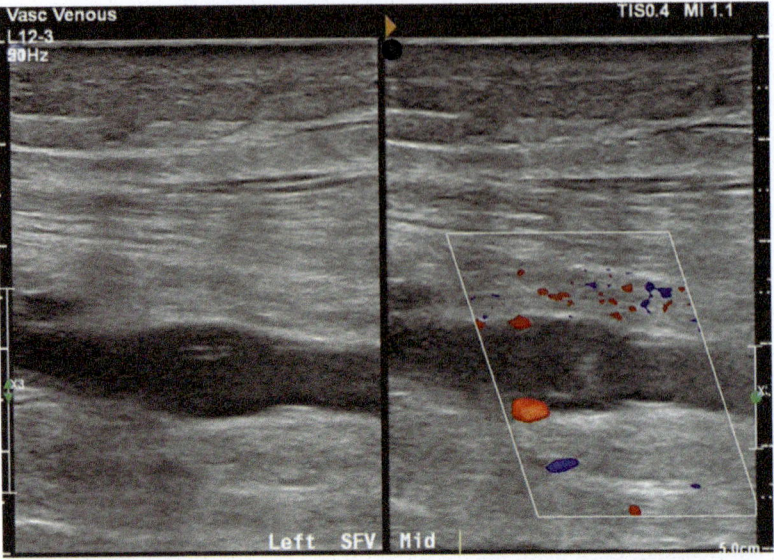

Fig. 3.4 Ultrasound of the left lower leg demonstrates thrombosis of the common femoral vein with no flow

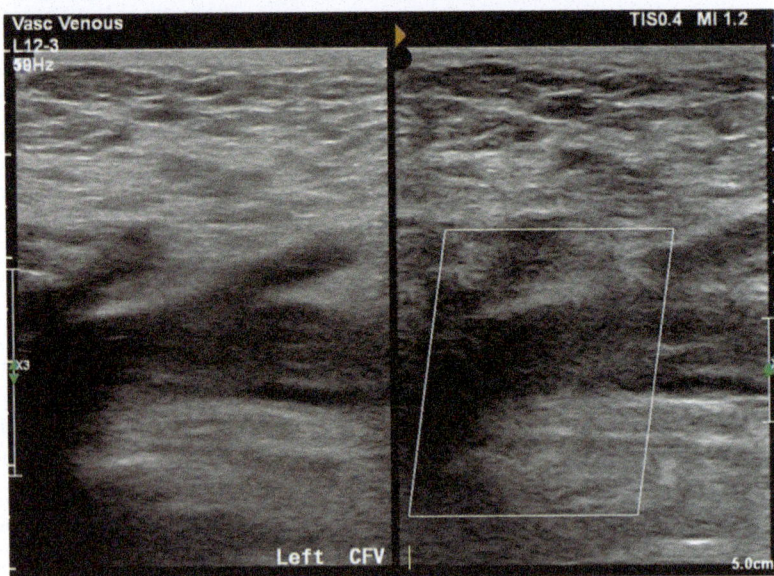

predisposition of left-sided DVT in pregnant patients (Fig. 3.4).

This is presumably due to compression of the left common iliac vein by the crossing right iliac artery and/or the gravid uterus, and is seen in approximately 75–96% of cases [24]. Table 3.3 summarizes the symptoms of DVT and PE.

Although without risk, inexpensive, and readily available, sonography is less accurate for pel-

vic vein thrombosis because of their deep location. Secondly, the size of the gravid uterus in the latter half of pregnancy, coupled with the technical difficulty of performing graded compression in the pelvis, makes it extremely difficult to image these veins. Studies show that pelvic MRI is of value in these patients, as it shows better detail and extent of the thrombosis, and complements the role of ultrasound in

Table 3.3 Symptoms of DVT and/or PE

	DVT	PE
Symptoms (in decreasing order of frequency)	Swelling (88%)	Dyspnea
	Extremity discomfort (79%)	Tachypnea
	Difficulty walking (21%)	Tachycardia
	Lower abdominal pain, back pain and whole leg swelling—think of isolated iliac vein thrombosis	Chest pain

pregnant patients [26]. Also, a negative examination does not exclude pulmonary embolism and warrants additional investigation, typically with computed tomography [10, 23].

3.5.1.5 Computed Tomography

Computed tomography is performed as a definitive test in patients where the radiograph is normal, and the patient is symptomatic. It has advantages and disadvantages enumerated in Table 3.4.

CT pulmonary angiography is an important diagnostic imaging examination which gives clinicians a definitive diagnosis in most pregnant patients and provides an alternate diagnosis in patients without imaging evidence of PE (Fig. 3.5).

A role of dual energy CT has been established in assessing for pulmonary embolism and looking for areas of pulmonary infarction on ventilation–perfusion mismatch maps (Fig. 3.6).

Radiation exposure to maternal breast and fetus, and potential risks to iodinated contrast material, are the relative disadvantages of CT, although the latter is a relatively minor disadvantage in pregnant patients. Physiological changes of increased circulatory volume and altered cardiac output can directly affect the quality of the examination and increase flow artifacts, thereby reducing the diagnostic quality [25]. In cases where the CT is non-diagnostic, patients may need serial ultrasound or repeat CT.

Table 3.4 CT pulmonary angiography: advantages, disadvantages, and clinical implications

Component	Description
Advantages	High sensitivity and specificity based on multiple trials in the general population. Easy access, short acquisition time, and interpretation Definitively depicts clot and provides alternate diagnosis in negative cases Negative test effectively excludes diagnosis of pulmonary embolism in most low- to intermediate-risk populations
Disadvantages	Physiologic changes of pregnancy may increase the non-diagnostic rate High maternal breast radiation dose Inherent false-positive and false-negative rates, especially in low- and high-risk patients, respectively, according to clinical risk criteria Risk associated with use of iodinated contrast material
Clinical implications	Provides confident diagnosis Estimation of clot burden may be useful for comparison to future examinations. Alternative diagnosis (e.g., pneumonia) may stop work-up Non-diagnostic results may require repeat examination or serial US

Reference: Adapted from [10]

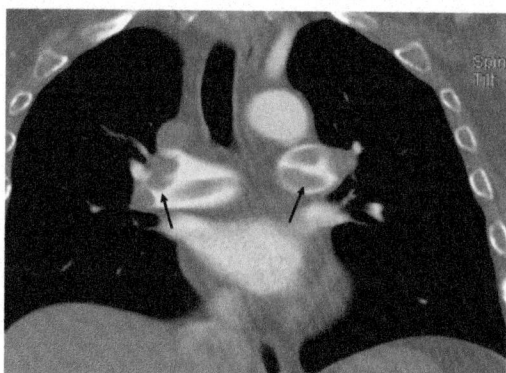

Fig. 3.5 Coronal IV contrast-enhanced CT image of a young pregnant woman shows filling defects in both main pulmonary arteries (arrows) which are saddle pulmonary emboli

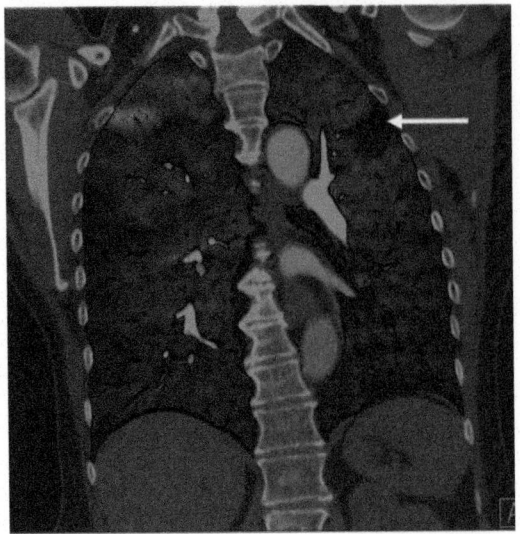

Fig. 3.6 Coronal ventilation–perfusion maps obtained using the lung algorithm for this young pregnant woman, the V/Q mismatch aided in detecting PE. On the source CT pulmonary angiogram images, no definite filling defect was detected

Table 3.5 Reducing radiation dose to maternal breast and fetus in CT pulmonary angiography

Modifiable CT factors	External factors	Workflow modification
Reduction in tube current Reduction in tube voltage Increase in pitch Increase in detector collimation thickness Reduction of z-axis	Thin-layer bismuth breast shield Lead shielding Oral barium preparation	Elimination of lateral scout image Fixed injection timing rather than test run

Reference: [10, 27–29]

Radiation Dose Reduction Techniques in CT

The radiologist has an important role to play when pregnant patients are imaged, and familiarity with available radiation dose reduction methods used in CT pulmonary angiography is of paramount importance, and should be guided by the "as low as reasonably achievable" principle. Table 3.5 summarizes the currently available dose reduction methods.

3.5.1.6 Ventilation-Perfusion Scan

Scintigraphy may be diagnostic when the radiographs are normal, if the results are indicative of a high probability of pulmonary embolism. In a study by Scarsbrook et al., 73–92% of V/Q scans in pregnant patients demonstrated normal findings (Fig. 3.7) [25].

Studies have recommended that the diagnostic accuracy of a V/Q scan increases upwards of 97% in patients with normal chest radiographs, and with no history of asthma or chronic lung disease (Fig. 3.8) [20, 29, 30]. Compared to the V/Q scan, which has a sensitivity of 41%, CT angiography has an overall higher sensitivity (81–91%) and a specificity (93–97%) for the identification of emboli in the main, lobar, and segmental pulmonary arteries as compared to the V/Q scan [30]. Studies have demonstrated that both have comparable performance in the diagnosis of PE, with no statistically significant difference across trimesters between the proportions of positive, negative, and indeterminate results. All studies conclusively demonstrated that maternal dose was consistently higher with CT angiography, whereas the fetal dose was less across all trimesters [29, 31–33].

Table 3.6 summarizes the salient features of lung scintigraphy.

Radiation Dose Reduction Techniques Used for V/Q Scans

Table 3.7 enumerates some commonly used fetal dose reduction techniques.

Centers around the world routinely eliminate the ventilation component of the scan and reduce the dose of the perfusion component to 50%, without compromising the accuracy of the examination, and significantly reducing the maternal and fetal radiation dose [30, 32]. Repeated studies have proven the ability to make an accurate diagnosis on perfusion scans alone [34, 35].

Finally, we have included a summary table (Table 3.8) comparing the radiation doses of various modalities used in the detection of pulmonary embolism.

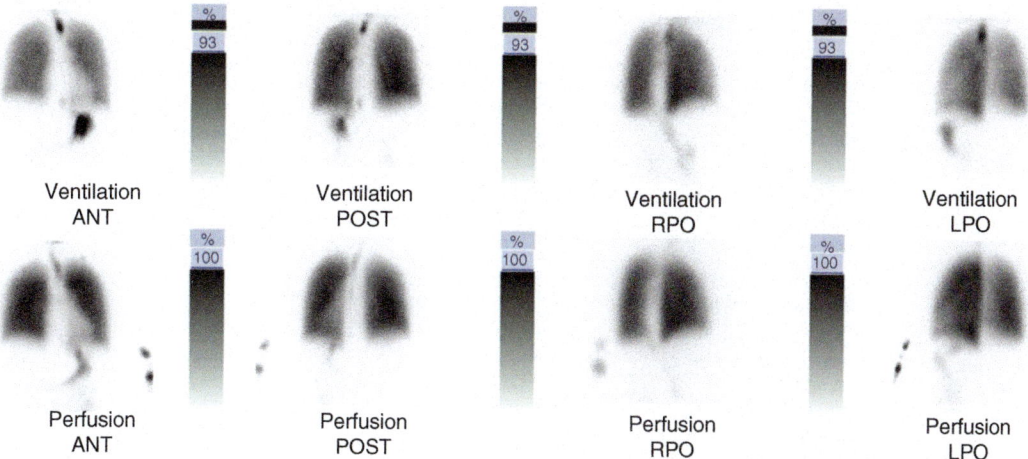

Fig. 3.7 Tc-99m DTPA ventilation scan and Tc-99m MAA perfusion scan was performed on this young pregnant woman presenting with acute onset dyspnea and an intravenous iodinated contrast allergy. No evidence of V-Q mismatch was detected

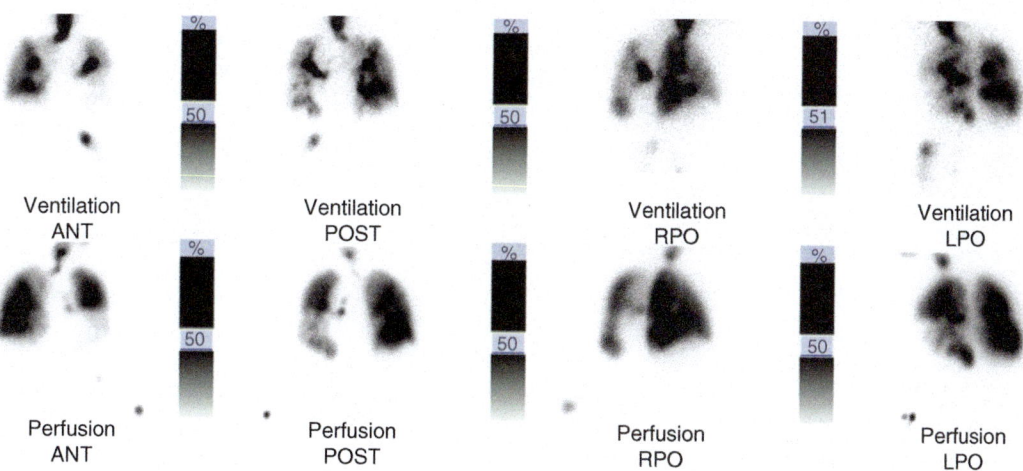

Fig. 3.8 Tc-99m DTPA ventilation scan and Tc-99m MAA perfusion scan were performed on this young pregnant woman presenting with acute onset dyspnea. Ventilation scan shows mostly central tracer deposition, probably related to suboptimal ventilatory effort. Small size perfusion defects are seen in the left lower lobe, involving the lateral and anteromedial basal segments. A small perfusion defect is also noted in the right lower lobe, superior segment. Overall, the examination was interpreted as intermediate probability of pulmonary embolism, according to PIOPED criteria

3.5.1.7 Magnetic Resonance Imaging

Magnetic resonance imaging (MRI) has a limited role in thoracic emergencies in general, particularly in the evaluation of suspected pulmonary embolism in pregnant patients. There have been a few studies which have looked at the role of MR angiography using modified techniques for improving spatial resolution, shortened acquisition time, and motion artifacts in the general population. Protocols which combine true fast imaging with steady-state precession and gadolinium-enhanced perfusion MR angiography (MRPA) performed with a parallel acquisition technique have demonstrated high specificity and sensitivity for PE (93% and 100%), respectively, in the general population compared to

Table 3.6 Ventilation–perfusion scan advantages, disadvantages, and clinical implications

Component	Description
Advantages	Radionuclides used are considered safe in pregnancy and pose minimal inherent risk
	Low maternal breast radiation (30- to 630-fold less than with CT pulmonary angiography)
	Age and health status of majority of pregnant population minimizes non-diagnostic rate compared with the general population
Disadvantages	Inability to provide an alternative diagnosis in the absence of pulmonary embolism
	Limited access and interpretability after hours at some centers
	Long acquisition time
	3–25% non-diagnostic rate leading to further imaging
Clinical implications	Clinically helpful only if normal probability, low probability, or high probability
	Withholding treatment in low-risk patients with non-diagnostic results may be acceptable
	Non-diagnostic rate reduced by excluding patients with lung disease or abnormal chest radiographs
	Fetal dose minimized with use of low-dose perfusion—only technique without compromising accuracy
	Can be used in patients with contrast material allergy or impaired renal function
Future	Mixed recommendations as initial second-line test favored by PIOPED II investigators as a means of imaging in pregnancy
	Lower breast dose and lower non-diagnostic rate in the pregnant population may suggest a role later during pregnancy or the post-partum period, when the radiation risk to glandular breast tissue is presumed higher

Reference: Adapted from Pahade et al. [10]

Table 3.7 Fetal dose reduction in V/Q scan

Reduce dose of ventilation agent
Reduce dose of perfusion agent
Eliminate ventilation portion of the scan
Increase patient hydration
Encourage frequent voiding or insert Foley catheter to reduce fetal exposure to radiotracer accumulation in the bladder

Table 3.8 Summary of effective dose of various imaging modalities to mother and fetus

Examination	Effective whole-body dose (mSv)	Fetal dose (mGy)	Effective dose/breast (mGy)
PA chest radiograph	0.06–0.25	0.01	
Low radiation dose perfusion scintigraphy	0.6–1.0	0.1–0.37	0.11–0.3
V/Q scintigraphy	1.2–6.8	0.1–0.8	0.22–0.28
Pulmonary CTA	2–20	0.01–0.66	10–70
Background radiation	2.5	1.1–2.5	

Reference: Adapted from [10]

16-detector CT pulmonary angiography [36, 37]. However, there are not enough studies to evaluate the role of non-contrast MRPA for the detection of PE, much less the role of IV contrast-enhanced MRPA due to the contraindication of gadolinium during pregnancy [38, 39].

MR has a very limited role in the evaluation of pulmonary infections, and a secondary role in the evaluation of suspected aortic dissection, and will be discussed in the relevant sections.

3.5.2 Infection

Pneumonia along with pulmonary embolism was one of the commonest causes of fatality in the pregnant population in the United States between 1974 and 1978 [40]. There have been concerns that due to known physiological and immunological changes in pregnancy, these patients may be more predisposed pneumonia, have recurrent infections, have atypical features, and run a longer course than the usual population. It has been widely reported that during pregnancy there is a change in the cellular immunity which is protective to the fetus [41]. There are a host of hormonal changes in pregnancy involving progesterone, human chorionic gonadotrophin, cortisol, and alpha-fetoprotein, which may inhibit the cell-mediated immune system, and theoretically increase the risk of infection, especially fungal and viral [41–43]. During pregnancy, the gravid uterus elevates the diaphragm by up to 4 cm, and splays the thoracic cage by up to 5–7 cm. This is turn reduces the ability to clear secretions, reduces the functional residual capacity, and increases oxygen consumption, overall increasing vulnerability to lung infection [44].

The incidence of pneumonia in pregnancy is difficult to estimate, as there are multiple factors including geographic location, socioeconomic status of the patient, and other considerations [45].

The diagnosis of pneumonia in a healthy woman with no prior cardiorespiratory disease is usually straightforward in patients presenting with symptoms of cough, dyspnea, and fever. Usual initial testing includes bloodwork and a postero-anterior chest radiograph. The role of the lateral radiograph is limited in a pregnant patient due to the higher maternal dose and limited diagnostic benefit, although studies have shown that the dose to conceptus is negligible [46, 47]. Chest radiographic findings range from peribronchial thickening, increased bronchovascular markings, and air-space disease in earlier stages, to dense consolidation with or without pleural effusions in frank pneumonia. Patients can also have lobar collapse secondary to mucus plugging (Figs 3.9 and 3.10).

CT is usually reserved for problem solving or to exclude complications including lung abscess formation and/or empyema, where the manage-

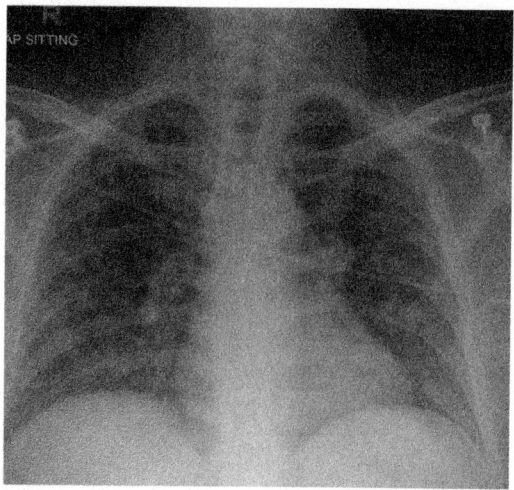

Fig. 3.9 Chest radiograph demonstrates multifocal areas of consolidation in this young pregnant woman who presented with shortness of breath and fever of a few days' duration

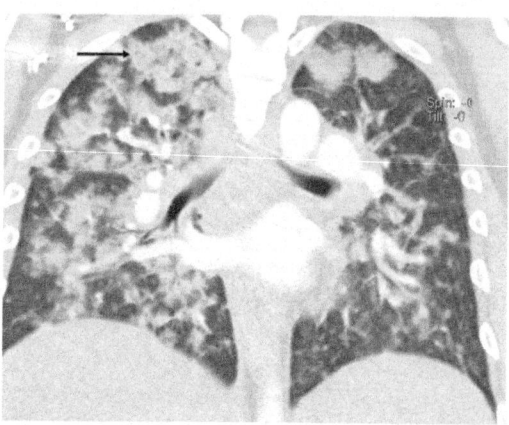

Fig. 3.10 Chest CT coronal projection of the same patient demonstrates multi-focal pneumonia ranging from patchy air-space disease to dense consolidation (black arrow)

ment of the patient may change substantially. While imaging these patients, it should be remembered to follow the CT dose reduction techniques as discussed in Table 3.5.

The CT features of viral and bacterial pneumonia do not vary much due to the basic similarity in the underlying pathologic process. The broad spectrum of CT findings of viral pneumonia includes: (a) disturbance in parenchymal attenuation; (b) ground-glass opacity and air-space disease; (c) nodules and tree-in-bud opacities; (d) interlobular septal thickening; and (e) bronchial wall thickening (Figs. 3.11 and 3.12) [43].

The role of chest MRI in the diagnosis of pneumonia was reported by Syrjala et al.; the authors reported an accuracy comparable to chest radiography, and almost similar accuracy compared with HRCT [48]. However, the results have

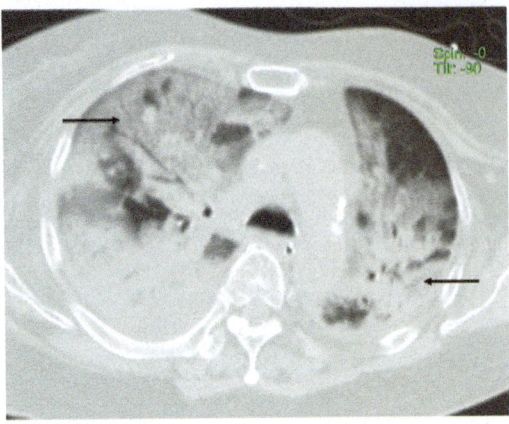

Fig. 3.11 Axial CT image, lung window, demonstrates bilateral lobar consolidation, interlobular septal thickening (arrow), and ground-glass opacities, findings which are consistent with pneumonia in this pregnant patient who presented with shortness of breath and fever. The differential diagnosis would primarily be pulmonary hemorrhage, especially in post-partum patients

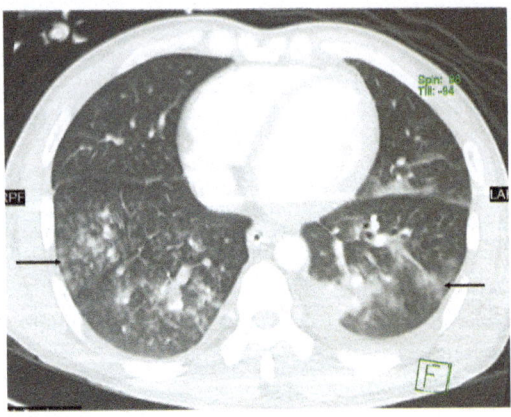

Fig. 3.12 Axial CT image, lung window, of this pregnant woman demonstrates scattered areas of "tree-in bud" opacities associated with interlobar septal thickening (black arrows). There is also dense consolidation seen in the posterobasal segment of the left lower lobe

not been replicated in any other major studies, and further studies need to be conducted on pregnant patients to establish its role. Another potential role of MRI of the chest is in patients with tuberculosis and especially in the assessment of treatment, to avoid additional radiation exposure in this subset of patients who may require repeated follow-up imaging examinations. Imaging findings of consolidation in the lung are inhomogeneous signal intensity on T1- and T2-weighted images, compared with the normal lung which shows no visible signal [48, 49].

3.5.3 Pulmonary Arteriovenous Malformations (PAVMs)

PAVMs are rare anomalous direct communications between arteries and veins of the pulmonary vasculature. They are usually associated with hereditary hemorrhagic telangiectasia (HHT), an autosomal dominant vascular disorder, whereas only 10–20% of cases are sporadic [50]. The natural history of these conditions is to increase in size. This is, however, accelerated in certain conditions, including puberty, pulmonary arterial hypertension, and pregnancy. Usually asymptomatic, in pregnancy due to the physiological hemodynamic changes and enhanced right-to-left shunting, it is quite common for patients to become symptomatic and to be diagnosed with this condition for the first time, usually in the first or second trimesters [51]. The symptoms are usually dyspnea, hypoxia, and pulmonary hypertension. Due to overlap of symptoms, these patients are initially thought to have a pulmonary embolism, a far more common cause of respiratory distress in pregnancy. Chest radiographs are the first line of investigation in patients presenting with these symptoms, and although the chest radiographic appearance may not be specific, careful examination reveals focal tubular/nodular opacities in the lungs (Fig. 3.13).

More definitive imaging is performed with CT without and/or with IV contrast [51, 52]. CT demonstrates the detailed anatomic location and type of PAVM, which are most commonly seen in the lower lobes [53]. On IV contrast-enhanced CT images, PAVMs are a cluster of serpiginous vessels with enhancement of the feeding artery, a central area, and a draining vein or veins, all demonstrated on early-phase images (Fig. 3.14).

Radionuclide perfusion scanning has a selected role in the diagnosis of this condition (Fig. 3.15).

Table 3.9 summarizes the imaging findings of a simple-type PAVM.

The presence of a single or multiple untreated PAVM during pregnancy has been associated with a high risk of life-threatening complications, including hemoptysis, rupture, hemothorax, hypovolemic shock, and rarely death, with significant increase in morbidity and mortality [51, 55]. Although not followed in all countries, detection and treatment of asymptomatic pregnant women is recommended [56]. Patients with HHT should be considered a high-risk group. The treatment of PAVM is usually the same as general population guidelines. After initial diagnosis, symptomatic patients should be treated with transcatheter angioembolization to prevent the complications arising in late pregnancy or post-partum. International consensus guidelines recommends the selection of PAVMs for embolization based on feeding artery diameter, generally 3 mm or greater, although targeting PAVMs with feeding artery diameter as low as 2 mm may be appropriate (Fig. 3.16) [57].

Surgical resection or lobectomy is reserved for more florid cases and when there is hemodynamic instability. Post-delivery, these patients should be followed up lifelong as per established guidelines. Patients with suspected HHT should be referred to a geneticist for further evaluation [51, 58, 59].

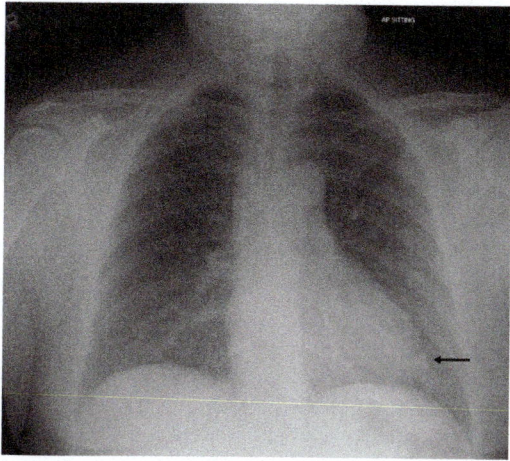

Fig. 3.13 Chest radiograph demonstrates nodular opacities in the left lower zone, retrocardiac location (black arrow). The patient subsequently had an IV contrast-enhanced CT thorax performed, which revealed a pulmonary arteriovenous malformation

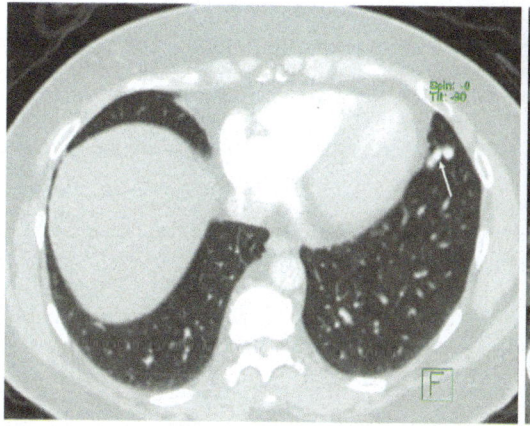
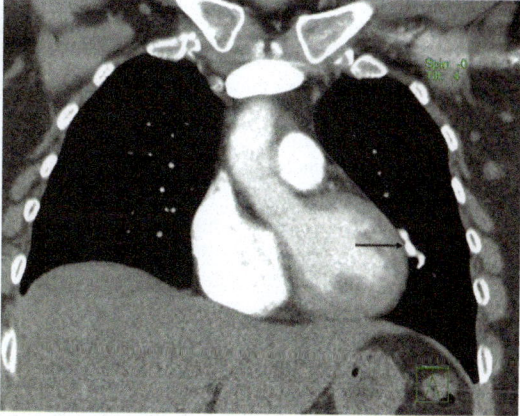

Fig. 3.14 IV contrast-enhanced chest computed tomography axial (left) and coronal images (right) of this young pregnant woman demonstrate a high-density large nodular focus with dilated and serpiginous connecting vessels in the inferior lingular segment (white arrow on axial and the black arrow on coronal images)

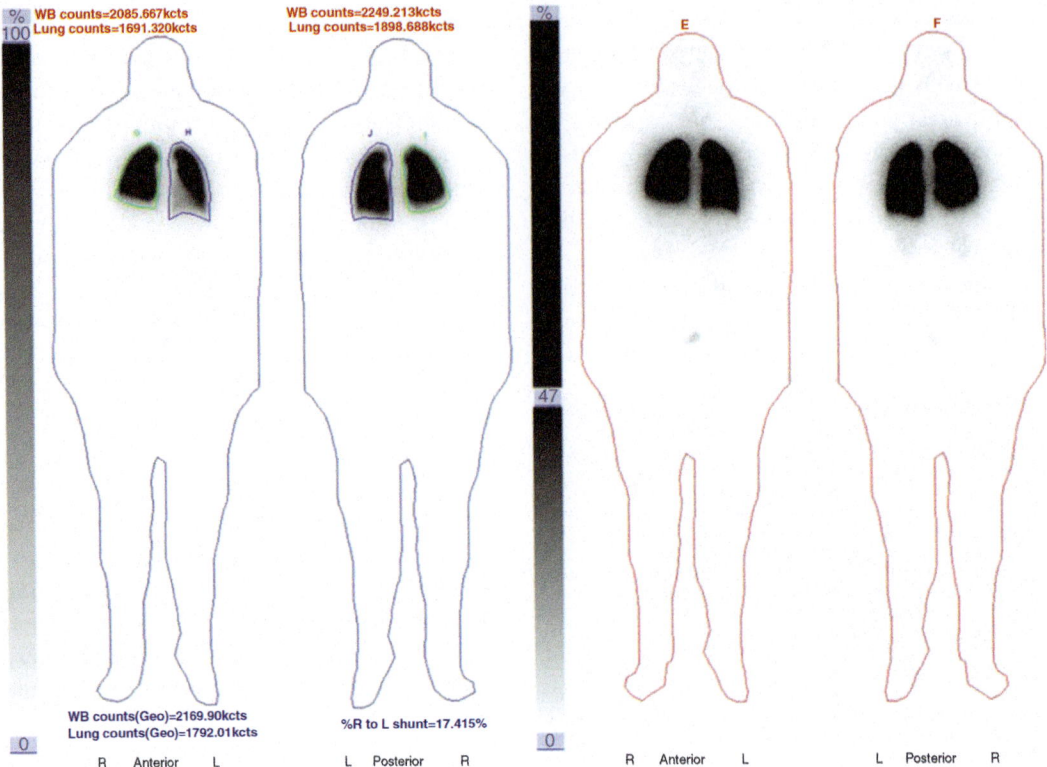

Fig. 3.15 Whole-body imaging and planar images of the lung were performed following injection of Tc-99m-MAA. There is a normal uniform distribution of Tc-99m-MAA in both lungs. There was visible localization of Tc-99m-MAA in brain, kidneys, and bladder (not shown for the purpose of this chapter). A calculated systemic component of the total injected Tc-99m-MAA is 17.4%. This examination indicated mild arteriovenous shunting in the lungs, with a right-to-left shunt fraction of 17.4%

Table 3.9 Imaging features of pulmonary arteriovenous malformations

Modality	Findings
Chest radiograph	Solitary or cluster of nodular opacities, usually in the lower lobes; sometimes seen as a soft-tissue opacity, occasionally calcifications/phleboliths may be seen
Computed tomography	Homogeneous, well-circumscribed, non-calcified nodule measuring up to several centimeters in diameter or the presence of a serpiginous mass that is connected to blood vessels; contrast is not mandatory to make a diagnosis or anatomic visualization [54] Post-contrast: enhancing serpiginous mass with a demonstration of feeder artery, aneurysm component, with draining vein or veins Images should be acquired in the arterial phase
Perfusion scintigraphy	Tc-99m MAA in the brain pre-treatment demonstrates right-to-left shunts, appears as matched V/Q defects, and corresponds to radiographic opacity.; post-treatment of AVM, brain uptake is not seen
Catheter angiography	Used for treatment of PAVMs

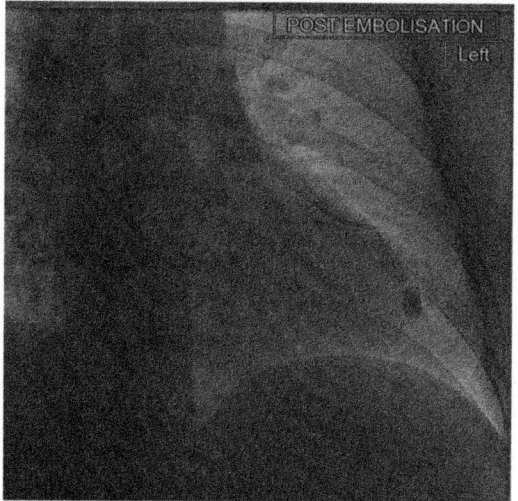

Fig. 3.16 Post-PAVM embolization image of a PAVM in the inferior lingular segment shown earlier in Fig. 3.14

3.5.4 Amniotic Fluid Embolism

Amniotic fluid embolism is a rare, highly fatal complication of pregnancy and childbirth, with a reported maternal mortality rate of 80% [60]. AFE is a non-thrombotic pulmonary embolism and develops when the amniotic fluid is forced into the bloodstream through tears in the uterine veins during normal labor. It has been reported that some cases may occur when the placenta is disrupted during surgery or trauma [61]. Table 3.10 summarizes the symptoms, signs, and imaging features of this condition.

The management of AFE is usually supportive, and involves a multi-disciplinary approach.

3.6 Cardiac Emergencies

3.6.1 Myocardial Infarction

The incidence of acute myocardial infarction (AMI) and coronary artery disease (CAD) is quite low in women of reproductive age group, approximately 0.6–1 per 10,000 pregnancies, as has been shown by population-based studies in the United States [65, 66]. In pregnancy, the risk of AMI increases up to threefold compared to women of

Table 3.10 Symptoms, signs, and imaging characteristics of amniotic fluid embolism

Symptoms and signs	Dyspnea, shock, cyanosis with rapid progression to cardiopulmonary collapse, and fulminant pulmonary edema Occasionally features of disseminated intravascular coagulation Central nervous system symptoms—convulsions and hyperreflexia can occur [61–63]
Imaging findings	
Chest radiographs	Diffuse bilateral heterogeneous and homogeneous areas of increased opacity, which are indistinguishable from acute pulmonary edema from other causes (Fig. 3.17) [64]; pulmonary edema Pearl: Look for cardiomegaly to distinguish from ARDS
CT	Non-specific findings—ill-defined centrilobular ground-glass opacities with a predilection for the lower lobes (Fig. 3.18); detection of micro-emboli on CT is almost never possible CT is very helpful in evaluating for alternative causes, including ARDS, diffuse pulmonary hemorrhage, and aspiration pneumonia (Fig. 3.19) [63]

the same age group who are not pregnant, ranging between 5% and 37% [67, 68]. Most maternal fatalities occur at the time or within 2 weeks of infarction, usually in the peri-partum period. Fetal death, usually associated with maternal death, occurs in 12–34% patients [69]. As always, hormonal and hemodynamic changes, and changes in autoimmune status, have been implicated as possible etiological factors [70].

After initial preliminary diagnosis with electrocardiography, patients usually undergo CT coronary angiography. Cardiac catheterization is reserved for urgent circumstances, for therapy after diagnostic findings on CT coronary angiography, or when non-invasive imaging is non-diagnostic and there is continued clinical concern [71]. Coronary arterial dissection, which is discussed in detail in the next section, is the most common cause of AMI in pregnant patients, followed by atherosclerosis, clots, and occasionally coronary arterial spasm [70].

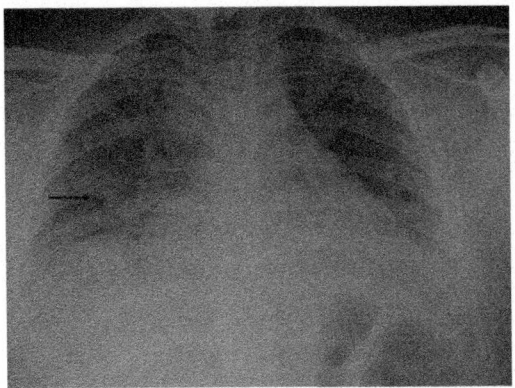

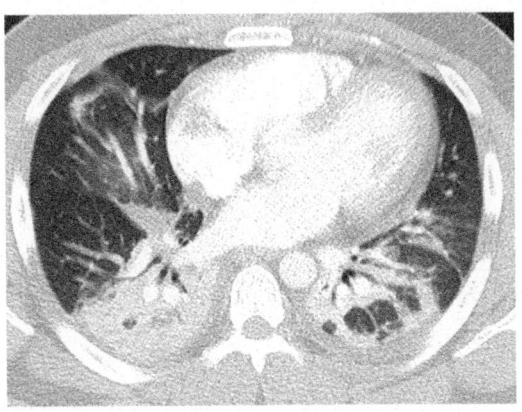

Fig. 3.17 Chest radiograph of this 33-year-old woman presenting with acute shortness of breath and mild fever, 4 days after delivery, shows bilateral air-space disease (black arrow) and pleural effusions. The heart is enlarged. The findings are strongly suggestive of ARDS

Fig. 3.19 Axial CT pulmonary angiogram, lung window image of this 33-year-old woman presenting with acute shortness of breath and mild fever, 4 days after delivery, shows bilateral basilar dense consolidation. The diagnosis in this patient was ARDS

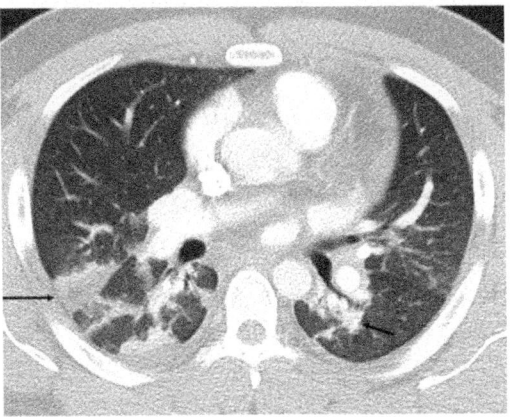

3.6.2 Pregnancy-Associated Spontaneous Coronary Artery Disease (P-SCAD)

P-SCAD is defined as a non-traumatic separation within the arterial wall by intramural hematoma, with the creation of a false lumen, with or without an intimal tear [72, 73]. It is a rare cause of acute coronary syndrome, accounting for 0.1–4% of all cases of ACS [74]. It is an even rarer and often underdiagnosed condition affecting young and pregnant women, with approximately 118 patients reported in the literature, to our knowledge. Patients are typically young and otherwise healthy young women, presenting with acute coronary syndrome, but the range of presentations can be from chest discomfort, unstable angina, to acute ST elevation myocardial infarction (STEMI) and cardiogenic shock, with a reported mortality of up to 50% in patients presenting in the acute phase in late pregnancy [75]. Patients with a history of smoking, a family history of CAD, hypercholesterolemia, and pre-eclampsia have been reported to have a greater risk for SCAD [76]. Rare risk factors including strenuous exercise, cocaine use, and an association with fibromuscular dysplasia

Fig. 3.18 Axial CT image lung window of this 37-year-old woman presenting with sudden acute shortness of breath who underwent CT pulmonary angiography in the immediate post-partum period shows right basilar consolidation and segmental collapse (long arrow), and several ill-defined ground-glass nodular and confluent air-space opacities (short arrow). One of the key CT findings of amniotic fluid emboli is ground-glass nodules associated with the terminal arterioles, which was the diagnosis strongly suggested based on CT combined with the clinical features in this patient. These represent the sequela of chemical pneumonitis from the embolized fluid. Intra-arterial filling defects are almost never large enough to be identified on CT pulmonary angiography in this condition. The main differential diagnosis for these imaging findings is ARDS (Fig. 3.19)

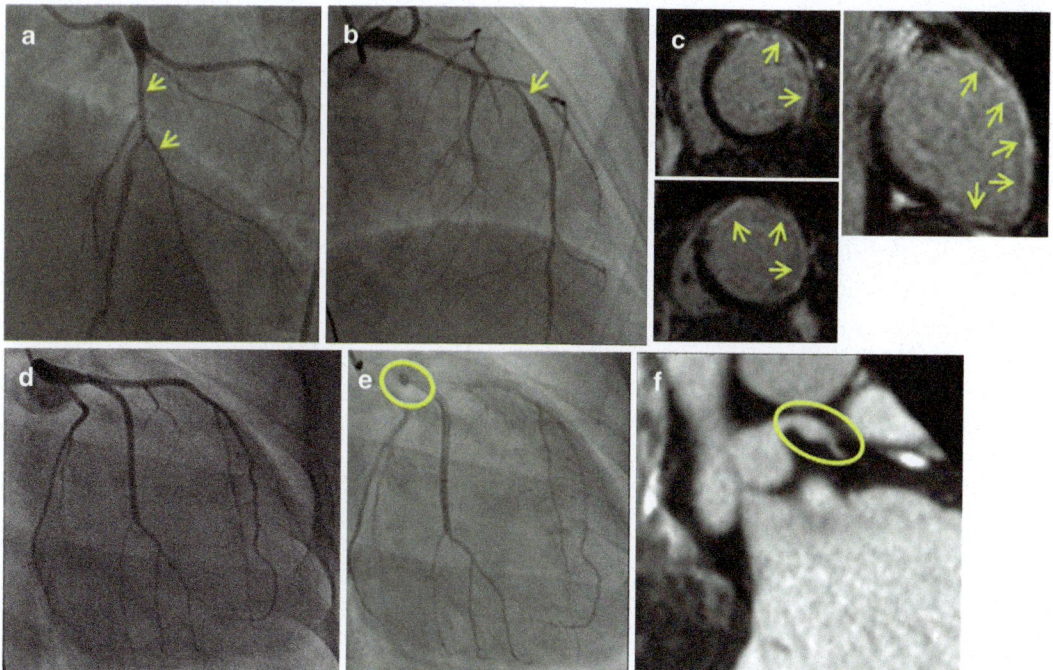

Fig. 3.20 Post-partum spontaneous coronary artery dissection: 10-day myocardial infarction coronary angiogram from a 31-year-old woman with myocardial infarction 10-day post-partum with a history of peripartum cardiomyopathy (left ventricular ejection fraction 30–40% after the third pregnancy, recovering to 60% before the fourth pregnancy). (**a**, **b**) There was spontaneous coronary artery dissection of the left main coronary artery extending into the left anterior descending and diagonal coronary arteries (arrows). (**c**) Cardiac magnetic resonance imaging showed extensive myocardial delayed enhancement (arrows), consistent with infarction of the anterior wall and septum (left ventricular ejection fraction 27%). (**d**) Follow-up angiography showed improved coronary caliber. Region of persistent contrast (**e**) correlated with distal left main aneurysmal changes on (**f**) computed tomography (ovals indicate corresponding regions). (Courtesy: Reprinted with permission from Dr. Marysia S. Tweet [77])

have also been reported [75]. The postulated pathophysiology suggests increased weakening of the elastin in the media of the coronary arteries due to excess progesterone [6].

Imaging currently plays a substantial role in the diagnosis of SCAD. Ideally, patients with high suspicion of SCAD should undergo urgent catheter angiography (Fig. 3.20).

Electrocardiographic-gated (ECG-gated) CT coronary angiography is reserved for the low-to-medium suspicion patients [78]. ECG gating helps in substantially reducing the motion artifacts. Table 3.11 enumerates the imaging features

and dose reduction techniques of CT coronary angiography for the diagnosis of SCAD in pregnant patients.

MRI and ultrasound have no proven role in the diagnosis of P-SCAD to our knowledge, although transesophageal echocardiography is helpful in evaluating for complications of the disease. MR angiography is helpful in evaluating for fibromuscular dysplasia in other parts of the body, which has a strong association with non-atherosclerotic SCAD [79].

Finally, the diagnosis of this condition is of paramount importance, as the treatment options

Table 3.11 Imaging features, pitfalls, and dose reduction techniques for CT coronary angiography in pregnancy

Dose reduction techniques	Heart rate control Patient positioning in center of scan field Increase pitch and collimation
CT features	Intimo-medial flap, with linear filling defect In the absence of above, narrowed lumen/total occlusion by thrombosed false lumen or intramural hematoma; occurs in normal coronary vessels
Pitfalls	1. Flow artifacts cause false-positive diagnosis Pearl: true intimo-medial flaps have distinct borders and would be continuous with the vessels wall, as opposed to flow artifacts which are not continuous with the vessel wall; multi-planar reformations are helpful to distinguish between the two 2. Overlapping vessels Pearl: MPRs, maximum intensity projections, and volume-rendered CT angiographic images are helpful

Reference: [78]

for myocardial infarction as a result of atherosclerosis are different from SCAD, and this condition should always be considered in pregnant and immediate post-partum patients [80].

3.6.3 Peri-partum Cardiomyopathy

Peri-partum cardiomyopathy is a rare, potentially life-threatening cardiac condition affecting pregnant women, usually in the late pregnancy and early puerperium [81]. The term was coined in 1971 after a 20-year experience in patients who developed cardiomegaly in the post-partum [82]. Geographic variations have been reported in the incidence of this disorder, ranging from 1 in 300 live births in Haiti, to 1 in 3000 live births in Europe and the United States [81]. The etiology of this condition is still not known, to our knowledge. The diagnosis of this condition requires the following criteria: (1) onset of heart failure in the last month of pregnancy or within first 5 months post-partum; (2) absence of documented heart disease during the pregnancy; and (3) the absence of an identifiable cause of heart failure [82, 83].

Although echocardiography is the initial modality used for evaluating cardiac conditions, cardiac magnetic resonance imaging (CMRI) is more accurate for the evaluation of chamber size and left ventricular function [84]. Myocardial damage and fibrosis translates to late gadolinium enhancement (LGE) on MRI, and is directly related to a worse prognosis of patients with heart failure [85, 86]. Left ventricular ejection fraction (LVEF) is an important independent predictor of

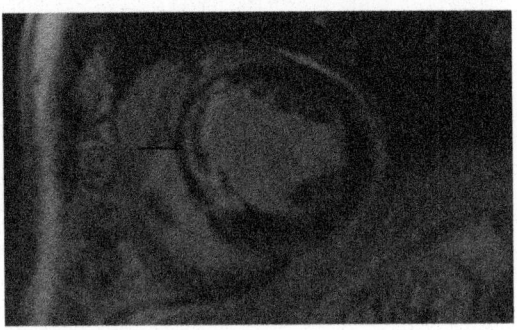

Fig. 3.21 Two-chamber MR image of this primigravida woman presenting with chest pain shows a large area of late gadolinium (15 min) transmural enhancement (black arrow) in the anterior, anteroseptal, and inferior septal walls of the left ventricle mid-cavity

survival in cardiac patients, especially in those with coronary artery disease [85].

Patients with PCM do not demonstrate any specific MRI pattern and can have LGE of the myocardium. LGE, if present, is a poor prognostic marker, is indicative of myocardial fibrosis or death, and is associated with delayed recovery [86]. Figure 3.21 demonstrates LGE in the anteroseptal myocardium in this 33-year-old pregnant woman who presented with cardiac failure.

3.6.4 Mitral Stenosis

Pregnancy unmasks underlying asymptomatic mitral valve disease in young women due to the increase hemodynamic stress. Among the mitral valve disorders, mitral stenosis (MS) is the most common form seen in pregnancy, with an overall

Table 3.12 Role of imaging in MS

Modality	Findings
Chest radiography	1. Left atrial enlargement Double-density sign: right side of enlarged left atrium pushes into adjacent lung and creates an additional contour superimposed over the right heart (Fig. 3.22) Elevation of the left main bronchus and splaying of the carina 2. Upper zone venous diversion 3. Pulmonary edema 4. Diffuse alveolar hemorrhage
Echocardiography	Role is to assess the MV area, pressure gradients, and LV and grade mitral stenosis Assess MV anatomy—leaflets/ mobility/architecture/calcification
CT	Same as radiography, albeit in greater detail (Figs. 3.23 and 3.24)
MRI	Cine MRI may be used for functional assessment and for better assessment of structural anatomy

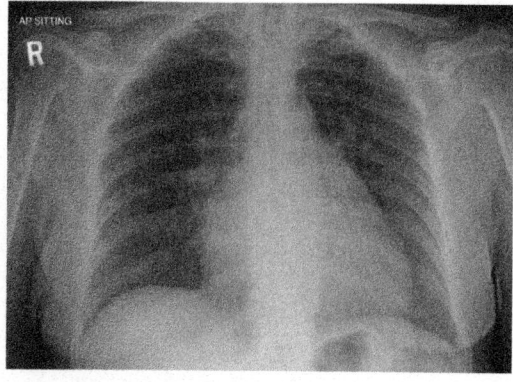

Fig. 3.22 Frontal chest radiograph of this young pregnant female presenting with shortness of breath and chest discomfort shows cardiomegaly and splaying of the carina due to left atrial enlargement

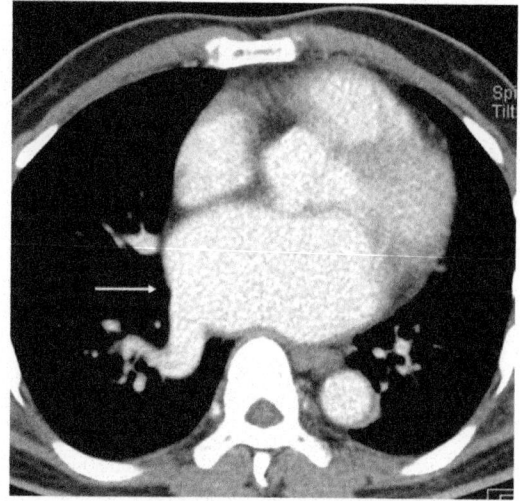

Fig. 3.23 IV contrast-enhanced axial CT image in the same patient as in Fig. 3.22 shows severe left atrial enlargement (white arrow) following mitral valve stenosis

estimated prevalence of 1–2% in developed countries, and up to 40–50% in developing countries [87, 88]. The prevalence of MS in pregnancy is associated with a marked increase in maternal morbidity and adverse fetal outcome, and has been shown to be related to the severity of the disease [89]. The adverse maternal events associated with MS include pulmonary edema, arrythmia, stroke, and thromboembolism. Multiple multi-center studies have shown that the complication rates are related to the severity of mitral stenosis and the patient's functional class [90].

The first line of radiological investigation of patients presenting with symptoms of suspected MS during pregnancy is chest radiography, followed by echocardiography when valvular heart disease is suspected. Table 3.12 enumerates the role and imaging findings of MS.

3.7 Chest Trauma

Trauma is the leading cause of maternal death from non-obstetrical causes, and affects 5–7% of all pregnancies. Road traffic collisions involving motor vehicles account for more than half of these cases, and the rest constitute falls, domestic violence, and other types of trauma [63, 91, 92]. The incidence and complications related to trauma have been covered in another chapter in this book. Therefore, we will focus only on specific thoracic complications of trauma affecting the pregnant woman in this section.

Table 3.13 broadly classifies thoracic injuries into compartments.

Broadly, causes of trauma are classified into blunt trauma and penetrating trauma. Motor vehicle collisions (MVCs), assaults, and falls consti-

Fig. 3.24 IV contrast-enhanced coronal CT image shows mitral valve calcifications (black arrow) in this pregnant woman who was diagnosed with mitral stenosis. Note the left atrial enlargement (white asterisk)

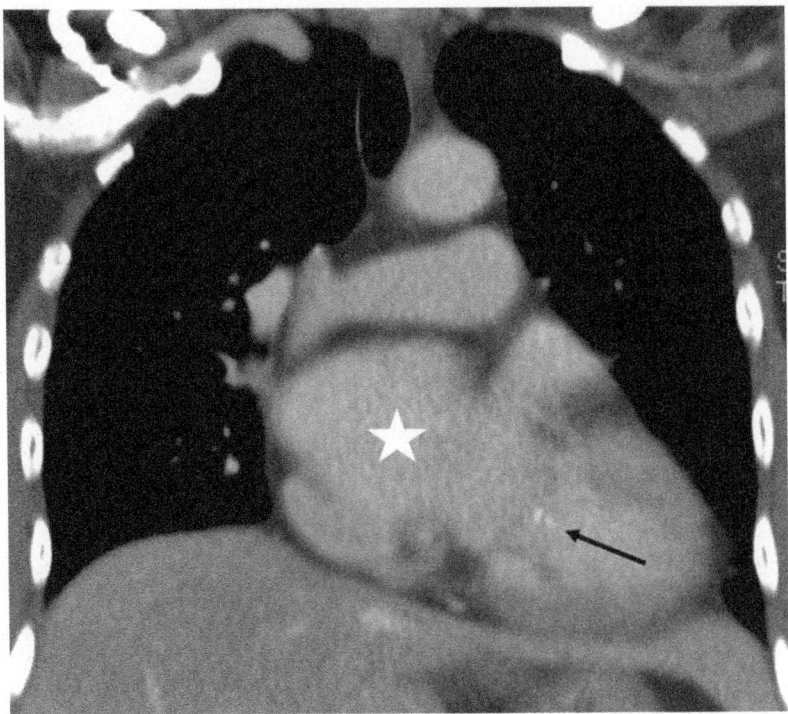

Table 3.13 Compartmentalized classification of thoracic injuries

Compartment	Anatomical structures involved
Extra-thoracic	• Soft-tissue lacerations/burns • Foreign bodies
Thoracic	
Bony cage	• Sternal injuries—look for sternoclavicular joint dissociation, mediastinal hematoma, and aortic dissection—significantly changes morbidity • Rib fractures—look hard for "flail segments", first rib fracture • Clavicle fracture (look for underlying vascular injuries)
Mediastinum	• Heart and great vessels: dissections, aneurysm, pericardial effusion, mediastinal hematoma
Airway injuries	• Tracheobronchial • Esophagus
Lung parenchyma	• Contusions • Pneumothorax and hemothorax
Diaphragm	• Diaphragmatic rupture/eventration with/without herniation of abdominal contents into the thoracic cavity

tute the former category, with MVCs topping the list at approximately 50% [91]. Gunshot and stab wounds constitute most of the penetrating injuries.

Radiographs are of limited importance in the setting of trauma in pregnant patients, because of their inability to reveal vital internal injuries. CT is the preferred imaging modality, even in pregnancy, as it obviates the need for additional radiographs, is a quick imaging modality, and provides accurate and vital information to rapidly manage patients and to minimize harm to the fetus.

3.8 Thoracic Cage Injuries

Blunt trauma to the thoracic cage can give rise to serious injuries. One of the commonly missed or overlooked injuries are subtle fractures of the sternum. Sagittal reformations of CT images (Fig. 3.25) are of importance in evaluating for these fractures, in pregnant as well as in non-pregnant patients. The radiologist must look for

Fig. 3.25 Sagittal bone reformatted image of a CT of the thorax performed with IV contrast demonstrates a subtle non-displaced sternal body fracture (black arrow)

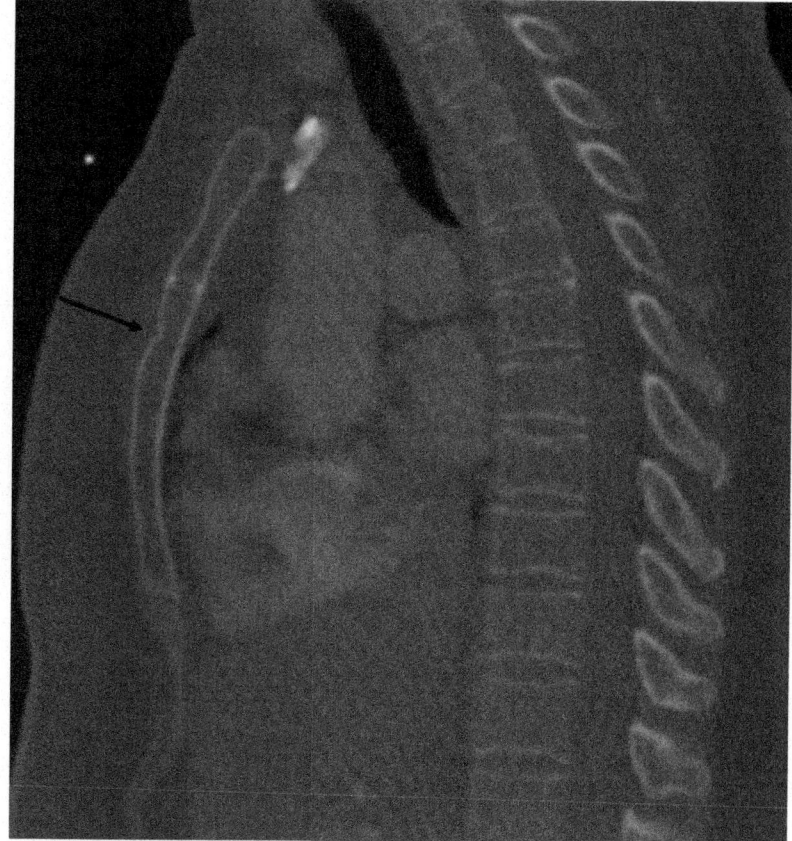

Fig. 3.26 Coned-down serendipity view of the left sternoclavicular joint demonstrates a posterior dislocation of the medial head of the left clavicle (black arrow). This was subsequently proven on the CT images (Fig. 3.27)

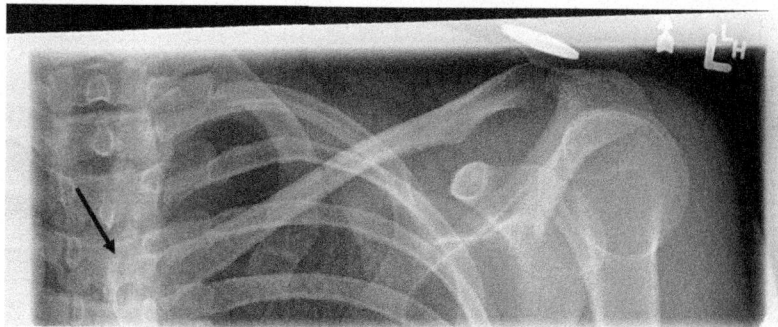

other associated injuries, including sternoclavicular joint dislocation, particularly posterior dislocation (Fig. 3.26). Axial CT images and three-dimensional reformations (Figs. 3.27 and 3.28) are particularly helpful in evaluating for these injuries. These are usually associated with anterior mediastinal hematoma, lung contusions, and subtle pneumothoraces (Fig. 3.29). Posterior dislocation of the sternoclavicular joint is an orthopedic emergency, as it can compress vital structures, i.e., the trachea, great vessels, and central nerves, and the trauma team should be made aware of the CT findings and pertinent negatives immediately after the scan is performed. Costochondral junctions should also be assessed carefully for on CT as well as for concomitant injuries.

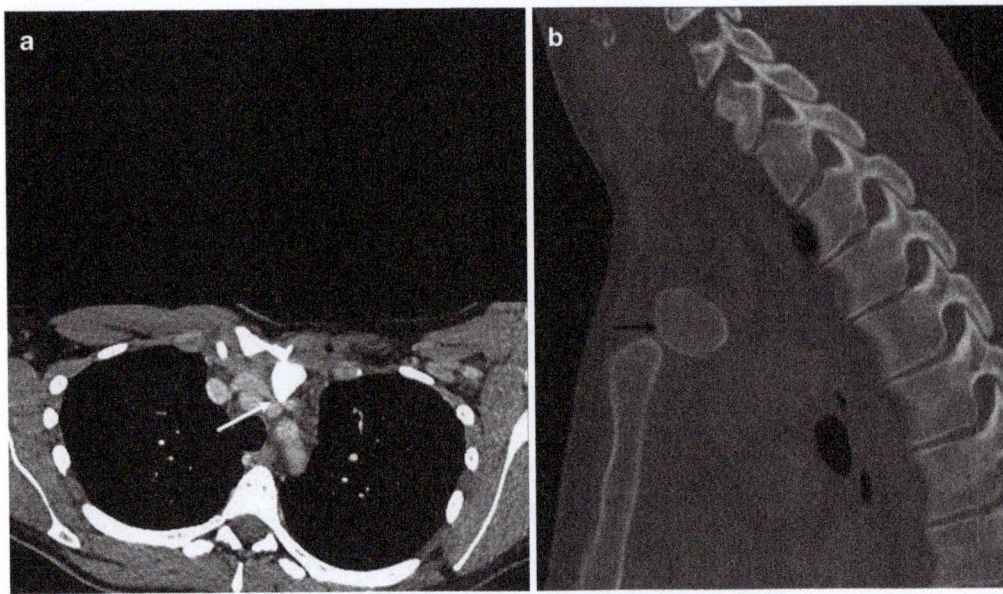

Fig. 3.27 IV contrast-enhanced axial image (**a**) and sagittal bone reformation (**b**) of the same patient as in Fig. 3.26 confirm the radiographic finding of posterior dislocation of the left sternoclavicular joint (black arrow). Note the vascular compression of the left brachiocephalic trunk by the dislocated medial end of the clavicle (white arrow). No thrombosis was detected (not shown)

Fig. 3.28 A 3D reconstruction of the same patient shows posterior dislocation of the medial head of the left clavicle (white asterisk) relative to the manubrium of the sternum. The opposite SC joint is intact

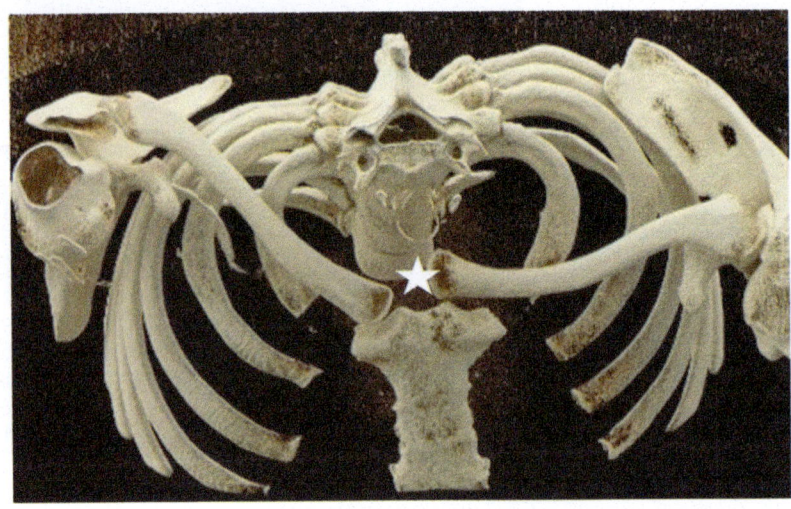

Rib fractures are one of the most common findings in patients with blunt chest trauma, and each rib must be evaluated with radiographs and with CT, to look for subtle non-displaced fractures (Fig. 3.30) [93]. "Flail chest" is a condition in which three or more consecutive ribs are fractured at two of more locations [92]. It is seen in up to 76% patients who had an MVC [94]. It is a marker of severe chest trauma and potential underlying vascular injuries. In one study, the researchers found that six or more rib fractures are independent predictors of overall mortality [95]. Table 3.14 enumerates the possible injuries associated with the location of rib fractures.

Fig. 3.29 IV contrast-enhanced axial CT image lung window of this young female pregnant patient involved in poly-trauma shows a small pneumothorax (long black arrow) in the left lung. Pulmonary contusions are noted in the lower lobes (short arrows)

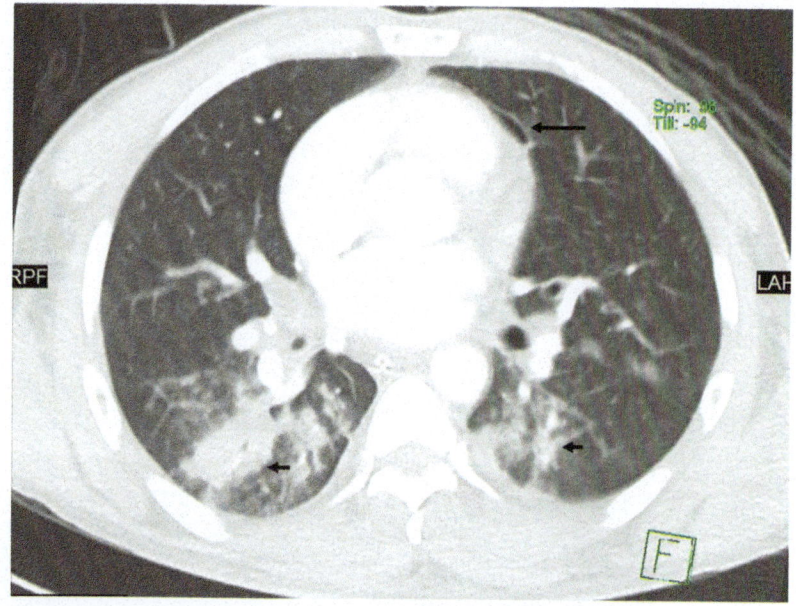

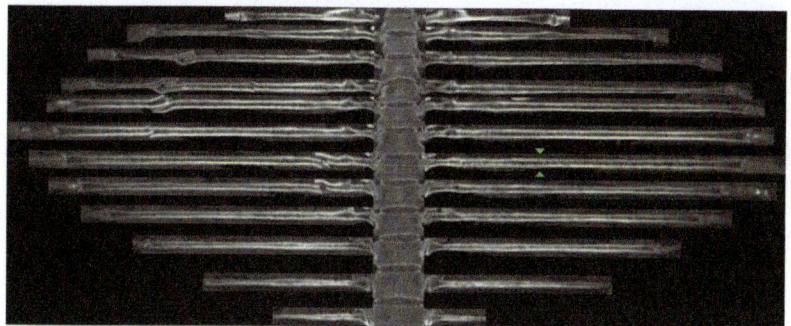

Fig. 3.30 Virtually rendered unfolded view of the ribs using the CT-Bone-Reading software tool. Ribs are labelled automatically. This was a 37-year-old pregnant woman involved in a motor vehicle collision. The patient had multiple displaced rib fractures on the right. This is useful in detecting non-displaced rib fractures which may be difficult to identify while interpreting conventional axial and multi-planar reconstructions

Table 3.14 Location of rib fractures and associated injuries

Location of rib	Injury site
1st	Subclavian vessel
1st to 3rd	Vascular, brachial plexus
4th to 9th	Cardiovascular and pulmonary
9th to 12th	Liver—right ribs Spleen—left ribs Diaphragmatic injuries

Reference: Adapted from [96]

Bedside ultrasound with a high-frequency probe is useful in assessing from intercostal hematomas, pleural effusions, and pneumothoraces. However, hemodynamically unstable patients with demonstrable rib fractures and lung opacification on chest radiography (Fig. 3.31) will benefit from IV contrast-enhanced CT imaging in the arterial phase, if their condition permits such emergency scanning, to detect active

Fig. 3.31 Frontal
radiograph of this
poly-trauma pregnant
patient shows a left
apical cap (black arrow)
secondary to upper rib
fracture. The patient also
had a fracture of the
lateral end of the left
clavicle (not shown)

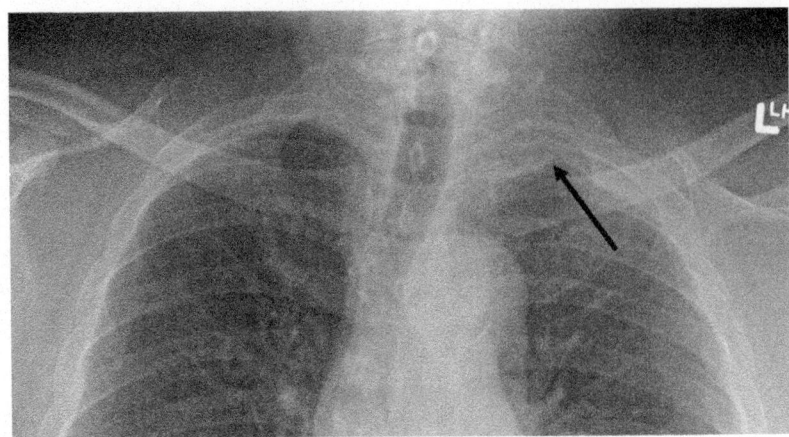

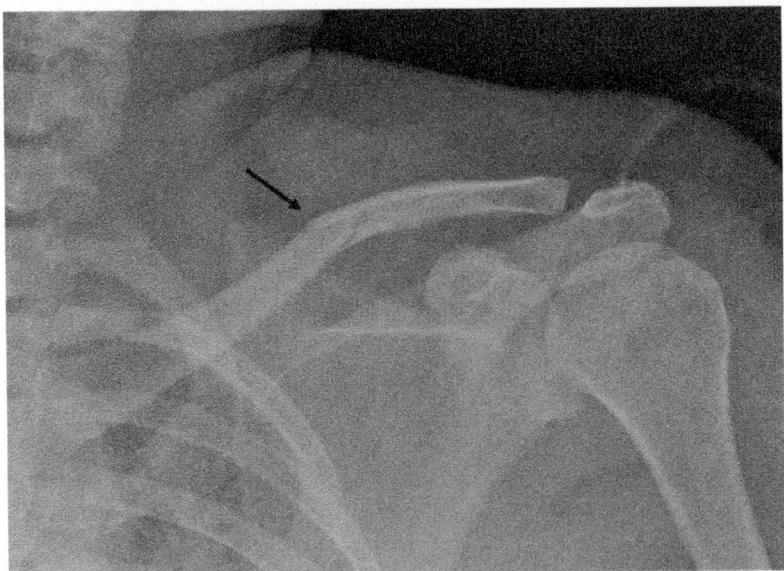

Fig. 3.32 Frontal projection of the left shoulder joint shows a minimally displaced fracture of the mid-shaft of the left clavicle (arrow). The patient also had non-displaced left second and third rib fractures (not shown). Sudden hemodynamic deterioration and development of a left side hemothorax prompted a CT trauma angiogram to be performed, which demonstrated an arterial blush (see Fig. 3.33) adjacent to the left second and third rib fractures. The patient subsequently underwent angioembolization of the bleeding vessel and was stabilized

bleeding (Figs. 3.32 and 3.33) arising from rupture of intercostal vessels. Early detection and intervention improve the overall outcome of these patients and potentially provides a better fetal outcome. Misdiagnosis of intercostal artery injury is associated with prolonged symptoms of chest pain, and with the development of traumatic pseudoaneurysms which delay fracture healing [97].

Hemothorax is defined as the presence of blood in the pleural space. On chest radiography, in the setting of trauma, a pleural effusion is hemorrhagic by definition and is only detectable if the volume exceeds 500 mL [96]. CT is more helpful in diagnosing and quantifying the hemothorax, and at the same time revealing or helping to exclude active contrast extravasation.

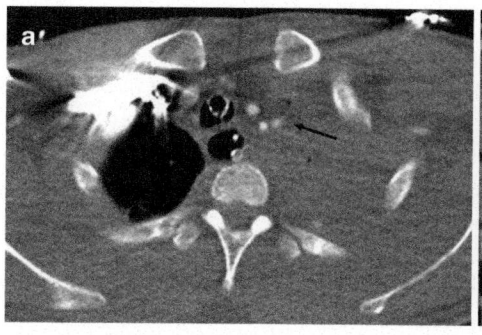
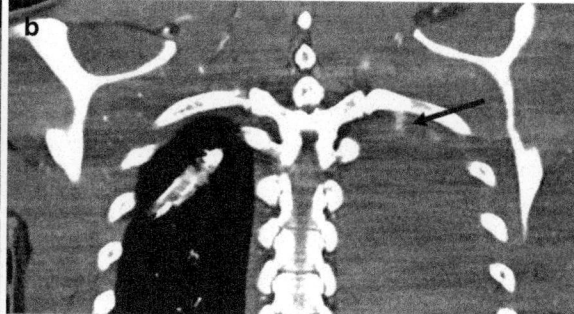

Fig. 3.33 Axial (**a**) and coronal (**b**) CT arterial-phase images, in this young pregnant woman who was involved in a motor vehicle collision, show an arterial blush (black arrow) subjacent to the left second rib, likely from ruptured intercostal vessels. The patient had left second and third rib fractures and a left hemothorax

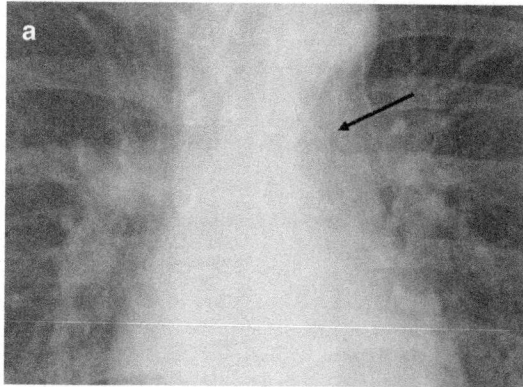
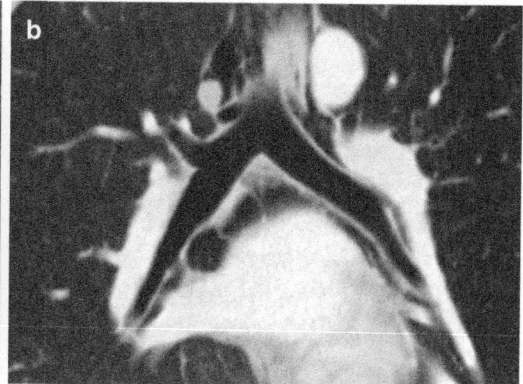

Fig. 3.34 A middle aged pregnant woman who presented with sudden chest pain and tightness. (**a**) Frontal radiograph shows a "double bronchial wall" sign (black arrow). Note the paratracheal emphysema. (**b**) Coronal CT reconstruction reveals that there is mediastinal air at the outer aspect of left bronchus, outlining the wall of bronchus, resulting in a "double wall" sign

3.9   Pneumothorax

Pneumothorax is one of the commonest complications arising from chest wall trauma. It is also considered in the differential diagnosis of patients presenting with chest pain and dyspnea. Spontaneous pneumothorax arising in pregnancy is a potentially life-threatening albeit rare entity, and only a few case reports have been reported in the literature to date, to our knowledge [98].

Pneumothorax, as in non-pregnant patients, is usually first diagnosed with chest radiographs, except in the supine projection, where a small-volume pneumothorax may elude diag-nosis. The radiologist should look for signs of tension pneumothorax, as it warrants immediate treatment. Well-managed patients with pneumothorax have a good prognosis, with no adverse fetal or maternal outcomes [99]. Primary management involves chest drainage in all patients with pneumothoraces irrespective of the size [100].

3.10   Pneumomediastinum

Also known as mediastinal emphysema, pneumomediastinum is associated with sternal fractures, flail chest, and with blunt thoracic injury without

Table 3.15 Radiographic signs of pneumomediastinum

Continuous diaphragm sign
Double bronchial sign
Left paracardial air
Tubular artery sign
Naclerio's V sign
Paratracheal air
Chest wall emphysema
Extra-pleural air sign

Reference: [102]

Table 3.16 Radiographic findings in pulmonary contusion

Modality	Findings	Pearls
Chest radiography	Patchy areas of cloud-like fluffy consolidation	Look for rib fractures and subtle pneumothorax and pneumomediastinum
CT	Non-segmental patchy consolidation	Usually at site of rib fracture or in contra-coup locations and in the paraspinal region

any associated bony trauma. It is also associated with injuries to the esophageal wall or to the tracheal–bronchial tract [101]. It is also seen in association with pneumothorax. One must be aware of the various radiographic signs of pneumomediastinum (Fig. 3.34; Table 3.15). The management of pneumomediastinum is usually conservative.

3.11 Parenchymal Contusions

Trauma to alveoli and hemorrhage into the airspaces constitutes the radiographic findings of pulmonary contusion. It is a common finding in post blunt trauma patients, with an incidence of up to 20–70% in severe trauma, and has a stronger association with rib fractures [103]. Table 3.16 summarizes the modality-specific radiographic findings of pulmonary contusion.

3.12 Conclusion

In this chapter, we have gone through the various thoracic emergencies that pregnant women may present with, some of which are particularly common in these women due to the physiological changes and have discussed the appropriate imaging necessary to evaluate them. We have categorized the emergencies into broader categories for easy reading and have discussed briefly the management of these conditions.

References

1. Wallace A, Hayton A, Marks P, Revell MA, Russell PG, Goergen APS. Radiation risk of medical imaging during pregnancy. Insid Radiol. 1997:1–7.
2. Wagner LK, Lester R, Saldana L. Chapter 4: Prenatal risks from ionizing radiations, ultrasound, magnetic fields and radiofrequency waves. In: Exposure of the pregnant patient to diagnostic radiations. A guide to medical anagement. 2nd ed. Madison WI: Medical Physics Publishing; 1997.
3. Clark SL, Belfort MA, Dildy GA, Herbst MA, Meyers JA, Hankins GD. Maternal death in the 21st century: causes, prevention, and relationship to cesarean delivery. Am J Obstet Gynecol. 2008;199:36.e1. https://doi.org/10.1016/j.ajog.2008.03.007.
4. Katz J, Shear TD, Murphy GS, Alspach D, Greenberg SB, Szokol J, Benson J. Cardiovascular collapse in the pregnant patient. Resc Transesophag Echocardiogr Open Heart Surg. 2017;31:203–6.
5. Dreizin D, Khati NJ, Akin EA, Zeman RK. Imaging pregnant and lactating patients 1. Radiographics. 2015;35:1751–65.
6. Plowman RS, Javidan-Nejad C, Raptis CA, Katz DS, Mellnick VM, Bhalla S, Cornejo P, Menias CO. Imaging of pregnancy-related vascular complications. Radiographics. 2017;37:1270–89.
7. Soma-Pillay P, Nelson-Piercy C, Tolppanen H, Mebazaa A. Physiological changes in pregnancy. Cardiovasc J Afr. 2016;27(2):89–94.
8. Troiano NH. Physiologic and hemodynamic changes during pregnancy. AACN Adv Crit Care. 2018;29:273–83.
9. Rodger M, Sheppard D, Gandara E, Tinmouth A. Haematological problems in obstetrics. Best Pract Res Clin Obstet Gynaecol. 2015;29:671–84.
10. Pahade JK, Litmanovich D, Pedrosa I, Romero J, Bankier AA, Boisella PM. Imaging pregnant patients with suspected pulmonary embolism: what the radiologist needs to know. Radiographics. 2009;29:639–54.
11. Knight M. Antenatal pulmonary embolism: risk factors, management and outcomes. BJOG. 2008;115:453–61.
12. British Thoracic Society Standards of Care Commitee Pulmonary Embolism Guideline Development Group. British Thoracic Society guidelines for the management of suspected acute pulmonary embolism. Thorax. 2003;58:470–83.

13. Schuster M, Fishman J, Copeland J, Hatabu H, Boiselle P. Pulmonary embolism in pregnant patients: a survey of practices and policies for CT pulmonary angiography. AJR Am J Roentgenol. 2003;181:1495–8.

14. Stein PD, Woodard PK, Weg JG, et al. Diagnostic pathways in acute pulmonary embolism: recommendations of the PIOPED II investigators. Radiology. 2007;242:15–21.

15. Refuerzo JS, Hechtman JL, Redman ME, Whitty JE. Venous thromboembolism during pregnancy: clinical suspicion warrants evaluation. J Reprod Med. 2003;48:767–70.

16. Stein PD, Fowler SE, Goodman LR, et al. Multidetector computed tomography for acute pulmonary embolism. N Engl J Med. 2006;354:2317–27.

17. Fidler JL, Patz EF Jr, Ravin CE. Cardiopulmonary complications of pregnancy: radiographic findings. AJR Am J Roentgenol. 1993;161:937–42.

18. Levy MS, Spencer F, Ginsberg JS, Anderson JA. Reading between the (guidelines): management of submassive pulmonary embolism in the first trimester of pregnancy. Thromb Res. 2008;121:705–7.

19. Hedengran KK, Andersen MR, Stender S, Szecsi PB. Large D-dimer fluctuation in normal pregnancy: a longitudinal cohort study of 4,117 samples from 714 healthy danish women. Obstet Gynecol Int. 2016;2016:3561675.

20. Forbes KP, Reid JH, Murchison JT. Do preliminary chest X-ray findings define the optimum role of pulmonary scintigraphy in suspected pulmonary embolism? Clin Radiol. 2001;56:397–400.

21. Cascio V, Hon M, Haramati LB, Gour A, Spiegler P, Bhalla S, Katz DS. Imaging of suspected pulmonary embolism and deep venous thrombosis in obese patients. Br J Radiol. 2018;91:20170956.

22. Devis P, Knuttinen MG. Deep venous thrombosis in pregnancy: incidence, pathogenesis and endovascular management. Cardiovasc Diagn Ther. 2017;7(Suppl 3):S309–19.

23. Kearon C, Julian JA, Newman TE, Ginsberg JS. Noninvasive diagnosis of deep venous thrombosis. McMaster Diagnostic Imaging Practice Guidelines Initiative. Ann Intern Med. 1998;128:663–77.

24. Pomp ER, Lenselink A, Rosendaal FR, Doggen CJ. Pregnancy, the postpartum period and prothrombotic defects: risk of venous thrombosis in the MEGA study. J Thromb Haemost. 2008;6:632–7.

25. Scarsbrook AF, Evans AL, Owen AR, Gleeson FV. Diagnosis of suspected venous thromboembolic disease in pregnancy. Clin Radiol. 2006;61:1–12.

26. Torkzad MR, Bremme K, Hellgren M, Eriksson MJ, Hagman A, Jorgensen T, Lund K, Sandgren G, Blomqvist L, Kalebo P. Magnetic resonance imaging and ultrasonography in diagnosis of pelvic vein thrombosis during pregnancy. Thromb Res. 2010;126:107–12.

27. Wang PI, Chong ST, Kielar AZ, Knoepp UD, Mazza MB, Goodsitt MM. Imaging of pregnant and lactating patients: Part 2, Evidence-based review and recommendations. AJR Am J Roentgenol. 2012;198:785–92.

28. Barnawi RA, Alrefai WM, Qari F, Aljefri A, Hagi SK, Khafaji M. Doctors' knowledge of the doses and risks of radiological investigations performed in the emergency department. Saudi Med J. 2018; 39:1130.

29. Revel M-P, Meyer G, Frija G. Pulmonary embolism during pregnancy:diagnosis with lung scintigraphy or CT angiography? Radiology. 2011;258:590. https://doi.org/10.1148/radiol.10100986.

30. Scarsbrook AF, Bradley KM, Gleeson FV. Perfusion scintigraphy: diagnostic utility in pregnant women with suspected pulmonary embolic disease. Eur Radiol. 2007;17:2554–60.

31. Winer-Muram HT, Boone JM, Brown HL, Jennings SG, Mabie WC, Lombardo GT. Pulmonary embolism in pregnant patients: fetal radiation dose with helical CT. Radiology. 2002;224:487–92.

32. Investigators P. Value of the ventilation/perfusion scan in acute pulmonary embolism: results of the Prospective Investigation of Pulmonary Embolism Diagnosis (PIOPED) study. JAMA. 1990;263:2753–9.

33. Parker MS, Hui FK, Camacho MA, Chung JK, Broga DW, Sethi NN. Female breast radiation exposure during CT pulmonary angiography. AJR Am J Roentgenol. 2005;185:1228–33.

34. Stein PD, Terrin ML, Gottschalk A, Alavi A, Henry JW. Value of ventilation/perfusion scans versus perfusion scans alone in acute pulmonary embolism. Am J Cardiol. 1992;69:1239–41.

35. Remy-Jardin M, Pistolesi M, Goodman LR, et al. Management of suspected acute pulmonary embolism in the era of CT angiography: a statement from the Fleischner Society. Radiology. 2007;245:315–29.

36. Kluge A, Luboldt W, Bachmann G. Acute pulmonary embolism to the subsegmental level: diagnostic accuracy of three MRI techniques compared with 16-MDCT. AJR Am J Roentgenol. 2006;187:W7–14.

37. Meaney JF, Weg JG, Chenevert TL, Stafford-Johnson D, Hamilton BH, Prince MR. Diagnosis of pulmonary embolism with magnetic resonance angiography. N Engl J Med. 1997;336:1422–7.

38. Heredia V, Altun E, Ramalho M, de Campos R, Azevedo R, Pamuklar E, Semelka RC. MRI of pregnant patients for suspected pulmonary embolism: steady-state free precession vs postgadolinium 3D-GRE. Acta Med Port. 2012;25:359–67.

39. Webb JA, Thomsen HS, Morcos SK, Members of Contrast Media Safety Committee of European Society of Urogenital Radiology (ESUR). The use of iodinated and gadolinium contrast media during pregnancy and lactation. Eur Radiol. 2005;15:1234–40.

40. Kaunitz AM, Hughes JM, Grimes DA, et al. Causes of maternal mortality in the United States. Obstet Gynecol. 1985;65:605–12.

41. Sridama V, Pacini F, Yang SL, et al. Decreased levels of helper T cells: a possible cause of immunodeficiency in pregnancy. N Engl J Med. 1982;307:352–6.

42. MacLennan FM. Maternal mortality from Mendelson's syndrome: an explanation? Lancet. 1986;1:587–9.

43. Franquet T. Imaging of pulmonary viral pneumonia. Radiology. 2011;260:18–39.

44. Murray JF, Nadel JA. The lungs and gynaecologic and obstetric disease. In: Textbook of respiratory medicine. 2nd ed. Philadelphia, PA: WB Saunders; 1994.

45. LA Berkowitz K. Risk factors associated with the increasing prevalence of pneumonia during pregnancy. Am J Obstet Gynecol. 1990;163:981–5.

46. Chaparian A, Aghabagheri M. Fetal radiation doses and subsequent risks from X-ray examinations: should we be concerned? Iran J Reprod Med. 2013;11:899–904.

47. Lim WS, Macfarlane JT, Colthorpe CL. Pneumonia and pregnancy. Thorax. 2001;56:398–405.

48. Syrjala H, Broas M, Ohtonen P, Jartti A, Pääkkö E. Chest magnetic resonance imaging for pneumonia diagnosis in outpatients with lower respiratory tract infection. Eur Respir J. 2017;49:1–7.

49. Schloß M, Heckrodt J, Schneider C, Discher T, Krombach GA. Magnetic resonance imaging of the lung as an alternative for a pregnant woman with pulmonary. Tuberculosis. 2015;9:7–13.

50. Di Guardo F, Viviana Lo Presti GC. Pulmonary arteriovenous malformations (PAVMs) and pregnancy: a rare case of hemothorax and review of the literature. Case Rep Obstet Gynecol. 2019;2019: 8165791.

51. Esplin MS, Varner MW. Progression of pulmonary arteriovenous malformation during pregnancy: case report and review of the literature. Obstet Gynecol Surv. 1997;52:248–53.

52. Khurshid I, Downie GH. Pulmonary arteriovenous malformation. Postgrad Med J. 2002;78:191–7.

53. Remy J, Remy-Jardin M, Giraud F, Wattinne L. Angioarchitecture of pulmonary arteriovenous malformations: clinical utility of three-dimensional helical CT. Radiology. 1994;191:657–64.

54. Remy J, Remy-Jardin M, Wattinne L, Deffontaines C. Pulmonary arteriovenous malformations: evaluation with CT of the chest before and after treatment. Radiology. 1992;182:809–16.

55. Chao H, Chern M, Chen Y, Chang S. Recurrence of pulmonary arteriovenous malformations in a female with hereditary hemorrhagic telangiectasia. Am J Med Sci. 2004;327:294–8.

56. Shovlin CL, Sodhi V, McCarthy A, Lasjaunias P, Jackson JE, Sheppard MN. Estimates of maternal risks of pregnancy for women with hereditary haemorrhagic telangiectasia (Osler-Weber-Rendu syndrome): suggested approach for obstetric services. BJOG. 2008;115:1108–15.

57. Faughnan ME, Palda VA, Garcia-Tsao G, et al. International guidelines for the diagnosis and management of hereditary haemorrhagic telangiectasia. J Med Genet. 2011;48:73–87.

58. Lacombe P, Lacout A, et al. Diagnosis and treatment of pulmonary arteriovenous malformations in hered-

itary hemorrhagic telangiectasia: an overview. Diagn Interv Imaging. 2013;94:835–48.

59. Anin SR, Ogunnoiki W, Sabharwal T, Harrison-phipps K. Pulmonary arteriovenous malformation unmasked in pregnancy: a case report. Obstet Med. 2013;6:179–81.

60. Montagnana M, Cervellin G, Franchini M, Lippi G. Pathophysiology, clinics and diagnostics of non-thrombotic pulmonary embolism. J Thromb Thrombolysis. 2011;31:436–44.

61. Burrows A, Khoo SK. The amniotic fluid embolism syndrome: 10 years' experience at a major teaching hospital. Aust New Zeal J Obstet Gynaecol. 1995;35:245–50.

62. Peterson EP, Taylor HB. Amniotic fluid embolism. An analysis of 40 cases. Obstet Gynecol. 1970;35:787–93.

63. Müller NL, Fraser RS, Colman NC, Pare D. Radiologic diagnosis of diseases of the chest. 1st ed. Philadelphia, PA: Saunders; 2001.

64. Fidler JL, Patz EF, Ravin CE. Cardiopulmonary complications of pregnancy: radiographic findings. Am J Roentgenol. 1993;161:937–42.

65. James AH, Jamison MG, Biswas MS, Brancazio LR, Swamy GK, Myers ER. Acute myocardial infarction in pregnancy: a United States population-based study. Circulation. 2006;113:1564–71.

66. Petitti DB, Sidney S, Quesenberry CP Jr, Bernstein A. Incidence of stroke and myocardial infarction in women of reproductive age. Stroke. 1997;28: 280–3.

67. Ladner HE, Danielsen B, Gilbert WM. Acute myocardial infarction in pregnancy and the puerperium: a population-based study. Obstet Gynecol. 2005;105:480–4.

68. Berg CJ, Callaghan WM, Syverson C, Henderson Z. Pregnancy-related mortality in the United States, 1998 to 2005. Obstet Gynecol. 2010;116:1302–9.

69. Hankins GD, Wendel GD Jr, Leveno KJ, Stoneham J. Myocardial infarction during pregnancy: a review. Obstet Gynecol. 1985;65:139–46.

70. Elkayam U, Jalnapurkar S, Barakkat MN, Katri N, Kealey AJ, Mehra A, Roth A. Pregnancy-associated acute myocardial infarction. Cardiovasc Manag Pregnancy. 2014;129:1695–702.

71. Kealey A. Coronary artery disease and myocardial infarction in pregnancy: a review of epidemiology, diagnosis, and medical and surgical management. Can J Cardiol. 2010;26:185–9.

72. Saw J. Spontaneous coronary artery dissection. Can J Cardiol. 2013;29:1027–33.

73. Maehara A, Mintz GS, Castagna MT, Pichard AD, Satler LF, Waksman R, Suddath WO, Kent KM, Weissman NJ. Intravascular ultrasound assessment of spontaneous coronary artery dissection. Am J Cardiol. 2002;89:466–8.

74. Mortensen KH, Thuesen L, Kristensen IB, Christiansen EH. Spontaneous coronary artery dissection: a western Denmark heart registry study. Catheter Cardiovasc Interv. 2009;74:710–7.

75. Sheikh AS, O'Sullivan M. Pregnancy-related spontaneous coronary artery dissection: two case reports and a comprehensive review of literature. Hear Views. 2012;13:53–65.

76. Koul AK, Hollander G, Moskovits N, Frankel R, Herrera L, Shani J. Coronary artery dissection during pregnancy and the postpartum period: two case reports and review of literature. Catheter Cardiovasc Interv. 2001;52:88–94.

77. Tweet MS, Hayes SN, Codsi E, Gulati R, Rose CH, Best PJM. Spontaneous coronary artery dissection associated with pregnancy. J Am Coll Cardiol. 2017;70:426–35.

78. Kim JJ, Dillon WP, Glastonbury CM, Provenzale JM, Wintermark M. Sixty-four-section multidetector CT angiography of carotid arteries: a systematic analysis of image quality and artifacts. Am J Neuroradiol. 2010;31:91–9.

79. Jacqueline S, Eve A, Tara S, et al. Spontaneous coronary artery dissection. Circ Cardiovasc Interv. 2014;7:645–55.

80. Codsi E, Tweet MS, Rose CH, Arendt KW, Best PJM, Hayes SN. Spontaneous coronary artery dissection in pregnancy: what every obstetrician should know. Obstet Gynecol. 2016;128:731.

81. Sliwa K, Fett J, Elkayam U. Peripartum cardiomyopathy. Lancet. 2006;368:687–93.

82. Demakis JG, Rahimtoola SH. Peripartum cardiomyopathy. Circulation. 1971;44:964–8.

83. Homans DC. Peripartum cardiomyopathy. N Engl J Med. 1985;312:1432–7.

84. Mouquet F, Lions C, de Groote P, Bouabdallaoui N, Willoteaux S, Dagorn J, Deruelle P, Lamblin N, Bauters C, Beregi JP. Characterisation of peripartum cardiomyopathy by cardiac magnetic resonance imaging. Eur Radiol. 2008;18:2765–9.

85. Igor K, et al. Prognostic value of routine cardiac magnetic resonance assessment of left ventricular ejection fraction and myocardial damage. Circ Cardiovasc Imaging. 2011;4:610–9.

86. Schelbert EB, Elkayam U, Cooper LT, et al. Myocardial damage detected by late gadolinium enhancement cardiac magnetic resonance is uncommon in peripartum cardiomyopathy. J Am Heart Assoc. 2017;6:e005472. https://doi.org/10.1161/JAHA.117.005472.

87. Kannan M, Vijayanand G. Mitral stenosis and pregnancy: current concepts in anaesthetic practice. Indian J Anaesth. 2010;54:439–44.

88. Movahed M-R, Ahmadi-Kashani M, Kasravi B, Saito Y. Increased prevalence of mitral stenosis in women. J Am Soc Echocardiogr. 2006;19:911–3.

89. Hameed A, Karaalp IS, Tummala PP, Wani OR, Canetti M, Akhter MW, Goodwin I, Zapadinsky N, Elkayam U. The effect of valvular heart disease on maternal and fetal outcome of pregnancy. J Am Coll Cardiol. 2001;37:893–9.

90. Tsiaras S, Poppas A. Mitral valve disease in pregnancy: outcomes and management. Obstet Med. 2009;2:6–10.

91. Mattox KL, Goetzl L. Trauma in pregnancy. Crit Care Med. 2005;33:S385–9.

92. Connolly AM, Katz VL, Bash KL, McMahon MJ, Hansen WF. Trauma and pregnancy. Am J Perinatol. 1997;14:331–6.

93. Weiser TG. Overview of thoracic trauma. Kenilworth, NJ: Merck; 2014.

94. Borman JB, Aharonson-Daniel L, Savitsky B, Peleg K. Unilateral flail chest is seldom a lethal injury. Emerg Med J. 2006;23:903–5.

95. Flagel BT, Luchette FA, Reed RL, Esposito TJ, Davis KA, Santaniello JM, Gamelli RL. Half-a-dozen ribs: the breakpoint for mortality. Surgery. 2005;138:717–25.

96. Talbot BS, Gange CP, Chaturvedi A, Klionsky N, Hobbs SK, Chaturvedi A. Traumatic rib injury: patterns, imaging pitfalls, complications, and treatment. Radiographics. 2017;37:628–51.

97. Chemelli AP, Thauerer M, Wiedermann F, Strasak A, Klocker J, Chemelli-Steingruber IE. Transcatheter arterial embolization for the management of iatrogenic and blunt traumatic intercostal artery injuries. J Vasc Surg. 2009;49:1505–13.

98. Pinto RM, Mahankali S, Prasanna BS, Ramkumar MM. Spontaneous pneumothorax in pregnancy: a challenge for anaesthesiologist. J Obstet Anaesth Crit Care. 2017;7:106–8.

99. Jain P, Goswami K. Recurrent spontaneous pneumothorax during pregnancy: a case report. J Med Case Reports. 2009;3:81. https://doi.org/10.1186/1752-1947-3-81.

100. Garg R, Sanjay, Das V, Usman K, Rungta S, Prasad R. Spontaneous pneumothorax: an unusual complication of pregnancy--a case report and review of literature. Ann Thorac Med. 2008;3:104–5.

101. Chawla A. Thoracic imaging basic to advanced. 1st ed. New York, NY: Springer; 2019.

102. Zylak CM, Standen JR, Barnes GR, Zylak CJ. cPneumomediastinum revisited. Radiographics. 2000;20:1043–57.

103. Cohn SM. Pulmonary contusion: review of the clinical entity. J Trauma. 1997;42:973–9.

Non-traumatic Abdominal and Pelvic Emergencies in Pregnant Patients: Role of Ultrasound

4

Raffaella Basilico, Andrea Delli Pizzi,
Erica Mincuzzi, Roberta Danzi,
Alessandra Ricciardulli,
and Luiza Grzycka-Kowalczyk

Contents

R. Basilico (✉) · A. D. Pizzi · E. Mincuzzi
Department of Neurosciences, Imaging and Clinical
Sciences, G. d'Annunzio University of Chieti-
Pescara, Chieti, Italy

R. Danzi
Department of Diagnostic Imaging,
Pineta Grande Hospital, Castel Volturno, Italy

A. Ricciardulli
Department of Obstetrics and Gynaecology,
G. d'Annunzio University of Chieti-Pescara,
Chieti, Italy

L. Grzycka-Kowalczyk
Department of Radiology,
Medical University of Lublin, Lublin, Poland

© Springer Nature Switzerland AG 2020
M. N. Patlas et al. (eds.), *Emergency Imaging of Pregnant Patients*,
https://doi.org/10.1007/978-3-030-42722-1_4

4.1 Acute Appendicitis

Acute appendicitis is considered the most common non-obstetric, non-traumatic surgical emergency during pregnancy, followed by cholecystitis, ovarian torsion, and bowel obstruction [1]. Moreover, it accounts for 25% of non-obstetrical surgical intervention performed during pregnancy, being the prevalent cause of such interventions [2]. The reported incidence of acute appendicitis in pregnancy is between 0.04% and 0.2% [3], i.e. occurring in approximately 1/800 pregnant women, and it can occur in any of the three trimesters, although the highest incidence has been reported during the second trimester, with a frequency of 35–50% [4]. However, appendiceal perforation is more frequent during the third trimester. If the diagnosis is delayed, the complication rate is much higher, particularly that of perforation, with associated peritonitis and septicemia, potentially leading to substantial adverse maternal and fetal outcomes, including miscarriage, preterm labor, and intrauterine death. In case of uncomplicated appendicitis, fetal loss rate has been reported to be 3–5%, without a significant effect on maternal mortality. However, in perforated appendicitis, the fetal loss rate increases to 20–25%, and maternal mortality rate rises to around 4% [5]. Although non-operative treatment of acute appendicitis continues to be attempted with mixed success at present in the general population, appendectomy remains the mainstay of acute appendicitis treatment in pregnant women, and should be performed in a timely manner to reduce the risks of complicated appendicitis to the mother and the fetus. Laparoscopic appendectomy is the preferred approach for the treatment of acute appendicitis in this patient population [6].

4.1.1 Etiology/Pathology

The relatively high incidence of appendicitis during pregnancy may be explained by many factors. One of the main mechanisms involved in the rapid development of appendicitis in pregnancy is that increased pelvic vascularity and displacement of the appendix by the uterus may accelerate necrosis and perforation; moreover, the growth of local lymphatic drainage associated with interference with omental migration may favor systemic spread of the inflammatory process. In fact, particularly, the changing position of the appendix limits the ability of the omentum to wall off the inflammation [7].

4.1.2 Diagnosis

4.1.2.1 Clinical Signs

Pregnancy can obscure the signs and symptoms of acute appendicitis, and markers of inflammation are normally somewhat elevated in otherwise normal pregnancy. Leukocytosis, elevated C-reactive protein (CRP) levels, and symptoms including nausea, vomiting, and anorexia are frequently present during pregnancy, especially in the first trimester. Moreover, the clinical examination is quite difficult due to often-delayed peritoneal signs caused by the laxity of the anterior abdominal wall. The most common symptom is constant abdominal pain, whereas right lower quadrant pain is the most predictable symptom of acute appendicitis, particularly during the first trimester. Due to the displacement of the appendix caused by uterus enlargement, after the third month of pregnancy, the pain may change location, and typically moves progressively upwards and laterally up to and above the level of the right iliac crest at the end of the sixth month of pregnancy [8] (Fig. 4.1).

4.1.2.2 Ultrasound

Ultrasound is the first-line imaging modality for investigating suspected appendicitis in pregnancy, using the same parameters for non-pregnant patients, including visualization of a blind-ending, dilated (>6–7 mm in diameter), aperistaltic and non-compressible tubular structure arising from the medial aspect of the cecum, 1–3 cm below the ileocecal valve, which corresponds to the patient's site of pain. Associated sonographic findings including appendiceal wall

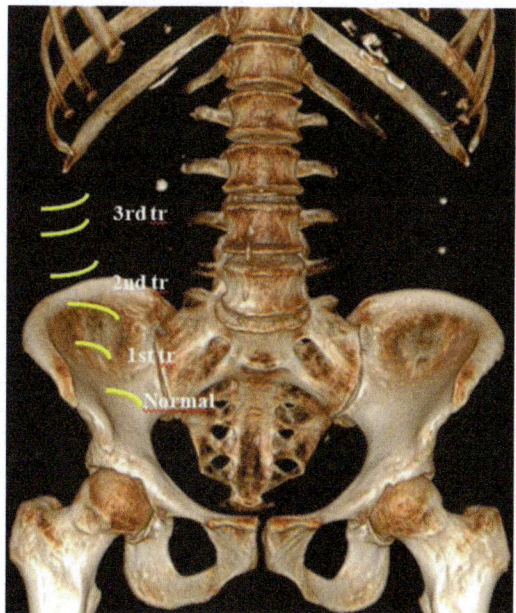

Fig. 4.1 Coronal 3D CT reformation: displacement of the appendix during pregnancy, according to Baer et al. [9]

thickening (>2 mm), appendicolith(s), increased echogenicity of the surrounding fat due to inflammation, hypoechoic free fluid, and periappendiceal fluid, and discrete fluid collections, which must all be carefully searched for (Fig. 4.2). In patients with gangrenous or perforated appendicitis, hyperechoic spots consistent with air bubbles may be seen in the appendiceal wall or outside the appendix, respectively (Fig. 4.3).

There are no guidelines regarding the use of transvaginal ultrasound in this clinical setting, to our knowledge. This technique can be used to look for the presence and size of adnexal or uterine disorders, which can also be used to diagnose or exclude acute appendicitis, and to detect free fluid in the pouch of Douglas.

Transabdominal ultrasound with the graded-compression technique is the diagnostic procedure of choice for suspected acute appendicitis, but this technique is difficult to perform with the patient in a supine position during the late second trimester and in the third trimester of pregnancy, because the enlarged gravid uterus does not allow adequate compression. For women in the late

second trimester or third trimester, it is recommended that patient be scanned in the left lateral decubitus position, which allows displacement of the gravid uterus, so that the graded-compression technique can be used without difficulty.

No further examination is recommended when US is positive for appendicitis, negative with a low clinical suspicion, or shows an alternative diagnosis that explains the clinical presentation such as ovarian torsion or nephrolithiasis [10].

However, the displacement of the appendix according to the stages of pregnancy makes the sonographic evaluation more difficult in pregnant women than in normal individuals. Its efficacy can decrease after the 32nd week of gestation, due to the narrow field of view owing to the enlarged uterus and placenta [11]. The reported sensitivity and specificity of US in the diagnosis of appendicitis during pregnancy vary from 67% to 100%, and from 83% to 96%, respectively [12]. This variability mostly depends on the operator experience combined with the stage of pregnancy. Moreover, unfortunately a large number of indeterminate results for the diagnosis of appendicitis in pregnancy have been reported by many studies, ranging from 71% to upwards of 98.4% [13, 14]. This high rate of inconclusive results is partly due to the upward shift of the appendix with the progression of the pregnancy, and graded-compression US is very difficult to perform as pregnancy progresses.

Another explanation is that sonologists are more unwilling to make a positive or negative diagnosis of appendicitis utilizing US in pregnancy, because of the potential consequences of an incorrect diagnosis in this group of patients. A false-negative result may delay necessary surgical intervention, with increased risks for the mother and the fetus, whereas a false-positive result will expose the fetus to the risks of unnecessary anesthesia and surgery. These reasons led the European Society of Urogenital Radiology and the American College of Radiology to recommend magnetic resonance imaging (MRI) as the second-line imaging modality after an inconclusive US, and to only perform CT when MRI is not available [15–17].

A very recent study from Poletti [18] demonstrated that non-contrast low radiation dose CT with oral contrast performed after indeterminate US in 29 of 37 pregnant women had a sensitivity of 100% and a specificity of 92% in the diagnosis of appendicitis; this algorithm reduces the need for standard CT when MRI is not available, which is often the case after hours or on weekends at many centers in Europe.

4.2 Acute Biliary Disorders in Pregnancy

Acute biliary disease represents the second most common cause of a non-traumatic acute abdomen, after appendicitis, in pregnant patients, occurring in approximately 1 in 1600–10,000 pregnancies [19]. About 3–10% of pregnant patients have cholelithiasis, which is the cause of 90% cases of acute biliary disorders [20].

During pregnancy, physiologic changes are encountered in the gastrointestinal tract, which

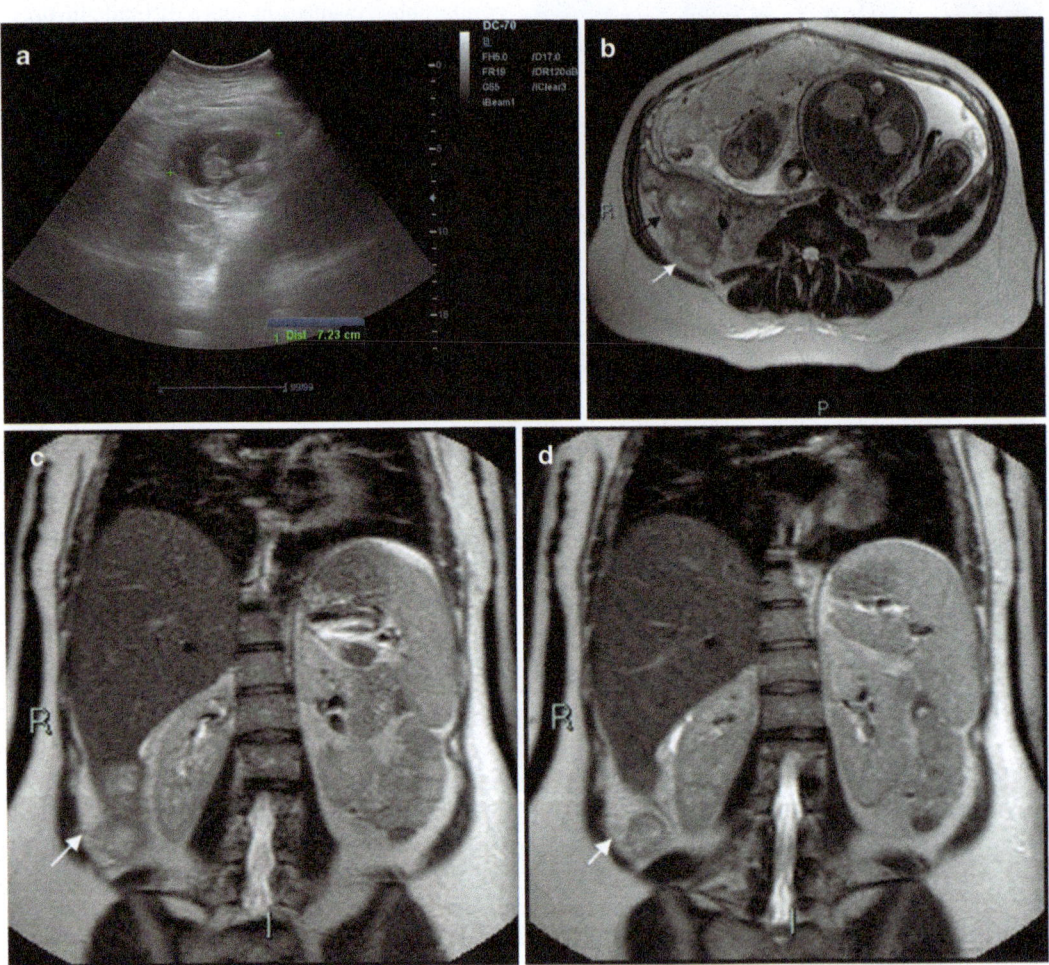

Fig. 4.2 Thirty-two-year-old woman at 16 weeks' gestation, presenting with right upper quadrant pain and nausea. Ultrasound shows an inhomogeneous mass-like area in the right mid abdomen posteriorly, representing the proximal portion of a substantially dilated appendix (**a**). Axial (**b**) and coronal T2-weighted TSE MR images (**c, d**) better demonstrate a markedly thickened fluid-filled appendix (white arrow) arising from the base of the cecum (black arrow), with periappendiceal inflammatory changes (arrows in **c** and **d**), located just below the inferior aspect of the right hepatic lobe. Surgery confirmed the diagnosis of acute appendicitis (**e**)

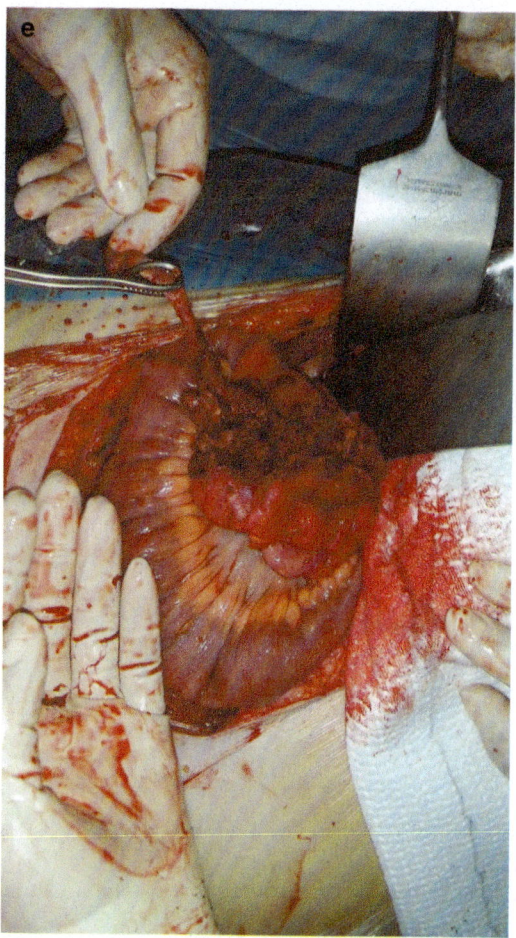

Fig. 4.2 (continued)

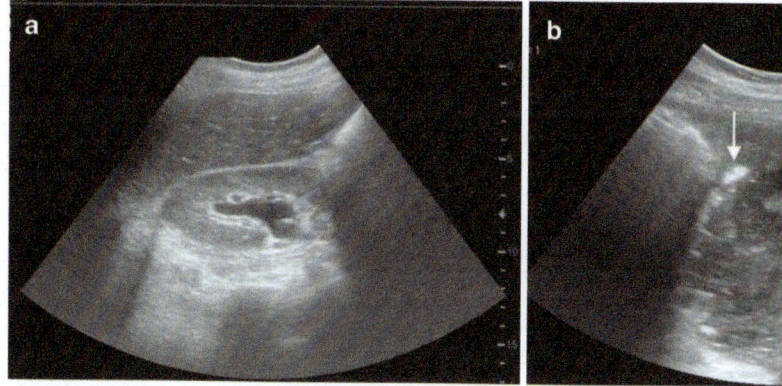

Fig. 4.3 Twenty-eight-year-old woman, pregnant at 30 weeks, presenting with right upper quadrant pain. Ultrasound showed mild to moderate right hydronephrosis, and a stent was placed into the right urinary tract for presumed urolithiasis (**a**). One week later, due to worsening pain and abdominal tenderness, the patient underwent additional sonography, which showed a dilated, sausage-like, blind-ending tubular structure with endoluminal echoes, representing an inflamed appendix (**b**). Hyperechoic foci indicating air bubbles were seen in the appendiceal wall (arrow) (**b**). After removal of the appendix, the pathological diagnosis was gangrenous appendicitis

increases the risk of cholelithiasis and biliary sludge formation. In particular, the sex steroid hormones of pregnancy induce alteration of gallbladder motility and biliary lipid composition; progesterone represents the sex steroid hormone with the greatest potential to alter biliary motility. In fact, it induces smooth muscle relaxation of the gallbladder and decreased gallbladder contractility, which boosts the gallbladder volume and promotes the formation of biliary sludge, a precursor of gallstone formation, Moreover, the high levels of estrogen increase the lithogenicity of bile, due to the high cholesterol saturation of bile [21, 22]. Finally, obesity, or a BMI of 30 mm/kg^2 or more, higher triglyceride levels, and low HDL levels may be associated with gallbladder disease during pregnancy [23].

Acute biliary disease includes a spectrum of pathology, with lithiasis of the gallbladder, cholecystitis, choledocholithiasis, cholangitis, and acute pancreatitis; all of these disorders can have a substantial impact on fetal morbidity and mortality [24]. Imaging should be used to confirm the diagnosis of cholecystitis based on clinical data, and to identify any complications which require prompt and adequate treatment.

An adequate US examination requires a careful evaluation of the liver, gallbladder, biliary tract, and pancreas, with the patient in multiple positions; evaluation with color Doppler is also helpful for the assessment of the flow of the gallbladder wall and the portal vein, in order to exclude secondary portal venous thrombosis. In equivocal or challenging cases in which US remains indeterminate (i.e., a dilated common bile duct with no clear evidence of calculi), non-contrast magnetic resonance with cholangio-pancreatography sequences (MRCP) should be considered in pregnant women, especially after the 16th week of gestation, to assess for associated choledocholithiasis, pancreatitis, and other complications.

4.2.1 Gallbladder Lithiasis

The incidence of gallstone formation increases with parity, from 5.1% in the first pregnancy to 12.3% to after three or more pregnancies, and also during the pregnancy and the post-partum period (4–6 weeks after birth) from 5.1% to 10.2% post-partum [25, 26].

The characteristic symptoms of gallstones are episodic attacks of severe pain in the right upper abdominal quadrant (biliary colic) for at least 15–30 min, with radiation to the right back or shoulder, and pain relief with analgesics. Most attacks resolve spontaneously.

US examination may show as in non-pregnant patients:

- Highly reflective echogenic foci within gallbladder lumen from the anterior surface of the gallstone(s).
- Marked posterior acoustic shadowing.
- Mobility of the gallstone with a change of patient position (gravity-dependent movement).
- Color Doppler examination may demonstrate a twinkling artifact (useful for identification of small stones).

4.2.2 Acute Cholecystitis

Cholecystitis is one of the most common causes of biliary surgery during pregnancy, following repeated biliary colic [27]. It is defined as an acute inflammation of the gallbladder wall, regardless of the cause. In the majority of patients, the underlying etiology is obstruction of the cystic duct by an impacted stone in either the neck of the gallbladder or the cystic duct. If cystic duct patency is re-established, acute cholecystitis may resolve spontaneously within 5–7 days after the onset of symptoms, while obstruction and dilatation of cystic duct may provide a progressive disease course and predispose to a higher chance of developing complications.

The process usually begins with a stone located in the gallbladder neck or cystic duct, causing impaired drainage of bile into the extrahepatic ducts and duodenum. Consequently, there is progressive gallbladder dilatation and increased intraluminal pressure, wall inflammatory thickening, and bacterial super-infection. The increase in the intraluminal pressure prevents arterial perfusion, causing wall ischemia and then necrosis, and ultimately perforation [28].

The symptomatology of acute cholecystitis is almost identical in pregnant patients and non-pregnant women; it includes nausea, vomiting, dyspepsia with intolerance of fat-containing food, and acute onset of a colicky or stabbing pain which begins in the epigastrium or right upper abdominal quadrant and radiates to the back. Physical examination may reveal a Murphy's sign, but this depends largely on gestational age and body habitus. Serum levels of direct bilirubin and transaminases may be elevated, as in non-pregnant women, while serum alkaline phosphatase is less helpful during pregnancy because levels can be double, caused by high estrogen levels [29].

The primary US findings of acute cholecystitis may include, as in non-pregnant patients:

- The presence of gallstones or biliary sludge
- Gallbladder distension (transverse diameter ≥5 cm)
- Gallbladder wall thickening (>3 mm)
- Pericholecystic fluid
- Hyperemic wall upon evaluation with color Doppler, which shows increased arterial flow
- Hyperechogenic pericholecystic fat

MR with MRCP may be requested to identify or exclude co-existing bile duct calculi in patients with known or suspected acute cholecystitis, as in non-pregnant patients, particularly if the liver function tests/bilirubin levels are elevated, and/or there is dilatation of the common duct and/or central bile ducts on initial US (Fig. 4.4).

The differential diagnosis in pregnant women is very broad, and includes myocardial infarction, acute fatty liver, HELLP syndrome (hemolysis, elevated liver enzymes, and low platelet count), acute appendicitis, pre-eclampsia, acute hepatitis, pancreatitis, peptic ulcer disease, pyelonephritis, pneumonia, and even herpes zoster.

Potential complications of untreated acute cholecystitis include the following:

- Gallbladder empyema, which results when purulent material distends the gallbladder lumen.

- Gangrenous cholecystitis, whose typical US features are a thickened wall with a multi-layered, striated appearance; Doppler US may demonstrate absent perfusion either focally or diffusely.
- Emphysematous cholecystitis, which occurs as a result of ischemia with necrosis of the gallbladder wall; US shows asymmetrical wall thickness with gas within the gallbladder wall and lumen, corresponding to necrosis and the presence of gas-forming bacteria, and gas may be seen also in the pericholecystic soft tissues or elsewhere in the biliary tract.
- Gallbladder perforation (GBP), which is a potentially life-threatening complication of acute cholecystitis, occurring in approximately 2–11% of patients, which requires surgical intervention [30].

The most frequent site of perforation is the gallbladder fundus, due to the relatively lower blood supply in this region. Niemeier in 1934 [31] classified free gallbladder perforation, which is still in use, and generalized biliary peritonitis as type I GBP, pericholecystic abscess, and localized peritonitis as subacute or type II GBP, and cholecystoenteric fistula as chronic or type III GBP.

US examination may reveal:

- Discontinuity of the gallbladder wall, with or without the gallbladder lumen collapsed
- Pericholecystic fluid with or without ascites
- Pericholecystic abscess (intrahepatic or extrahepatic) with defined margins and a pseudo-wall
- Pneumatosis in the gallbladder and/or in the biliary system
- Adhesion of the gallbladder to the duodenum or intestinal loop

4.2.3 Choledocholithiasis

The presence of choledocholithiasis contributes to increased morbidity and mortality associated with gallstone disease, and particularly in pregnancy. If there is a clinical suspicion of choledocholithiasis, patient workup and management are more complex compared with that for suspected simple cholelithiasis, leading to additional diagnostic and

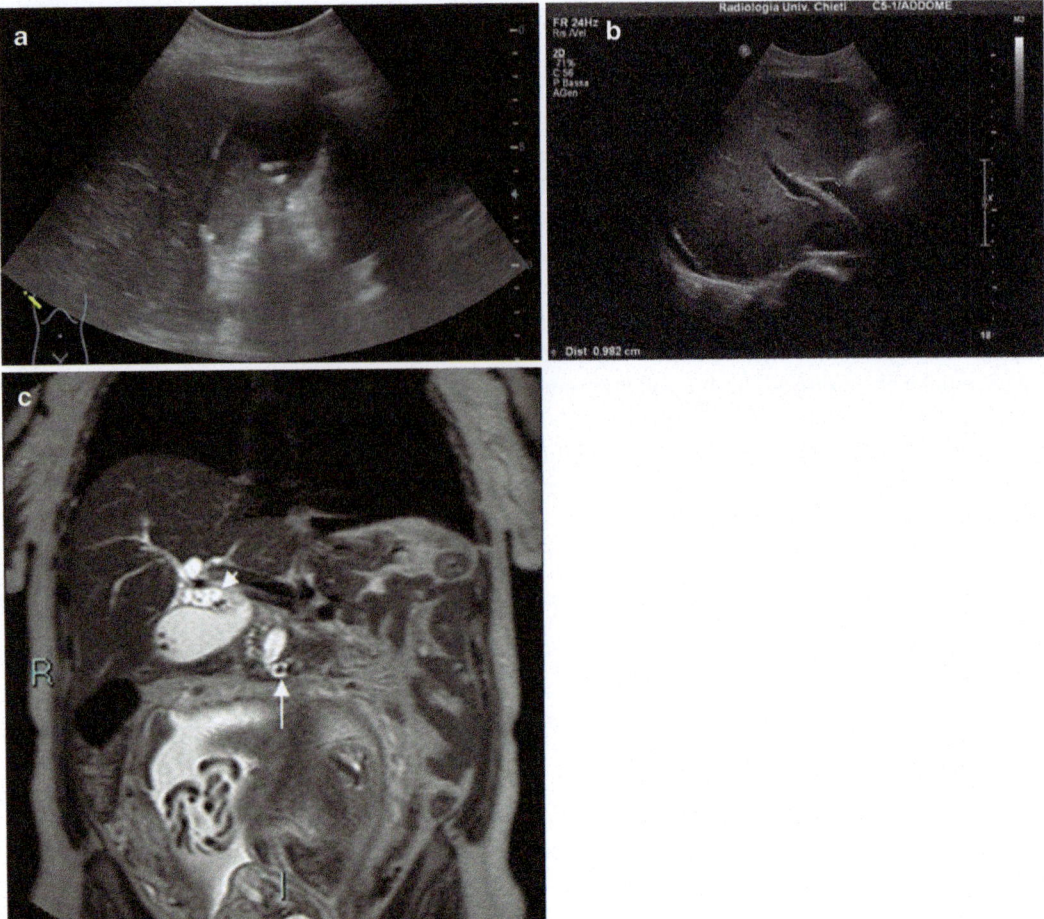

Fig. 4.4 Pregnant woman at 30 weeks' gestation with acute right upper quadrant pain and vomiting. Ultrasound showed a distended gallbladder with a thickened wall, biliary sludge, and multiple gallstones (**a**). These features were highly consistent with acute cholecystitis. Ultrasound also showed mild dilatation of the common bile duct, which is visualized only in its proximal portion (**b**). Coronal T2-weighted TSE MR image then demonstrated an obstructing calculus in the distal portion of the common bile duct (arrow). Dilated cystic duct with calculi is also present (arrowhead) (**c**)

therapeutic procedures. The vast majority of cases of choledocholithiasis occur as a result of the passage of stones from the gallbladder through the cystic duct into the main biliary duct.

Laboratory tests, including elevated bilirubin, alkaline phosphatase, and c-glutamyl transpeptidase levels, can suggest biliary obstruction, but unfortunately are not specific. The white blood cell count is elevated in patients with associated ascending cholangitis.

Although US is highly accurate for the diagnosis of biliary ductal dilatation, the direct depiction of bile duct stones as intraductal echogenic foci with acoustic shadowing is often suboptimal due to duodenal gas which frequently limits the ability to visualize the distal common bile duct. Changes in anatomy and patient size in pregnancy may further complicate diagnosis with US.

MRCP is the most accurate non-invasive imaging examination for the detection of bile duct stones. It has high sensitivity and very high specificity (approximately 84–96%, comparable to ERCP) [32].

4.2.4 Cholangitis

In 80% of patients, the pathogenesis of ascending cholangitis is an impacted stone in the common bile duct, with resultant biliary obstruction, increased intraluminal pressure, and super-infection of the bile by the retrograde ascent of bacteria from the duodenum and/or portal venous system. Increased biliary pressure pushes the infection into the biliary canaliculi, the hepatic veins, and the perihepatic lymphatics, potentially leading to suppurative infection and bacteremia [33].

The diagnosis is based on clinical and laboratory data. Patients with acute cholangitis present with right upper quadrant pain, high fever, jaundice, and, at the last stage, with sepsis.

The role of imaging is the identification of biliary dilatation with associated duct calculi and thickening of the wall of the duct. MRCP is the most sensitive imaging modality and provides more information on the evaluation of biliary system as dilatation of the intrahepatic bile ducts, alteration of the signal of ductal contents, and the presence of multi-loculated collections.

4.3 Acute Urinary Tract Disease

4.3.1 Hydronephrosis and Stone Disease in Pregnancy

Renal colic is one of the most frequent non-obstetric causes of abdominal and/or pelvic pain in pregnancy and subsequent indication for hospitalization [15, 16]. However, the incidence of symptomatic cases of nephrolithiasis and urolithiasis is somewhat uncommon: It is estimated to be up 1 in 1500 pregnancy, involving most frequently multi-parous women without a previous history of ureteral calculi [15, 16].

4.3.1.1 Etiology
During pregnancy, anatomical and physiological changes represent risk factors for stone development. Anatomical factors include dilatation of the renal calyces, of the renal pelvis, and of the ureters, especially on the right, due to the extrinsic compression of the mid and distal tract of the ureter between the gravid uterus and the iliopsoas muscle, and the effect of progesterone on ureteral smooth muscle.

Physiological changes, including the effect of the increased cardiac output and subsequent increase in glomerular filtration rate and decreased systemic vascular resistance, lead to hydronephrosis and hydroureter. During pregnancy, there is also increased production of lithogenic factors (oxalate, uric acid, sodium, and calcium), and of inhibitory factors such as urinary citrate simultaneously. This latter causes a rise in urinary pH, which promotes calcium phosphate crystallization [34]. As noted, the dilatation of the collecting system has a right-sided predominance compared with the left, reflecting the "physiologic hydronephrosis of pregnancy," which frequently occurs more often without consequences such as calculi formation and/or urinary tract infection, and during the second and third trimester causing urinary stasis [35].

4.3.1.2 Clinical Signs and Diagnosis
The most frequent symptoms of urinary calculi in pregnant women are colicky flank pain and hematuria. The pain is generally associated with nausea and vomiting.

Urinary stasis can increase the risk of urinary infections, and for this reason, patients may present fever, lower urinary tract symptoms, and rarely eclampsia [34].

Ultrasound (US) is the first-line imaging examination in the diagnosis of nephrolithiasis and symptomatic ureteral stones during pregnancy, in association with blood chemistry tests and urinalysis. US shows the renal parenchyma, pelvocaliceal system, the upper portions of the ureter(s), if dilated, and potentially dilated lower ureters, and the bladder.

Although recommended as the initial imaging examination for a variety of reasons (low cost, safety, portability, ease of repeatability), US also has several important disadvantages, which limit its accuracy, especially later in pregnancy. First, it has poor sensitivity for the detection of ureteral calculi, in pregnancy in particular, due to the deep position of the retroperitoneal ureters. Second, US is nonspecific because of its inability to readily provide differentiation between ureteral obstruction secondary to calculi, and physiological hydronephrosis and hydroureter. In physiologic hydronephrosis, however, usually the ureteral dilatation is not seen below the level of the pelvic rim/iliac artery, and the dilatation is usually bilateral, especially in the later stages of gestation (Fig. 4.5). On the other hand, if dilatation is detected, it may suggest the presence of a lower ureteral calculus, if present [34] (Fig. 4.6).

Transvaginal US is very useful for the assessment of the ureterovesical junction. Color Doppler can be used to detect the passage of the urine at the ureterovesical junction, i.e., "ureteral jets." In non-pregnant patients, the absence of this sign is relatively sensitive and specific for obstruction. The diagnostic value of this sign is reduced in pregnant women because the ureteral jets may be absent in 15% of asymptomatic pregnant patients. Hydration and contralateral decubitus position may decrease false-positive results distending the

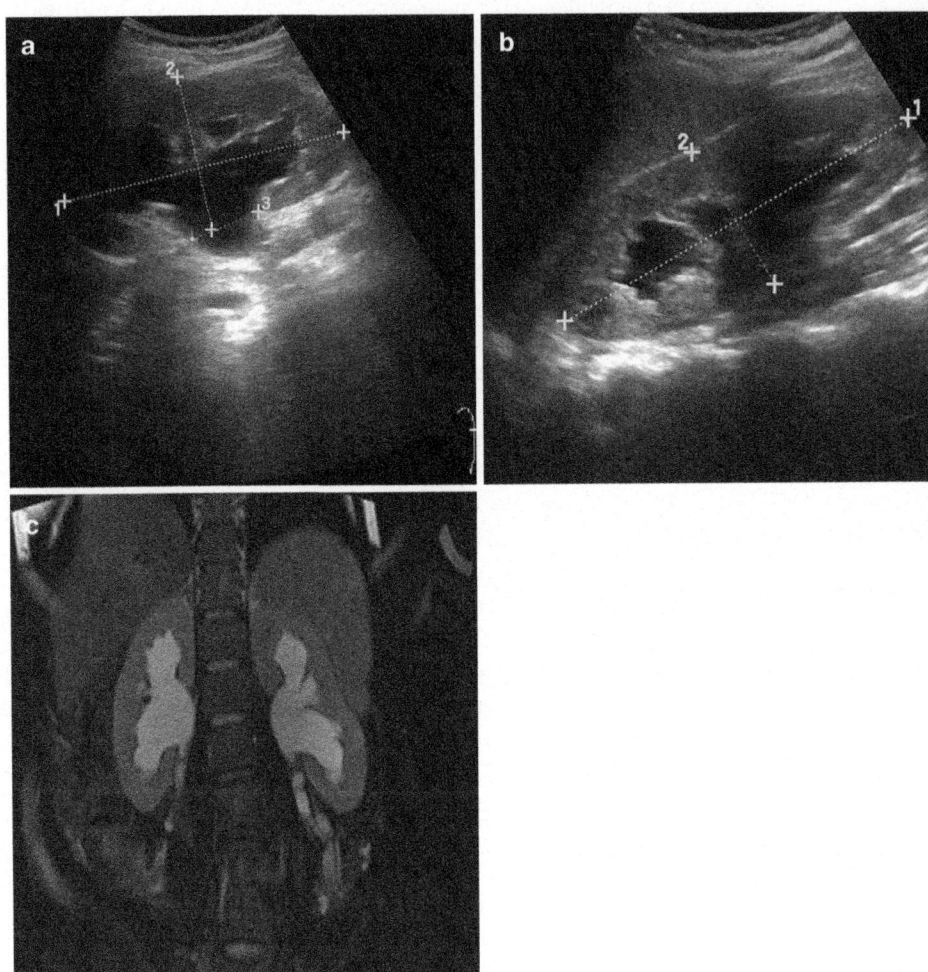

Fig. 4.5 Ultrasound of bilateral physiologic hydronephrosis and hydroureter in a 35-year-old pregnant patient at 27 weeks' gestation (**a, b**) with renal enlargement, dilatation of each renal pelvis and of the calyces (**a**), as well as of the proximal-most ureters (**b**). Subsequent coronal T2-weighted MR image shows dilation of the collecting systems of both kidneys in the same patient (**c**)

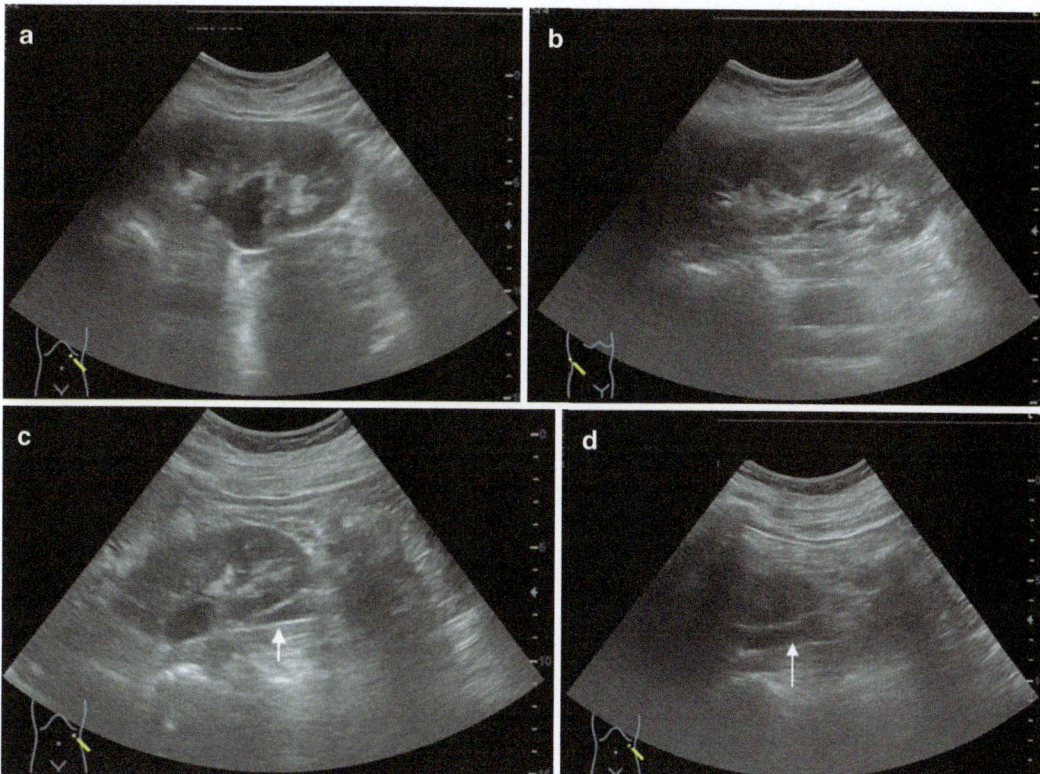

Fig. 4.6 Pregnant woman at 28 weeks' gestation presented to the emergency department with right flank pain. Ultrasound shows mild verging on moderate left hydronephrosis (**a**), and no dilatation of the right renal pelvis or calices (**b**). Ultrasound also demonstrates dilatation of the left proximal ureter (arrows in **c** and **d**), but a ureteral calculus is not seen. This unilateral hydronephrosis and ureteral dilatation is suspicious for the presence of pelvic ureteral obstruction, particularly due to a calculus, which was then definitively diagnosed on MRI (not shown)

bladder, reducing the degree of physiological dilatation and optimizing evaluation for ureteral jets [36].

When US fails to help establish a diagnosis or in case of persistent symptoms with conservative patient management, MRI is the second-line imaging examination, because it helps in differentiating physiologic from obstructive hydronephrosis and hydroureter.

CT uses ionizing radiation, and should be avoided during pregnancy if possible; however, in patients without a clear diagnosis, low radiation dose CT is recommended (<50 Gy), because it is the best imaging examination for characterizing the exact size and shape of a calculus, if present, and is superior to MR, especially for the evaluation of smaller calculi. Low-dose radiation CT is considered safe if used selectively [34].

4.3.1.3 Therapy

The initial management of colicky flank pain in nephrolithiasis and urolithiasis is conservative, using pain medications, antibiotics, and hydration, as smaller and more distal ureteral calculi may pass spontaneously, as in non-pregnant individuals. Second-line management should be implemented when conservative therapy fails, in patients with fever, uncontrolled pain, and/or large calculi. These include temporizing drainage with percutaneous nephrostomy or double-J stenting, and stone extraction with ureteroscopy [34].

4.3.2   Upper Urinary Tract Infections

Pyelonephritis refers to upper urinary (renal) tract infection, usually with associated ascending infection affecting the bladder, ureters, and the renal pelvis and calyces, although alternatively it can be caused by infection seeded from the blood. Infection of the upper urinary must be detected and distinguished from infection of the lower urinary tract, because the first one requires radiological investigation. The aim of imaging is to detect and then treat any potential complications (e.g., obstruction, abscess, perirenal fluid collection) with drainage.

The most frequent infections are community acquired, caused by enterobacteria (*Escherichia coli*) and other gram-negative bacilli. Less frequent are hospital-acquired infections caused by *Pseudomonas aeruginosa* and other agents which are more virulent and are often resistant to multiple antibiotics. Urinary tract infections are most commonly seen in young women. Pregnant women have a higher risk of pyelonephritis. However, the development of a frank renal abscess, secondary to pyelonephritis, is very uncommon [35].

The development of upper urinary infection is based on two pathophysiological mechanisms: ascending infection and hematogenous infection. In ascending infection, bacteria in the infected urine directly reach the papillae and collecting ducts.

4.3.2.1 Clinical Signs and Diagnosis

The most frequent signs and symptoms are fever and lumbar fossa region pain. Other clinical criteria are urine dipstick positive for leukocytes and nitrites, and positive urinalysis.

Ultrasound is the first-line imaging examination for the evaluation of dilatation of pelvicalyceal system, obstruction, suspected urinary tract infection, and the associated complications including abscess, although it has poor sensitivity for the detection of foci of pyelonephritis [35]. Most patients have a normal examination; possible abnormalities which can be identified, however, including focal hypoechoic regions, renal enlargement, loss of the normal renal sinus fat appearance due to edema, and parenchymal hyperechogenicity [37]. US is also helpful for demonstrating dilatation of the pelvicalyceal system and other

findings of obstruction. On the other hand, it is not specific because of its inability, as already noted, to help differentiate between ureteral obstruction which may require emergency drainage, and the physiological hydronephrosis and hydroureter of pregnancy. However, the role of sonography may be improved by using high-frequency and color Doppler imaging. Particularly, color Doppler can better reveal foci of pyelonephritis as perfusion defects, compared with gray-scale imaging [35].

A renal abscess appears on sonography as a well-defined hypoechoic area contained within the cortex or in the corticomedullary parenchyma. It demonstrates internal echoes and can be associated with a diffusely hypoechoic kidney due to acute pyelonephritis. Perinephric fluid collections may also be seen [38].

In some patients, pyelonephritis may be associated with an infected parenchymal cyst, when it is present. At US, this infected cyst appears as an avascular, round mass, with tiny internal echoes and wall thickening, which needs to be differentiated from a renal abscess (Fig. 4.7).

Conservative management is based on antibiotic therapy. Percutaneous drainage or surgery has to be performed in patients not responding to conservative measures.

4.4   Adnexal Torsion

Adnexal torsion is a serious pathological condition which can give rise to pain of varying degrees. This is the fifth among the most common gynecological surgical emergencies, with a prevalence of 2.7%. The incidence of ovarian torsion in pregnancy is relatively rare, with a reported incidence of 1–10 per 10,000 spontaneous pregnancies [39].

Adnexal torsion is caused by the partial or complete rotation of the ovarian pedicle on its axis. This event can interrupt the normal artery flow and venous drainage, causing ischemia and necrosis. If torsion persists over 36 or 48 h, it is considered a surgical emergency due to the risk of irreversible damage to functional ovarian

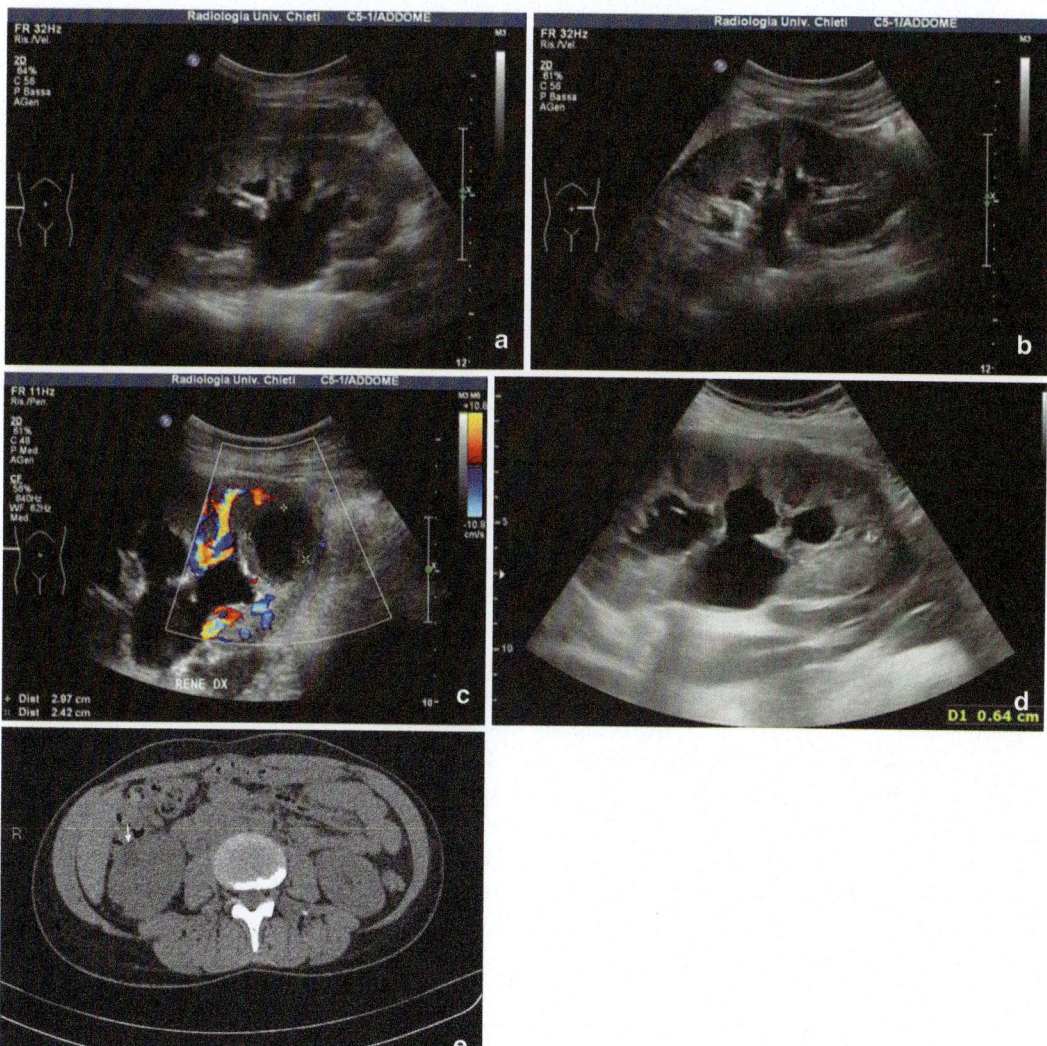

Fig. 4.7 Thirty-three-year-old woman at 25 weeks' gestation presenting with right flank pain, fever, and leukocytosis. Ultrasound shows right renal enlargement with substantial hydronephrosis (**a**) and a normal left kidney (**b**). In the right lower pole of the right kidney, an anechoic cystic mass with a thickened wall but no color Doppler signal is seen (**c**). Three weeks after antibiotic therapy, repeat ultrasound shows persistence of right renal enlargement and hydronephrosis, and the disappearance of the cystic mass, and at the same site a small calcification is detected (**d**). The final diagnosis was pyelonephritis with an associated infected cyst. A cyst of the right renal lower pole anteriorly was noted on CT 3 years earlier (**e**)

tissue [40]. The torsion generally involves both structures but can involve only the ovary, and more rarely only the fallopian tube. Torsion may be caused by an underlying cyst or mass, but it can also arise in normal-appearing ovaries, especially in premenarchal girls as well as in pregnant patients with or without an underlying cyst or mass.

Possible risk factors include the following:

• Ovulation induction and ovarian hyperstimulation syndrome (OHSS) in preparation for assisted fertilization; the risk of torsion with ovarian hyperstimulation syndrome further increases with successful hyperstimulation cycles [41].

- History of adnexal torsion.
- Polycystic ovarian syndrome.
- Pregnancy; 12–25% of adnexal torsion cases occur during pregnancy [42], when both ligamentous laxity related to hormonal changes of pregnancy and mass effect from physiologic corpus luteal cysts may contribute to torsion.
- Ovary size increasing beyond 4–6 cm.

Common cysts associated with torsion include corpus luteal cysts, benign teratomas, follicular cysts, and cystoadenomas. Endometriomas and malignant ovarian tumors which are often associated with adhesions and therefore make the ovary much less mobile are rare cause of torsion (2%).

In most patients, the adnexal torsion of the ovary and its associated tube is unilateral, while it is very rarely bilateral and synchronous. The torsion causes an intense, sudden, and unilateral pelvic pain, which can last for several hours. At the same time, nausea and vomiting, and sometimes diarrhea or constipation, may also occur. In some cases, there may be a history of waxing and waning pain if the adnexa has been twisting and untwisting, i.e., the torsion can also be intermittent. The pain is due to occlusion of the vascular pedicle, with subsequent hypoxia. If torsion is prolonged, the adnexa can become necrotic and even infected, and the patient may exhibit signs of peritonitis. Delayed intervention can lead to irreversible damage to the tube and/or ovary. Laparoscopic detorsion of adnexal torsion is recommended as the definitive treatment in the first and second trimesters of pregnancy [8].

4.4.1 Ultrasound

Sonography is the most commonly used imaging examination for the diagnosis of adnexal torsion, if an ovarian/adnexal process is suspected prospectively. The diagnosis requires a high index of suspicion by the radiologist, but some sonographic signs are suggestive or highly suggestive [43]:

- Increase in the volume of the ovary, which appears as a solid or predominantly solid mass

- Edema of the ovarian parenchyma, which appears blurred with a hypoechoic echostructure compared to the normal ovary
- "String of pearls": ovarian follicles displaced peripherally due to edema
- Pelvic fluid
- Abnormal ovarian location

If a normal ovary is involved in the torsion, the edema causes enlargement of the ovary, which generally loses its oval shape, and become round or globular. Multiple small follicles at the periphery of the ovary are often identified as well, as a result of stromal edema and disruption of venous flow and are very characteristic, and particularly when the associated findings of ovarian swelling, heterogeneity, and decreased blood flow are also identified. As the arterial blood supply is compromised, hemorrhage and infarction occur, and the infarcted ovary may appear with an anechoic halo [44]. The location of the ovary can also be medio-superior to its usual location, in the pouch of Douglas, anterior to the uterus, or over to the contralateral side. Other common findings on sonography (or on MR or CT) are the presence of free fluid in the pelvic cavity, and the deviation of the uterus toward the side where the torsion occurred.

In 40–60% of cases of torsion, the vascularization of the ovary is completely absent. The torsion of the vascular pedicle can produce a specific artifact, which is not always identifiable, the "whirlpool sign." This sign is a unique, direct sign which represents the twisted pedicle—the torsion itself (Fig. 4.8). In partial or early torsion, both arterial and venous flow can be seen, within viable ovarian tissue. If spontaneous detorsion occurs, which is relatively common, the flow to the ovary may be increased, not decreased or eliminated, so the radiologist must carefully consider the sonographic findings in the context of the patient's history.

The diagnosis of maternal adnexal torsion is missed in upwards of 15–35% of patients, because of the non-specific clinical features and uncommon ultrasound findings, especially in cases with OHSS [45]. In this setting, emergent MRI of the abdomen and pelvis can be used for

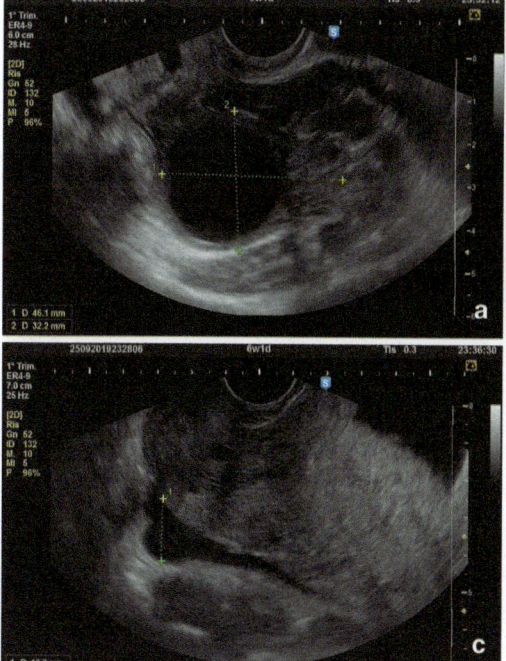

Fig. 4.8 Woman at 16 weeks' gestation with acute pelvic pain, primarily in the right lower quadrant. Transvaginal ultrasound shows an enlarged right ovary with a cystic mass and follicles displaced at its periphery (**a**). A twisted vascular pedicle (whirlpool sign) is noted just cranial to the ovary, indicating ovarian torsion (**b**). Free fluid is also present in the pelvis (**c**)

the diagnosis of adnexal torsion [46] (Lourenco et al. 2014; Asch et al. 2017).

4.5   Pelvic Masses Presenting Emergently in Pregnancy

Adnexal masses occur in approximately 2–10% of all pregnancies and are not a usual cause of pain, unless they are complicated by torsion, hemorrhage, or rupture [47]. The most common ovarian mass found in pregnancy is a benign ovarian cyst [48]. There are many types of benign ovarian cysts, including corpus luteal, follicular, hemorrhagic, and endometriotic cysts.

4.5.1   Functional or Simple Cyst

A functional cyst is a developing follicle and is commonly observed during ultrasound examination in pregnancy, especially earlier in the gesta-

tion. They usually appear as a 0.2- to 3-cm-anechoic cyst with a thin wall (<3 mm) and posterior acoustic enhancement. Follicular cysts usually disappear within 4–8 weeks, including in pregnancy [49, 50].

The corpus luteum develops from a follicle after ovulation, when the granulosa cells become luteinized. It contains blood, which accumulates in its central cavity. The US appearance is that of a cyst with a thick echogenic wall and peripheral vascularization on Doppler [51].

4.5.2   Ovarian Hyperstimulation Syndrome (OHSS) and Hyperreactioluteinalis

Ovarian hyperstimulation syndrome, hyperreactioluteinalis, and gestational trophoblastic disease are the three main conditions correlated with the clinical setting of high hCG levels. OHSS is an iatrogenic complication of ovula-

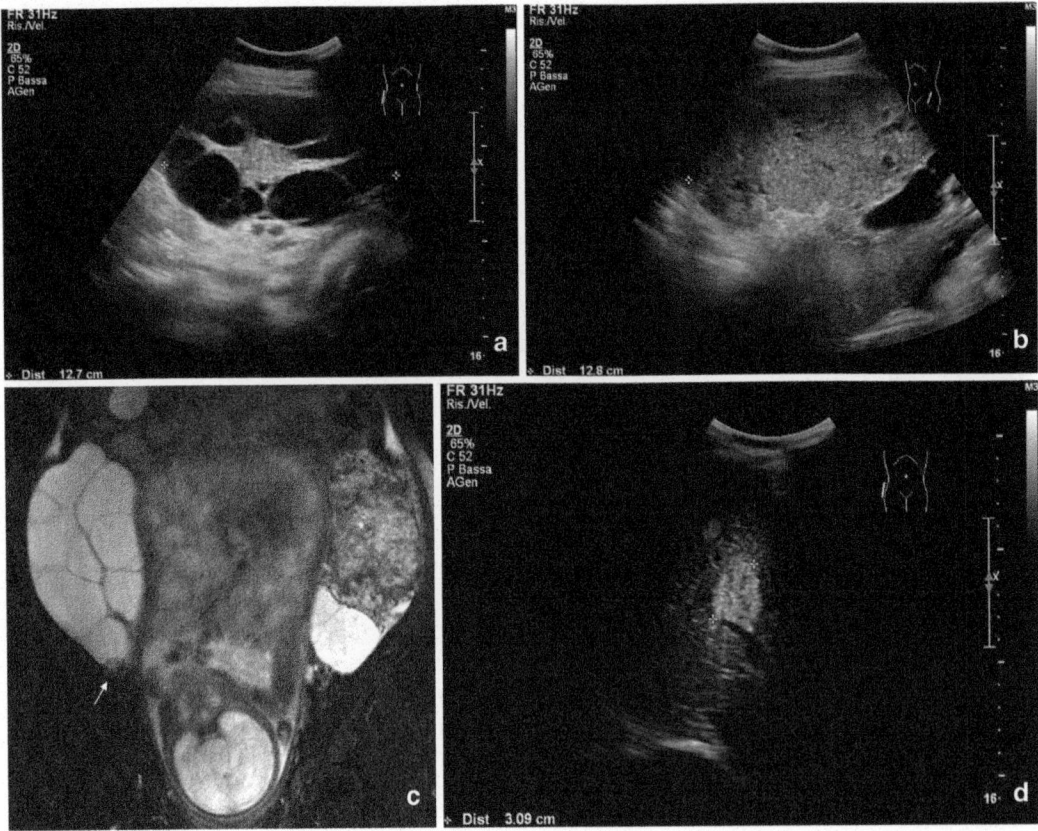

Fig. 4.9 Twenty-eight-year-old woman at 25 weeks' gestation who had not undergone ovulation induction, presenting with intermittent acute pelvic pain. Abdominal ultrasound shows bilateral enlarged ovaries (**a, b**). The right ovary has multiple thin-walled cysts of varying size (**a**). The left ovary appears as a solid mass with a few peripheral cysts (**b**). The solid component of the left ovary is difficult to differentiate between normal ovarian parenchyma and solid tissue. Coronal T2-weighted TSE MR image better demonstrates the presence of inhomogeneous solid tissue in the central part of the left ovary and the lower part of the right ovary (arrow) (**c**). The final diagnosis was bilateral ovarian choriocarcinoma with hyperechoic liver metastases (**d**)

tion induction, and occurs during early pregnancy or during the luteal phase. If high circulating serum hCG levels are associated with gestational trophoblastic disease, polycystic ovarian disease, and triplet pregnancies, the condition is called hyperreactioluteinalis. Most cases regress spontaneously later in pregnancy or after delivery [52]. US findings in patients with OHSS or hyperreactioluteinalis include markedly enlarged ovaries containing multiple, large, peripherally located, thin-walled cysts. The large ovaries are at risk of torsion, and must be differentiated from ovarian tumors including choriocarcinoma, which can also produce high hCG levels; in equivocal or problematic patients,

MRI can provide better characterization of the ovarian process (Fig. 4.9).

4.5.3 Hemorrhagic Ovarian Cyst

Hemorrhagic ovarian cyst is usually symptomatic with acute lower abdominal pain. In some patients, ascites can be present, while blood tests often show normocytic anemia with mild elevation of inflammatory markers [53]. The main differential diagnosis is with ectopic pregnancy, and determining and monitoring the HCG levels is mandatory [54, 55].

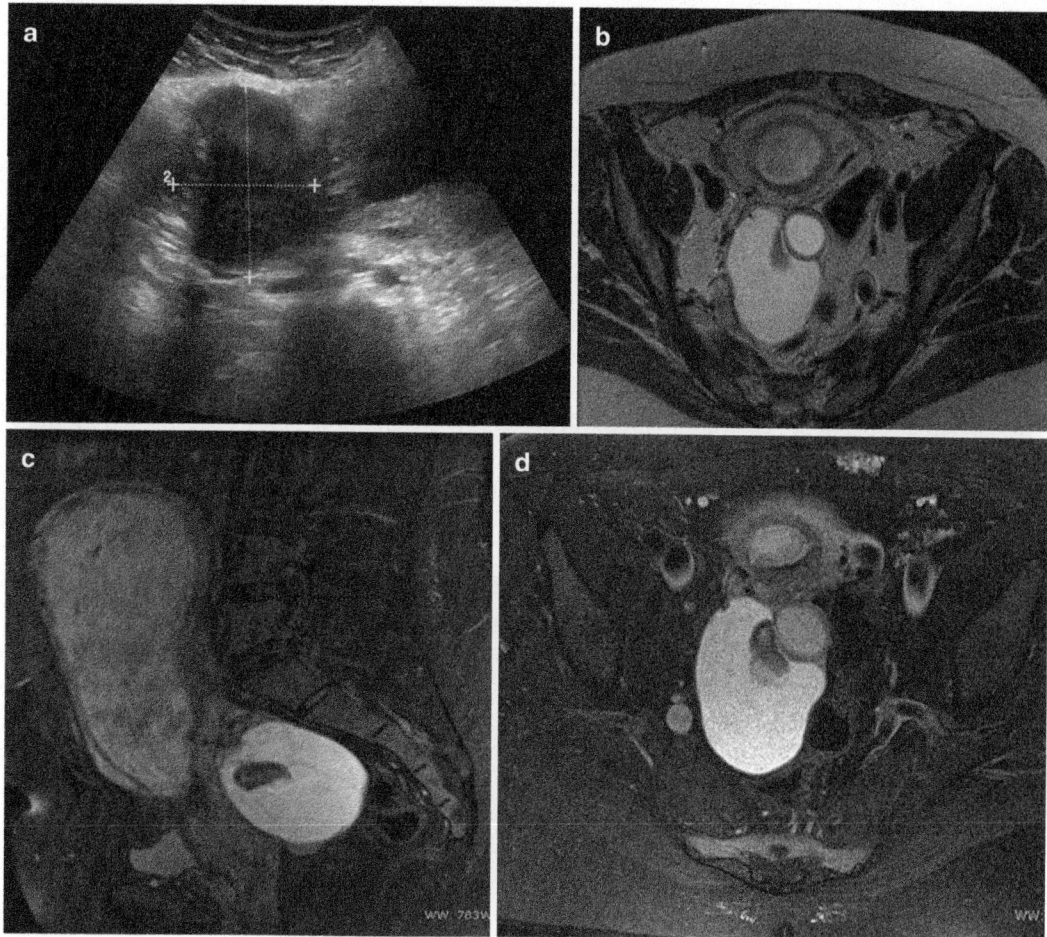

Fig. 4.10 Twenty-five-year-old woman, 15 weeks pregnant, presented with abdominal pain. Abdominal ultrasound shows a unilocular ovarian cyst with "spider web" contents and blood clots, representing a hemorrhagic cyst (**a**). The same patient on MRI, which was subsequently performed, shows a large (7.1 × 5.4 × 6.5 cm) hemorrhagic cyst containing blood and blood clots, with high signal intensity on a T2-weighted axial image (**b**), and on sagittal and axial T2 fat-saturated images, representing subacute clot (**c**, **d**)

In the acute stage, the hemorrhage appears isoechoic to the stroma, and this can often be misinterpreted as an enlarged ovary. Over time, the clot forms and there is the typical "spider-web" appearance (Fig. 4.10). The presence of intra-abdominal fluid should always be assessed in order to exclude rupture of the cyst [56]. Urgent surgery may very occasionally (for example in case of underlying coagulopathy or anticoagulant treatment) be required in patients with hemorrhagic cyst rupture and on-going hemoperitoneum.

A particular type of hemorrhagic cyst is the hemorrhagic corpus luteal cyst. It usually shows a vascularized wall and an avascular internal lace-like pattern [57], and can be distinguished from other hemorrhagic cysts because it typically has a ring-of-fire appearance at the periphery.

4.5.4 Dermoid Cyst Rupture

Dermoid cyst (mature cystic teratoma) represents the most common ovarian neoplasm. Most of them are asymptomatic, but in 3% it can cause torsion, and even more rarely it undergoes to rupture (with or without associated torsion). Symptomatic patients usually show acute pelvic pain, nausea, and vomiting [58].On ultrasound, a cystic teratoma usually appears as a cystic mass with hyperechoic areas due to the fat content [59].

4.5.5 Endometriotic Cyst

The cyclical bleeding of endometrial hormonally responsive cells placed outside the myometrium is responsible for endometriosis development. This situation leads to the growth of blood-filled cyst(s) ("chocolate" cysts or endometriomas) within one or both ovaries (80% cases), and there may also be associated hemorrhagic ascites, less commonly. When the inflammation became chronic, fibrosis and adhesions within the pelvis may develop [60].

Symptoms often include chronic pelvic pain, dyspareunia, dysmenorrhea, and infertility. On ultrasound, endometriomas usually show low-level echogenicity (also called a "ground-glass pattern") (Fig. 4.11). The differential diagnosis includes hemorrhagic cysts, which are more common. Moreover, compared to endometriomas, they tend to be unilateral and unilocular, disappear over time, and usually do not show a "T2 dark spot" [61, 62]. The rupture of an endometriotic cyst is very uncommon but may require emergency surgery [63].

4.5.6 Cystadenomas and Cystadenocarcinomas

When an ovarian cyst is complex (and not hemorrhagic), a cystadenoma or cystadenocarcinoma must be considered in the differential diagnosis. Serous cystadenoma usually appears as anechoic cystic mass or with thin septations, whereas mucinous tumors have corpuscular content. Irregular septations and mural nodules substantially increase the likelihood of a cystadenocarcinoma being present (Figs. 4.12 and 4.13). When malignancy is suspected in utero, a mini-laparotomy is typically performed in the second trimester; if diagnosis is not made

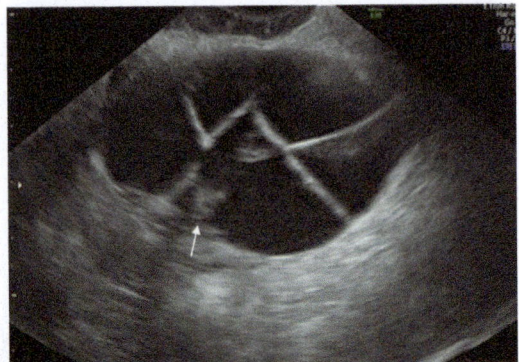

Fig. 4.12 Thirty-three-year old woman at 30 weeks' gestation. Transvaginal ultrasound shows a large cyst with thick and irregular septations and a small mural node (arrow). The final diagnosis was cystadenocarcinoma

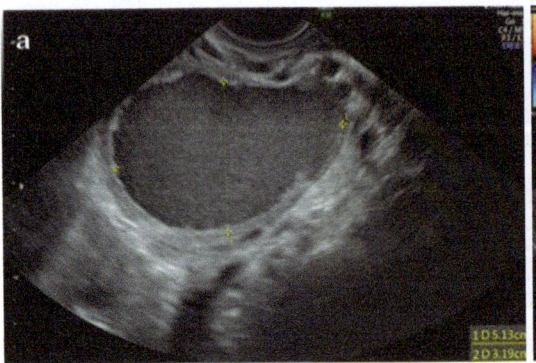
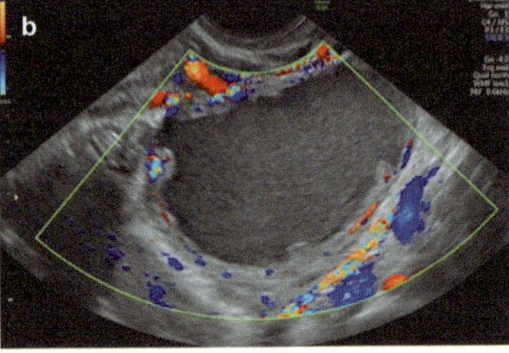

Fig. 4.11 Twenty-two-year old woman at 18 weeks' gestation. Transvaginal ultrasound shows a large ovarian cyst with diffuse low-level internal echoes, with the classic appearance of a "chocolate cyst" (**a**). No color flow signal is present inside the cyst, which is highly consistent with an endometrioma (**b**)

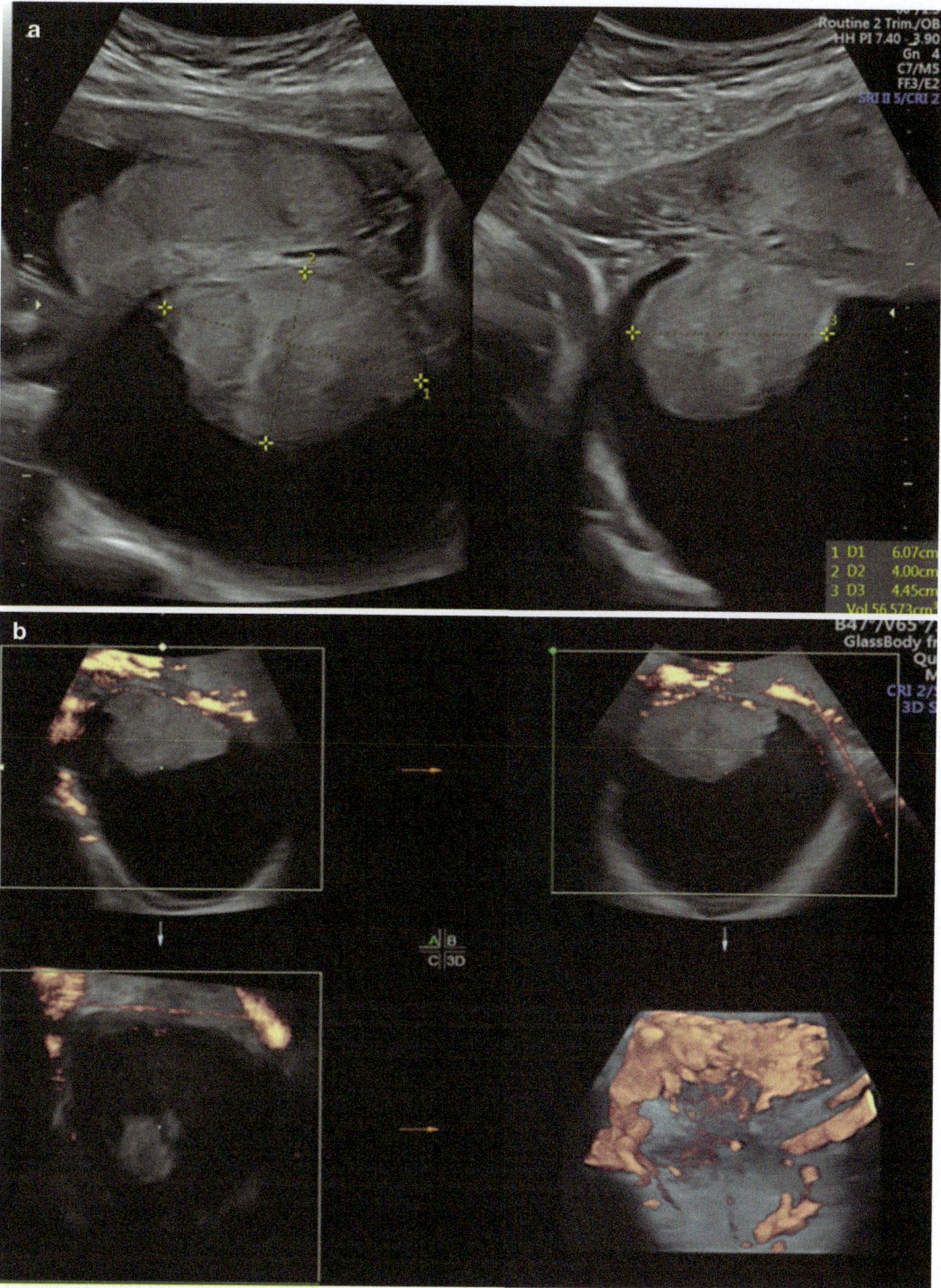

Fig. 4.13 Twenty-nine-year-old woman at 16 weeks' gestation, who presented with lower abdominal pain. On abdominal ultrasound, a cystic mass with a solid, mural nodule was visualized (**a**), with increased blood flow on Doppler images (**b**), which proved to be a cystadenocarcinoma after removal. MRI performed after sonography but prior to surgery confirmed the findings of a complex cystic mass, on a sagittal T2-weighted image with fat suppression (**c**), and on a coronal T2-weighted image (**d**). On sagittal T2-weighted fat-sat image (**c**) and on axial T2-weighted image (**e**), please note enlarged, gravid uterus consistent with 16GW

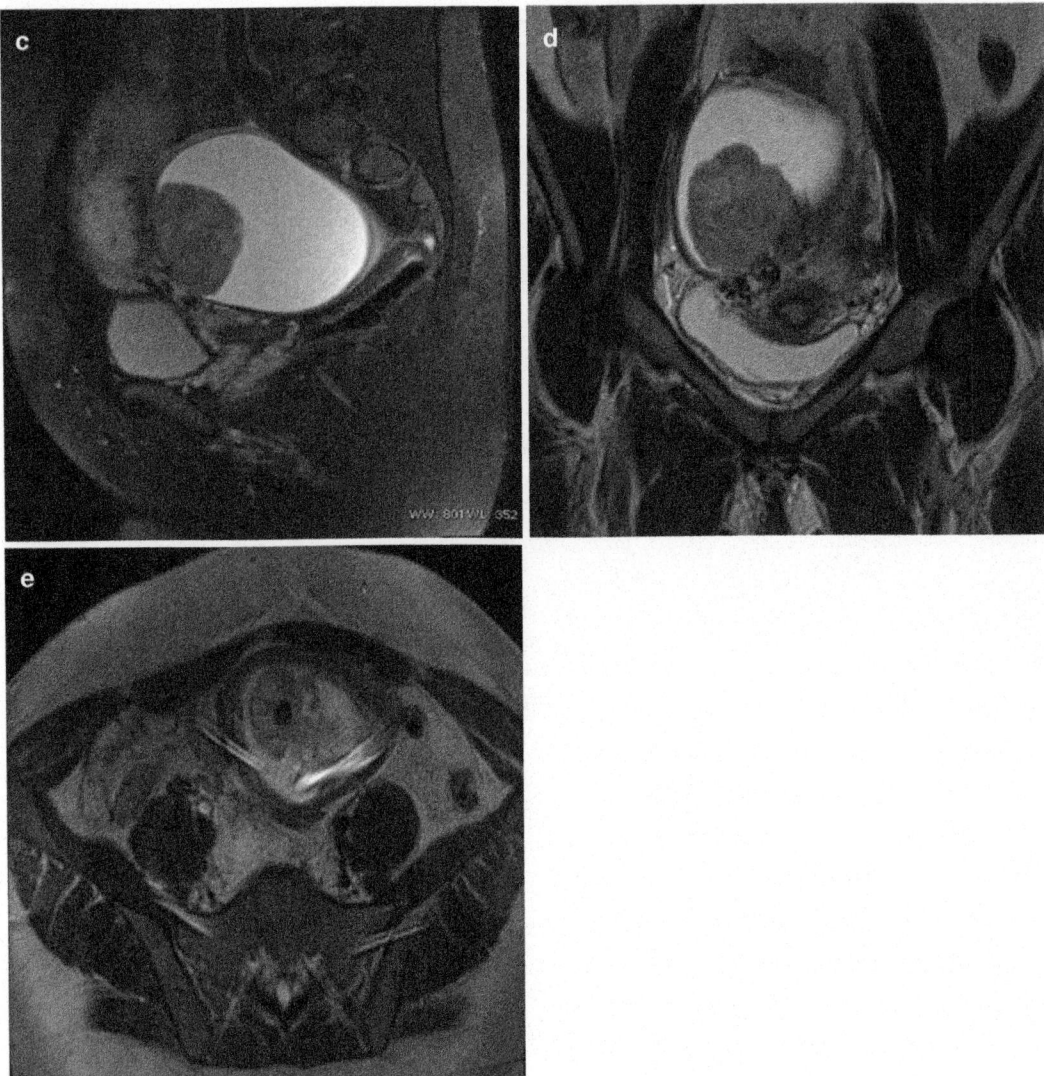

Fig. 4.13 (continued)

until late in gestation, removal of the ovary can be performed at the time of Cesarean delivery [64].

4.5.7 Fibroids

Fibroids, a.k.a. leiomyomas, are the most common pelvic tumors in fertile age females. In fact, they occur in a percentage ranging between 20% and 30% of women 30 years of age or older. They are benign smooth muscle tumors that are sensi-

tive to estrogens, and may became symptomatic (acute pain) during the fourth decade [65], or during pregnancy. Acute pain may be due to the following reasons:

- Degeneration of a fibroid outgrowing its blood supply
- Torsion of a pedunculated fibroid
- Prolapse of a submucosal fibroid
- Hemorrhagic infarction caused by thrombosis of the venous outflow (oral contraceptive pill, pregnancy)

Acute complications of fibroids are fortunately rare, but acute bleeding can very rarely lead to hypovolemic shock and death. Ultrasound usually represents the first-line imaging modality for the identification of fibroids and any associated suspected complications. They typically appear as well-defined hypoechoic masses arising within the surrounding myometrium, with or without posterior acoustic enhancement, and/or calcifications. On the other hand, the degeneration of fibroids appears with a more complex US pattern, showing cystic areas and circumferential vascularity on Doppler. The absence of flow on Doppler is very suggestive of necrosis [66].

4.5.8 Pelvic Inflammatory Disease

Pelvic inflammatory disease (PID) includes endometritis, salpingitis, and tubo-ovarian abscesses. From a pathological point of view, it represents the spread of inflammation from the endometrial cavity (*Chlamydia trachomatis* and *Neisseria gonorrhoea* are frequently responsible for ascending cervicitis) into the fallopian tubes and then elsewhere in the pelvis and abdomen. Potential causes of secondary PID include diverticulitis, appendicitis, and tuberculosis. It accounts for 25% of emergency visits due to gynecological pain. Patients usually have leukocytosis, increased inflammatory markers, and have fever [67]. Complications of PID can be serious and disabling, including infertility, ectopic pregnancy, chronic abdominal and pelvic pain, and the development of tubo-ovarian abscesses which may occasionally be drained by interventional radiologists or may surgery [68]. In the early phase of infection, the US appearance can be normal. When the disease advances, it may show uterine enlargement with loss of tissue planes and endometrial thickening. Hydrosalpinx or pyosalpinx represent two possible complications of salpingitis. The tubes may appear folded with echogenic material inside. Pyosalpinx can evolve into tubo-ovarian abscesses. In this case, in the fallopian tubes and ovaries, echogenic debris representing inflammatory exudates, blood, and pus are appreciable.

Ovarian cancer should always be considered among the differential diagnoses of a tubo-ovarian mass. The clinical presentation plays an important role, and follow-up imaging following treatment usually confirms the diagnosis [69].

References

1. Zachariah SK, Fenn M, Jacob K, et al. Management of acute abdomen in pregnancy: current perspectives. Int J Womens Health. 2019;11:119–34.
2. Mourad J, Elliott JP, Erickson L, Lisboa L. Appendicitis in pregnancy: new information that contradicts long-held clinical beliefs. Am J Obstet Gynecol. 2000;182:1027–9.
3. Choi JJ, Mustafa R, Lynn ET, Divino CM. Appendectomy during pregnancy: follow-up of progeny. J Am Coll Surg. 2011;213(5):627–32.
4. Ueberrueck T, Koch A, Meyer L, et al. Ninety-four appendectomies for suspected acute appendicitis during pregnancy. World J Surg. 2004;28:508–11.
5. Doberneck RC. Appendectomy during pregnancy. Am Surg. 1985;51(5):265–8.
6. Selzer DJ, Stefanidis D. Surgical emergencies in the pregnant patient. Adv Surg. 2019;53:61–177.
7. Koepsell TD. In serach of the causes of appendicitis. Epidemiology. 1991;2(5):319–21.
8. Augustin G. Acute abdomen during pregnancy. New York: Springer; 2014.
9. Baer JL, Reis RA, Arens RA. Appendicitis in pregnancy: with changes in position and axis of the normal appendix in pregnancy. J Am Med Assoc. 1932;98:1359–64.
10. Freeland M, King E, Safcsak K, et al. Diagnosis of appendicitis in pregnancy. 2009;198(5):753–8.
11. Woodfield CA, Lazarus E, Chen KC, Mayo-Smith WW. Abdominal pain in pregnancy: diagnoses and imaging unique to pregnancy – review. AJR Am J Roentgenol. 2010;194(6 Suppl):WS14–30.
12. Williams R, Shaw J. Ultrasound scanning in the diagnosis of acute appendicitis in pregnancy. Emerg Med J. 2007;24(5):359–60.
13. Lehnert BE, Gross JA, Linnau KF, Moshiri M. Utility of ultrasound for evaluating the appendix during the second and third trimester of pregnancy. Emerg Radiol. 2012;19:293–9.
14. Ramalingam V, LeBedis C, Kelly JR, et al. Evaluation of a sequential multi-modality imaging algorithm for the diagnosis of acute appendicitis in the pregnant female. Emerg Radiol. 2015;22:125–32.
15. Masselli G, Derchi L, McHugo J, et al. Acute abdominal and pelvic pain in pregnancy: ESUR recommendations. Eur Radiol. 2013a;23:3485–500.
16. Masselli G, Derme M, Laghi F, et al. Imaging of stone disease in pregnancy. Abdom Imaging. 2013b;38(6):1409–14.

17. Smith MP, Katz DS, Lalani T, et al. ACR appropriateness Criteria® right lower quadrant pain—suspected appendicitis. Ultrasound Q. 2015;31:85–91.

18. Poletti PA, Botsikas D, Becker M, et al. Suspicion of appendicitis in pregnant women:emergency evaluatioon by sonography and low-dose CT and oral contrast. Eur Radiol. 2019;29(1):345–52.

19. Kammerer W. Nonobstetric surgery during pregnancy. Med Clin North Am. 1979;63:1157–64.

20. Basso L, McCollum P, Darling M, et al. A study of cholelithiasis during pregnancy and its relationship with age, parity, menarche, breastfeeding, dysmenorrhea, oral contraception and a maternal history of cholelithiasis. Gynecol Obstet. 1992;175:41–6.

21. Everson GT. Gastrointestinal motility in pregnancy. Gastroenterol Clin North Am. 1992;21:751.

22. Scott LD. Gallstone disease and pancreatitis in pregnancy. Gastroenterol Clin North Am. 1992;21:803.

23. Littlefield A, et al. Cholelithiasis: presentation and management. J Midwifery Womens Health. 2019;64(3):289–97.

24. Ramin K, Richey S, Ramin S, et al. Acute pancreatitis in pregnancy. Am J Obstet Gynecol. 1995;173:187–91.

25. Dhiman RK, Chawla YK. Is there a link between estrogen therapy and gallbladder disease? Expert Opin Drug Saf. 2006;5(1):117–29.

26. Pearl J, Price R, Richardson W, Fanelli R, Society of American Gastrointestinal Endoscopic Surgeons. Guidelines for diagnosis, treatment, and use of laparoscopy for surgical problems during pregnancy. Surg Endosc. 2011;25(11):3479–92.

27. Ghumman E, Barry M, Grace PA. Management of gallstones in pregnancy. Br J Surg. 1997;84(12):1646–50.

28. O'Connor OJ, Maher MM. Imaging of cholecystitis. AJR Am J Roentgenol. 2011;196:W367–74.

29. Hiatt JR, Hiatt JC, Williams RA, et al. Biliary disease in pregnancy: strategy for surgical management. Am J Surg. 1986;151:263–5.

30. Ausania F, Guzman Suarez S, Alvarez Garcia H, Senra del Rio P, Casal Nunez E. Gallbladder perforation: morbidity, mortality and preoperative risk prediction. Surg Endosc. 2015;29:955–60.

31. Niemeier OW. Acute free perforation of the gallbladder. Ann Surg. 1934;99(6):922–4.

32. Griffin N, Wastle M, Dunn W, et al. Magnetic resonance cholangiopancreatography versus endoscopic retrograde cholangiopancreatography in the diagnosis of choledocholithiasis. Eur J Gastroenterol Hepatol. 2003;15(7):809–8126.

33. Catalano OA, Sahani DV, Forcione DG, et al. Biliary infections: spectrum of imaging findings and management. Radiographics. 2009;29(7):2059–80.

34. Masselli G, Weston M, Spencer J. The role of imaging in the diagnosis and management of renal stone disease in pregnancy. Clin Radiol. 2015;70(12):1462–71.

35. Ifergan J, Pommier R, Brion MC, Glas L, Rocher L, Bellin MF. Imaging in upper urinary tract infections. Diagn Interv Imaging. 2012;93(6):509–19.

36. Wachsberg RH. Unilateral absence of ureteral jets in the third trimester of pregnancy: pitfall in color Doppler US diagnosis of urinary obstruction. Radiology. 1998;209(1);279–81.

37. Craig W, Wagner B, Travis M. Pyelonephritis: radiologic-pathologic correlations. Radiographics. 2008;28:255–76.

38. Peces R, Peces C, Benítez A, Sánchez Villanueva R, Cuesta E. Pregnant patient with acute pyelonephritis and renal corticomedullary abscess: ultrasound and MRI imaging. Nefrologia. 2009;29(5):492–4.

39. Hasson J, Tsafrir Z, Azem F, et al. Comparison of adnexal torsion between pregnant and nonpregnant women. Am J Obstet Gynecol. 2010;202:536 e.1–.e.6.

40. Tobiume T, Shiota M, Umemoto M, Kotani Y, Hoshiai H. Predictive factors for ovarian necrosis in torsion of ovarian tumor. Tokoku J Exp Med. 2012;225(3):203–5.

41. Mashiach S, Bider D, Moran O, Goldenberg M, Ben Rafael Z. Adnexal torsion of hyperstimulated ovaries in pregnancies after gonadotropin Therapy. Fertil Steril. 1990;53:76–80.

42. Desai S, Allahbadia G, Dulal A. Ovarian torsion: diagnosis by color Doppler ultrasonography. Obstet Gynecol. 1994;84:699–701.

43. Chang H, Bhatt S, Dogra V. Pearls and pitfalls in diagnosis of ovarian torsion. Radiographics. 2008;28 (5):1355–68.

44. Bowen A. Ovarian torsion diagnosed by ultrasonography. South Med J. 1985;78:1376–9.

45. Chang SD, Yen CF, Lo LM, et al. Surgical intervention for maternal ovarian torsion in pregnancy. Taiwan J Obstet Gynecol. 2011;50:458–62.

46. Rha SE, Byun JY, Jung SE, et al. CT and MR imaging features of adnexal torsion. Radiographics. 2002;22:283–94.

47. Schwartz N, Timor-Tritsch IE, Wang E. Adnexal masses in pregnancy. Clin Obstet Gynecol. 2009;52(4):570–85.

48. Cappell MS, Friedel D. Abdominal pain during pregnancy. Gastroenterol Clin North Am. 2003;32(1):1–58.

49. Stenchever M. Comprehensive gynaecology. 2nd ed. Philadelphia: Mosby; 2001.

50. de Haan J, Verheecke M, Amant F. Management of ovarian cysts and cancer in pregnancy. Facts Views Vis Obgyn. 2015;7(1):25–31.

51. Vandermeer FQ, Wong-You-Cheong JJ. Imaging of acute pelvic pain. Clin Obstet Gynecol. 2009;52:2–20.

52. Park SB, Han BH, Lee YH. Ultrasonographic evaluation in acute pelvic pain in pregnant and postpartum period. Med Ultrason. 2017;19(2):218–23.

53. Hertzberg BS, Kliewer MA, Bowie JD, et al. Adnexal ring sign and hemoperitoneum caused by hemorrhagic ovarian cyst: pitfall in the sonographic diagnosis of ectopic pregnancy. AJR Am J Roentgenol. 1999;173:1301–2.

54. Kaakaji Y, Nghiem HV, Nodell C, Winter TC. Sonography of obstetric and gynecologic emergencies: Part II, Gynecologic emergencies. AJR Am J Roentgenol. 2000a;174:651–6.

55. Kaakaji Y, Nghiem HV, Nodell C, Winter TC. Sonography of obstetric and gynecologic emergencies: Part I, Obstetric emergencies. AJR Am J Roentgenol. 2000b;174:641–9.
56. Jeong YY, Outwater EK, Kang HK. Imaging evaluation of ovarian masses. Radiographics. 2000;20:1445–70.
57. Valentin L. Use of morphology to characterize and manage common adnexal masses. Best Pract Res Clin Obstet Gynaecol. 2004;18:71–89.
58. Kalish GM, Patel MD, Gunn ML, Dubinsky TJ. Computed tomographic and magnetic resonance features of gynecologic abnormalities in women presenting with acute or chronic abdominal pain. Ultrasound Q. 2007;23:167–75.
59. Comerci JT, Licciardi F, Bergh PA, Gregori C, Breen JC. Mature cystic teratoma: a clinicopathologic evaluation of 517 cases and review of the literature. Obstet Gynecol. 1994;84:22–8.
60. Busard MP, Pieters-van den Bos IC, Mijatovic V, Van Kuijk C, Bleeker MC, van Waesberghe JH. Evaluation of MR diffusion-weighted imaging in differentiating endometriosis infiltrating the bowel from colorectal carcinoma. Eur J Radiol. 2012;81(6):1376–80.
61. Corwin MT, Gerscovich EO, Lamba R. et al. Differentiation of ovarian endometriomas from hemorrhagic cysts at MR imaging: utility of the T2 dark spot sign. Radiology. 2015;271(1):126–32.
62. Foti PV, Farina R, Palmucci S, et al. Endometriosis: clinical features, MR imaging findings and pathologic correlation. Insights Imaging. 2018;9(2):149–72.
63. Huang YH, Liou JD, Hsieh CL, et al. Long-term follow-up of patients surgically treated for ruptured ovarian endometriotic cysts. Taiwan J Obstet Gynecol. 2011;50(3):306–11.
64. Chiang G, Levine D. Imaging of adnexal masses in pregnancy. J Ultrasound Med. 2004;23:805–81.
65. Webb EM, Green GE, Scoutt LM. Adnexal mass with pelvic pain. Radiol Clin North Am. 2004;42(2):329–48.
66. Vercellini P, Maddalena S, de Giorgi O, Aimi G, Crosignani PG. Abdominal myomectomy for infertility: a comprehensive review. Hum Reprod. 1998;13:873–9.
67. Roche O, Chavan N, Aquilina J, et al. Radiological appearances of gynaecological emergencies. Insights Imaging. 2012;3:265. https://doi.org/10.1007/s13244-012-0157-0.
68. Dohke M, Watanabe Y, Okumura A. Comprehensive MR imaging of acute gynecologic diseases. Radiographics. 2000;20:1551–66.
69. Sam JW, Jacobs JE, Birnbaum BA. Spectrum of CT findings in acute pyogenic pelvic inflammatory disease. Radiographics. 2002;22:1327–34.

MRI Evaluation of the Pregnant Patient with Suspected Appendicitis: Imaging Considerations and Alternative Explanations for Abdominal and Pelvic Pain

5

Daniel R. Ludwig, Richard Tsai,
Demetrios A. Raptis, and Vincent M. Mellnick

Contents

5.1   Introduction

Appendicitis is the most common non-obstetrical condition necessitating emergency surgery in the pregnant patient, and is estimated to complicate 1/1000 pregnancies [1–3]. Abdominal pain, nausea, and vomiting are common complaints during normal pregnancy, confounding the diagnosis of acute intra-abdominal and intra-pelvic pathology [4, 5]. Additionally, pregnant patients often have a non-specific leukocytosis which renders laboratory evaluation less useful [4], although a substantially elevated serum white blood cell count (i.e., >18,000) can be a helpful clinical feature [6]. In comparison, leukocytosis has a relatively higher positive predictive value, although a somewhat limited negative predictive value, for appendicitis in the non-pregnant adult patient in the correct clinical setting [7, 8]. The clinical presentation of

D. R. Ludwig (✉) · D. A. Raptis · V. M. Mellnick
Mallinckrodt Institute of Radiology,
Washington University School of Medicine,
Saint Louis, MO, USA
e-mail: ludwigd@wustl.edu;
d.raptis@wustl.edu; mellnickv@wustl.edu

R. Tsai
Advanced Radiology Consultants,
Leawood, KS, USA

© Springer Nature Switzerland AG 2020
M. N. Patlas et al. (eds.), *Emergency Imaging of Pregnant Patients*,
https://doi.org/10.1007/978-3-030-42722-1_5

appendicitis can also be masked in pregnancy, in part due to upward displacement of the appendix by the gravid uterus [9], and loss of the guarding response in the setting of peritonitis as a result of physiologic changes to the abdominal wall musculature [5, 10]. A delay in diagnosis can lead to perforation of the appendix, which substantially increases the risk for early delivery and fetal loss [11–13]. Conversely, just the act of performing surgery such as diagnostic laparoscopy, whether there is or is not appendicitis, is also associated with early delivery and fetal loss [14]. Given the non-specific clinical presentation and the risk of adverse outcomes with delayed or misdiagnosis, imaging plays an essential role in directing timely and effective patient care.

Computed tomography (CT) with intravenous (IV) contrast has emerged as the preferred imaging modality in adult non-pregnant patients with suspected appendicitis [15, 16]. In the pregnant patient, cross-sectional imaging modalities which do not expose the patient to ionizing radiation, i.e., ultrasound and magnetic resonance (MR) imaging, are strongly preferred [17, 18]. A recent revision to the American College of Radiology's Appropriateness Criteria in 2018 supported the use of either non-contrast MR imaging or ultrasound for the initial evaluation of suspected appendicitis in pregnancy [19]. Given the high non-visualization rate of ultrasound in the pregnant patient reported in multiple publications [18, 20], MR imaging is currently performed as the first-line diagnostic test at our institution. MR imaging has the added advantage of simultaneous evaluation for alternative explanations for abdominal and pelvic pain [21].

In this chapter, we will first review MR imaging techniques and special considerations for imaging the pregnant patient. Next, we will illustrate the MR findings of acute appendicitis and review the performance of MR imaging for the diagnosis of appendicitis in pregnancy. Finally, we will briefly review the MR imaging appearance of multiple additional entities which can result in abdominal and/or pelvic pain in the pregnant patient, many of which can mimic appendicitis. These include hepatobiliary, gastrointestinal, genitourinary, and obstetrical and gynecologic pathologies.

5.2 MR Imaging Technique and Considerations in Pregnancy

MR imaging of the abdomen is performed at 1.5 Tesla (T) for all pregnant patients at our institution due to the increased radiofrequency energy deposition (specific absorption rate; SAR) and the resultant increased tissue heating at 3 T [22]. While higher field strengths do provide increased signal-to-noise, resulting in improved spatial resolution and tissue contrast, the added benefit may not justify the added theoretical risk [22]. Furthermore, scanning at 1.5 T, in our experience, is sufficient to provide an examination of high diagnostic quality. Although not performed at our institution, 3 T MR imaging is currently considered safe during the second and third trimesters of pregnancy; however, the use of 3 T MR in pregnancy remains slightly controversial [23, 24]. Three Tesla MR is more commonly used in fetal imaging, in which a higher signal-to-noise may be needed.

Gadolinium-based IV contrast crosses the placental barrier, and in utero exposure is associated with adverse fetal outcomes in large recent human epidemiologic studies, with exposure during the second and third trimesters thought to confer the greatest risk [25, 26]. A recent meta-analysis found no difference in the diagnostic accuracy of MR imaging performed without versus with IV contrast for the diagnosis of acute appendicitis [27]. Thus, gadolinium-based IV contrast is not indicated for the evaluation of the pregnant patient with suspected appendicitis. In rare situations in which the use of gadolinium-based contrast is deemed necessary, the benefits and risks should be discussed, and informed consent should be obtained prior to the MRI examination.

No study has systematically compared the diagnostic accuracy of MR imaging performed without versus with oral contrast for the diagnosis of appendicitis, to our knowledge, in pregnancy or in non-pregnant patients. The delay introduced by the oral contrast preparation increases the time to diagnosis, which increases the risk for perforation. As a result, oral contrast is avoided as part of our routine MR imaging protocol. However, oral contrast (e.g., a dilute barium sulfate suspension) may be helpful for simultaneous evaluation of the small bowel if the differential diagnosis also includes inflammatory bowel disease (IBD). Specifically, MR enterography utilizing oral contrast improves the depiction of active small bowel inflammation and interloop abscesses [28–30].

The patient is positioned supine and is imaged with a phased-array body coil, which is centered over the iliac crests. The field of view extends from the liver hilum to the pubic symphysis. Left lateral tilt or decubitus positioning is selectively used to improve patient comfort and hemodynamics [31]. Our multi-planar multi-weighted imaging protocol includes single-shot T2-weighted images, T2-weighted images with fat saturation (FS), balanced steady-state free-precession (bSSFP) gradient-echo images, and fast low-angle shot T1-weighted gradient-echo images with FS (Table 5.1).

Each sequence performed plays a key role in evaluation for acute appendicitis. Single-shot T2-weighted images serve as the workhorse sequence, allowing for rapid imaging which minimizes the effect of peristalsis. T2-weighted FS images are used to identify free fluid and to increase the conspicuity of periappendiceal fat stranding. bSSFP gradient-echo images are useful for evaluating the abdominopelvic vasculature and to assist in differentiating the appendix from the right gonadal vein. T1-weighted images

with FS are useful for evaluation of appendiceal contents and for identifying hemorrhagic processes in the pelvis.

5.3   MR Findings of Appendicitis

The appendix is a blind-ending, tubular loop of bowel connected to the cecum, which may play a role in the gastrointestinal immune system [32]. The etiology of appendicitis still remains poorly understood, to our knowledge; however, luminal obstruction is generally a requisite feature, resulting in appendiceal distention, bacterial overgrowth, and ischemic change related to venous outflow obstruction [33, 34]. Causes of luminal obstruction include impaction of an appendicolith or fecal material, lymphoid hyperplasia, and rarely a tumor such as carcinoid [33, 35]. Acute appendicitis is defined histopathologically by the presence of transmural inflammation, ulceration, or thrombosis, and is often accompanied by the findings of intraluminal pus [33, 36]. Simple appendicitis has the potential to progress to gangrenous or perforated appendicitis, which can result in intra-abdominal and intra-pelvic abscess formation [33].

Findings of acute appendicitis on MR imaging include appendiceal distention (size ≥8 mm), a fluid-filled appendix, periappendiceal soft-tissue stranding and adjacent free fluid, thickening of the appendiceal wall, and the presence of an appendicolith or appendicoliths (Fig. 5.1). A combination of these imaging findings is diagnostic of acute appendicitis in the appropriate clinical setting (Fig. 5.2). Of these findings, the most reliable features of appendicitis are periappendiceal soft-tissue stranding and appendiceal wall thickening [37]. Despite the substantial inter-radiologist agreement for appendiceal size [37], distention alone should not be used to make the diagnosis of appendicitis, as the size of a normal appendix can frequently fall in the 8–10 mm range [38, 39].

When present, an appendicolith is associated with a higher rate of complicated appendicitis and/or perforation [40, 41]. Periappendiceal abscess formation can be diagnosed without IV

Table 5.1 MR imaging protocol for suspected appendicitis in pregnancy

Technique	Basic sequences
Field strength: 1.5 T Intravenous contrast: None Oral contrast: None Coverage: Liver hilum to pubic symphysis	• Variable scout • Axial, coronal, and sagittal single-shot T2-weighted imaging • Axial single-shot T2-weighted imaging with fat saturation • Axial and coronal bSSFP gradient-echo imaging • Axial fast low-angle shot T1-weighted gradient-echo imaging with fat saturation (pelvis only)

bSSFP balanced steady-state free precession

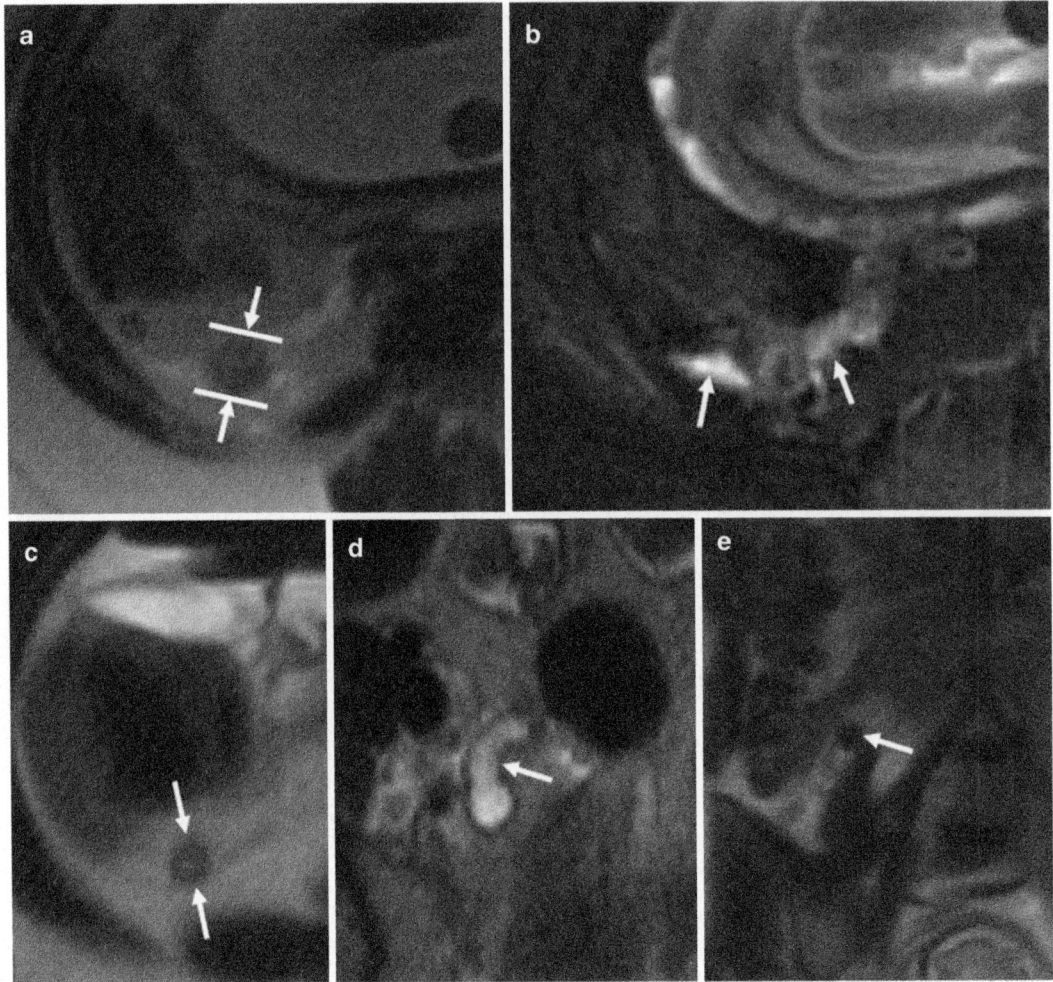

Fig. 5.1 MRI findings of acute appendicitis in pregnancy. Findings of acute appendicitis include an appendiceal diameter ≥8 mm (**a**, arrows; axial T2-weighted MR image), periappendiceal soft-tissue stranding, and free fluid (**b**, arrows; axial T2-weighted fat-suppressed MR image), thickening of the appendiceal wall (**c**, arrows; axial T2-weighted MR image), a fluid-filled appendix (**d**, arrow; coronal T2-weighted MR image), and the presence of an appendicolith, which is hypointense on a T2-weighted image (**e**, arrow; coronal T2-weighted MR image)

contrast on MR imaging by the presence of a periappendiceal fluid collection with mass effect, extra-luminal gas within the collection, and/or a defect in the wall of the appendix [42, 43]. The addition of diffusion-weighted sequences may often help in differentiating a noninfected periappendiceal fluid collection from an abscess [42].

Air within the appendix can be appreciated as blooming artifact on the T1-weighted gradient-echo images, and may be a helpful feature to exclude appendicitis, when present [44, 45] (Fig. 5.3). Occasionally, intraluminal gas can be seen in patients with appendicitis, especially in the setting of appendicitis involving only the appendiceal tip [43, 46, 47]. T1 hyperintensity within the appendix (i.e., the T1-bright appendix sign), attributed to the presence of intraluminal stool, is helpful to exclude appendicitis, as it has been demonstrated to have a high specificity but low sensitivity for a normal appendix [48] (Fig. 5.4).

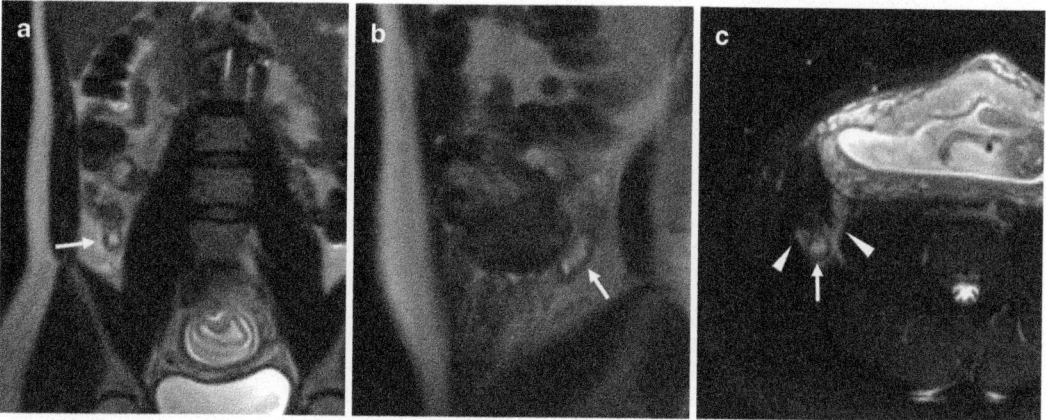

Fig. 5.2 Acute appendicitis in a 35-year-old pregnant woman at 24 weeks gestation presenting with right lower quadrant pain. Coronal T2-weighted (**a**), sagittal T2-weighted (**b**), and axial fat-suppressed T2-weighted (**c**) MR images show an enlarged, fluid-filled appendix with thickening of the appendiceal wall (arrows). Surrounding periappendiceal soft-tissue stranding is best appreciated on T2-weighted fat-suppressed images (arrowheads)

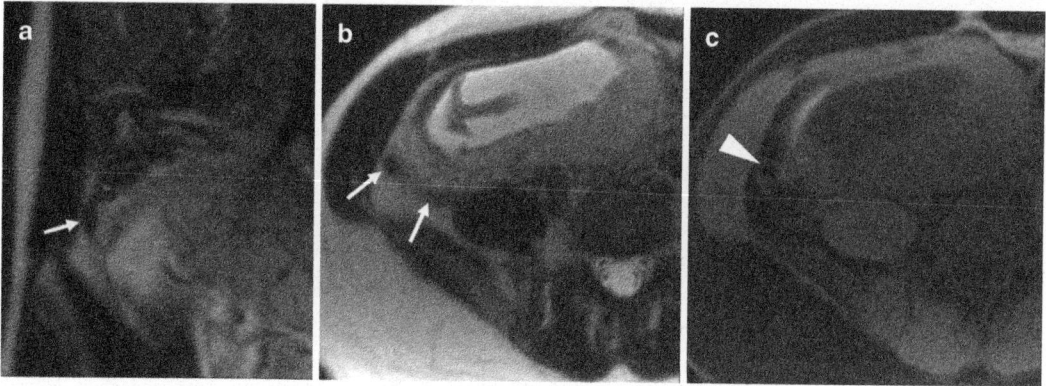

Fig. 5.3 Normal appendix with intraluminal gas in a 20-year-old pregnant woman at 16 weeks gestation with right lower quadrant pain. Coronal and axial T2-weighted MR images (**a**, **b**, respectively) show a normal appearing appendix, without wall thickening or periappendiceal stranding (arrows). On the corresponding axial T1-weighted gradient-echo MR image (**c**), blooming is seen within the appendiceal lumen (arrowhead), which is consistent with intraluminal gas

The interpreting radiologist should assess for each of these features and provide an interpretation of the MR examination as positive, indeterminate, or negative for appendicitis. In support of this notion, the final interpretation has been shown to have near perfect agreement in an inter-radiologist reliability study, and provides the highest level of diagnostic accuracy when compared to individual features interpreted in isolation [27, 37]. A meta-analysis aggregating the results of 30 studies found a sensitivity of 94% and a specificity 97% for the diagnosis of appendicitis on MR imaging in the pregnant patient [27]. Notably, a single-institution series found that no patient with an MR examination interpreted as indeterminate had progressive appendicitis requiring surgical management [37]. Mild or self-limited appendicitis was possible in some of these patients, and conservative management proved effective in this subgroup.

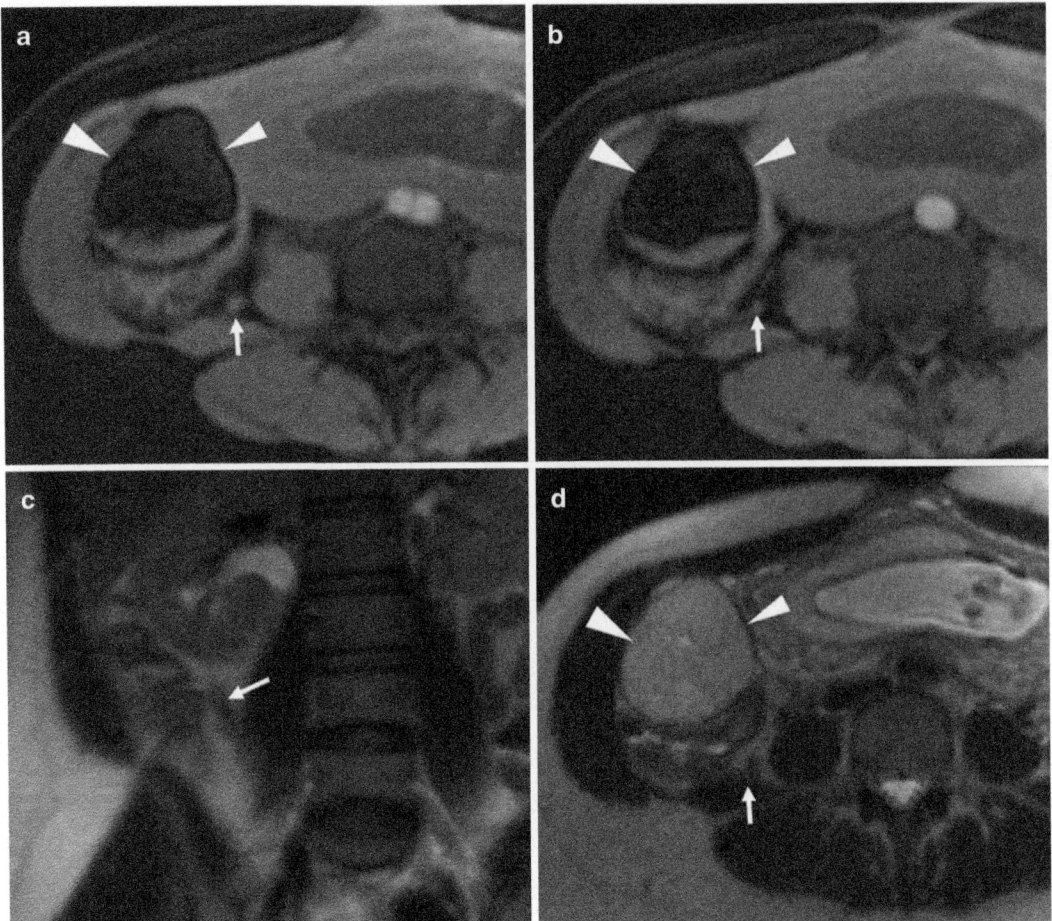

Fig. 5.4 Normal appendix with a T1-bright appendix sign, and an incidental dermoid cyst, in a 25-year-old pregnant woman with right lower quadrant pain. Sequential T1-weighted MR images with fat saturation (**a, b**) show high signal intensity within the appendiceal lumen filling more than half its length (arrows), indicating the T1-bright appendix sign. Coronal and axial T2-weighted MR images (**c, d**, respectively) show a normal-sized appendix, without wall thickening or periappendiceal stranding (arrows). Incidental note is made of a T2-hyperintense mass arising from the right adnexa (arrowheads), which parallels the intensity of fat on all sequences and suppressed on T1-weighted imaging with fat saturation (arrowheads), and which is highly consistent with a dermoid cyst

In the gravid patient, the appendix is often displaced upwards from its normal location in the right lower quadrant with the degree of displacement proportional to the gestational age [9]. Due to the abnormal location and dilated vascular structures related to pregnancy, the appendix can be difficult to visualize on MR imaging, with reported visualization rates of 60–95% in pregnant patients [37, 49–51]. Furthermore, inter-radiologist reliability studies show only a fair to moderate

agreement for appendix visualization [37, 49]. Several studies have shown non-visualization of the appendix on MR imaging has a negative predictive value that approaches 100% in the absence of secondary signs of appendicitis, similar to the negative predictive value of visualization of a normal appendix [37, 49, 50]. Conversely, the appendix is almost always visualized in pregnant patients who actually have appendicitis. By contrast, ultrasound has a markedly limited negative predictive value when the appendix is not visualized [18, 20, 52]. As a result, non-visualization of the appendix on MR with the absence of inflammatory changes within the right lower quadrant should be interpreted as negative rather than indeterminate.

Occasionally, a dilated right gonadal vein can mimic an enlarged appendix on MR imaging (Fig. 5.5). Both the right gonadal vein and the appendix may appear as a rounded or tubular structure in the right lower quadrant. The gonadal vein can be identified by its connection to the inferior cava, and is usually hyperintense on bSSFP images.

CT of the abdomen and pelvis may be appropriate in the pregnant patient with suspected appendicitis when MRI is not available or is

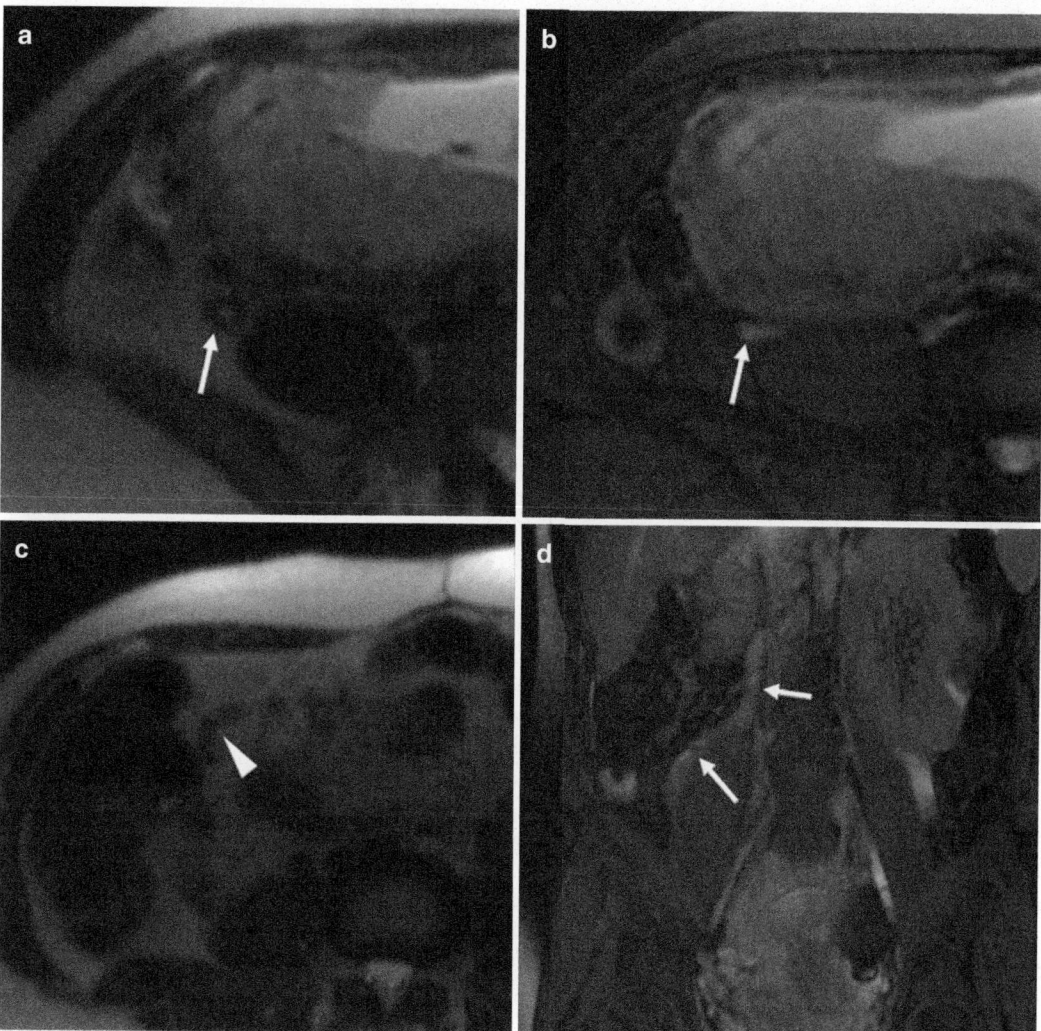

Fig. 5.5 Enlarged right gonadal vein mimicking appendicitis in a 26-year-old pregnant woman at 28 weeks gestation with right lower quadrant pain. Axial T2-weighted MR image (**a**) demonstrates a rounded structure in the right lower quadrant which has the appearance of a thick-walled appendix (arrow). This structure is hyperintense on axial (**b**) and coronal (**d**) bSSFP MR images, and connects to the inferior vena cava (arrows), representing the right gonadal vein. Axial T2-weighted MR image (**c**) demonstrates a normal appendix in the right lower quadrant (arrowhead)

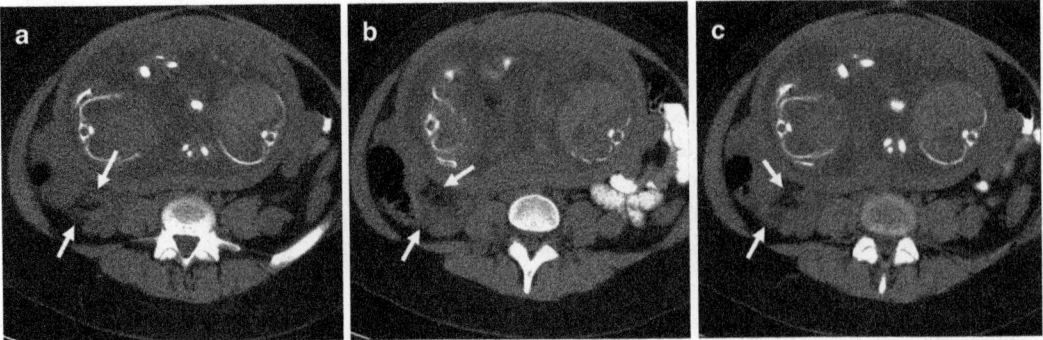

Fig. 5.6 Acute appendicitis in a 25-year-old woman at 32 weeks gestation who underwent low-dose CT with oral but without IV contrast. Sequential non-enhanced axial CT images (**a–c**, cranial to caudal) depict a retrocecal tubular structure with mild surrounding inflammation (arrows), likely representing the inflamed appendix that was found at the time of surgery. The use of a low-dose non-enhanced CT protocol makes evaluation more difficult

inconclusive [19, 53]. IV iodinated contrast is safe to administer in pregnancy (i.e., U.S. FDA category B), and should be used when appendicitis is suspected [54, 55]. Low-radiation-dose CT has the potential to reduce fetal radiation dose when incorporated into diagnostic imaging algorithms [56]. However, dose reduction techniques also have the potential to render an examination of limited quality or even non-diagnostic (Fig. 5.6). Low-dose protocols, if employed, should be thoroughly vetted prior to use, as limited quality examination may need to be repeated, effectively resulting in an increased dose to the fetus. A sensible approach should be used for fetal dose reduction, specifically avoiding unnecessary or multi-phasic CT examinations. Appendicitis is depicted similarly on CT and MRI, and the CT findings of appendicitis include appendiceal wall thickening, distention, and periappendiceal soft-tissue stranding, as in the non-pregnant patient [57].

5.4 Hepatobiliary Causes of Abdominal Pain

Ultrasound is the imaging modality of choice for the evaluation of the pregnant patient with right upper quadrant abdominal pain [58], as it depicts the gallbladder and other hepatobiliary findings with a high degree of accuracy [59]. Due to upward displacement of the appendix by the gravid uterus [9], and the potential symptomatic overlap between appendicitis and hepatobiliary causes of abdominal pain, hepatobiliary pathology may be encountered during MR imaging evaluation for suspected appendicitis.

Gallstones are more frequent in pregnancy due to increased levels of reproductive hormones, as a result of increased biliary secretion of cholesterol and delayed gallbladder emptying [60–62]. Accordingly, gallstones occur in approximately 1 in 10 pregnancies, and symptomatic gallbladder disease complicates approximately 1 in 300 pregnancies [63]. Patients with symptomatic gallstones present with post-prandial epigastric or right upper quadrant pain, lasting several hours at a time. If these symptoms persist and are accompanied by constitutional symptoms including fever, nausea, and vomiting, cholecystitis should be considered [64].

On MR imaging, gallstones appear as rounded areas of low signal intensity on T2-weighted images. Findings of acute cholecystitis include the presence of gallstones, accompanied by gallbladder wall thickening, pericholecystic fluid and/or fat stranding, and gallbladder distention [65] (Fig. 5.7). Additionally, complications of cholecystitis, including gangrenous cholecystitis and perforation, are readily depicted on MR imaging [66]. Acute cholecystitis is typically managed surgically in the pregnant patient [67].

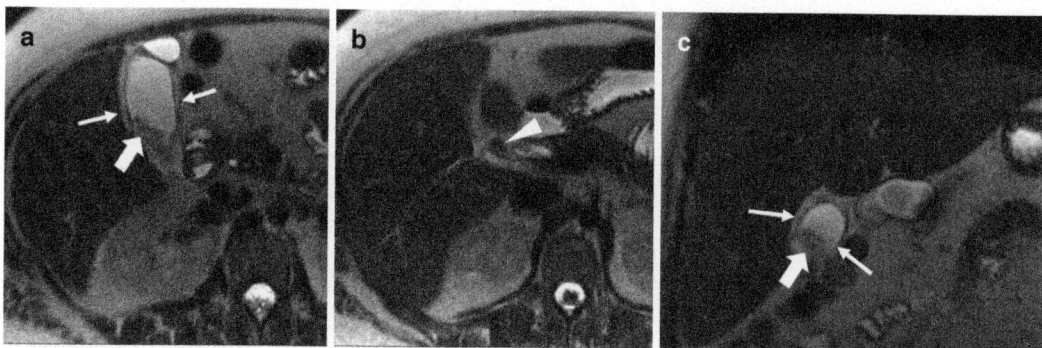

Fig. 5.7 Acute cholecystitis in a 23-year-old pregnant woman at 19 weeks gestation with right upper quadrant abdominal pain and fever. Sequential axial T2-weighted MR images (**a, b**) and coronal T2-weighted MR image (**c**) show a distended gallbladder with circumferential wall thickening (thin arrows). Gallstones are seen within the dependent portion of the gallbladder (thick arrows). Additionally, a T2-hypointense gallstone is seen within the cystic duct (arrowhead). This constellation of findings is highly consistent with acute calculus cholecystitis, which was managed conservatively after the patient experienced a perioperative medication-induced anaphylactic reaction

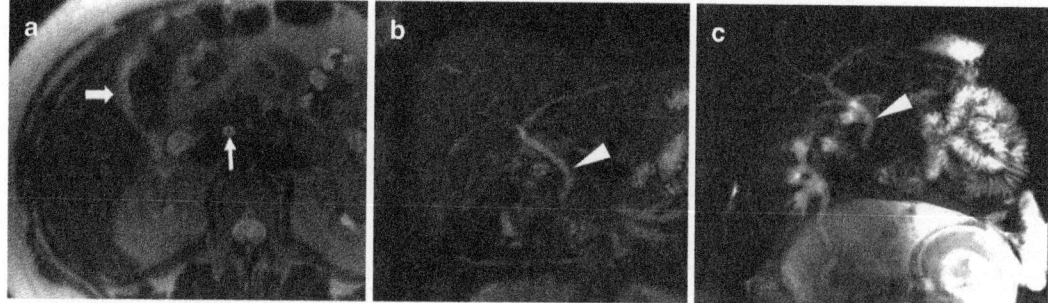

Fig. 5.8 Flow void mimicking a common bile duct calculus in 23-year-old woman at 25 weeks gestation, with right upper quadrant abdominal pain and elevated liver function tests, 1 week after undergoing a laparoscopic cholecystectomy for biliary colic. Axial T2-weighted MR image (**a**) shows a central filling defect in the distal common bile duct (thin arrow). A small amount of fluid is seen within the gallbladder fossa, which is expected after very recent cholecystectomy (thick arrow). Axial T2-weighted MR image with fat saturation (**b**) and thick-slab MR cholangiopancreatography image (**c**) show no associated calculus in the common bile duct (arrowheads). Thus, the filling defect is most consistent with a flow-related artifact; the patient was managed conservatively, and her liver function tests improved without intervention

Choledocholithiasis occurs when a gallstone passes into the common bile duct, or occasionally after in situ formation such as in patients with prior cholecystectomy, and can be complicated by superimposed cholangitis. Patients with choledocholithiasis present with right upper quadrant abdominal pain, jaundice, abnormal liver function tests with an elevated serum bilirubin, and superimposed fever and leukocytosis when cholangitis occurs. MR imaging has higher sensitivity than ultrasound for the diagnosis of choledocholithiasis, especially when MR cholangiopancreatography is performed [68]. Typical MR findings of choledocholithiasis include gallstones in the common bile duct and intrahepatic and extrahepatic biliary duct dilation [69]. Due to the speed of the single-shot T2-weighted acquisition, flow-related artifact, which manifest as a signal void centrally within a bile duct, has the potential to mimic a bile duct calculus [70] (Fig. 5.8). A signal void within the biliary tract should be evaluated in multiple

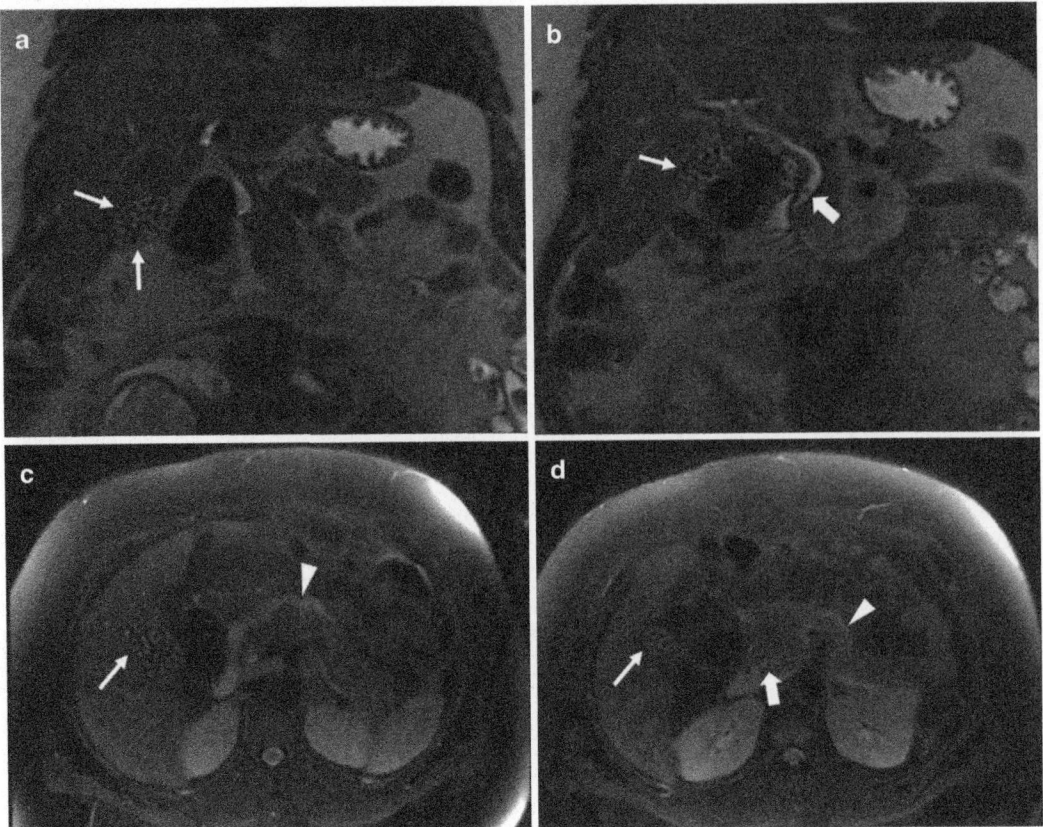

Fig. 5.9 Choledocholithiasis with gallstone pancreatitis in a 30-year-old pregnant woman at 23 weeks gestation with upper abdominal pain. Sequential coronal T2-weighted MR images (**a**, **b**) demonstrate numerous small gallstones filling the gallbladder (thin arrows). Additionally, a calculus is present in the distal common bile duct (thick arrows). Sequential axial T2-weighted fat-suppressed MR images (**c**, **d**) also demonstrate pancreatic edema with peripancreatic fluid (arrowheads), indicating gallstone pancreatitis

planes, as a calculus will persist across multiple series and projections.

Choledocholithiasis infrequently results in pancreatitis, occurring as a result of ampullary obstruction [71]. Other etiologies of pancreatitis do occur in pregnancy, but gallstone pancreatitis is by far the most common [71]. Clinical features of pancreatitis include epigastric abdominal pain, nausea, vomiting, and elevated lipase. Pancreatitis manifests as pancreatic edema and peripancreatic fluid on MR imaging, with potential but very rare complications including pancreatic necrosis, peripancreatic collections, pseudoaneurysm formation, and venous thrombosis [72, 73] (Fig. 5.9).

HELLP syndrome (hemolysis, elevated liver enzyme levels, and low platelet count) occurs exclu-sively in pregnancy and is a complication of pre-ecclampsia, affecting approximately 1 in 1500 pregnancies [74]. Features of HELLP syndrome on imaging include hepatomegaly, hepatic edema, ascites, and pleural effusions. MR imaging can depict complications of HELLP syndrome, includ-ing hepatic necrosis, intrahepatic hematoma, and extrahepatic hematoma [75] (Fig. 5.10).

5.5 Gastrointestinal Causes of Abdominal Pain

A variety of non-appendiceal gastrointestinal pathologies occur in the pregnant patient, most of which occur at a similar incidence to in the

Fig. 5.10 HELLP syndrome resulting in subcapsular hepatic hematoma in a 35-year-old pregnant woman who underwent urgent delivery 2 days prior to MRI evaluation. Coronal T2-weighted MR image (**a**) demonstrates a subcapsular hepatic collection which is heterogeneous but predominantly isointense to the liver (arrows). Axial T1-weighted fat-suppressed MR image (**b**) demonstrates areas of high signal intensity within the collection (arrows), indicating a subcapsular hematoma

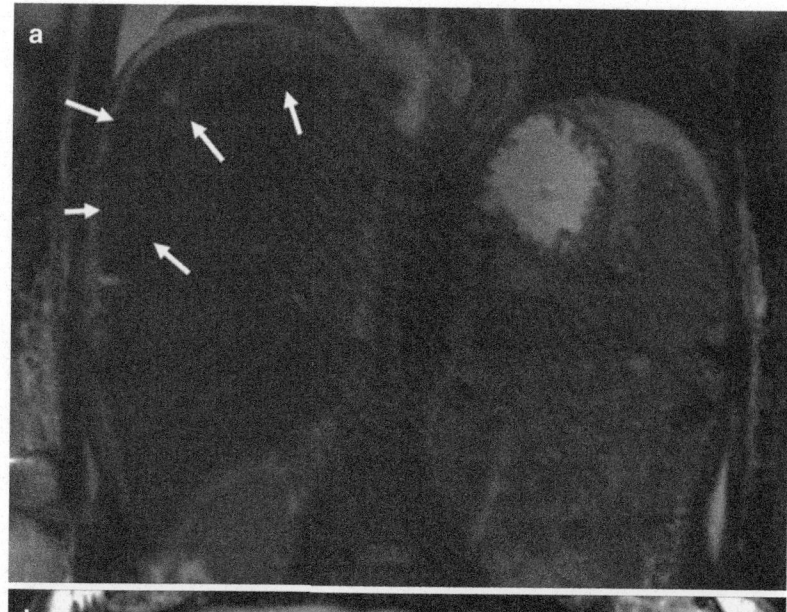

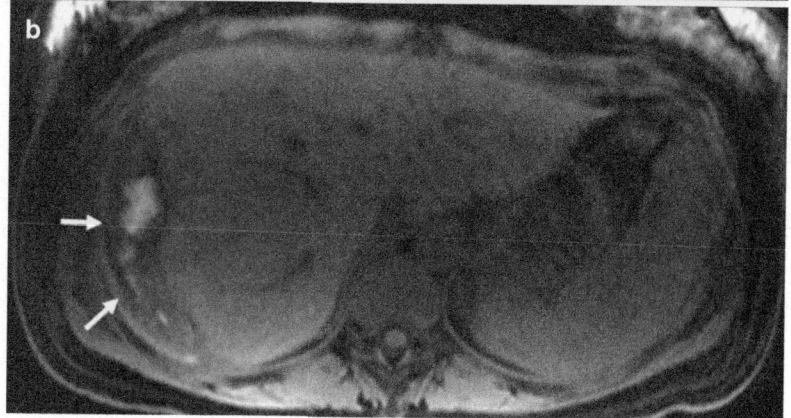

non-pregnant patient [76]. Many of these pathologies result in abdominal (and/or pelvic) pain, nausea, and vomiting, and have the potential to mimic appendicitis in the pregnant patient. MR imaging performed for appendicitis may therefore depict one of these alternative gastrointestinal etiologies of abdominal and/or pelvic pain.

Small bowel obstruction is a relatively rare cause of abdominal pain in pregnancy, and most commonly occurs secondary to adhesions from prior surgery [77, 78]. Less common causes include volvulus, intussusception, and hernias, such as those related to prior gastric bypass surgery [79]. In general, most etiologies of small bowel obstruction in the non-pregnant patient

also occur in the pregnant patient. Clinical manifestations of small bowel obstruction include nausea, vomiting, and crampy abdominal pain. MR imaging can readily depict the presence of a small bowel obstruction, which appears as multiple distended fluid-filled loops of proximal small bowel, with a transition zone to decompressed distal small bowel (Fig. 5.11). MR imaging can also be used to identify the potential etiology and to help select patients for non-operative management, including those with small bowel obstruction secondary to adhesions, which is lower-grade without evidence of immediate complications such as closed-loop obstruction, peritonitis, ischemia, or perforation [77].

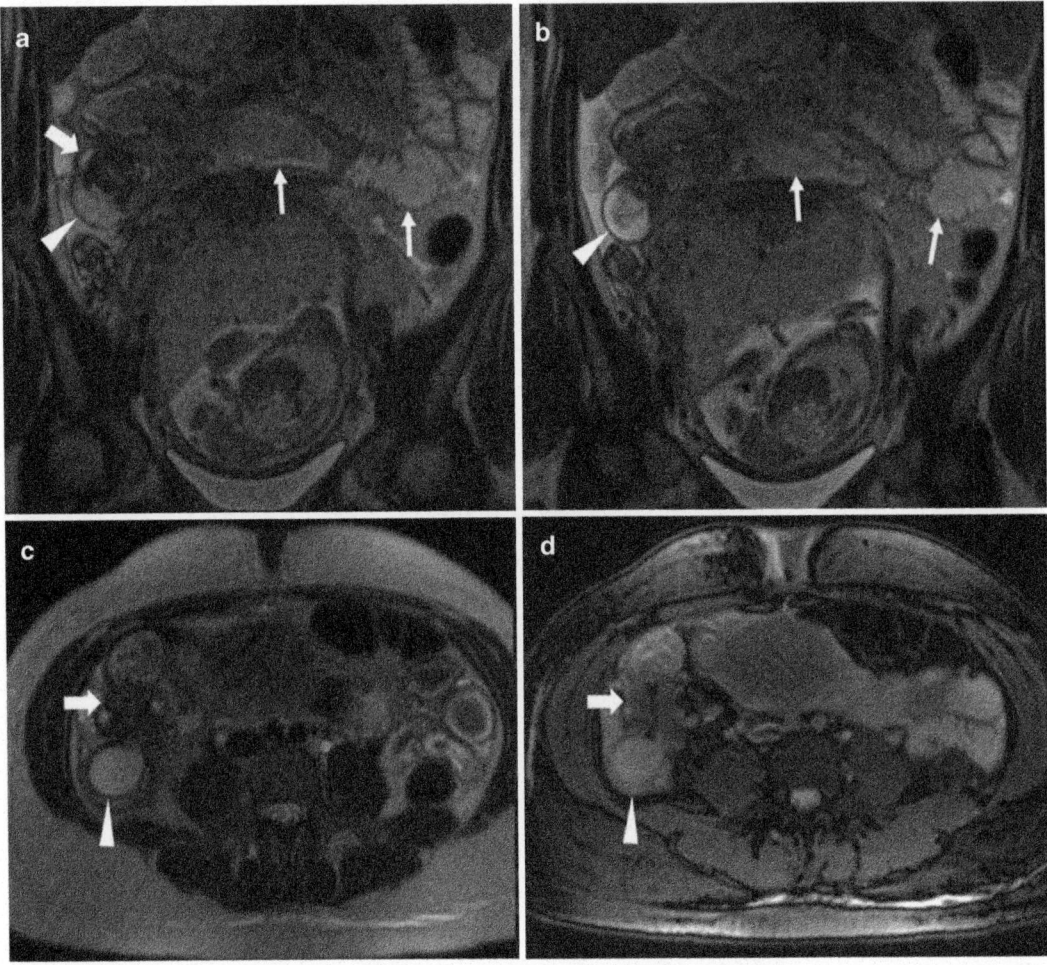

Fig. 5.11 Small bowel obstruction secondary to intussusception related to a Meckel's diverticulum in a 28-year-old pregnant woman at 21 weeks gestation with presenting with diffuse abdominal pain. Sequential coronal T2-weighted MR images (**a**, **b**) demonstrate multiple dilated loops of small bowel (thin arrows), representing a small bowel obstruction. In the right lower quadrant, there is an ileocolic intussusception (thick arrows) secondary to a cystic point lead mass (arrowheads), shown to better advantage on axial T2-weighted (**c**) and bSSFP (**d**) MR images. Surgery confirmed the presence of an ileocolic intussusception, and a Meckel's diverticulum was identified as the lead point

Another possible cause of abdominal pain in this patient population is inflammatory bowel disease (IBD), a condition which frequently affects younger patients, many of whom are of reproductive age. Moreover, Crohn's disease, in particular, has a slight female predominance [80]. The incidence of IBD in the pregnant patient is similar to in the non-pregnant patient, and approximately 20% of female patients with IBD who conceive with their disease in remission will experience a disease flare during pregnancy [81]. However, the severity of IBD flares may be worse in pregnant compared to non-pregnant women [82]. Common presenting symptoms of an IBD flare include abdominal pain, diarrhea, and occasionally fever; because of Crohn's disease's predilection for the terminal ileum, right

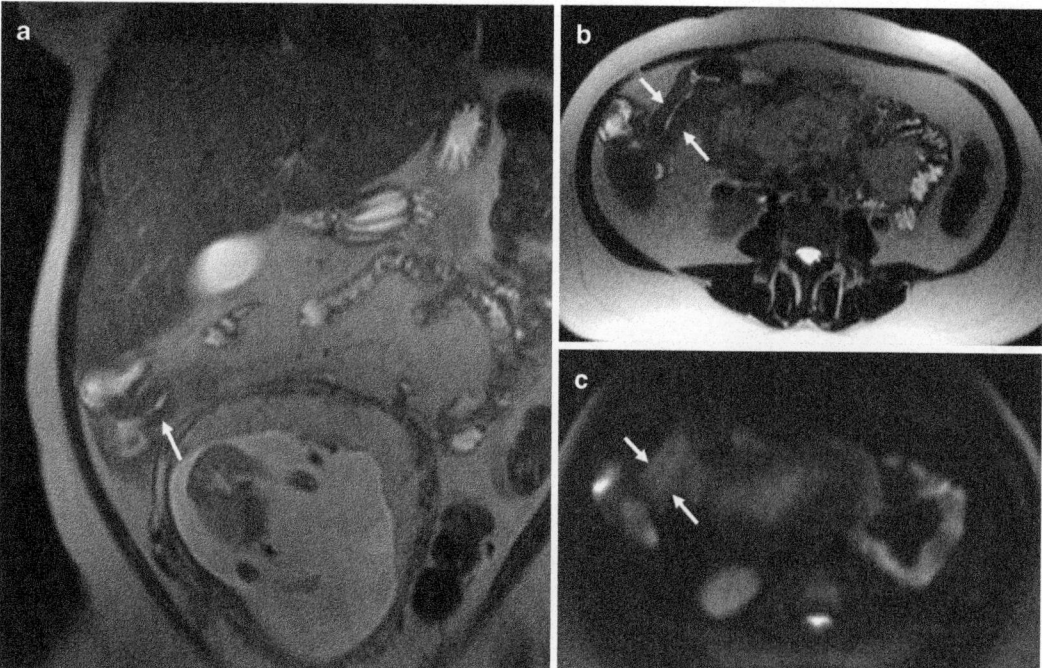

Fig. 5.12 Terminal ileitis secondary to inflammatory bowel disease in a 24-year-old pregnant woman at 22 weeks gestation, with Crohn's disease, who presented with right lower quadrant abdominal pain. Coronal T2-weighted (**a**) and axial T2-weighted (**b**) MR images demonstrate wall thickening of the terminal ileum with associated submucosal edema (arrows). Axial diffusion-weighted MR image (**c**) demonstrates increased signal intensity within the wall of the terminal ileum (arrows), which is consistent with acute inflammation

lower quadrant pain is the common presenting symptom, and may be misconstrued clinically as primary appendicitis, and particularly if the patient is not known to have IBD.

On MR imaging, active inflammation in IBD manifests as bowel wall thickening, submucosal edema, and perienteric stranding [28] (Fig. 5.12). If performed, diffusion-weighted imaging may show restricted diffusion within the segments of inflamed bowel, which implies the presence of moderate to severe disease. Complications of Crohn's disease are readily detected on MR imaging, and include fibrostenotic disease, abscess formation, and fistulization [83]. Fibrostenotic disease, a consequence of chronic inflammation, resultant fibrosis of the bowel wall, and stricture formation, can result in small- and large-bowel obstruction (Fig. 5.13).

Diverticulitis is rather uncommon in younger pregnant patients, and has been reported to complicate approximately 1 in 6000 pregnancies [76]. Presenting symptoms include fever and left lower quadrant pain, as in non-pregnant patients, although the location of pain is dependent on the affected segment of colon. Diverticulitis manifests as colonic wall thickening and pericolonic fat stranding surrounding a site of diverticulosis, and is readily seen on MR imaging, which can also be used to identify complications including perforation/abscess formation [84] (Fig. 5.14).

A well-known mimic of diverticulitis, epiploic appendagitis, is a relatively common entity which also has the potential to mimic acute appendicitis (although it occurs more frequently in non-pregnant individuals on the left), and is caused by torsion of an epiploic appendage and/

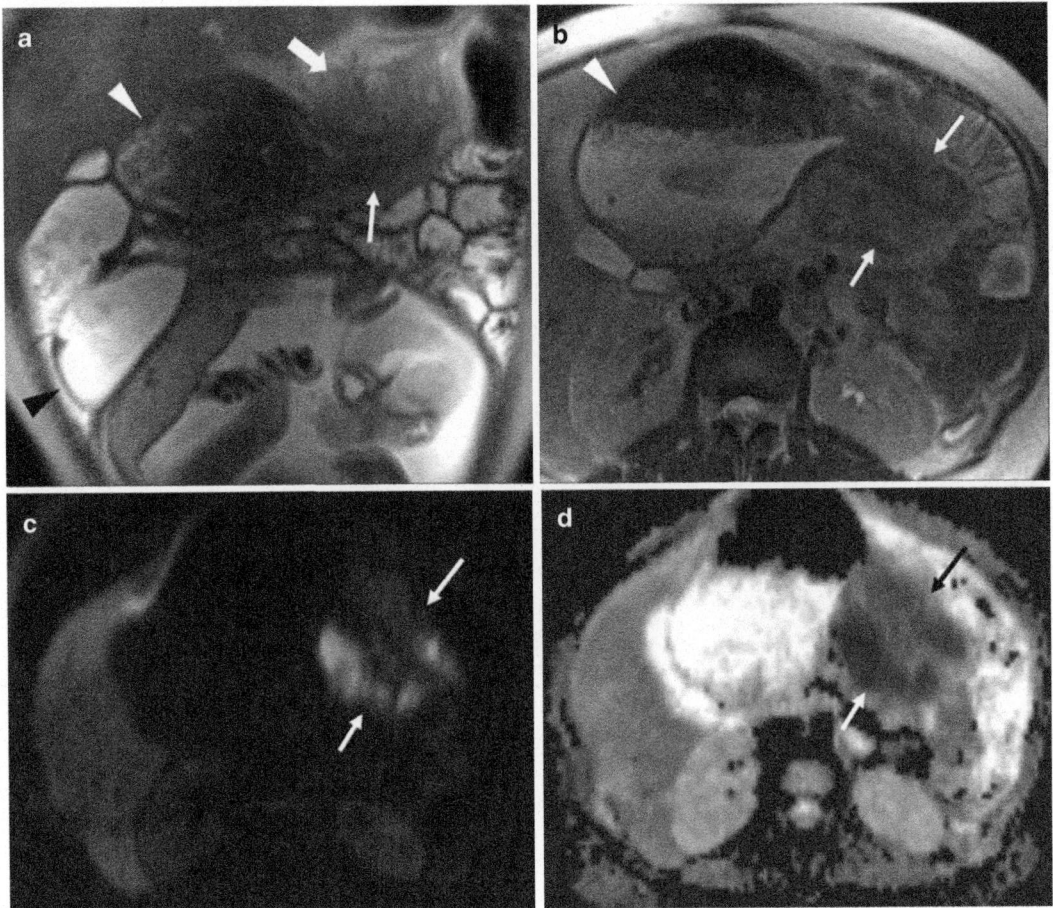

Fig. 5.13 Large bowel obstruction in a 30-year-old pregnant woman with Crohn's disease. Coronal and axial T2-weighted MR images (**a, b**, respectively) show marked wall thickening of the distal transverse colon (thin arrows) with associated pericolonic fat stranding (thick arrow). There is dilation of the proximal large bowel (arrow-heads), which is consistent with large bowel obstruction. Axial diffusion-weighted MR image and corresponding apparent diffusion coefficient image (**c, d**, respectively) demonstrate extensive diffusion restriction within the thickened segment of transverse colon (thin arrows), a feature of acute inflammation

or spontaneous thrombosis of its draining vein [85]. On MR imaging, epiploic appendagitis appears as fat stranding and inflammatory change surrounding a fat-intensity small ovoid mass adjacent to the colon (Fig. 5.15).

5.6 Genitourinary Causes of Abdominal Pain

Due to the potential symptomatic overlap between renal colic and appendicitis, it is relatively common to encounter genitourinary pathology on an

abdominal MR imaging examination performed for suspected appendicitis. Obstructive urolithiasis occurs at a similar rate in both pregnant and non-pregnant patients, and is estimated to complicate 1 in 1500 pregnancies, frequently with concurrent infection, or there may be urinary tract infection alone [86, 87]. Ultrasound is the modality of choice for evaluation of the pregnant patient with acute onset of flank pain and suspected urolithiasis [88]. While ultrasound readily depicts the presence of hydronephrosis, it has a rather low sensitivity for the demonstration of ureteral calculi [89]. Furthermore, the physiologic hydrone-

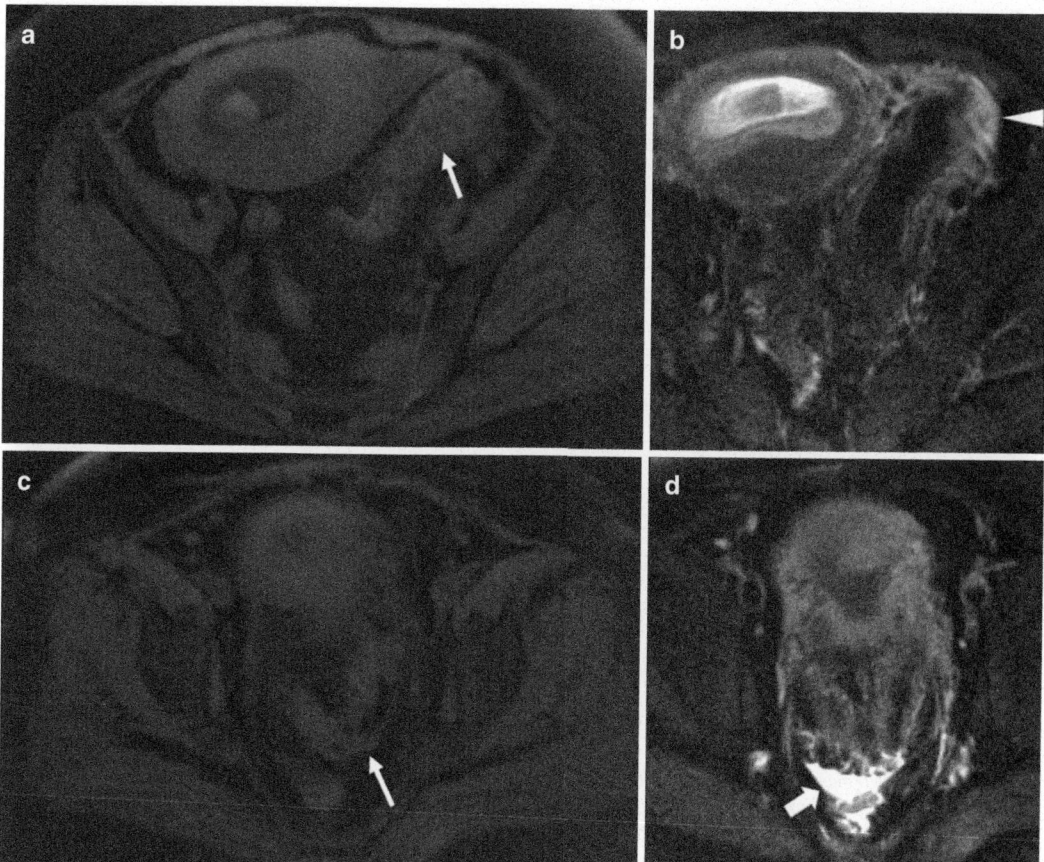

Fig. 5.14 Uncomplicated sigmoid diverticulitis in a 37-year-old pregnant woman in her first trimester presenting with nausea, vomiting, and left lower quadrant abdominal pain. Axial T1-weighted fat-suppressed MR images (**a, c**) demonstrate bowel wall thickening involving the sigmoid colon (thin arrows). Axial T2-weighted fat-suppressed MR images (**b, d**) demonstrate pericolonic fat stranding (arrowhead) and a small amount of free fluid in the dependent portion of the pelvis (thick arrow). These findings are diagnostic of acute sigmoid diverticulitis, and the patient was managed conservatively with antibiotic therapy

phrosis of pregnancy, caused by compression of the ureters between the gravid uterus and pelvic brim, affects more than 80% of pregnancies in the latter stages of gestation, right more often than left [90]. Thus, the finding of hydronephrosis on ultrasound has limited positive predictive value for the presence of a ureteral calculus. MR imaging may be helpful for demonstrating urolithiasis, especially using MR urography, which can be performed without contrast in the pregnant patient [91–93]. Whereas physiologic hydronephrosis is characterized by smooth tapering of the mid to distal ureter at the level of the pelvic brim, obstructive hydronephrosis manifests as a T2-hypointense calculus in the ureter, with an abrupt transition from distended to normal caliber ureter. MR imaging can also depict complications of urolithiasis, including forniceal rupture (Fig. 5.16).

5.7 Obstetrical and Gynecologic Causes of Abdominal Pain

In the pregnant patient, obstetrical and gynecologic causes are relatively frequent sources of abdominal and pelvic pain [94]. Pelvic ultrasound is the preferred technique when these enti-

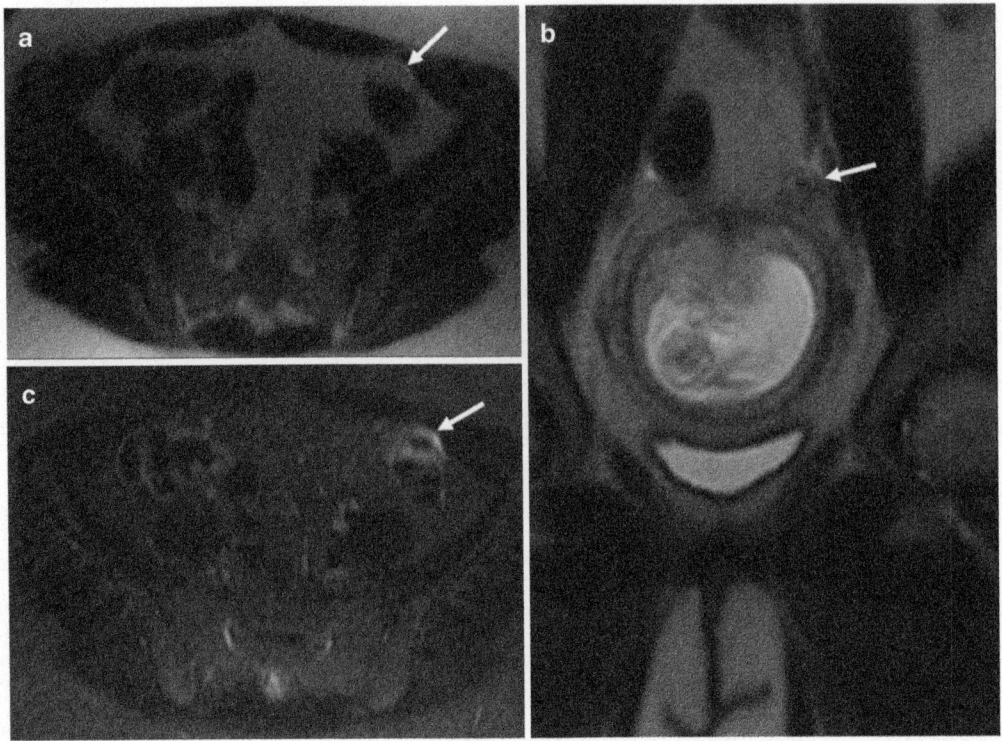

Fig. 5.15 Epiploic appendagitis in a 27-year-old pregnant woman at 9 weeks gestational age with left lower quadrant pain. Axial (**a**) and coronal (**b**) T2-weighted, and axial T2-weighted fat-suppressed (**c**) MR images demonstrate an oval, fat-intensity small ovoid mass associated with the sigmoid colon and surrounding stranding, representing epiploic appendagitis

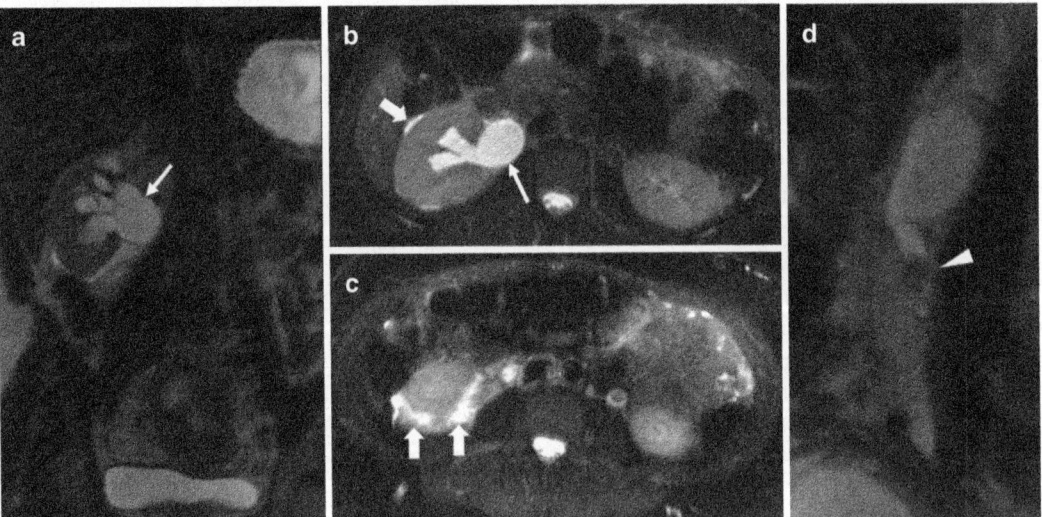

Fig. 5.16 Ureterolithiasis with forniceal rupture in a 35-year-old pregnant woman at 10 weeks gestation presenting with right lower quadrant and right flank pain. Coronal T2-weighted MR image (**a**) demonstrates right hydronephrosis (thin arrow). Sequential axial T2-weighted fat-suppressed MR image (**b**, **c**) show fluid tracking around the right kidney, indicating forniceal rupture, as well as right hydronephrosis (thin arrow). An obstructing calculus was identified in the mid right ureter (arrowhead), best demonstrated on a sagittal T2-weighted MR image (**d**)

ties are suspected [95]. However, it is important to be aware of the MR imaging appearance of these entities, as the clinical presentation can overlap with that of appendicitis and be quite non-specific, and these entities may be encountered during MR evaluation.

Ectopic pregnancy affects up to 2% of all pregnancies, and is the leading cause of maternal mortality during the first trimester of pregnancy [96]. Patients with ectopic pregnancy commonly present in the first trimester with abdominal pain and vaginal bleeding [97]. Prior to rupture, ectopic pregnancy may be asymptomatic and encountered incidentally. MR imaging findings of ectopic pregnancy include a lack of an intrauterine gestational sac, an adnexal or tubal mass, and hemoperitoneum [98] (Fig. 5.17). It is unclear the precise point in pregnancy in which

an intrauterine gestational sac should be identified on MR imaging, to our knowledge [98]. Additionally, heterotopic pregnancies, i.e., the presence of a concurrent intrauterine and an extrauterine gestation, while overall very rare, complicate as many as 1 in 100 pregnancies after ovulation induction or in vitro fertilization [99, 100]. Thus, care should be taken to assess for an ectopic pregnancy in every patient, regardless of whether an intrauterine gestational sac is visualized or not.

Endometriosis, a condition among women of child-bearing age, is characterized by endometrial-like tissue outside of the uterus [101]. Due its association with infertility, endometriosis is uncommonly encountered during pregnancy. Furthermore, in the pregnant patient, endometriosis often symptomatically improves due to the

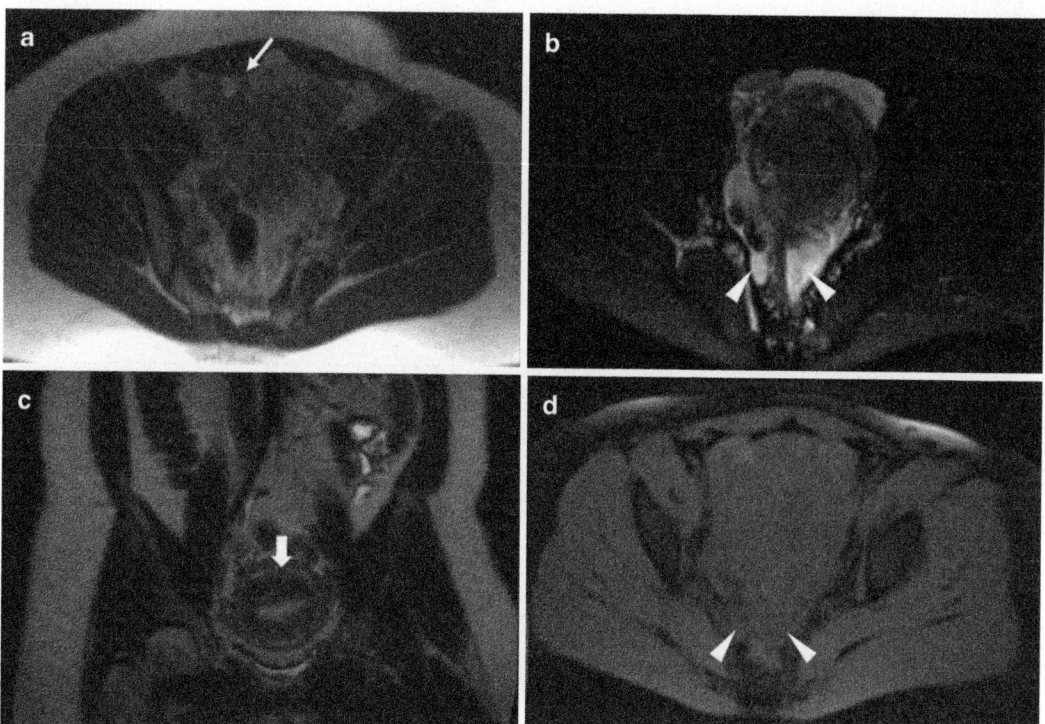

Fig. 5.17 Right-sided tubal ectopic in a 37-year-old woman with prior tubal ligation who presented with right lower quadrant pain and positive HCG. Axial (**a**) and coronal (**c**) T2-weighted MR images demonstrates a complex cystic mass in the right adnexa (thin arrow) and an empty uterus (thick arrow). Axial T2-weighted fat-suppressed (**b**) and T1-weighted fat-suppressed (**d**) MR images demonstrate free fluid in the pelvis with increased signal on T1-weighted images, diagnostic of hemoperitoneum. A ruptured right tubal ectopic pregnancy was confirmed at surgery

hormonal changes occurring in pregnancy [102]. However, endometriosis may still be symptomatic during pregnancy and has the potential to mimic appendicitis by causing lower abdominal pain. The MR findings of endometriosis include hemorrhagic masses in the pelvis, hematosalpinx, and hemoperitoneum (Fig. 5.18). Adnexal masses which are T1-hypertense and demonstrate T2-hypointensity (i.e., T2 "shading") are relatively characteristic for endometriomas, although the differential diagnosis for T2 shading also includes a hemorrhagic cyst [103]. Endometriosis most commonly involves the adnexa; however,

deposits can occur within the peritoneal cavity, along serosal surfaces of gastrointestinal and genitourinary structures, and even within the soft tissues of the abdominal wall after abdominal surgery [104]. T1-weighted imaging is performed with fat saturation to aid in the distinction between an endometrioma and a dermoid cyst, both of which are bright on T1-weighted imaging, but the latter of which suppresses with fat suppression due to the presence of macroscopic fat (Fig. 5.4).

Adnexal torsion is relatively rarely encountered during pregnancy, complicating approximately

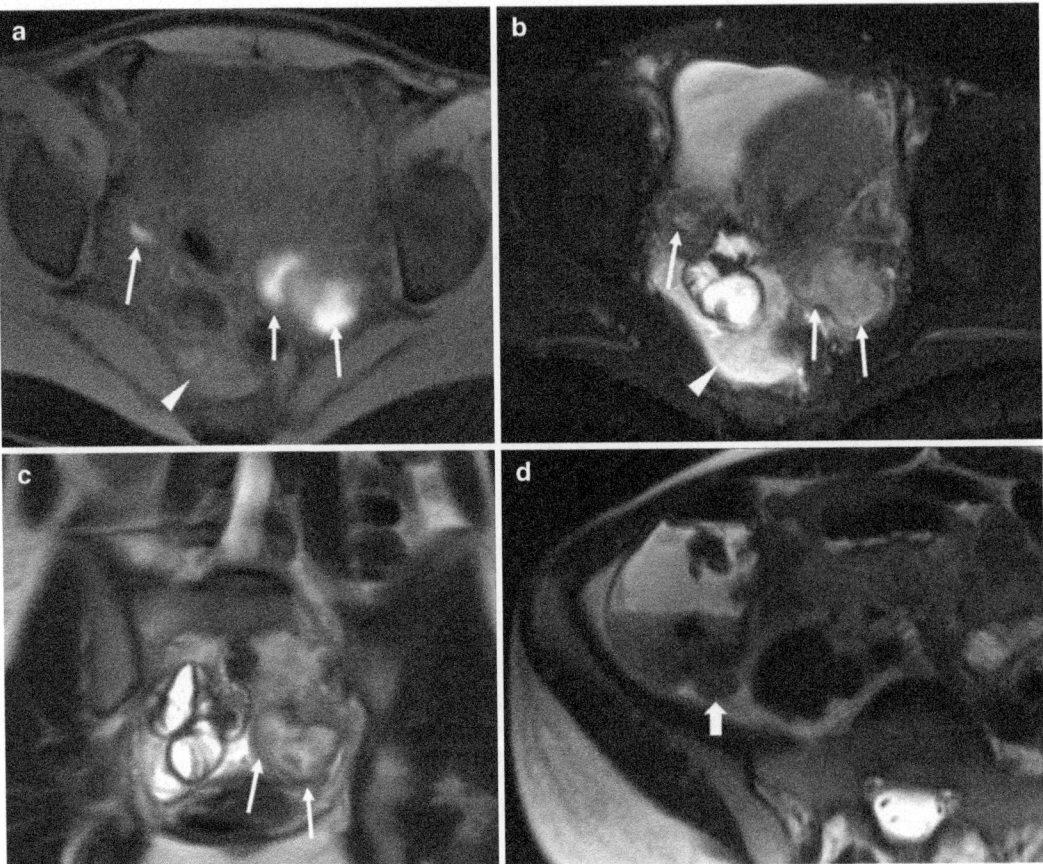

Fig. 5.18 Endometriosis with secondary inflammation of the appendix in a 24-year-old woman with right lower quadrant abdominal pain. Axial T1-weighted fat-suppressed MR image (**a**) demonstrates multiple T1-hyperintense hemorrhagic masses in the pelvis (arrows) with intermediate signal intensity on corresponding axial T2-weighted fat-suppressed (**b**) and coronal T2-weighted (**c**) MR images (arrows), indicative of T2 shading and consistent with endometriosis. Additionally, there was free fluid in the pelvis (arrowheads) which showed intermediate signal intensity on T1-weighted images, consistent with hemoperitoneum. Axial T2-weighted MR image at the level of the appendix (**d**) demonstrated thickening of the wall of the appendix which was normal in size, likely representing secondary inflammation

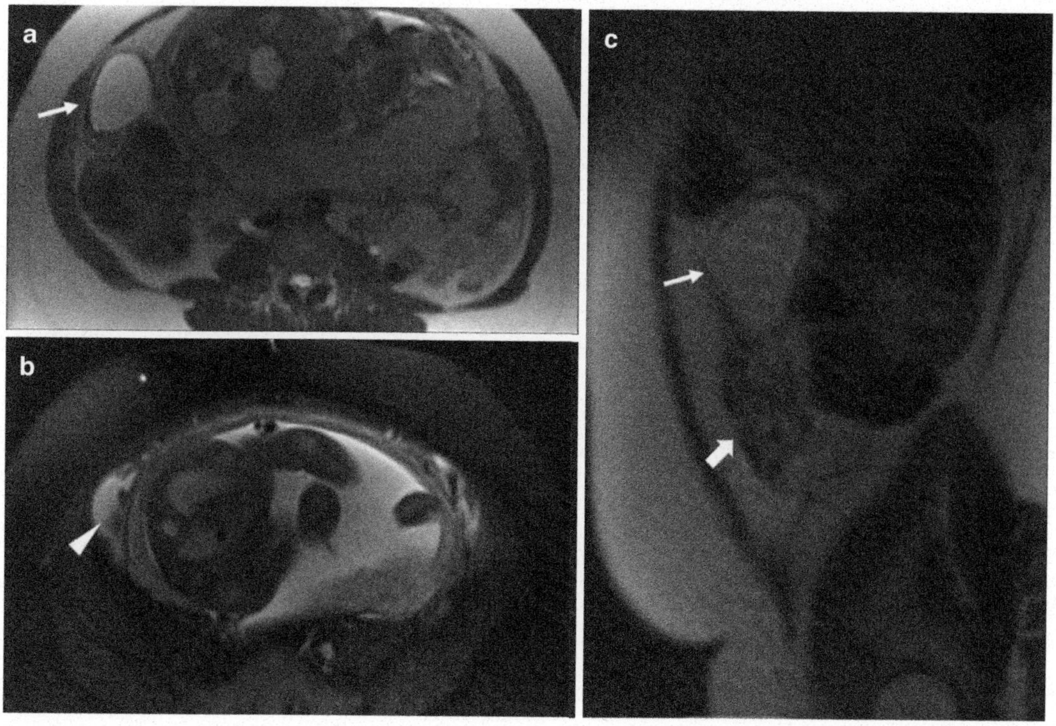

Fig. 5.19 Ovarian torsion secondary to a serous cystadenoma in a 22-year-old pregnant woman at 36 weeks gestation who presented with severe right lower quadrant abdominal pain. Axial (**a**) and sagittal (**c**) T2-weighted MR images demonstrate a cystic mass arising from the right adnexa (thin arrows). Right gonadal vessels just inferior to the right adnexa were engorged (thick arrow). Transaxial T2-weighted fat-suppressed MR image (**b**) demonstrates a small amount of free fluid in the right lower quadrant. The patient was taken urgently to the operating room, and right ovarian torsion secondary to a serous cystadenoma was confirmed at surgery

1–5 in 10,000 spontaneous pregnancies [105]; however, the incidence of torsion increases markedly to nearly 1 in 10 pregnant women with ovarian hyperstimulation syndrome, in the setting of ovulation induction [106]. Rotation of the adnexa around its ligamentous support and twisting of the vascular pedicle are defining features of torsion, which result in vascular compromise of the ovary and/or fallopian tube, and resultant hemorrhagic necrosis [107]. An underlying adnexal mass which serves as a lead point is a finding in the majority of patients [108]. Woman with adnexal torsion commonly present with acute, sharp, and constant or intermittent abdominal/pelvic pain. MR imaging features of adnexal torsion include ipsilateral adnexal enlargement, deviation of the uterus towards the torsed side, fat stranding surrounding the torsed adnexa, twisting of the vascular pedicle, and engorgement of the adnexal vessels distal to the twist [109]. When present, an associated ovarian mass may be identified on MR imaging (Fig. 5.19).

5.8 Conclusion

Appendicitis can be difficult to diagnose clinically in the pregnant patient, and thus imaging plays an essential role in directing patient care. MRI is the preferred diagnostic examination at our institution, due to its lack of ionizing radiation and the high non-visualization rate of the appendix using ultrasound. In the pregnant patient, MRI is performed at 1.5 T without oral or intravenous contrast, and our comprehensive imaging protocol includes single-shot T2-weighted images, T2-weighted images with fat saturation, balanced steady-state free precession gradient-echo images, and T1-weighted gradient-echo images with fat saturation. MRI, especially when interpreted by experienced radiologists, has high diagnostic accuracy for the diagnosis or exclusion of acute appendicitis in pregnancy. The MR findings of appendicitis include an enlarged (size ≥ 8 mm) appendix with a thickened wall, periappendiceal inflammation, and the presence of one or multiple appendicoliths. MRI can be used to simultaneously evaluate for an alternative explanation for abdominal and/or pelvic pain in the pregnant patient. MRI should be considered the first-line diagnostic test in the pregnant patient with abdominal and/or pelvic pain and suspected appendicitis.

Acknowledgements *Disclosure of Conflicts of Interest*: The authors have no relevant relationships to disclose.

References

1. Tracey M, Fletcher HS. Appendicitis in pregnancy. Am Surg. 2000;66(6):555–9.
2. Abbasi N, Patenaude V, Abenhaim HA. Management and outcomes of acute appendicitis in pregnancy-population-based study of over 7000 cases. BJOG. 2014;121(12):1509–14.
3. Mourad J, Elliott JP, Erickson L, Lisboa L. Appendicitis in pregnancy: new information that contradicts long-held clinical beliefs. Am J Obstet Gynecol. 2000;182(5):1027–9.
4. Cappell MS, Friedel D. Abdominal pain during pregnancy. Gastroenterol Clin North Am. 2003;32(1):1–58.
5. Mayer IE, Hussain H. Abdominal pain during pregnancy. Gastroenterol Clin North Am. 1998;27(1):1–36.
6. Theilen L, Mellnick V, Shanks A, Tuuli M, Odibo A, Macones G, et al. Acute appendicitis in pregnancy: predictive clinical factors and pregnancy outcomes. Am J Perinatol. 2016;34(6):523–8.
7. Lee SL, Walsh AJ, Ho HS. Computed tomography and ultrasonography do not improve and may delay the diagnosis and treatment of acute appendicitis. Arch Surg. 2001;136(5):556–62.
8. Kessler N, Cyteval C, Gallix B, Lesnik A, Blayac P-M, Pujol J, et al. Appendicitis: evaluation of sensitivity, specificity, and predictive values of US, Doppler US, and laboratory findings. Radiology. 2004;230(2):472–8.
9. Oto A, Srinivasan PN, Ernst RD, Koroglu M, Cesani F, Nishino T, et al. Revisiting MRI for appendix location during pregnancy. AJR Am J Roentgenol. 2006;186(3):883–7.
10. Wu V, Armson BA. Appendicitis in pregnancy: clinical presentation and perinatal outcome. J SOGC. 1999;21(14):1328–33.
11. Babaknia A, Parsa H, Woodruff JD. Appendicitis during pregnancy. Obstet Gynecol. 1977;50(1):40–4.
12. Tamir IL, Bongard FS, Klein SR. Acute appendicitis in the pregnant patient. Am J Surg. 1990;160(6):571–6.
13. Ueberrueck T, Koch A, Meyer L, Hinkel M, Gastinger I. Ninety-four appendectomies for suspected acute appendicitis during pregnancy. World J Surg. 2004;28(5):508–11.
14. McGory ML, Zingmond DS, Tillou A, Hiatt JR, Ko CY, Cryer HM. Negative appendectomy in pregnant women is associated with a substantial risk of fetal loss. J Am Coll Surg. 2007;205(4):534–40.
15. Bendeck SE, Nino-Murcia M, Berry GJ, Jeffrey RB. Imaging for suspected appendicitis: negative appendectomy and perforation rates. Radiology. 2002;225(1):131–6.
16. Coursey CA, Nelson RC, Patel MB, Cochran C, Dodd LG, DeLong DM, et al. Making the diagnosis of acute appendicitis: do more preoperative CT scans mean fewer negative appendectomies? A 10-year study. Radiology. 2010;254(2):460–8.
17. Patel SJ, Reede DL, Katz DS, Subramaniam R, Amorosa JK. Imaging the pregnant patient for non-obstetric conditions: algorithms and radiation dose considerations. Radiographics. 2007;27(6):1705–22.
18. Lehnert BE, Gross JA, Linnau KF, Moshiri M. Utility of ultrasound for evaluating the appendix during the second and third trimester of pregnancy. Emerg Radiol. 2012;19(4):293–9.
19. Garcia EM, Camacho MA, Karolyi DR, Kim DH, Cash BD, Chang KJ, et al. ACR appropriateness criteria® right lower quadrant pain-suspected appendicitis. J Am Coll Radiol. 2018;15(11):S373–87.
20. Israel GM, Malguria N, McCarthy S, Copel J, Weinreb J. MRI vs. ultrasound for suspected appendicitis during pregnancy. J Magn Reson Imaging. 2008;28(2):428–33.
21. Spalluto LB, Woodfield CA, DeBenedectis CM, Lazarus E. MR imaging evaluation of abdominal pain during pregnancy: appendicitis and other nonobstetric causes. Radiographics. 2012;32(2):317–34.
22. Tocchio S, Kline-Fath B, Kanal E, Schmithorst VJ, Panigrahy A. MRI evaluation and safety in the developing brain. Semin Perinatol. 2015;39(2):73–104.
23. Patenaude Y, Pugash D, Lim K, Morin L, Lim K, Bly S, et al. The use of magnetic resonance imaging in the obstetric patient. J Obstet Gynaecol Can. 2014;36(4):349–55.
24. ACR. ACR–SPR practice parameter for the safe and optimal performance of fetal magnetic resonance imaging (MRI). 2014. https://www.acr.org/-/media/ACR/Files/Practice-Parameters/mr-fetal.pdf. Accessed 25 Mar 2019.
25. Ray JG, Vermeulen MJ, Bharatha A, Montanera WJ, Park AL. Association between MRI exposure during

pregnancy and fetal and childhood outcomes. JAMA. 2016;316(9):952–61.

26. Fraum TJ, Ludwig DR, Bashir MR, Fowler KJ. Gadolinium-based contrast agents: a comprehensive risk assessment. J Magn Reson Imaging. 2017;46(2):338–53.

27. Duke E, Kalb B, Arif-Tiwari H, Daye ZJ, Gilbertson-Dahdal D, Keim SM, et al. A systematic review and meta-analysis of diagnostic performance of MRI for evaluation of acute appendicitis. AJR Am J Roentgenol. 2016;206(3):508–17.

28. Kaushal P, Somwaru AS, Charabaty A, Levy AD. MR enterography of inflammatory bowel disease with endoscopic correlation. Radiographics. 2017;37(1):116–31.

29. Fidler JL, Guimaraes L, Einstein DM. MR imaging of the small bowel. Radiographics. 2009;29(6):1811–25.

30. Rimola J, Rodriguez S, García-Bosch O, Ordás I, Ayala E, Aceituno M, et al. Magnetic resonance for assessment of disease activity and severity in ileocolonic Crohn's disease. Gut. 2009;58(8):1113–20.

31. Kinsella SM, Lee A, Spencer JA. Maternal and fetal effects of the supine and pelvic tilt positions in late pregnancy. Eur J Obstet Gynecol Reprod Biol. 1990;36(1–2):11–7.

32. Yong FA, Alvarado AM, Wang H, Tsai J, Estes NC. Appendectomy: a risk factor for colectomy in patients with clostridium difficile. Am J Surg. 2015;209(3):532–5.

33. Bhangu A, Søreide K, Di Saverio S, Assarsson JH, Drake FT. Acute appendicitis: modern understanding of pathogenesis, diagnosis, and management. Lancet. 2015;386(10000):1278–87.

34. Baird DLH, Simillis C, Kontovounisios C, Rasheed S, Tekkis PP. Acute appendicitis. BMJ. 2017;357:j1703.

35. Swischuk LE, Chung DH, Hawkins HK, Jadhav SP, Radhakrishnan R. Non-fecalith-induced appendicitis: etiology, imaging, and pathology. Emerg Radiol. 2015;22(6):643–9.

36. Marudanayagam R, Williams GT, Rees BI. Review of the pathological results of 2660 appendicectomy specimens. J Gastroenterol. 2006;41(8):745–9.

37. Tsai R, Raptis C, Fowler KJ, Owen JW, Mellnick VM. MRI of suspected appendicitis during pregnancy: interradiologist agreement, indeterminate interpretation and the meaning of non-visualization of the appendix. Br J Radiol. 2017;90(1079):20170383.

38. Willekens I, Peeters E, Maeseneer MD, de Mey J. The normal appendix on CT: does size matter? PLoS One. 2014;9(5):e96476.

39. Jan Y-T, Yang F-S, Huang I-K. Visualization rate and pattern of normal appendix on multidetector computed tomography by using multiplanar reformation display. J Comput Assist Tomogr. 2005;29(4):446–51.

40. Atema JJ, van Rossem CC, Leeuwenburgh MM, Stoker J, Boermeester MA. Scoring system to distinguish uncomplicated from complicated acute appendicitis. Br J Surg. 2015;102(8):979–90.

41. Yoon HM, Kim JH, Lee JS, Ryu J-M, Kim DY, Lee J-Y. Pediatric appendicitis with appendicolith often presents with prolonged abdominal pain and a high risk of perforation. World J Pediatr. 2018;14(2):184–90.

42. Abdeen N, Naz F, Linthorst R, Khan U, Dominguez PC, Koujok K, et al. Clinical impact and cost-effectiveness of noncontrast MRI in the evaluation of suspected appendiceal abscesses in children. J Magn Reson Imaging. 2019;49(7):e241–9.

43. Kim HY, Park JH, Lee YJ, Lee SS, Jeon J-J, Lee KH. Systematic review and meta-analysis of CT features for differentiating complicated and uncomplicated appendicitis. Radiology. 2017;287(1):104–15.

44. Pedrosa I, Levine D, Eyvazzadeh AD, Siewert B, Ngo L, Rofsky NM. MR imaging evaluation of acute appendicitis in pregnancy. Radiology. 2006;238(3):891–9.

45. Rettenbacher T, Hollerweger A, Macheiner P, Rettenbacher L, Frass R, Schneider B, et al. Presence or absence of gas in the appendix: additional criteria to rule out or confirm acute appendicitis—evaluation with US. Radiology. 2000;214(1):183–7.

46. Hong H-S, Cho HS, Woo JY, Lee Y, Yang I, Hwang J-Y, et al. Intra-appendiceal air at CT: is it a useful or a confusing sign for the diagnosis of acute appendicitis? Korean J Radiol. 2016;17(1):39–46.

47. Chin CM, Lim KL. Appendicitis: atypical and challenging CT appearances: resident and fellow education feature. Radiographics. 2015;35(1):123–4.

48. Shin I, An C, Lim JS, Kim M-J, Chung YE. T1 bright appendix sign to exclude acute appendicitis in pregnant women. Eur Radiol. 2017;27(8):3310–6.

49. Al-Katib S, Sokhandon F, Farah M. MRI for appendicitis in pregnancy: is seeing believing? Clinical outcomes in cases of appendix nonvisualization. Abdom Radiol (NY). 2016;41(12):2455–9.

50. Kearl YL, Claudius I, Behar S, Cooper J, Dollbaum R, Hardasmalani M, et al. Accuracy of magnetic resonance imaging and ultrasound for appendicitis in diagnostic and nondiagnostic studies. Acad Emerg Med. 2016;23(2):179–85.

51. Kim DW, Suh CH, Yoon HM, Kim JR, Jung AY, Lee JS, et al. Visibility of normal Appendix on CT, MRI, and sonography: a systematic review and meta-analysis. AJR Am J Roentgenol. 2018;211(3):W140–50.

52. Vu L, Ambrose D, Vos P, Tiwari P, Rosengarten M, Wiseman S. Evaluation of MRI for the diagnosis of appendicitis during pregnancy when ultrasound is inconclusive. J Surg Res. 2009;156(1):145–9.

53. Ramalingam V, LeBedis C, Kelly JR, Uyeda J, Soto JA, Anderson SW. Evaluation of a sequential

multi-modality imaging algorithm for the diagnosis of acute appendicitis in the pregnant female. Emerg Radiol. 2015;22(2):125–32.

54. Tirada N, Dreizin D, Khati NJ, Akin EA, Zeman RK. Imaging pregnant and lactating patients. Radiographics. 2015;35(6):1751–65.

55. American College of Radiology, Committee on Drugs and Contrast Media. ACR manual on contrast media v10.3 [Internet]. 2018. https://www.acr.org/Clinical-Resources/Contrast-Manual. Accessed May 8 2019.

56. Poletti P-A, Botsikas D, Becker M, Picarra M, Rutschmann OT, Buchs NC, et al. Suspicion of appendicitis in pregnant women: emergency evaluation by sonography and low-dose CT with oral contrast. Eur Radiol. 2019;29(1):345–52.

57. Pinto Leite N, Pereira JM, Cunha R, Pinto P, Sirlin C. CT Evaluation of appendicitis and its complications: imaging techniques and key diagnostic findings. Am J Roentgenol. 2005;185(2):406–17.

58. Yarmish GM, Smith MP, Rosen MP, Baker ME, Blake MA, Cash BD, et al. ACR appropriateness criteria right upper quadrant pain. J Am Coll Radiol. 2014;11(3):316–22.

59. Bennett GL. Evaluating patients with right upper quadrant pain. Radiol Clin North Am. 2015;53(6):1093–130.

60. Valdivieso V, Covarrubias C, Siegel F, Cruz F. Pregnancy and cholelithiasis: pathogenesis and natural course of gallstones diagnosed in early puerperium. Hepatology. 1993;17(1):1–4.

61. Maringhini A. Biliary sludge and gallstones in pregnancy: incidence, risk factors, and natural history. Ann Intern Med. 1993;119(2):116.

62. Augustin G. Acute biliary tract diseases. In: Acute abdomen during pregnancy. Cham: Springer; 2014.

63. Mendez-Sanchez N, Chavez-Tapia NC, Uribe M. Pregnancy and gallbladder disease. Ann Hepatol. 2006;5(3):227–30.

64. Ghumman E, Barry M, Grace PA. Management of gallstones in pregnancy. Br J Surg. 1997;84(12):1646–50.

65. Kaura SH, Haghighi M, Matza BW, Hajdu CH, Rosenkrantz AB. Comparison of CT and MRI findings in the differentiation of acute from chronic cholecystitis. Clin Imaging. 2013;37(4):687–91.

66. Watanabe Y, Nagayama M, Okumura A, Amoh Y, Katsube T, Suga T, et al. MR imaging of acute biliary disorders. Radiographics. 2007;27(2):477–95.

67. Date RS, Kaushal M, Ramesh A. A review of the management of gallstone disease and its complications in pregnancy. Am J Surg. 2008;196(4):599–608.

68. Singh A, Mann HS, Thukral CL, Singh NR. Diagnostic accuracy of MRCP as compared to ultrasound/CT in patients with obstructive jaundice. J Clin Diagn Res. 2014;8(3):103–7.

69. Chen W, Mo J-J, Lin L, Li C-Q, Zhang J-F. Diagnostic value of magnetic resonance cholangiopancreatography in choledocholithiasis. World J Gastroenterol. 2015;21(11):3351–60.

70. Irie H, Honda H, Kuroiwa T, Yoshimitsu K, Aibe H, Shinozaki K, et al. Pitfalls in MR cholangiopancreatographic interpretation. Radiographics. 2001;21(1):23–37.

71. Mali P. Pancreatitis in pregnancy: etiology, diagnosis, treatment, and outcomes. Hepatobiliary Pancreat Dis Int. 2016;15(4):434–8.

72. Miller FH, Keppke AL, Dalal K, Ly JN, Kamler V-A, Sica GT. MRI of pancreatitis and its complications: part 1, acute pancreatitis. AJR Am J Roentgenol. 2004;183(6):1637–44.

73. Papadakis EP, Sarigianni M, Mikhailidis DP, Mamopoulos A, Karagiannis V. Acute pancreatitis in pregnancy: an overview. Eur J Obstet Gynecol Reprod Biol. 2011;159(2):261–6.

74. Haram K, Svendsen E, Abildgaard U. The HELLP syndrome: clinical issues and management. A review. BMC Pregnancy Childbirth. 2009;9(1):8.

75. Nunes JO, Turner MA, Fulcher AS. Abdominal imaging features of HELLP syndrome: a 10-Year retrospective review. AJR Am J Roentgenol. 2005;185(5):1205–10.

76. Longo SA, Moore RC, Canzoneri BJ, Robichaux A. Gastrointestinal conditions during pregnancy. Clin Colon Rectal Surg. 2010;23(2):80–9.

77. Webster P, Bailey M, Wilson J, Burke D. Small bowel obstruction in pregnancy is a complex surgical problem with a high risk of fetal loss. Ann R Coll Surg Engl. 2015;97(5):339–44.

78. Sivanesaratnam V. The acute abdomen and the obstetrician. Baillieres Best Pract Res Clin Obstet Gynaecol. 2000;14(1):89–102.

79. Kakarla N, Dailey C, Marino T, Shikora SA, Chelmow D. Pregnancy after gastric bypass surgery and internal hernia formation. Obstet Gynecol. 2005;105(5 Pt 2):1195–8.

80. Munkholm P, Langholz E, Nielsen OH, Kreiner S, Binder V. Incidence and prevalence of Crohn's disease in the county of Copenhagen, 1962-87: a sixfold increase in incidence. Scand J Gastroenterol. 1992;27(7):609–14.

81. Hashash JG, Kane S. Pregnancy and inflammatory bowel disease. Gastroenterol Hepatol. 2015;11(2):96–102.

82. Hatch Q, Champagne BJ, Maykel JA, Davis BR, Johnson EK, Bleier JI, et al. The impact of pregnancy on surgical Crohn disease: an analysis of the nationwide inpatient sample. J Surg Res. 2014;190(1):41–6.

83. Gauci J, Sammut L, Sciberras M, Piscopo N, Micallef K, Cortis K, et al. Small bowel imaging in Crohn's disease patients. Ann Gastroenterol. 2018;31(4):395–405.

84. Heverhagen JT, Ishaque N, Zielke A, Bohrer T, Sitter H, Berthold LD, et al. Feasibility of MRI in the diagnosis of acute diverticulitis: initial results. MAGMA. 2001;12(1):4–9.

85. Rao PM, Rhea JT, Wittenberg J, Warshaw AL. Misdiagnosis of primary epiploic appendagitis. Am J Surg. 1998;176(1):81–5.

86. Meher S, Gibbons N, DasGupta R. Renal stones in pregnancy. Obstet Med. 2014;7(3):103–10.
87. Semins MJ, Matlaga BR. Management of urolithiasis in pregnancy. Int J Womens Health. 2013;5:599–604.
88. Coursey CA, Casalino DD, Remer EM, Arellano RS, Bishoff JT, Dighe M, et al. ACR appropriateness criteria® acute onset flank pain--suspicion of stone disease. Ultrasound Q. 2012;28(3):227–33.
89. Butler EL, Cox SM, Eberts EG, Cunningham FG. Symptomatic nephrolithiasis complicating pregnancy. Obstet Gynecol. 2000;96(5 Pt 1):753–6.
90. Rasmussen PE, Nielsen FR. Hydronephrosis during pregnancy: a literature survey. Eur J Obstet Gynecol Reprod Biol. 1988;27(3):249–59.
91. Spencer JA, Chahal R, Kelly A, Taylor K, Eardley I, Lloyd SN. Evaluation of painful hydronephrosis in pregnancy: magnetic resonance urographic patterns in physiological dilatation versus calculous obstruction. J Urol. 2004;171(1):256–60.
92. Muthusami P, Bhuvaneswari V, Elangovan S, Dorairajan LN, Ramesh A. The role of static magnetic resonance urography in the evaluation of obstructive uropathy. Urology. 2013;81(3):623–7.
93. Mullins JK, Semins MJ, Hyams ES, Bohlman ME, Matlaga BR. Half Fourier single-shot turbo spin-echo magnetic resonance urography for the evaluation of suspected renal colic in pregnancy. Urology. 2012;79(6):1252–5.
94. Woodfield CA, Lazarus E, Chen KC, Mayo-Smith WW. Abdominal pain in pregnancy: diagnoses and imaging unique to pregnancy—review. AJR Am J Roentgenol. 2010;194(6 Suppl):WS14–30.
95. Rodgers SK, Chang C, DeBardeleben JT, Horrow MM. Normal and abnormal US findings in early first-trimester pregnancy: review of the society of radiologists in ultrasound 2012 consensus panel recommendations. Radiographics. 2015;35(7):2135–48.
96. Sivalingam VN, Duncan WC, Kirk E, Shephard LA, Horne AW. Diagnosis and management of ectopic pregnancy. J Fam Plann Reprod Health Care. 2011;37(4):231–40.
97. Alkatout I, Honemeyer U, Strauss A, Tinelli A, Malvasi A, Jonat W, et al. Clinical diagnosis and treatment of ectopic pregnancy. Obstet Gynecol Surv. 2013;68(8):571–81.
98. Parker RA, Yano M, Tai AW, Friedman M, Narra VR, Menias CO. MR imaging findings of ectopic pregnancy: a pictorial review. Radiographics. 2012;32(5):1445–60.
99. Wu Z, Zhang X, Xu P, Huang X. Clinical analysis of 50 patients with heterotopic pregnancy after ovulation induction or embryo transfer. Eur J Med Res. 2018;23(1):17.
100. Barrenetxea G, Barinaga-Rementeria L, Lopez de Larruzea A, Agirregoikoa JA, Mandiola M, Carbonero K. Heterotopic pregnancy: two cases and a comparative review. Fertil Steril. 2007;87(2):417. e9–417.e15.
101. Petresin J, Wolf J, Emir S, Müller A, Boosz AS. Endometriosis-associated maternal pregnancy complications – case report and literature review. Geburtshilfe Frauenheilkd. 2016;76(8):902–5.
102. Leone Roberti Maggiore U, Ferrero S, Mangili G, Bergamini A, Inversetti A, Giorgione V, et al. A systematic review on endometriosis during pregnancy: diagnosis, misdiagnosis, complications and outcomes. Hum Reprod Update. 2016;22(1):70–103.
103. Siegelman ES, Oliver ER. MR imaging of endometriosis: ten imaging pearls. Radiographics. 2012;32(6):1675–91.
104. Woodward PJ, Sohaey R, Mezzetti TP. Endometriosis: radiologic-pathologic correlation. Radiographics. 2001;21(1):193–216.
105. Hasson J, Tsafrir Z, Azem F, Bar-On S, Almog B, Mashiach R, et al. Comparison of adnexal torsion between pregnant and nonpregnant women. Am J Obstet Gynecol. 2010;202(6):536.e1–6.
106. Mashiach S, Bider D, Moran O, Goldenberg M, Ben-Rafael Z. Adnexal torsion of hyperstimulated ovaries in pregnancies after gonadotropin therapy. Fertil Steril. 1990;53(1):76–80.
107. Houry D, Abbott JT. Ovarian torsion: a fifteen-year review. Ann Emerg Med. 2001;38(2):156–9.
108. Bider D, Mashiach S, Dulitzky M, Kokia E, Lipitz S, Ben-Rafael Z. Clinical, surgical and pathologic findings of adnexal torsion in pregnant and nonpregnant women. Surg Gynecol Obstet. 1991;173(5):363–6.
109. Rha SE, Byun JY, Jung SE, Jung JI, Choi BG, Kim BS, et al. CT and MR imaging features of adnexal torsion. Radiographics. 2002;22(2):283–94.

Imaging of Non-obstetric Pelvic Emergencies

6

Joseph W. Owen and Karen Tran-Hardining

Contents

6.1 Gastrointestinal

6.1.1 Appendicitis

The most common cause of an emergency surgery in pregnancy is appendicitis, with an estimated prevalence of 50–70 incidents per 1000 patients [1]. Due to its high incidence and potential morbidity [2], appendicitis is often suspected in pregnant women presenting to the emergency department with abdominal pain, nausea, vomiting, fever, or leukocytosis.

The variable location of the appendix during pregnancy presents a diagnostic challenge compared to the nonpregnant patient. With advancing gestation, the cecum and appendix are increasingly elevated out of the pelvis by the gravid uterus, and may sometimes be found in the right upper quadrant [3]. This can result in appendicitis manifesting as upper abdominal pain, and can

J. W. Owen (✉)
Department of Radiology, University of Kentucky College of Medicine, Lexington, KY, USA
e-mail: joseph.owen@uky.edu

K. Tran Hardining
Department of Radiological Sciences, University of California Irvine, Irvine, CA, USA
e-mail: Karennt@hs.uci.edu

© Springer Nature Switzerland AG 2020
M. N. Patlas et al. (eds.), *Emergency Imaging of Pregnant Patients*,
https://doi.org/10.1007/978-3-030-42722-1_6

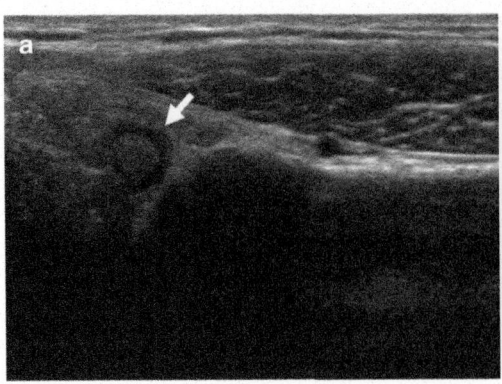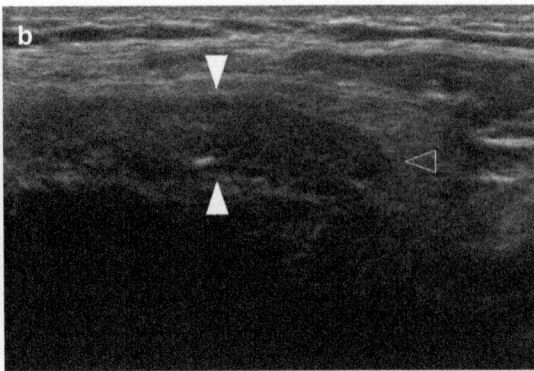

Fig. 6.1 Ultrasound images of a normal appendix. (**a**) Transverse grayscale US image of the right lower quadrant reveals a tubular structure with bowel wall signature (white arrow) overlying the psoas muscle. (**b**) Sagittal grayscale US image demonstrates the tubular structure is blind-ending (open arrowhead) and measures 6 mm in diameter (white arrowheads), confirming the presence of a normal appendix

make the appendix difficult to identify on ultrasound.

The traditional first-line modality for evaluating suspected appendicitis (Fig. 6.1) in a pregnant patient is ultrasound with graded compression [4]. As pregnancy advances and the uterus enlarges, graded compression becomes increasingly difficult, reducing ultrasound's ability to distinguish the appendix. Sonographic findings of acute appendicitis include a noncompressible tubular structure measuring greater than 6 mm with thickened hyperemic walls and surrounding inflammatory fat stranding [5]. Appendicoliths may be visualized as hyperechoic foci with posterior acoustic shadowing within the blind-ending tubular appendix. Nonperistaltic small bowel and small bowel wall thickening may be visualized in the right lower quadrant due to the adjacent appendiceal inflammation [6]. There is high variability in sonographic skills, and the appendix may not be visualized in 88–92% of examinations [7], even with experienced sonographers.

Due to the variable sensitivity of ultrasound and the increasing availability of MR in emergency departments, MR is increasingly used as the primary imaging modality for suspected appendicitis in pregnancy [8]. MR can assess for appendicitis without exposing pregnant patients to the ionizing radiation of CT, and studies have demonstrated the negative predictive value of

MR in the evaluation of appendicitis to be as high as 100% [9]. The variable location of the appendix in pregnancy does not pose as substantial a challenge for MR as for ultrasound, as long as a well-designed MR protocol provides an adequate field of view to cover the abdomen and the pelvis (Fig. 6.2). An MR field of view that includes the abdomen and pelvis also allows for the characterization of non-appendiceal pathology, which may not have been evident with a focused US (Table 6.1).

The MR features typically seen in acute appendicitis in pregnancy are like those seen in nonpregnant patients (Fig. 6.3). MR findings include a dilated appendix measuring 8 mm or more with a fluid-filled lumen (hyperintense on T2-weighted fat-suppressed images and hypointense on T1-weighted images) and a thickened (≥2 mm), edematous appendiceal wall (hypointense on T1-weighted images and slightly hyperintense on T2-weighted images) [10]. There may also be surrounding inflammation, seen as areas of high signal intensity on the T2-weighted fat-suppressed images and low signal intensity on the T1-weighted images. The absence of intraluminal blooming artifact on T2*-weighted images or on gradient-recalled echo T1-weighted images suggests a lack of intraluminal air [11].

Findings indeterminate for acute appendicitis include high signal intensity luminal contents on T2-weighted images, with a diameter of 6–7 mm,

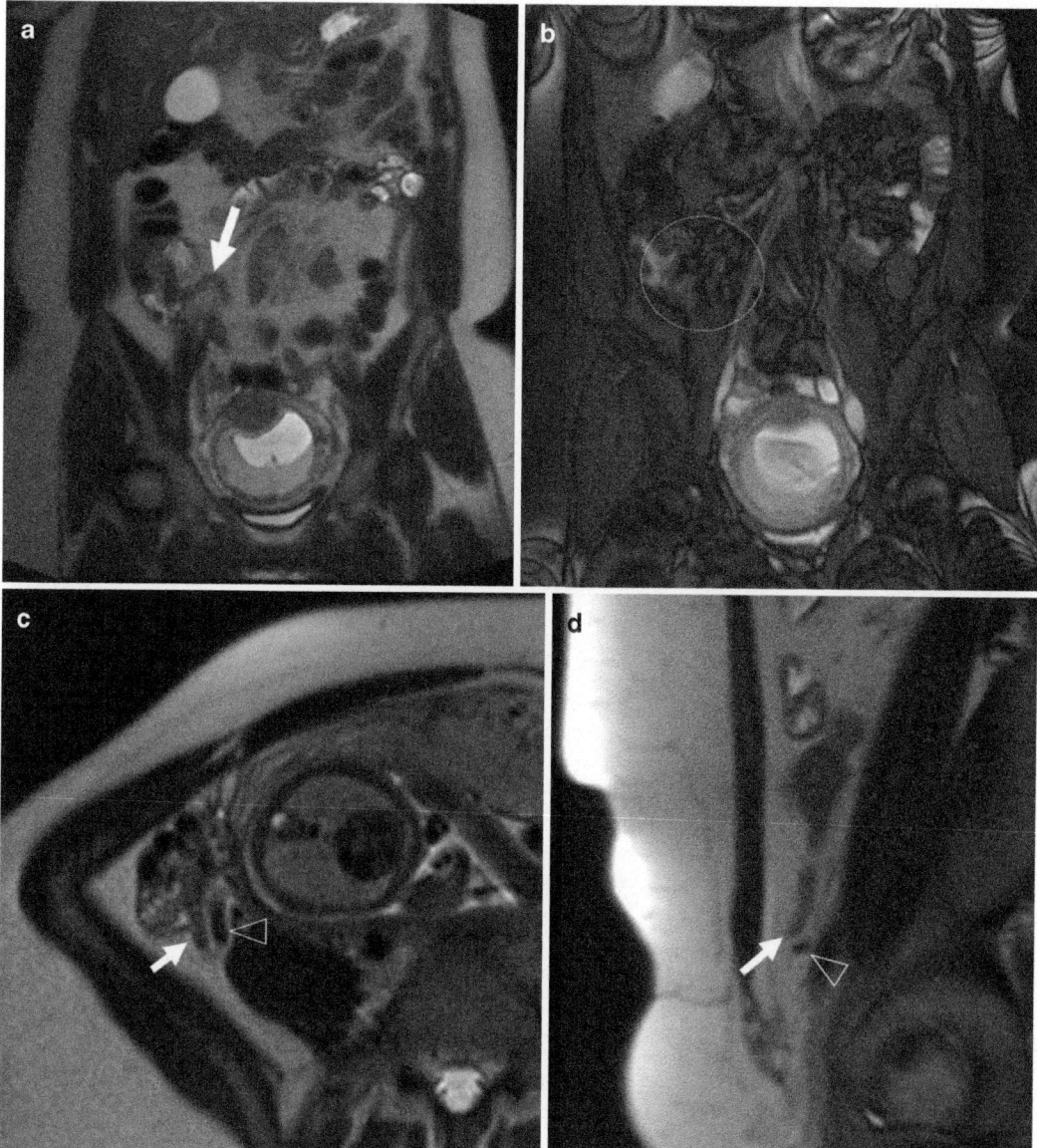

Fig. 6.2 MR images of a normal appendix. Twenty-seven-year-old pregnant woman, estimated gestational age 14 weeks, presents with abdominal pain. (**a**) Coronal T2-weighted single-shot turbo spin-echo MR image demonstrating a normal caliber tubular structure arising from the cecum (arrow) consistent with a normal appendix. (**b**) Coronal fat-suppressed steady-state free-procession MR image demonstrating no surrounding mesenteric inflammation (dotted circle). A different patient with estimated gestation age of 32 weeks presents with right lower quadrant abdominal pain. (**c**) Axial and (**d**) sagittal T2-weighted turbo spin-echo images show the normal appendix (arrow) arising from the cecum, with an adjacent ovarian vein (open arrowhead), which can be mistaken for the appendix. Note the hypointensity of the ovarian vein relative to the appendix due to a flow void within the vein

but without associated wall thickening, peri-appendiceal fat stranding, or fluid [3]. When findings for acute appendicitis are equivocal, pregnant patients may be observed and reimaged if abdominal pain persists. For most cases where the diagnosis of appendicitis is equivocal on MR, appendicitis is not present [12]. Nonvisualization of the appendix on MR has a

Table 6.1 Suspected appendicitis in pregnancy protocol

Sequence	Orientation	TR	TE	Matrix	Slices	Slice thickness (mm)	Voxel size	Concatenations	Acquisition time (s)
T2 single-shot turbo spin-echo	Coronal	1450	83	256 × 256	27	5	1.4 × 1.4 × 5.0 mm	2	39
T2 single-shot turbo spin-echo	Axial	1000	70	208 × 256	30	5	1.2 × 1.2 × 5.0 mm	3	50
T2 single-shot turbo spin-echo	Sagittal	1000	79	256 × 200	22	5	1.3 × 1.3 × 5.0 mm	2	30
T2 inversion recovery fat-suppression	Coronal	4120	104	512 × 512	27	5	0.7 × 0.7 × 5 mm	3	50
T1 spoiled gradient-recalled echo	Axial abdomen	119	4.76	384 × 512	22	6	0.6 × 0.6 × 6 mm	2	27
T1 spoiled gradient-recalled echo	Axial pelvis	119	4.76	384 × 512	22	6	0.6 × 0.6 × 6 mm	2	27
T2 fat-suppressed turbo spin-echo	Axial	4700	130	208 × 256	60	5	0.5 × 0.5 × 5 mm	4	94

T2-weighted turbo spin-echo sequences obtained in all three planes are the core sequences. Field of view should be anchored to the perineum and extend as far into the upper abdomen as your scanner geometry allows, ideally including the gallbladder, common bile duct, pancreas, and kidneys. Fat-suppressed T2-weighted images improve sensitivity for edema and free fluid. T1-weighted images increase sensitivity for blood

high negative predictive value for acute appendicitis [12]. Free fluid in the pelvis or right lower quadrant can be a normal finding in pregnancy, and should not be the basis for diagnosing acute appendicitis. One pitfall of MR imaging for suspected appendicitis in pregnancy is mistaking dilated ovarian veins for the appendix. Ovarian veins may be greater than 8 mm during pregnancy, and are often located in the right lower quadrant or abut the cecum. Veins should have flow voids on T2 weighted images, differentiating vessels from the T2 hyperintense lumen of a fluid-filled appendix (Fig. 6.3).

Studies have demonstrated that abdominal and pelvic CT have a 92% sensitivity, 99% specificity, and 99% negative predictive value for diagnosing appendicitis [13]. If MRI is contraindicated or unavailable, CT of the abdomen and pelvis should be considered the second-line

examination [11]. Both intravenous and oral contrast can greatly increase appendix visualization [11]. If possible, pregnant women should be scanned on modern CT equipment with high-pitch, dose modulation, and iterative reconstruction to minimize dose to the fetus and mother.

6.1.2 Cholelithiasis and Acute Cholecystitis

Cholelithiasis is a common finding in pregnant patients with abdominal pain. Two percent to 4% of pregnant patients have gallstones, and 5% of pregnant patients with gallstones develop symptoms [14]. Ultrasound is the method of choice for detecting gallstones, offering high sensitivity and accuracy of greater than 95% [15]. On US, gallstones are hyperechoic foci with posterior acoustic shadowing,

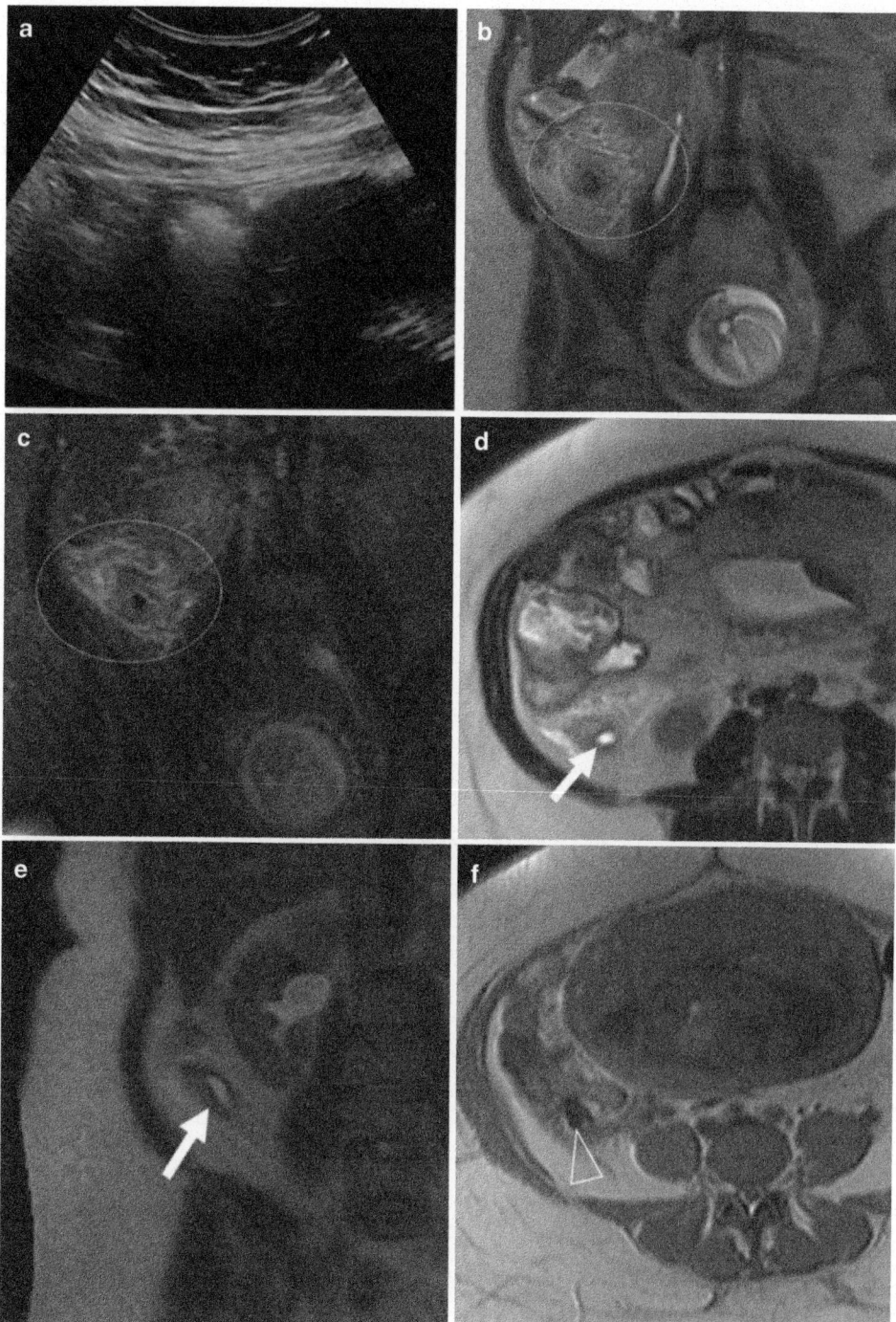

Fig. 6.3 Acute appendicitis. Twenty-eight-year-old pregnant woman, estimated gestational age 22 weeks, presents with right lower quadrant abdominal pain. (**a**) Grayscale US image shows gas-filled bowel with posterior acoustic shadowing obscuring the right lower quadrant. (**b**) Coronal T2-weighted single-shot turbo spin-echo and (**c**) fat-suppressed T2-weighted coronal single-shot turbo spin-echo images showing T2 hyperintense mesenteric edema (dotted circle) surrounding the inflamed appendix. (**d**) Axial and (**e**) coronal T2 weighted turbo spin-echo images showing a fluid filled, dilated appendix, with wall thickening (arrow). (**f**) Axial T1-weighted gradient-recalled echo images showing a signal void at the base of the appendix, consistent with an appendicolith (open arrowhead)

located in the gallbladder [15]. Gallstones and sludge can be differentiated from polyps by repositioning the patient into a decubitus position and assessing for mobility. Gallstones appear as signal voids within the gallbladder on T2-weighted MR images [3], and can be T1 hyperintense or signal voids on gradient-recalled echo T1-weighted images.

Acute cholecystitis is the second most common cause of an acute abdomen necessitating surgical intervention during pregnancy [16]. Detection of gallstones along with other US findings can lead to the diagnosis of acute cholecystitis. Ultrasound characteristics associated with acute cholecystitis include a positive Murphy's sign (maximum ten-derness during compression with the transducer directly over an incompressible gallbladder), a thickened gallbladder wall greater than 3 mm, and pericholecystic fluid [15]. It must be remembered that acalculous acute cholecystitis can less commonly occur, in the absence of gallstones.

MR has a high positive predictive value of up to 100% for the diagnosis of acute cholecystitis [17]. MR features include gallbladder wall thickening (>3 mm), gallbladder wall edema (T2 hyperintense gallbladder wall) (Fig. 6.4), and pericholecystic fluid [3]. Sometimes, a signal void may be seen in the cystic duct or gallbladder neck due to an obstruction from a

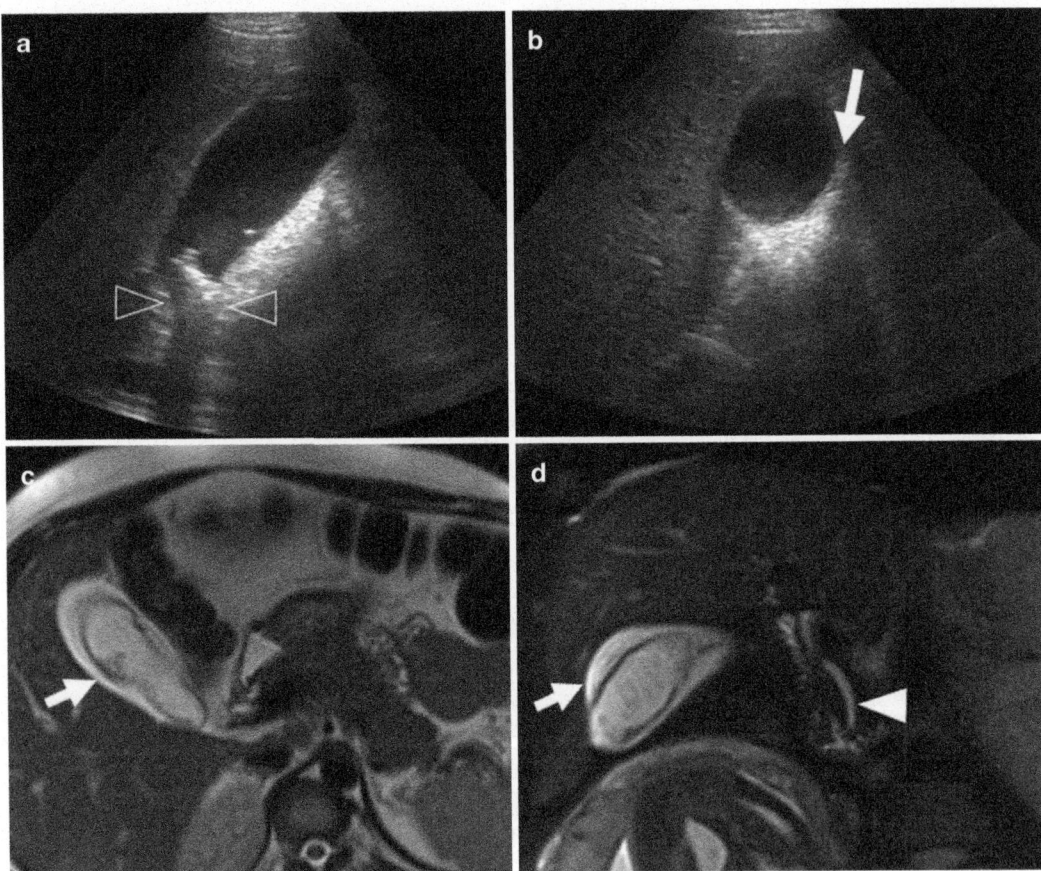

Fig. 6.4 Acute cholecystitis: Twenty-seven-year-old pregnant woman, estimated gestational age 27 weeks, presents with right upper quadrant pain, nausea, and leukocytosis. (**a**) Grayscale US long-axis image of the gallbladder shows echogenic foci with posterior acoustic shadowing (open arrowheads) in the neck of the gallbladder. (**b**) Short-axis US image of the gallbladder shows wall thickening greater than 3 mm (arrow). Sonographic Murphy's sign was positive. MRCP was performed to diagnose or exclude choledocolithiasis. (**c**) Axial T2-weighted single-shot turbo spin-echo image shows gallbladder wall thickening and mucosal irregularity (arrow). (**d**) Oblique coronal fat-suppressed single-shot turbo spin-echo image redemonstrates the gallbladder wall thickening and irregularity (arrow), with a normal caliber common bile duct (arrowhead) without filling defects. Acute cholecystitis was confirmed at laparoscopy

gallstone [3]. Complications of acute cholecystitis include perforation and abscess.

6.1.3 Pancreatitis

In the pregnant population, most cases of pancreatitis are due to gallstones and choledocholithiasis [18]. Patients typically present with abdominal pain, nausea, and vomiting. If clinical symptoms are suggestive of pancreatitis, but the serum amylase and/or lipase activity is less than three times the upper limit of normal, characteristic imaging findings are required to diagnose acute pancreatitis [19].

Ultrasound can be used to detect or exclude gallstones or bile duct dilatation [20] but may not be sensitive to choledocholithiasis or abnormalities of the pancreatic parenchyma (Fig. 6.5) due to obscuration by overlying bowel gas [20]. In some instances, ultrasound can demonstrate peripancreatic fluid collections, as a secondary sign of acute necrotizing pancreatitis [20].

MR imaging features of acute pancreatitis include parenchymal edema and peripancreatic fluid (Fig. 6.5). The edematous pancreatic parenchyma may have high signal intensity on T2-weighted images and low signal intensity on T1-weighted images. The normal pancreas has the highest T1-weighted signal intensity of the solid organs of the upper abdomen, and any decrease in signal intensity relative to the liver or spleen should warrant a close assessment for edema, inflammation, or neoplasia. Peripancreatic fluid manifests as high signal intensity within the peripancreatic retroperitoneum (Fig. 6.5) on T2-weighted images [3]. In cases of necrotizing pancreatitis, the pancreatic parenchyma can be replaced by necrosis, and acute collections can have variable signal intensity with a mixture of fat, fluid, and blood. T1 hyperintensity within a collection indicates hemorrhagic pancreatitis and should prompt close inspection for vascular complications. The presence of gas within a collection can be seen as multifocal T1 and T2 signal voids, with blooming artifact on T1-weighted in-phase images. Gas is a concerning feature that may indicate superinfection in the absence of recent intervention.

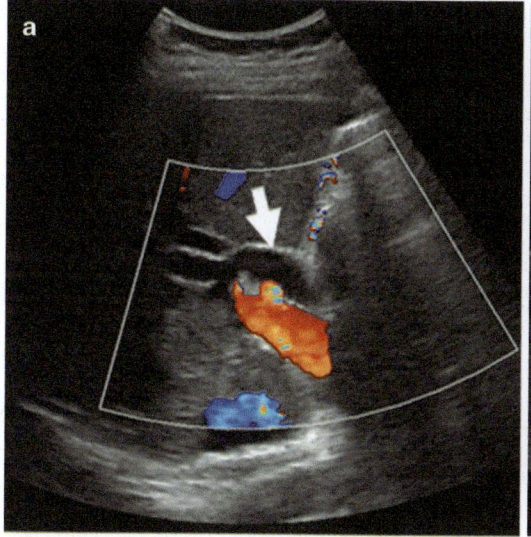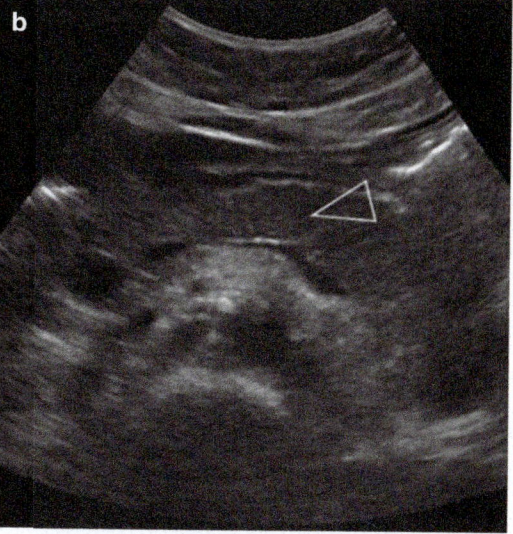

Fig. 6.5 Acute pancreatitis: Twenty-four-year-old woman, estimated gestational age 4 weeks, presents 5 weeks post-cholecystectomy with epigastric pain and elevated lipase. (**a**) Color Doppler US image of the right upper quadrant shows a dilated common bile duct. (**b**) Grayscale transverse US image of the pancreas shows no abnormality. MRCP was performed to assess for choledocolithiasis. (**c**) Axial fat-suppressed T2-weighted turbo spin-echo image shows peripancreatic edema (arrowhead) and common bile duct dilation (arrow). (**d**) Coronal T2-weighted single-shot turbo spin-echo image shows peripancreatic edema (arrowheads). (**e**) Thick-slab T2-weighted MRCP image shows a dilated common bile duct (arrow) without filling defect. Papillary stenosis was evident at ERCP, and was treated with sphincterotomy

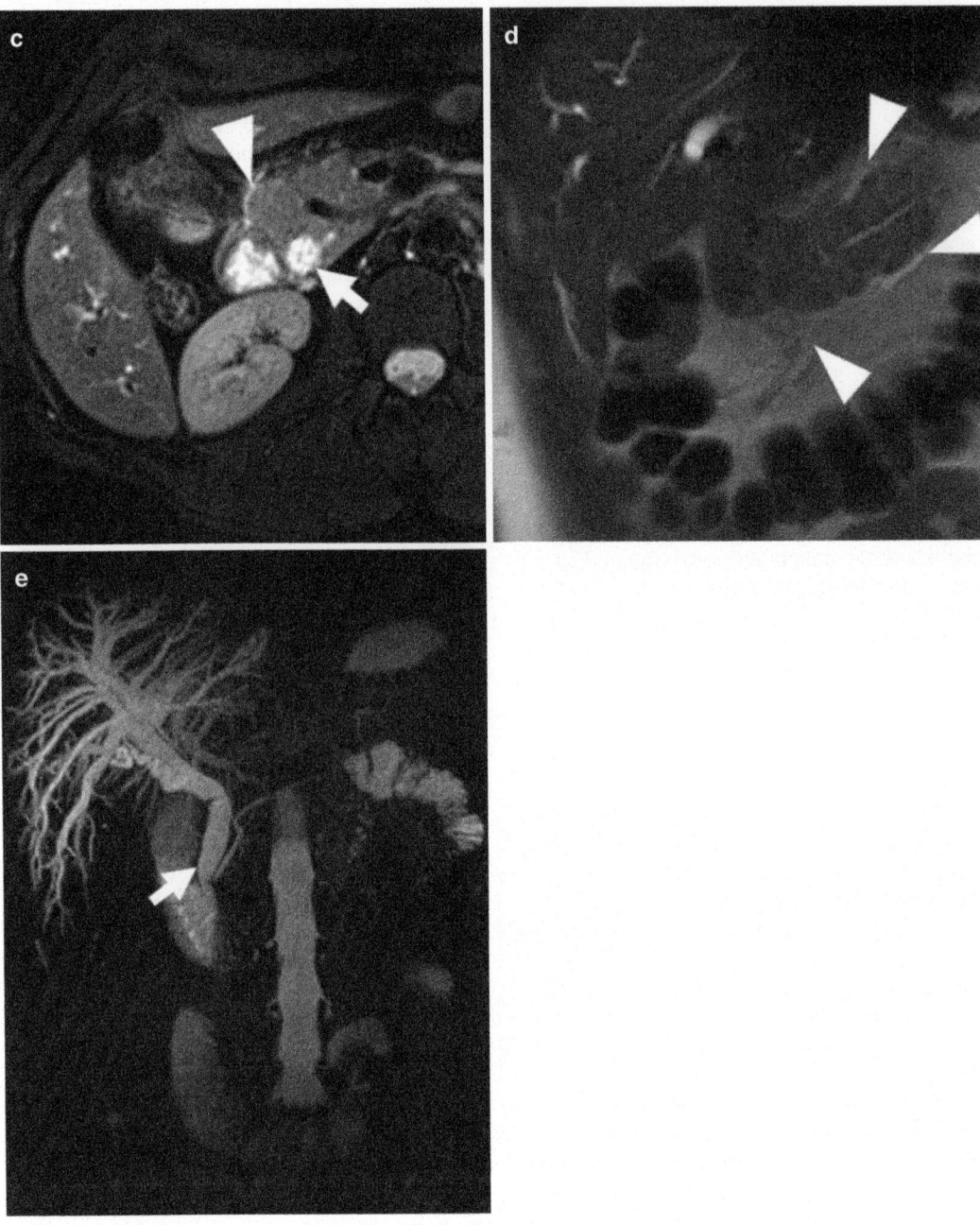

Fig. 6.5 (continued)

6.1.4 Inflammatory Bowel Disease

Pregnant women with inflammatory bowel disease (IBD) may present with abdominal pain in pregnancy. The peak incidence for IBD ranges from 15 to 25 years of age, which coincides with the common range of age for reproduction. Pregnant patients with IBD may present without a previously known diagnosis of IBD or with an acute exacerbation. The symptoms of IBD can mimic acute appendicitis, manifesting as right lower quadrant pain, nausea, and vomiting, as 80% of IBD cases involve the terminal ileum [21].

Ultrasound can detect active inflammation of IBD, and complications from penetrating disease, such as abscess. Grayscale unenhanced ultrasound may be used to localize and evaluate the length of the affected intestinal segments [22]. Thickening of the small bowel wall to greater than 3–4 mm [22] can be detected with ultrasound, although it is a nonspecific finding (Fig. 6.6). The inflamed bowel wall may show a thick hyperechoic central layer, the edematous submucosa, between the muscularis propria and inner mucosa. Segments of affected bowel may appear rigid with loss of normal peristaltic activity [22]. Color and power Doppler can be used to identify increased mural or extra-visceral vascularity related to active inflammation [22]. Ultrasound may also be a useful modality for detecting transmural complications including inflammatory masses, abscesses, or fistulas [22] (Fig. 6.7). IV contrast-enhanced ultrasound is

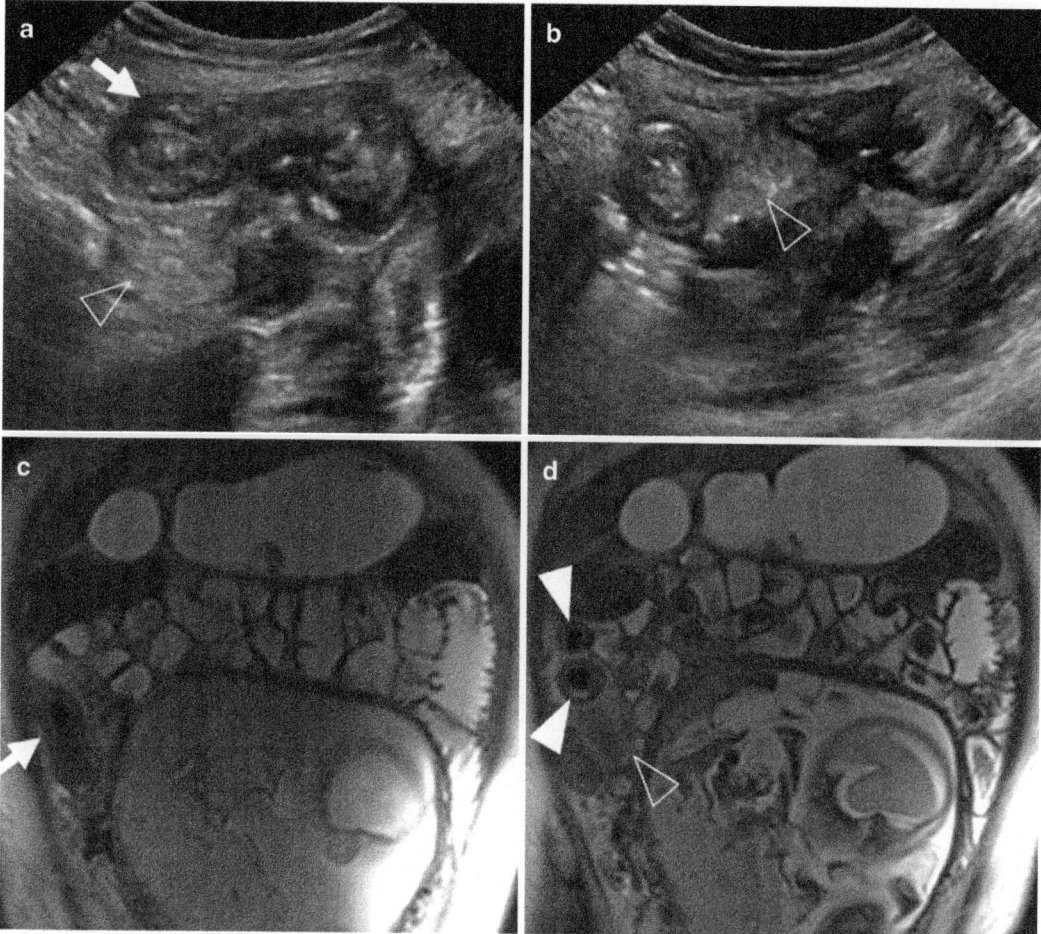

Fig. 6.6 Crohn's disease with active inflammation. Twenty-one-year-old pregnant woman, estimated gestational age 16 weeks, presents with abdominal pain and untreated Crohn's disease. (**a, b**) Grayscale US images show a loop of distal ileum with wall thickening (arrow) and adjacent echogenic mesenteric fat (open arrowhead). The thickened loop of bowel was aperistaltic on real-time US imaging. (**c, d**) Coronal T2-weighted single-shot turbo spin-echo images show the loop of distal ileum with wall thickening (arrow), T2-hyperintense submucosal edema (arrowheads), and adjacent mesenteric fat stranding (open arrow), corresponding to the ultrasound findings on active inflammation

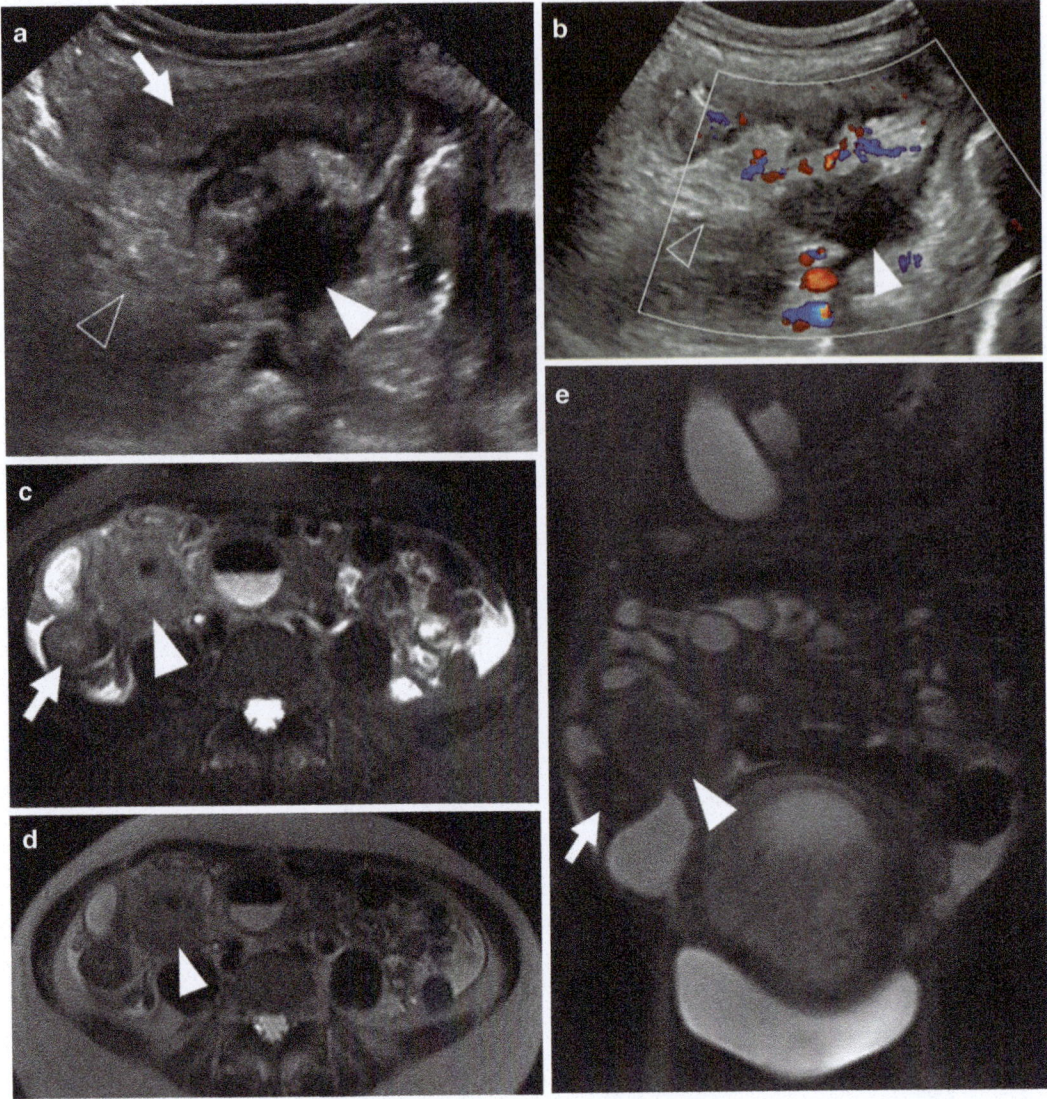

Fig. 6.7 Crohn's disease with penetrating disease. The same patient in Fig. 6.6. (**a**) Grayscale and (**b**) color Doppler sonographic images show a thickened distal ileum (arrow), echogenic mesenteric fat (open arrowhead), and a fluid collection with irregular margins consistent with an abscess (arrowhead). (**c**) Fat-suppressed and (**d**) unsuppressed axial T2 weighted turbo spin-echo, and (**e**) coronal fat-suppressed T2-weighted single-shot turbo spin-echo images show a thickened distal ileum (arrow) with a large inflammatory mesenteric mass (arrowhead) or phlegmon, corresponding to the ultrasound images. Note the drainable portion of the collection was more evident on US than on MR

increasingly used to evaluate patients with known IBD for the grading of disease activity and differentiating between inflammation or mural fibrosis [22]. While there are no known risks to the fetus, there are limited safety data for ultrasound contrast agents in pregnancy, and their use should be limited to cases of necessity [23].

MR enterography is the optimal modality for evaluating IBD in pregnancy. Although intravenous contrast is contraindicated, the large field of view and high contrast resolution of MR permit detection of the spectrum of disease findings associated with IBD. Active inflammation may manifest as wall thickening and mural stratification with T2 hyperintense submucosal edema in the bowel wall [3] (Fig. 6.6). An aperistaltic bowel segment can be identified with steady-state-free procession CINE imaging. Luminal narrowing with or without upstream dilation can be characterized without the use of intravenous contrast. Many neutral or negative enteric contrast agents are safe in pregnancy, and provide luminal distention of the bowel to improve the detection of luminal narrowing. T2-weighted sequences may reveal perienteric inflammation, such as T2 hyperintense mesenteric edema, fatty proliferation of the mesentery, mesenteric nodal enlargement, and free fluid [3]. MR enterography can be used to detect and characterize the complications of penetrating disease to guide management and intervention. Distortion of the mesentery, tethering of bowel to other bowel segments, other organs, or the abdominal wall may indicate a fistula. MR is also sensitive for the identification of inflammatory masses (phlegmon) and abscesses [24] (Fig. 6.7). MR enterography examinations with an adapted noncontrast protocol for pregnancy can help exclude IBD or establish disease activity and to help diagnose complications in pregnant patients [25].

6.1.5 Diverticulitis

Although diverticulitis is more common in an older population, it is occasionally diagnosed in patients of reproductive age.

Transabdominal sonography can be used to evaluate pregnant patients with suspected diverticulitis, but is not as widely used as a first-line imaging examination in the United States [26]. Graded compression should be employed to reduce overlying bowel gas shadowing [26]. US findings of acute diverticulitis include bowel wall thickening ($\geq$4–5 mm) and echogenic non-compressible fat surrounding one or more diverticula [27]. A "target sign" or "pseudo-kidney sign" may be seen as a hypoechoic wall surrounding a hyperechoic center [27]. Ultrasound can also demonstrate peri-colonic fat inflammation and to help identify complications such as an abscess [26] or perforation. In a meta-analysis, there were no significant differences in the diagnostic accuracy of US versus CT in diagnosing acute colonic diverticulitis [28], but this analysis did not focus on pregnant patients. Despite the reported sensitivity and specificity, US is operator dependent and may not be sufficient for preoperative planning if surgical intervention is required.

The sensitivity and specificity of MR imaging in the detection of diverticulitis in the nonpregnant population have been found to be 86–94% and 88–92%, respectively [26]. MRI is comparable in its ability to reveal alternative diagnoses as a CT scan [26], but in pregnant patients, intravenous MR contrast agents are contraindicated, which may slightly reduce sensitivity and specificity. MR imaging features include diverticula with adjacent focal bowel wall thickening and T2 hyperintense mesocolic edema [3]. Peri-colonic T2 hyperintense fluid may be detected adjacent to the affected bowel [3] (Fig. 6.8). MR imaging may also demonstrate complications of acute diverticulitis, including perforation, abscess, and colovesical fistula [3]. Perforation can be retroperitoneal or intraperitoneal and can be seen as signal voids, which bloom on T1 in-phase gradient-recalled echo or steady-state-free procession sequences. An abscess will manifest as a T2 hyperintense well-defined fluid collection with surrounding T2 hyperintense edema. Colovesical fistula may be seen as loss of the fat plane between the bladder and the colon with gas in the nondependent portion of the bladder. In some patients, a fluid-filled or a gas-filled tract may be seen connecting the colon and bladder. Overall, noncontrast MR imaging can be used to identify and characterize diverticulitis and its complications with similar specificity to CT, and without the need for ionizing radiation.

6.2 Gynecological

6.2.1 Torsion

Ovarian torsion occurs when the ovary or fallopian tube rotates around the vascular pedicle occluding the ovarian artery or vein [29]. Patients usually present with lower abdominal or pelvic pain. Ovarian torsion is rare, with an overall estimated incidence of 2–3% of gynecologic emergencies. However, there is an increased incidence in pregnant patients usually before 20 weeks of gestation, and this population makes up 17–20% of ovarian torsion cases [30, 31].

Diagnosing ovarian torsion on imaging can be difficult. Bar-on et al. found that preoperative

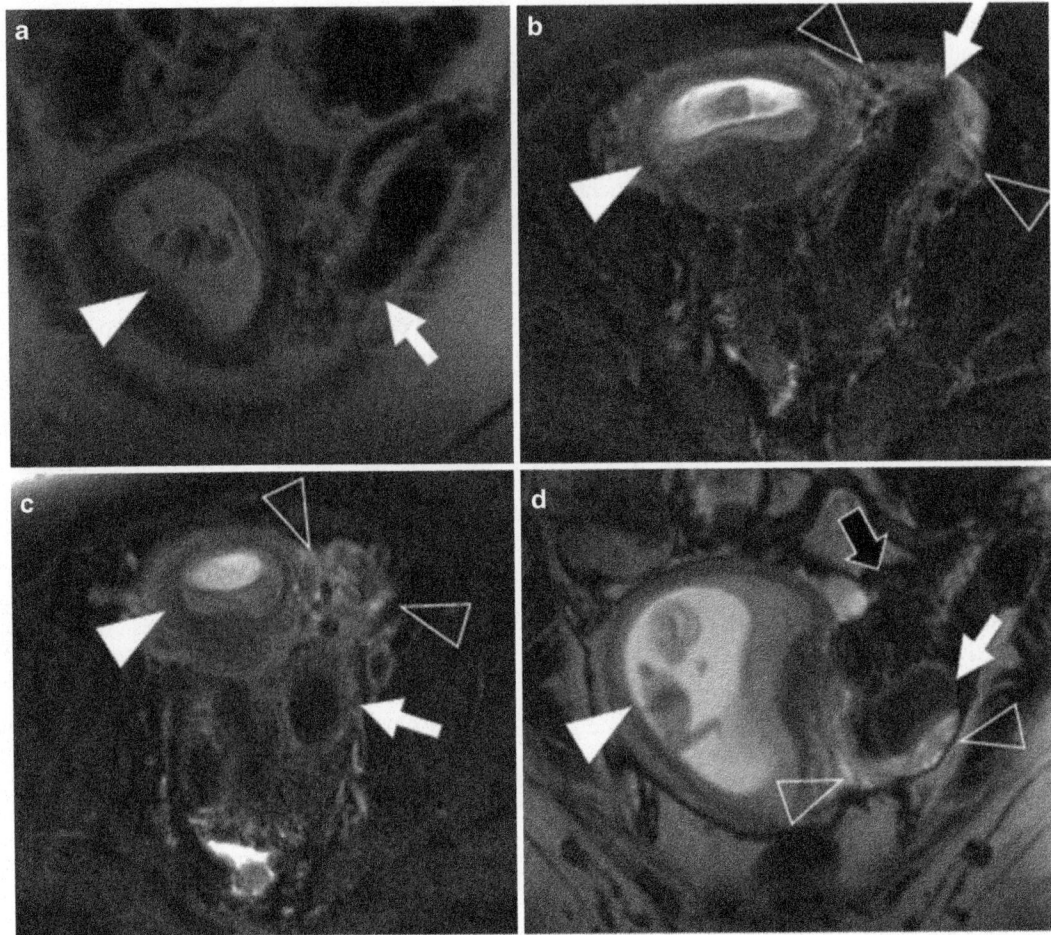

Fig. 6.8 Perforated diverticulitis. Thrity-seven-year-old pregnant woman, estimated gestational age 14 weeks, presents with acute abdominal pain, fever, and leukocytosis. (**a**) Coronal T2-weighted single-shot turbo spin-echo image shows the gravid uterus (arrowhead), and mild colonic wall thickening and free fluid (arrow). (**b, c**) Axial T2-weighted fat-suppressed turbo spin-echo images show the gravid uterus (arrowhead), the thick-walled colon (arrow), and surrounding fat stranding (open arrowheads). The inflamed diverticula was not seen, but (**d**) a steady-state-free procession image shows blooming artifact in the mesentery (black arrow) indicating the presence of extraluminal gas consistent with perforated diverticulitis. Colitis is in the differential diagnosis but less likely given the short segment of affected colon

diagnosis of ovarian torsion was confirmed in only 46% of patients [32]. Ultrasound is usually the initial imaging technique used when women present for suspected ovarian torsion. The ovary may be enlarged and edematous [29]. An ovarian mass, ascites, a twisted pedicle, or thickening of a cyst wall may also be seen on ultrasonography [30]. However, it has been found that between 9% and 26% of torsions occur in normal-appearing and normal-sized ovaries [31, 33].

MR imaging features also include an enlarged ovary, with or without an associated mass, and a twisted pedicle [30]. An enlarged edematous ovary is best seen on T2-weighted MRI [30]. Features that are better seen on MRI over ultrasonography include subacute ovarian hematoma best seen on T1-weighted images with fat saturation [30]. Free pelvic free fluid is also common [34]. The torsed ovary may show abnormal positioning anterior or posterior relative to the gravid uterus [29]. The fallopian tube may be thickened, engorged with heterogeneous fluid and debris, tortuous, or have a "knuckle." The fallopian tube may also appear twisted with a triangular shape (Fig. 6.9). Optimal

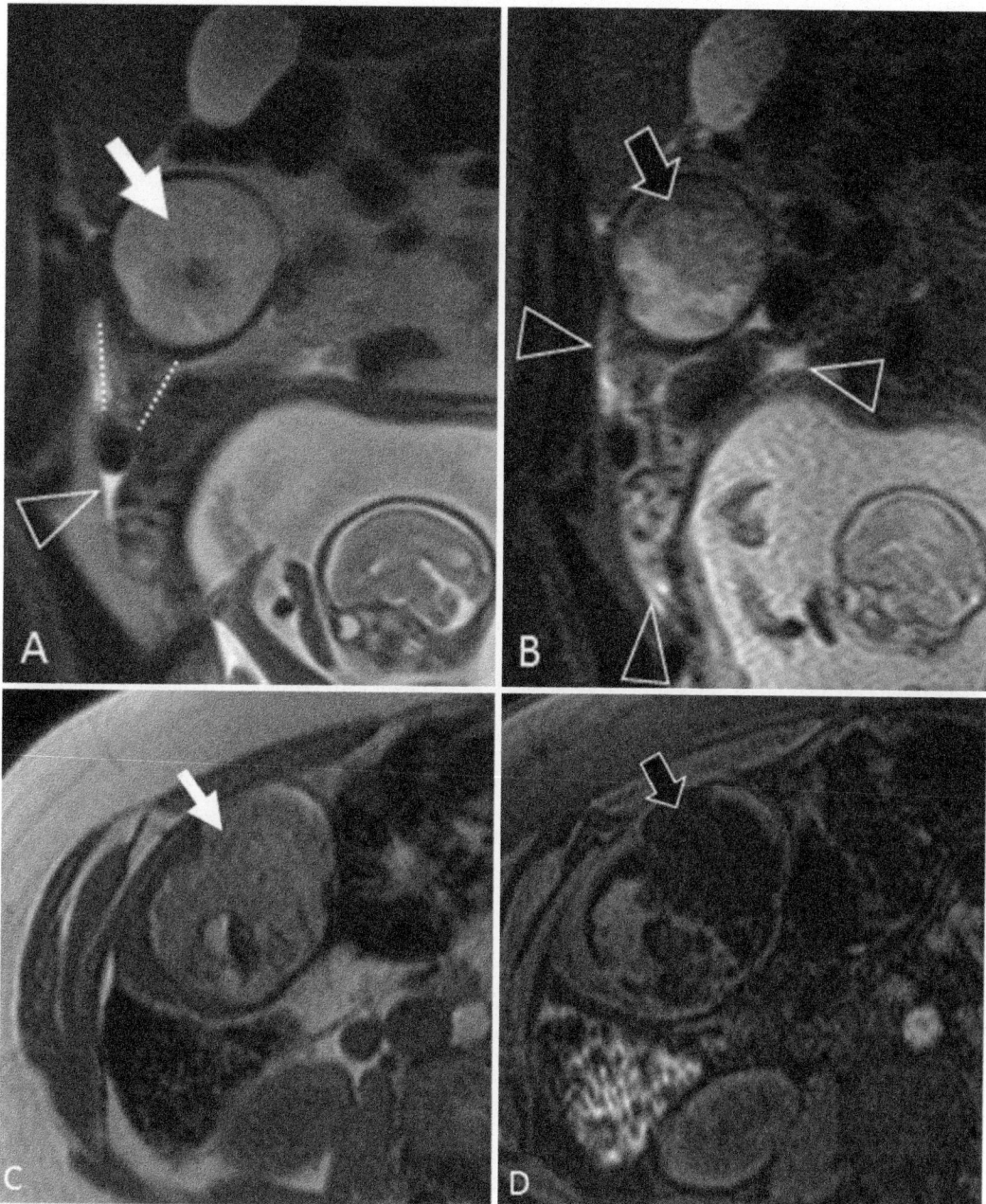

Fig. 6.9 Ovarian torsion. Twenty-five-year-old pregnant woman, estimated gestational age 20 weeks, presents with acute right lower quadrant abdominal pain. (**a**) Coronal T2-weighted single-shot turbo spin-echo image shows a cystic ovarian mass in the right mid abdomen cephalad to the uterus (arrow). The vascular pedicle is triangular and edematous (dotted lines). There is adjacent free fluid (open arrowhead). (**b**) Coronal fat-suppressed T2-weighted turbo spin-echo images show loss of signal in the cyst (black arrow) consistent with fat as well as T2 hyperintense edema and fluid in the right hemiabdomen. (**c**) T1-weighted and (**d**) fat-suppressed T1-weighted gradient-recalled echo images showing T1 hyperintense contents in the cyst (arrow) and loss of signal with fat suppression (black arrow), consistent with a teratoma, which predisposed the patient to ovarian torsion. Laparoscopic oophorectomy was performed confirming torsion and a mature cystic teratoma

detection of a twisted ovarian pedicle requires multiplanar MR acquisitions that are optimized for detection of the twisted pedicle, whose long-axis orientation can be variable [30].

Intervention for ovarian torsion should be prompt to preserve ovarian function. Laparoscopic de-torsion is the treatment of choice in women of reproductive age [29].

6.2.2 Pelvic Inflammatory Disease

Pelvic infection typically affects reproductive age women and can present in pregnant women. Pelvic inflammatory disease (PID) is inflammation of the endometrium, fallopian tubes, and the pelvis. It is common for patients to have abnormal vaginal discharge, fever, and leukocytosis [29].

Ultrasound findings of PID include indistinctness of the uterine serosal surface and increased echogenicity of peritoneal fat adjacent to pelvic structures [35]. More specific indicators of PID include fallopian tube swelling, wall thickening greater than 5 mm, incomplete septa from the tube folding on itself, or tube filling with echogenic, purulent material [35]. Doppler imaging may demonstrate hyperemia of the fallopian tube [35]. A tubo-ovarian abscess (TOA) may be seen on sonography as an inflammatory mass involving the fallopian tube and the ovary, with possible breakdown of separate tubal and ovarian architecture [35].

MRI protocol should include a T2-weighted, fat suppression sequence to improve sensitivity for detection of PID [36]. Fat-suppressed images allow distinction between intra-pelvic fat and inflammatory edema [36]. Imaging may be normal in the early phases of PID [37]. Subclinical PID may manifest as simple hydrosalpinx, with a thin-walled fluid-filled mass closely related to but separate from the ovary [29]. Hydrosalpinx often has a tubular or non-round C- or S-shaped configuration containing incomplete longitudinal folds [36]. Cervicitis and endometritis represent the earliest stage of infection in PID, and are seen as an increased

T2 signal in the cervical and uterine myometrium [36], and T2 hyperintense parametrial stranding. Gas in the endometrial cavity formed by gas-producing organisms will manifest as tiny T1 and T2 hypointense foci that demonstrate blooming artifact on in-phase T1-weighted dual-echo sequences [36]. Pyosalpinx manifests as fluid-filled, distended fallopian tubes [36], with variable T1 and T2 signal intensity depending on the presence of debris or pus in the fallopian tube. On MR imaging, a tubo-ovarian abscess typically appears as a complex fluid-containing pelvic mass with thick walls and septations and surrounding edema [36]. Other imaging findings include loss of fat planes between the mass and adjacent organs, thickening of the uterosacral ligaments, and fluid within the cul-de-sac [38].

When there is ascites, it can be difficult to differentiate a TOA from a cystic ovarian neoplasm. Significant surrounding inflammatory reaction associated with tubo-ovarian abscess can mimic other inflammatory disease processes such as ruptured appendicitis, or vice versa [29]. Key imaging features suggestive of appendicitis over a TOA include the presence of an appendicolith, cecal or rectosigmoid wall thickening, or cecal origin of a tubular structure [38]. In general, abscesses related to perforated diverticulitis tend to have thicker walls, extraluminal air, and fistula formation [38].

Management for the early pelvic inflammatory disease includes 14 days of empiric broad-spectrum antibiotics [39]. Surgical drainage or percutaneous intervention is typically reserved for patients who are septic or after failure of medical management, [39] unless the tubo-ovarian abscess exceeds 8–10 cm at presentation, and then primary drainage may be beneficial [29].

6.2.3 Degenerative Fibroids

The uterus enlarges during pregnancy, which can alter the blood supply to fibroids or leiomyomas, resulting in uterine fibroid degeneration. Pregnant patients with degenerating fibroids may present with fever, localized pain, and tenderness [40].

Ultrasound is usually the initial investigation, and both transabdominal (TA) and transvaginal (TV) US can provide important information [41]. A transvaginal technique is more sensitive for the diagnosis of small fibroids, but certain areas of the uterus may lie outside of the field of view [41]. In obese patients, a transabdominal technique may not adequately penetrate the pelvis to allow for visualization of the endometrium or entire uterus. Fibroids have a variable appearance on US, but are typically well-defined, solid masses with heterogeneous echogenicity. Fibroids often alter the normal outer uterine contour or impress on endometrium [41]. Fibroids are typically heterogeneous with echogenicity similar to hypoechoic to the myometrium [41]. Posterior acoustic shadowing is characteristic of calcified fibroids, but can also be seen in noncalcified fibroids [41]. Doppler US typically shows circumferential vascularity of the fibroid [41]. When fibroids degenerate, they transition from a solid mass, to a complex mass with areas of cystic necrosis, to a more simple-appearing cystic mass. Torsion can occur to pedunculated subserosal or submucosal fibroids, resulting in the absence of flow on Doppler imaging, and at times the separation of the fibroid from the uterine myometrium [41].

MRI is the preferred method for characterizing pelvic masses, as it is useful in differentiating the uterine origin of fibroids from masses of ovarian origin, and can demonstrate the uterine zonal anatomy [42]. MR imaging has been shown to be more sensitive for the identification of uterine fibroids than sonography [43]. Non-degenerate fibroids appear as well-defined masses demonstrating isointense signal to the myometrium on T1W images, and heterogeneous low signal intensity as compared to the myometrium on T2W images [44]. When fibroids degenerate, MR may demonstrate T2 hyperintense edema or

necrosis within the fibroid [3] (Fig. 6.10). A patient with multiple fibroids may have changes in only one fibroid, or in more than one of the fibroids, due to differences in their blood supply and location [45]. Degenerating fibroids usually demonstrate heterogeneous signal intensity on T1-weighted imaging, with central low signal intensity related to edema or cystic change, and areas of high signal intensity secondary to internal hemorrhage [46].

The diagnosis of degenerating fibroids as an etiology for abdominal pain in pregnancy may require close comparison of prior ultrasound examinations (or MR if available) to assess for interval change in the characteristics of the fibroid, and may necessitate MR for characterization, in addition to an initial US.

6.3 Genitourinary

6.3.1 Pyelonephritis

Urinary tract infections in pregnant patients are usually diagnosed based on clinical symptoms and laboratory findings. Classic symptoms of acute pyelonephritis include fever (temperature of 100 °F or greater), abrupt onset of chills, flank pain with costovertebral tenderness, dysuria, urinary frequency, and urgency [47]. When diagnosed, antibiotics are usually initiated, and diagnostic imaging is usually not required. However, imaging examinations can play a role when patients fail to respond to conservative therapy.

Ultrasound can be used as the first-line diagnostic tool to evaluate the urinary tract in pregnant patients with symptoms of pyelonephritis. Unfortunately, studies have reported that US demonstrated abnormalities in only 20–24% of patients with pyelonephritis [48]. Features of pyelonephritis include hydronephrosis, loss of corticomedullary differentiation, renal enlargement, and loss of renal sinus fat due to edema [49] (Fig. 6.11). There may be changes in the echogenicity of the renal parenchyma due to edema (hypoechoic) or hemorrhage (hyper-

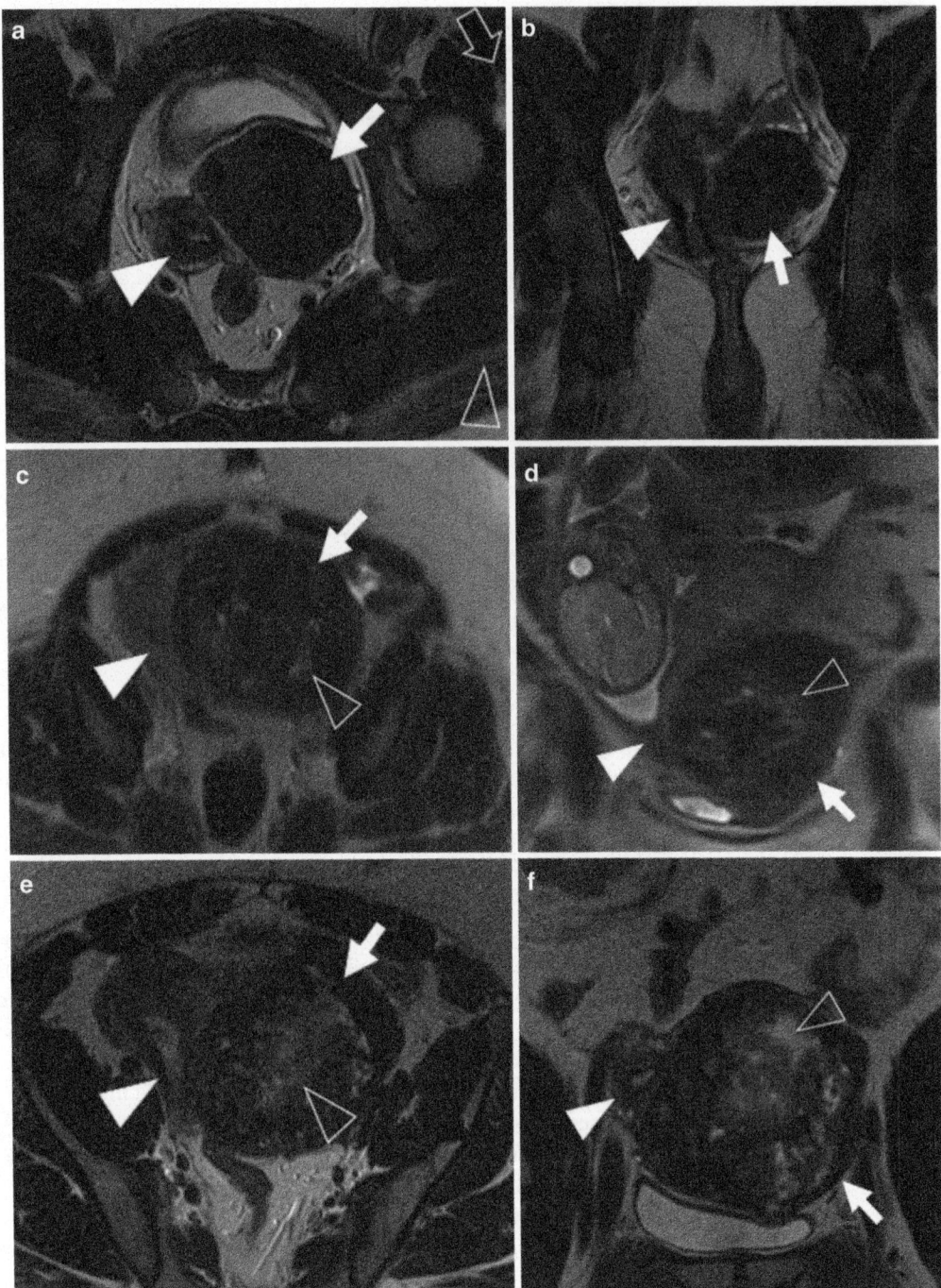

Fig. 6.10 Degenerating pedunculated fibroid. Thrity-six-year-old pregnant woman, estimated gestational age 34 weeks, presents due to pelvic pain. (**a**) Axial and (**b**) coronal T2-weighted images obtained 5 years prior to pregnancy demonstrated a submucosal fibroid (arrow) measuring 6 cm, abutting the cervix (arrowhead). (**c**) Axial and (**d**) coronal T2-weighted images at 34 weeks of EGA show enlargement of the fibroid to 12 cm (arrow), with areas of T2 hyperintensity consistent with necrosis or edema (open arrowheads), and with associated marked mass effect on the cervix. Cesarean section was required for delivery. (**e**) Axial and (**f**) coronal T2-weighted MR images obtained 6 months post-partum show continued enlargement of the fibroid (arrow), with increasing T2 hyperintense areas of degeneration (open arrowheads), and persistent mass effect on the cervix

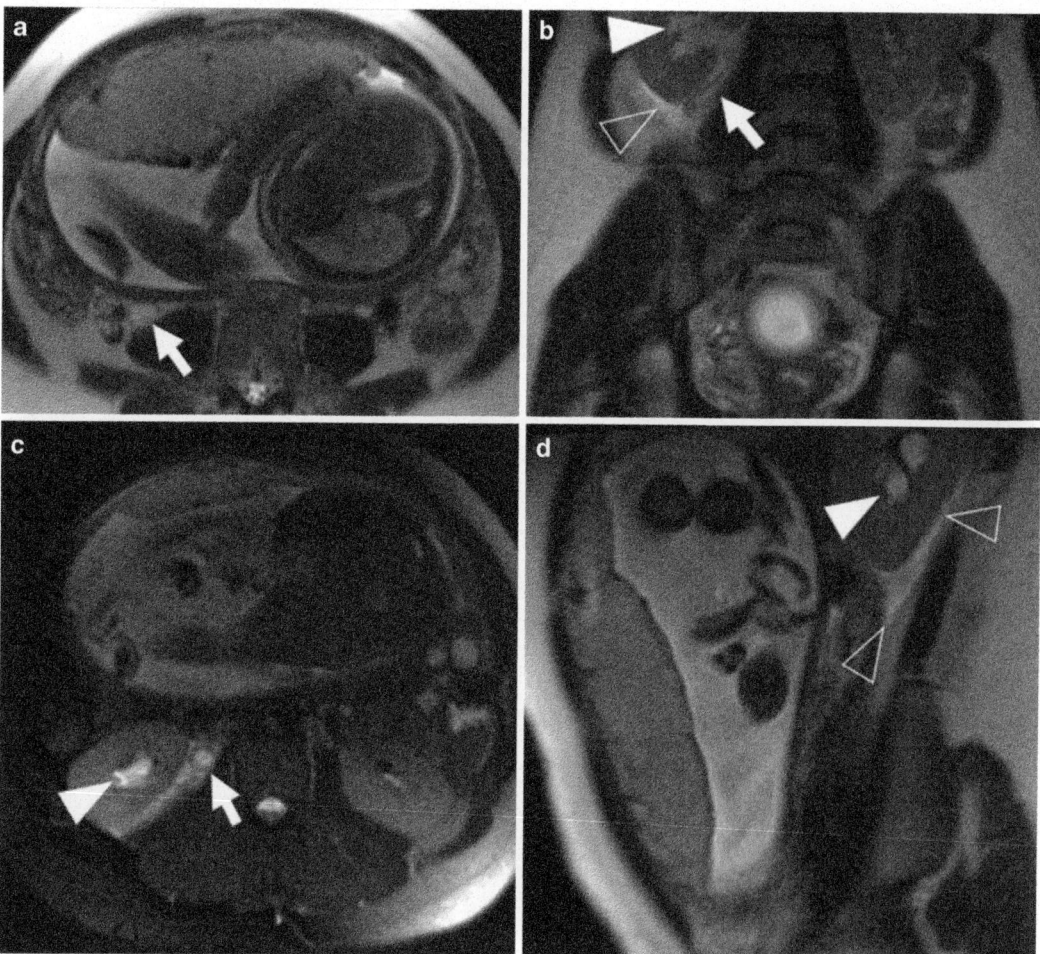

Fig. 6.11 Pyelonephritis. Twenty-five-year-old pregnant woman, estimated gestational age 37 weeks, presents with right lower quadrant pain. (**a**) Axial, (**b**) coronal, (**c**) axial fat-suppressed, and (**d**) sagittal T2-weighted single-shot turbo spin-echo images show right hydroureter (arrows), right hydronephrosis (arrowheads), and right perinephric fluid (open arrowheads). The patient was diagnosed with pyelonephritis and treated with antibiotics

echoic), both of which can have a mass-like appearance [50]. Doppler ultrasound interrogation may demonstrate areas of hypoperfusion [50]. Complications of acute pyelonephritis include collecting system gas seen as "dirty" shadowing with echoes and reverberations, perinephric extension of infection, and abscesses including microabscesses [50].

MR imaging findings of acute pyelonephritis include renal enlargement and edema (Fig. 6.12), areas of hemorrhage, intraparenchymal or perinephric abscesses, and surrounding fluid collections [51]. Inflammatory foci and fluid collections follow MRI characteristics of fluid, and are seen as low intensity signal on T1-weighted images, and high intensity signal on T2-weighted images [51]. Unlike simple cysts, abscesses may have a perceptible thick wall and adjacent T2 hyperintense perinephric edema.

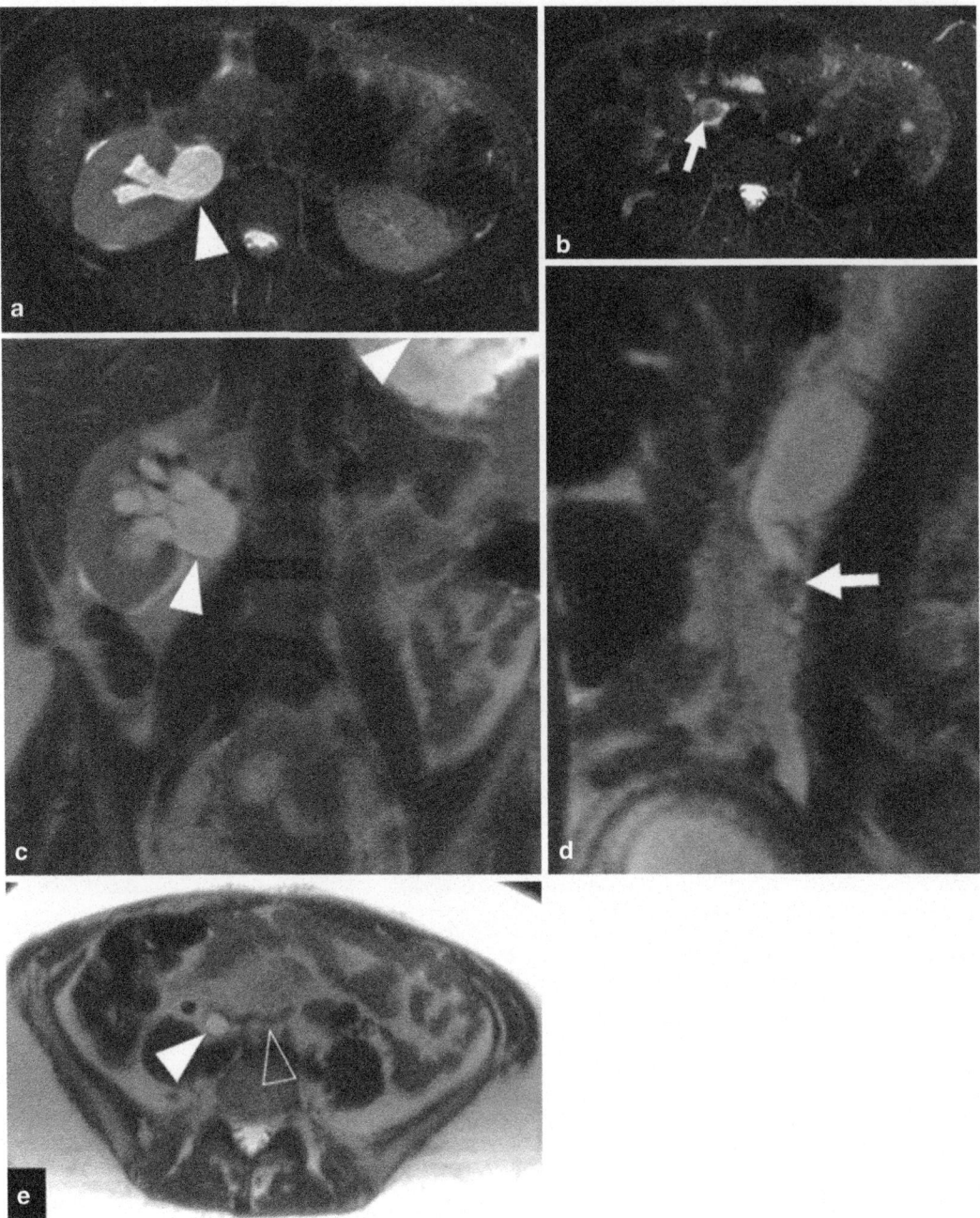

Fig. 6.12 Obstructive urolithiasis. Thirty-five-year-old pregnant woman, estimated gestational age 10 weeks, presents with acute right lower quadrant pain. (**a**, **b**) Axial T2-weighted fat-suppressed turbo spin-echo images show right hydronephrosis (arrowhead), and a hypointense filling defect in the proximal right ureter (arrow) consistent with a obstructing ureteral calculus. (**c**) Coronal and (**d**) sagittal T2-weighted single-shot turbo spin-echo images confirm the right hydronephrosis (arrowhead) and the hypointense calculus in the proximal right ureter (arrow). (**e**) Axial T2-weighted turbo spin-echo image shows a normal appendix (open arrowhead) and right hydroureter (arrowhead)

6.3.2 Urolithiasis

Although renal or ureteral calculi in pregnancy are uncommon, with a prevalence of 0.4–5 per 1000 pregnancies, urolithiasis is the most common painful reason for hospitalization in pregnant patients [7, 11]. However, surgical intervention is usually unnecessary, as 70–80% of ureteral calculi will spontaneously pass in pregnant patients [52].

Ultrasonography is typically the primary imaging modality for evaluation of hydronephrosis and urolithiasis in a pregnant patient [3]. However, the reported sensitivities for detection of genitourinary calculi with US range from 34% to 95.2% [52]. In addition, there can be difficulty in distinguishing hydronephrosis from physiologic dilatation in pregnancy, but an elevated intrarenal resistive index (RI) (>0.7) may help differentiate between these entities on Doppler US [53]. The absence of a ureteral jet on the suspected side of obstruction has been reported to have sensitivity of 100% and a specificity of 91% [54]. However, approximately 15% of asymptomatic pregnant women can have absent unilateral jets, and should be imaged in the contralateral decubitus position to prevent false-positive results [55]. Transvaginal US is the best method for the detection of distal ureteral calculi [11]. When intervention is necessary, intraoperative US can be used to confirm proper ureteral stent positioning after cystoscopic placement.

MR urography has a high reported sensitivity for the detection of urinary tract dilatation and for the identification of the site of obstruction. MR can be considered a second-line test when US fails to establish a diagnosis, if there are continued symptoms despite conservative management [11]. MR imaging demonstrates signs of obstructive hydronephrosis including enlargement of the affected kidney, dilated renal pelvis, perinephric fluid, and an abrupt change in ureteral caliber along its course [56]. An obstructing ureteral calculus on MRI appears as a signal void within the ureter [3] at the site of caliber change (Fig. 6.12). Physiologic hydronephrosis is seen as gradual, smooth tapering of the mid to distal ureter due to the gravid uterus and iliopsoas muscle causing extrinsic compression [56]. Perinephric fluid and renal enlargement are less common with hydronephrosis of pregnancy than with hydronephrosis from an obstructing calculus. Limitations of MR urography include relatively high cost, limited visualization of small renal calculi [11], poor signal-to-noise ratio, and susceptibility to motion artifact.

Physiologic hydronephrosis after the second trimester can be difficult to diagnose, and if MRI is unavailable or contraindicated, low-dose CT can be performed (Fig. 6.13) if there is a high suspicion for lower urinary tract calculi [57] or in an unstable patient. Low-dose CT has a much higher sensitivity than US, and can also be used to identify alternate sources of flank pain [11].

6.4 Conclusion

Pregnant women may present to the emergency department with non-specific clinical symptoms such as nausea, vomiting, and abdominal pain, which can be manifestations of obstetric, hepatobiliary, gastrointestinal, gynecologic, or urographic pathology. US is often the best initial imaging modality due to its widespread availability and lack of ionizing radiation, but MR, with its large field of view and excellent contrast resolution, can provide further characterization of a wide range of abdominal and pelvic emergencies. A well-designed abdominal and pelvic MR protocol tailored for pregnant patients can provide high sensitivity and specific for appendicitis, and will often help identify the numerous alternative diagnoses that can cause abdominal or pelvic pain. Computed tomography may be required in pregnancy but should be reserved for unstable patients, or for those for which MR is contraindicated, or unhelpful.

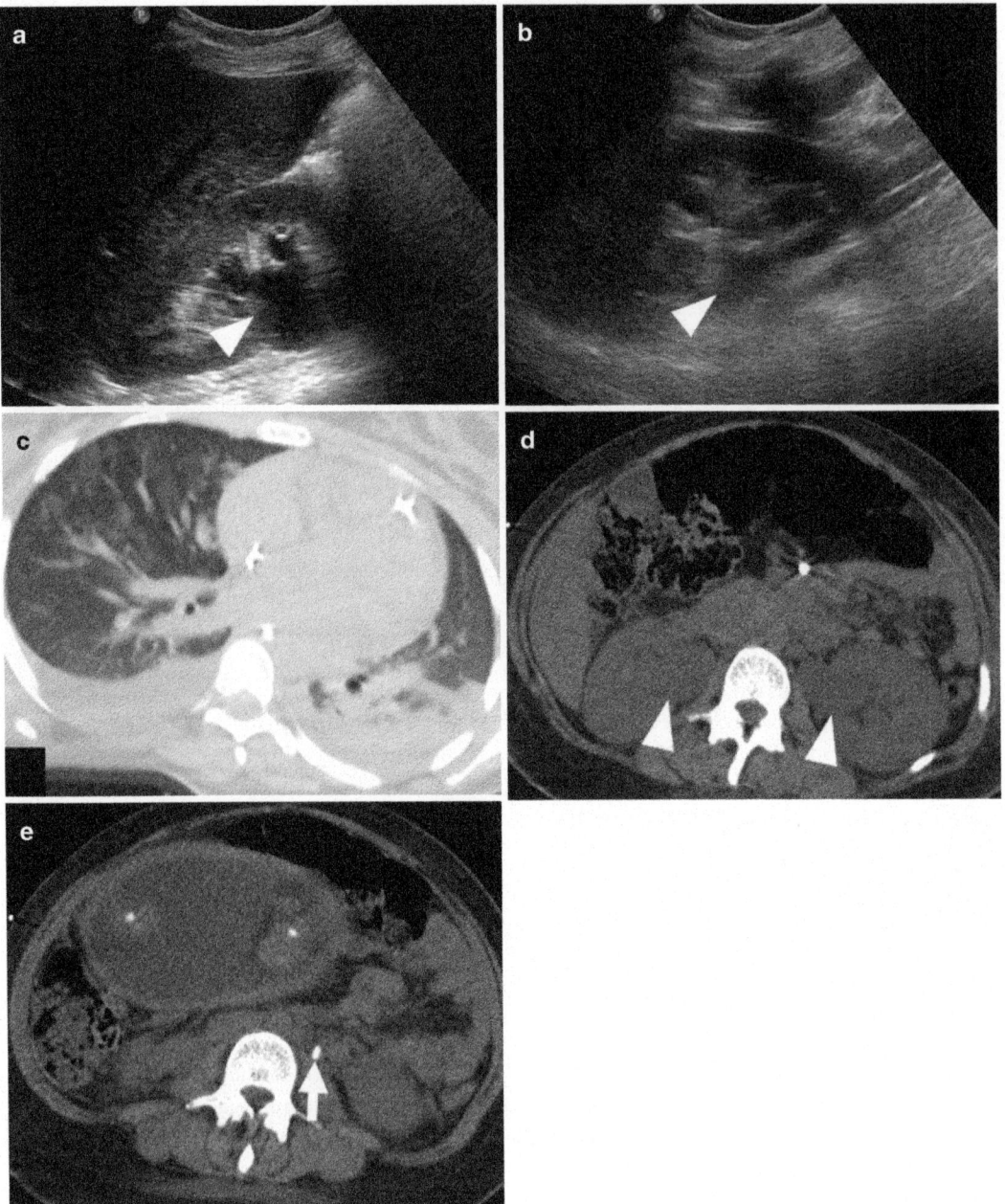

Fig. 6.13 Obstructive urolithiasis and urosepsis. Nineteen-year-old pregnant woman, estimated gestational age 27 weeks, presents in septic shock and was recently treated with oral antibiotics for urinary tract infection at an outside hospital. (**a**, **b**) Grayscale US images show right and left hydronephrosis (arrowhead). (**c**) Axial CT images of the lower lungs in lung window show bilateral effusions and patchy ground glass opacities consistent with pulmonary edema. (**d**) Axial CT image through the kidneys shows bilateral hydronephrosis (arrowheads). (**e**) Axial CT image through the midabdomen shows an obstructive left ureteral calculus. The patient was admitted to the ICU, intubated, and treated with IV antibiotics and ureteroscopic stone extraction

References

1. Tamir IL, Bongard FS, Klein SR. Acute appendicitis in the pregnant patient. Am J Surg. 1990;160(6):571–5; discussion 5–6.

2. Theilen LH, Mellnick VM, Shanks AL, Tuuli MG, Odibo AO, Macones GA, et al. Acute appendicitis in pregnancy: predictive clinical factors and pregnancy outcomes. Am J Perinatol. 2017;34(6):523–8.

3. Spalluto LB, Woodfield CA, DeBenedectis CM, Lazarus E. MR imaging evaluation of abdominal pain during pregnancy: appendicitis and other nonobstetric causes. Radiographics. 2012;32(2):317–34.

4. Lim HK, Bae SH, Seo GS. Diagnosis of acute appendicitis in pregnant women: value of sonography. AJR Am J Roentgenol. 1992;159(3):539–42.

5. Stone MB, Chao J. Emergency ultrasound diagnosis of acute appendicitis. Acad Emerg Med. 2010;17(1):E5.

6. Worrell JA, Drolshagen LF, Kelly TC, Hunton DW, Durmon GR, Fleischer AC. Graded compression ultrasound in the diagnosis of appendicitis. A comparison of diagnostic criteria. J Ultrasound Med. 1990;9(3):145–50.

7. Wieseler KM, Bhargava P, Kanal KM, Vaidya S, Stewart BK, Dighe MK. Imaging in pregnant patients: examination appropriateness. Radiographics. 2010;30(5):1215–29; discussion 30–3.

8. Theilen LH, Mellnick VM, Longman RE, Tuuli MG, Odibo AO, Macones GA, et al. Utility of magnetic resonance imaging for suspected appendicitis in pregnant women. Am J Obstet Gynecol. 2015;212(3):345e1–6.

9. Israel GM, Malguria N, McCarthy S, Copel J, Weinreb J. MRI vs. ultrasound for suspected appendicitis during pregnancy. J Magn Reson Imaging. 2008;28(2):428–33.

10. Pedrosa I, Levine D, Eyvazzadeh AD, Siewert B, Ngo L, Rofsky NM. MR imaging evaluation of acute appendicitis in pregnancy. Radiology. 2006;238(3):891–9.

11. Patel SJ, Reede DL, Katz DS, Subramaniam R, Amorosa JK. Imaging the pregnant patient for non-obstetric conditions: algorithms and radiation dose considerations. Radiographics. 2007;27(6):1705–22.

12. Tsai R, Raptis C, Fowler KJ, Owen JW, Mellnick VM. MRI of suspected appendicitis during pregnancy: interradiologist agreement, indeterminate interpretation and the meaning of non-visualization of the appendix. Br J Radiol. 2017;90(1079):20170383.

13. Lazarus E, Mayo-Smith WW, Mainiero MB, Spencer PK. CT in the evaluation of nontraumatic abdominal pain in pregnant women. Radiology. 2007;244(3):784–90.

14. Melnick DM, Wahl WL, Dalton VK. Management of general surgical problems in the pregnant patient. Am J Surg. 2004;187(2):170–80.

15. Bortoff GA, Chen MY, Ott DJ, Wolfman NT, Routh WD. Gallbladder stones: imaging and intervention. Radiographics. 2000;20(3):751–66.

16. Sharp HT. The acute abdomen during pregnancy. Clin Obstet Gynecol. 2002;45(2):405–13.

17. Catalano OA, Sahani DV, Kalva SP, Cushing MS, Hahn PF, Brown JJ, et al. MR imaging of the gallbladder: a pictorial essay. Radiographics. 2008;28(1):135–55; quiz 324.

18. Firstenberg MS, Malangoni MA. Gastrointestinal surgery during pregnancy. Gastroenterol Clin N Am. 1998;27(1):73–88.

19. Bollen TL. Imaging of acute pancreatitis: update of the revised Atlanta classification. Radiol Clin N Am. 2012;50(3):429–45.

20. Busireddy KK, AlObaidy M, Ramalho M, Kalubowila J, Baodong L, Santagostino I, et al. Pancreatitis-imaging approach. World J Gastrointest Pathophysiol. 2014;5(3):252–70.

21. Furukawa A, Saotome T, Yamasaki M, Maeda K, Nitta N, Takahashi M, et al. Cross-sectional imaging in Crohn disease. Radiographics. 2004;24(3):689–702.

22. Quaia E. Contrast-enhanced ultrasound of the small bowel in Crohn's disease. Abdom Imaging. 2013;38(5):1005–13.

23. Kodzwa R. Updates to the ACR manual on contrast media. Radiol Technol. 2017;89(2):186–9.

24. Bruining DH, Zimmermann EM, Loftus EV Jr, Sandborn WJ, Sauer CG, Strong SA, et al. Consensus recommendations for evaluation, interpretation, and utilization of computed tomography and magnetic resonance enterography in patients with small bowel Crohn's disease. Gastroenterology. 2018;154(4):1172–94.

25. Stern MD, Kopylov U, Ben-Horin S, Apter S, Amitai MM. Magnetic resonance enterography in pregnant women with Crohn's disease: case series and literature review. BMC Gastroenterol. 2014;14:146.

26. Destigter KK, Keating DP. Imaging update: acute colonic diverticulitis. Clin Colon Rectal Surg. 2009;22(3):147–55.

27. Abboud ME, Frasure SE, Stone MB. Ultrasound diagnosis of diverticulitis. World J Emerg Med. 2016;7(1):74–6.

28. Lameris W, van Randen A, Bipat S, Bossuyt PM, Boermeester MA, Stoker J. Graded compression ultrasonography and computed tomography in acute colonic diverticulitis: meta-analysis of test accuracy. Eur Radiol. 2008;18(11):2498–511.

29. Tran-Harding K, Lee JT, Owen J. Recognizing the CT manifestations of gynecologic conditions encountered in the emergency department. Curr Probl Diagn Radiol. 2019;48(5):473–81.

30. Duigenan S, Oliva E, Lee SI. Ovarian torsion: diagnostic features on CT and MRI with pathologic correlation. AJR Am J Roentgenol. 2012;198(2):W122–31.

31. Chang HC, Bhatt S, Dogra VS. Pearls and pitfalls in diagnosis of ovarian torsion. Radiographics. 2008;28(5):1355–68.

32. Bar-On S, Mashiach R, Stockheim D, Soriano D, Goldenberg M, Schiff E, et al. Emergency laparoscopy for suspected ovarian torsion: are we too hasty to operate? Fertil Steril. 2010;93(6):2012–5.

33. Bider D, Mashiach S, Dulitzky M, Kokia E, Lipitz S, Ben-Rafael Z. Clinical, surgical and pathologic findings of adnexal torsion in pregnant and nonpregnant women. Surg Gynecol Obstet. 1991;173(5):363–6.

34. Rha SE, Byun JY, Jung SE, Jung JI, Choi BG, Kim BS, et al. CT and MR imaging features of adnexal torsion. Radiographics. 2002;22(2):283–94.

35. Andreotti RF, Harvey SM. Sonographic evaluation of acute pelvic pain. J Ultrasound Med. 2012;31(11):1713–8.

36. Czeyda-Pommersheim F, Kalb B, Costello J, Liau J, Meshksar A, Arif Tiwari H, et al. MRI in pelvic inflammatory disease: a pictorial review. Abdom Radiol. 2017;42(3):935–50.

37. Roche O, Chavan N, Aquilina J, Rockall A. Radiological appearances of gynaecological emergencies. Insights Imaging. 2012;3(3):265–75.

38. Revzin MV, Mathur M, Dave HB, Macer ML, Spektor M. Pelvic inflammatory disease: multimodality imaging approach with clinical-pathologic correlation. Radiographics. 2016;36(5):1579–96.

39. Soper DE. Pelvic inflammatory disease. Obstet Gynecol. 2010;116(2 Pt 1):419–28.

40. Birchard KR, Brown MA, Hyslop WB, Firat Z, Semelka RC. MRI of acute abdominal and pelvic pain in pregnant patients. AJR Am J Roentgenol. 2005;184(2):452–8.

41. Wilde S, Scott-Barrett S. Radiological appearances of uterine fibroids. Indian J Radiol Imaging. 2009;19(3):222–31.

42. Dudiak CM, Turner DA, Patel SK, Archie JT, Silver B, Norusis M. Uterine leiomyomas in the infertile patient: preoperative localization with MR imaging versus US and hysterosalpingography. Radiology. 1988;167(3):627–30.

43. Dueholm M, Lundorf E, Hansen ES, Ledertoug S, Olesen F. Accuracy of magnetic resonance imaging and transvaginal ultrasonography in the diagnosis, mapping, and measurement of uterine myomas. Am J Obstet Gynecol. 2002;186(3):409–15.

44. Ueda H, Togashi K, Konishi I, Kataoka ML, Koyama T, Fujiwara T, et al. Unusual appearances of uterine leiomyomas: MR imaging findings and their histopathologic backgrounds. Radiographics. 1999;19 Spec No:S131–45.

45. Lev-Toaff AS, Coleman BG, Arger PH, Mintz MC, Arenson RL, Toaff ME. Leiomyomas in pregnancy: sonographic study. Radiology. 1987;164(2):375–80.

46. Leyendecker JR, Gorengaut V, Brown JJ. MR imaging of maternal diseases of the abdomen and pelvis during pregnancy and the immediate postpartum period. Radiographics. 2004;24(5):1301–16.

47. Campbell MF, Walsh PC, Retik AB. Campbell's urology. Philadelphia, PA: Saunders; 2002.

48. June CH, Browning MD, Smith LP, Wenzel DJ, Pyatt RS, Checchio LM, et al. Ultrasonography and computed tomography in severe urinary tract infection. Arch Intern Med. 1985;145(5):841–5.

49. Rigsby CM, Rosenfield AT, Glickman MG, Hodson J. Hemorrhagic focal bacterial nephritis: findings on gray-scale sonography and CT. AJR Am J Roentgenol. 1986;146(6):1173–7.

50. Craig WD, Wagner BJ, Travis MD. Pyelonephritis: radiologic-pathologic review. Radiographics. 2008;28(1):255–77; quiz 327–8.

51. Majd M, Nussbaum Blask AR, Markle BM, Shalaby-Rana E, Pohl HG, Park JS, et al. Acute pyelonephritis: comparison of diagnosis with 99mTc-DMSA, SPECT, spiral CT, MR imaging, and power Doppler US in an experimental pig model. Radiology. 2001;218(1):101–8.

52. Parulkar BG, Hopkins TB, Wollin MR, Howard PJ Jr, Lal A. Renal colic during pregnancy: a case for conservative treatment. J Urol. 1998;159(2):365–8.

53. Hertzberg BS, Carroll BA, Bowie JD, Paine SS, Kliewer MA, Paulson EK, et al. Doppler US assessment of maternal kidneys: analysis of intrarenal resistivity indexes in normal pregnancy and physiologic pelvicaliectasis. Radiology. 1993;186(3):689–92.

54. Deyoe LA, Cronan JJ, Breslaw BH, Ridlen MS. New techniques of ultrasound and color Doppler in the prospective evaluation of acute renal obstruction. Do they replace the intravenous urogram? Abdom Imaging. 1995;20(1):58–63.

55. Wachsberg RH. Unilateral absence of ureteral jets in the third trimester of pregnancy: pitfall in color Doppler US diagnosis of urinary obstruction. Radiology. 1998;209(1):279–81.

56. Spencer JA, Chahal R, Kelly A, Taylor K, Eardley I, Lloyd SN. Evaluation of painful hydronephrosis in pregnancy: magnetic resonance urographic patterns in physiological dilatation versus calculous obstruction. J Urol. 2004;171(1):256–60.

57. McAleer SJ, Loughlin KR. Nephrolithiasis and pregnancy. Curr Opin Urol. 2004;14(2):123–7.

Imaging of Abdominal and Pelvic Trauma in Pregnant Patients

7

Luiza Grzycka-Kowalczyk, Grzegorz Staśkiewicz,
Anna Drelich-Zbroja, Michał Kowalczyk,
and Mariano Scaglione

Contents

L. Grzycka-Kowalczyk (✉) · G. Staśkiewicz
1st Department of Radiology and Nuclear Medicine,
Medical University of Lublin, Lublin, Poland

A. Drelich-Zbroja
Department of Interventional Radiology and
Neuroradiology, Medical University in Lublin,
Lublin, Poland

M. Kowalczyk
1st Department of Anesthesiology and Intensive Care,
Medical University in Lublin, Lublin, Poland

M. Scaglione
Department of Radiology, Pineta Grande Hospital
Castel Volturno, Italy

James Cook University Hospital,
Middlesbrough, YSN, UK

Teeside University, School of health
and Life Sciences
Middlesbrough, YSN, UK

7.1   Introduction

Trauma during pregnancy can be associated with high fetal mortality rate as well as maternal morbidity. In this unique situation, a treating physician is dealing with two patients at once, thus, with increased responsibility as well as added anxiety of being aware of the potential effect of therapy for both patients at all times.

Trauma is considered the leading cause of nonobstetric maternal mortality. It has been estimated that even 25–27% women will be injured while pregnant. The most common cause of trauma is motor vehicle accidents, followed by falls from height, suicide attempts, and domestic violence [1, 2].

The leading cause of mother's mortality in trauma is head injury and hemorrhagic shock. Obstetric trauma has been associated with the risk factors such as young age, alcohol use, and drug use [3]. Some studies show pregnancy itself being a risk factor for trauma [4].

© Springer Nature Switzerland AG 2020

M. N. Patlas et al. (eds.), *Emergency Imaging of Pregnant Patients*,
https://doi.org/10.1007/978-3-030-42722-1_7

7.2   Imaging

Imaging investigations are of paramount importance in pregnant patients with trauma. Imaging allows for early diagnosis and complete assessment of all injuries, guiding the best management plan to surgeons, and helping to avoid unnecessary interventions and surgery [5].

First, the diagnosis of pregnancy may not be established or suspected at the time of patient presentation. However, in the settings of known pregnancy, fetal loss rates approach 40–50% in life-threatening trauma. While fetal loss occurs at a much lower rate with minor injuries (1–5%), minor injuries are much more common [6].

Maternal death almost always results in fetal death; therefore, the first goal of the medical team caring for the pregnant trauma patient is *to stabilize the mother*, keeping in mind that no mother that is alive means no fetus that is alive. Although there are reports of late third trimester pregnancies delivered by emergency cesarean section despite lethal maternal injuries, such cases are rare. The primary survey involves evaluation of airway, breathing, and circulation, and the secondary survey should focus on nonobstetric/obstetric injuries and fetal condition [7].

Concerns about fetal radiation exposure should neither deter nor delay radiologic evaluation.

The pregnant patient is predisposed to the same spectrum of injuries as the non-pregnant one, however, retroperitoneal hemorrhage is more common in pregnant women due to increased pelvic blood flow. The gravid uterus displaces the liver and spleen against the ribs and elevates the bladder out of the pelvis, making these more prone to injury. Moreover, as the kidneys and spleen enlarge, they are further susceptible to injury [1].

Certain injuries in pregnancy are associated with an increased risk of fetal loss. High maternal (9%) and even higher fetal (35%) mortality are associated with pelvic (and acetabular) fractures, which may increase up to 75% for severe fracture patterns [8].

In penetrating abdominal trauma, uterine and fetal injury increases as the gravid uterus enlarges, while providing greater maternal protection [1].

Complications of trauma to the gravid uterus include spontaneous abortion, preterm labor, premature rupture of membranes, placental abruption, placental laceration and infarction, and uterine laceration and rupture. Most injuries to the gravid uterus occur in the third trimester [7].

As the fetus is well protected by the mother's subcutaneous tissue, bony pelvis, uterus, and amniotic fluid, fetal injuries are relatively rare, most commonly skull fracture and head injury, seen in the late third trimester, and most often in the setting of a maternal pelvic fracture [9].

The use of *imaging examinations* to evaluate for specific maternal injuries has several important benefits. First, avoiding nonobstetrical laparotomy is beneficial, given that nonobstetrical laparotomy alone results in a 26% incidence of preterm labor in the second trimester and an 82% incidence of preterm labor in the third trimester. Thus, using imaging examinations to exclude injuries or to detect injuries that can be managed nonoperatively is beneficial. Furthermore, early diagnosis of maternal injuries is paramount because shock portends a poor outcome for both the mother and fetus, with fetal death rates approaching 80% [6].

7.2.1   Ultrasound Examination

In the acute setting, US is frequently used to evaluate the pregnant trauma patient. During initial evaluation, US allows for assessment of the fetus and estimation of its gestational age. For maternal evaluation, focused assessment with sonography in trauma (FAST) scans can be used to depict intraperitoneal, intrapleural, or pericardial fluid [6].

An example of ultrasound use in a trauma setting is presented in Fig. 7.1.

However, ultrasound in advanced pregnancy remains challenging, and its value declines in the third trimester, especially due to the technical difficulties resulting from the mechanical effects of the enlarging uterus. Hence, an adequate evaluation of the parenchymal organs, as well as free fluid, may be impaired due to the narrow field of view owing to the presence of overlying structures [10].

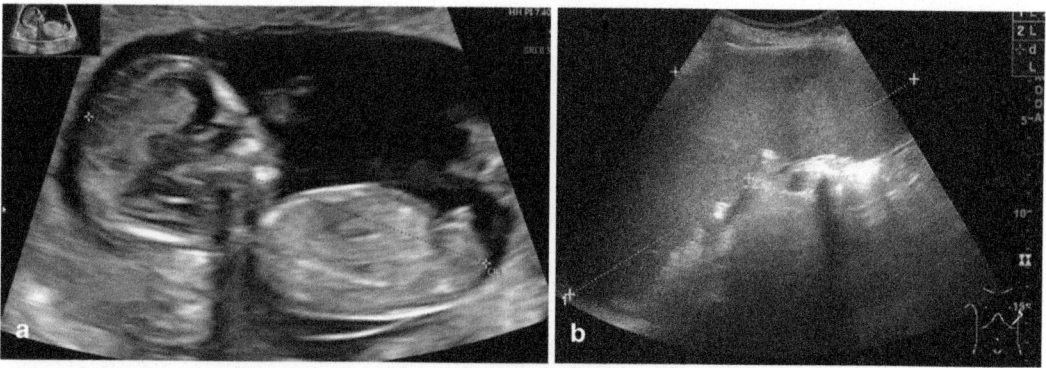

Fig. 7.1 Ultrasound images of 22-year-old patient in second trimester of her first pregnancy (**a**) after a motor vehicle collision. A (**b**) Hypoechoic region representing a splenic hematoma is depicted

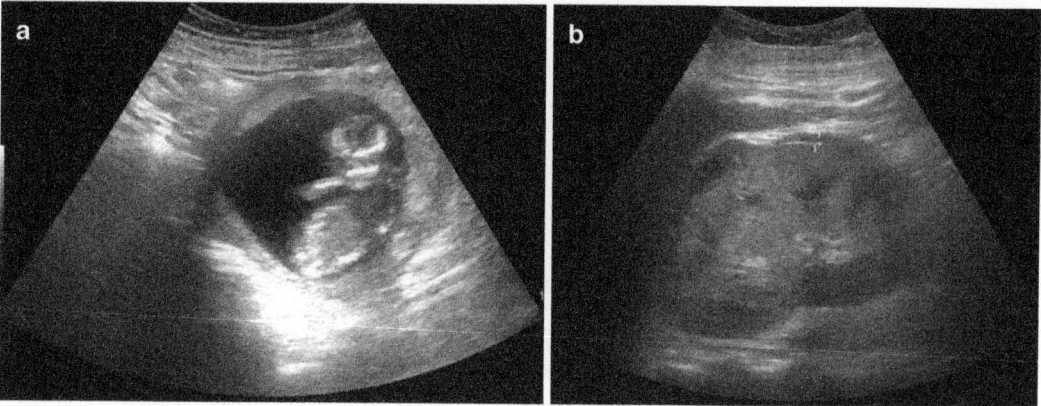

Fig. 7.2 Ultrasound images of a 28-year-old patient at 12 gestational weeks (**a**) with a subcapsular perirenal hematoma (**b**), as a result of a falling down the stairs

It is important to remember that US is not a substitute for a clinically needed diagnostic computed tomographic (CT) examination.

An example of ultrasound use in a trauma setting is presented in Fig. 7.2.

7.2.1.1 Safety of Ultrasound During Pregnancy

Ultrasound should be performed efficiently and only when clinically indicated, to minimize fetal exposure risk, keeping acoustic output levels As Low As Reasonably Achievable (commonly known as ALARA principle). Ultrasonography involves the use of sound waves and is not a form of ionizing radiation. There have been no reports of documented adverse fetal effects of diagnostic ultrasonography procedures, including from duplex Doppler imaging, to our knowledge [11].

The US Food and Drug Administration limits the spatial-peak temporal average intensity of ultrasound transducers to 720 mW/cm^2. At this intensity, the theoretical increase in temperature elevation for the fetus may be as high as 2 °C (35.6 °F). However, it is highly unlikely that any sustained temperature elevation will occur at any single fetal anatomic site. The temperature elevation is lowest with B-mode imaging, and is higher with color Doppler and spectral Doppler applications [12].

Ultrasonography should be used prudently, and only when its use is expected to answer a relevant clinical question or to otherwise provide potential medical benefit to the patient. When used in this manner and with machines that are configured correctly, ultrasonography does not pose a risk to the fetus or the pregnancy.

An example of ultrasound use in a trauma setting is presented in Fig. 7.3.

7.2.2 Computed Tomography

CT remains the "workhorse" modality for the imaging evaluation of trauma patients.

Although radiography, CT, and angiography utilize ionizing radiation, in major trauma, the risks of radiation to the pregnancy (mentioned in the introduction and discussed further in that chapter) are small compared with the risk of missed or delayed diagnosis of maternal injury. Therefore, CT scan is recommended as the first-line imaging modality in pregnant women who

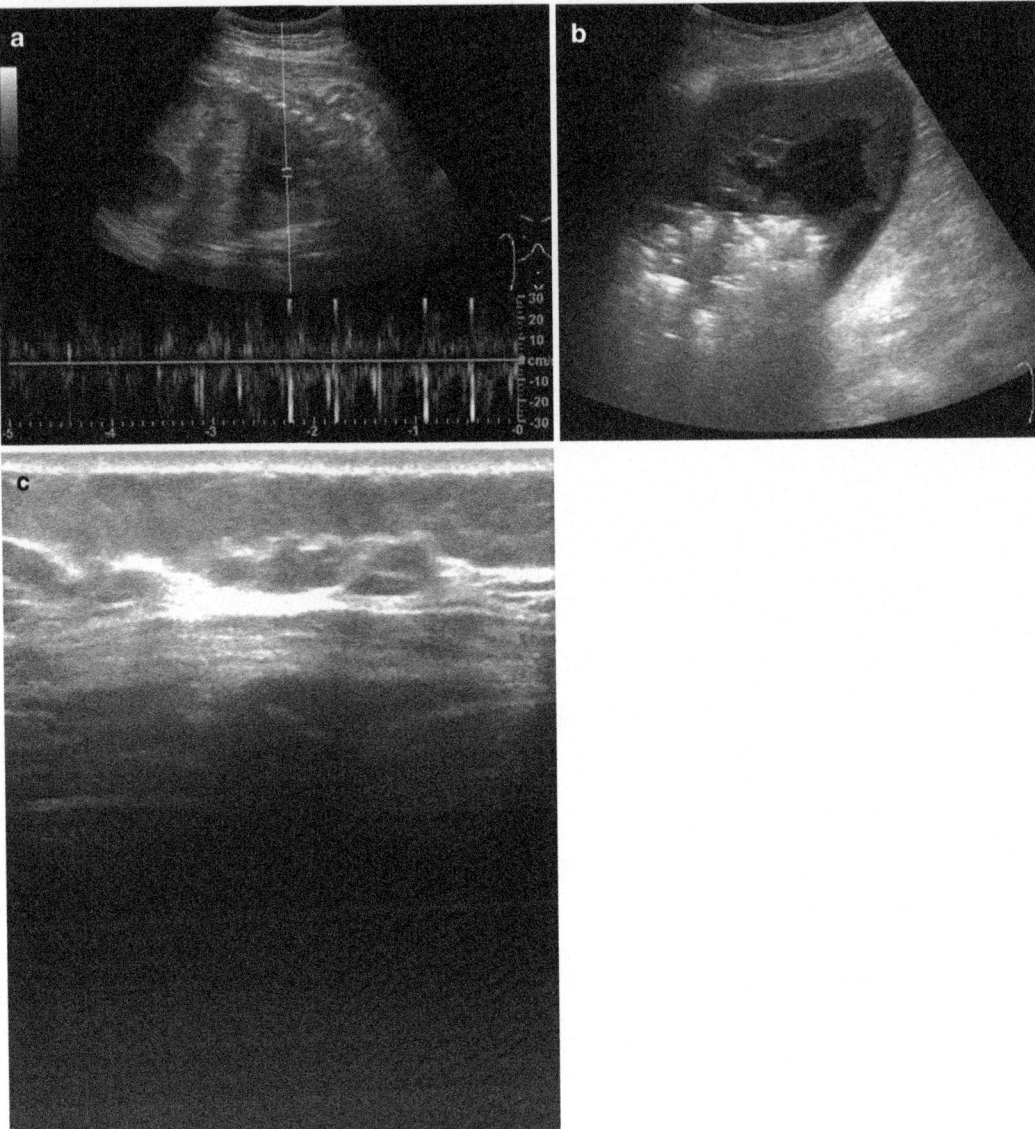

Fig. 7.3 Ultrasound images of a 32-year-old patient at 28 gestational weeks (**a**) admitted after a motor vehicle collision. Please note irregularly marginated hypoechoic areas within the spleen representing rupture, as well as a sub-capsular hematoma (**b**). Additional image with a linear transducer (**c**) revealed a rib fracture with cortical disruption and displacement

have sustained major trauma, especially high-energy traumas such as motor vehicle crashes, and the decision should be at the discretion of the treating physician.

However, efforts should be made to eliminate unnecessary scans, reduce overlap of body sec-tions, and avoid multiple passes where possible. It is important to generate a diagnostic test, and for that reason ultra low-dose protocols are not used [6].

An example of CT use in a trauma setting is presented in Fig. 7.4.

Fig. 7.4 A 20-year-old patient in the second trimester admitted after a motor vehicle collision. Whole-body CT was performed, scout (**a**). On axial IV contrast-enhanced images, apart from a gravid uterus, note high density free fluid, i.e., blood, in the presacral space (**b**), below the right hepatic lobe (**c**), and a displaced rib fracture on the left (**d**)

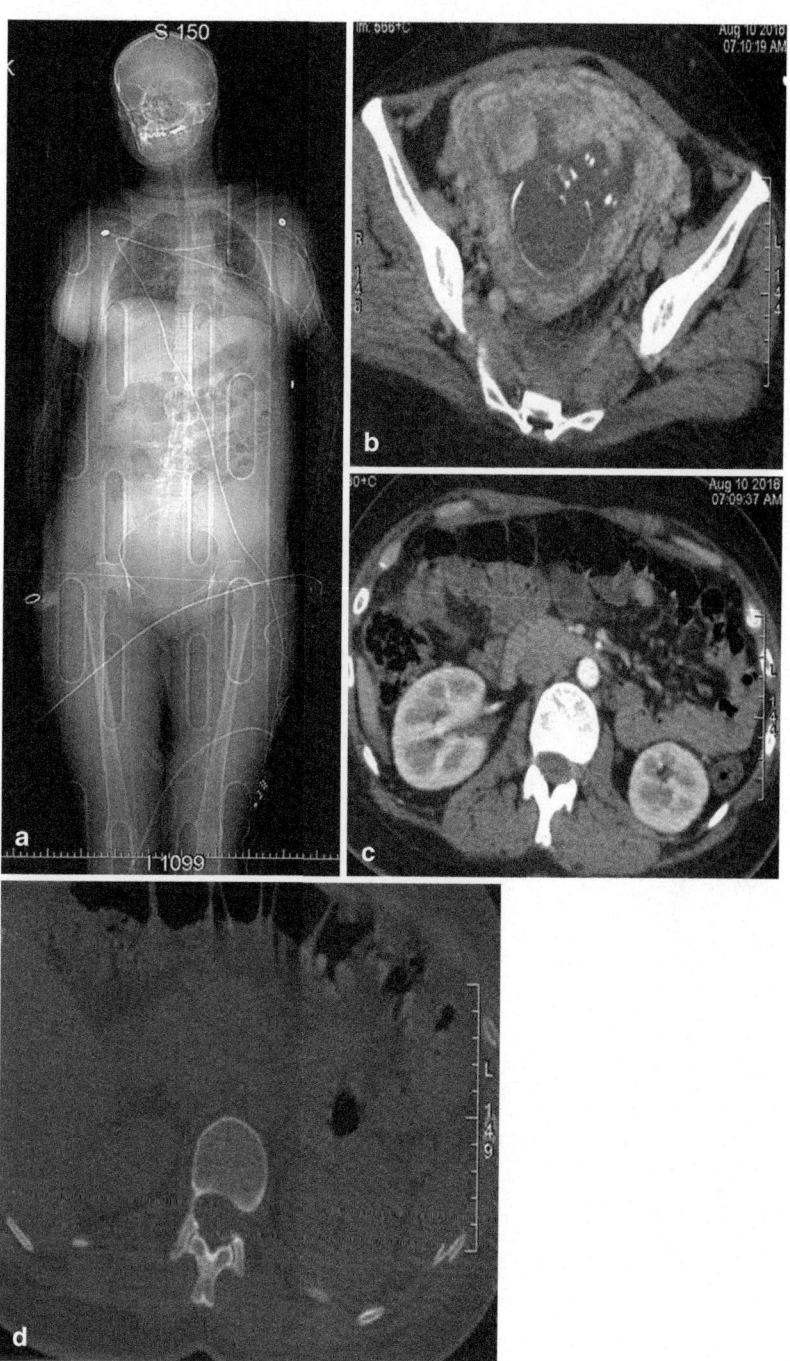

7.2.2.1 Safety of CT Imaging During Pregnancy

CT in the setting of pregnancy is something that we have to take all the measures to keep our radiation dose low and think whether we are doing the right thing in examining the patient.

Emergencies and non-emergencies are two settings which are quite different in the way CT should be used.

Emergencies require rapid and correct diagnosis as well as treatment decisions, and speed is an important factor. In such situation, CT has its big advantage over MR, as well as ultrasound, and in emergency settings the radiation dose is of secondary importance, especially when the emergency is potentially life threatening [12].

An example of CT use in a trauma setting is presented in Fig. 7.5.

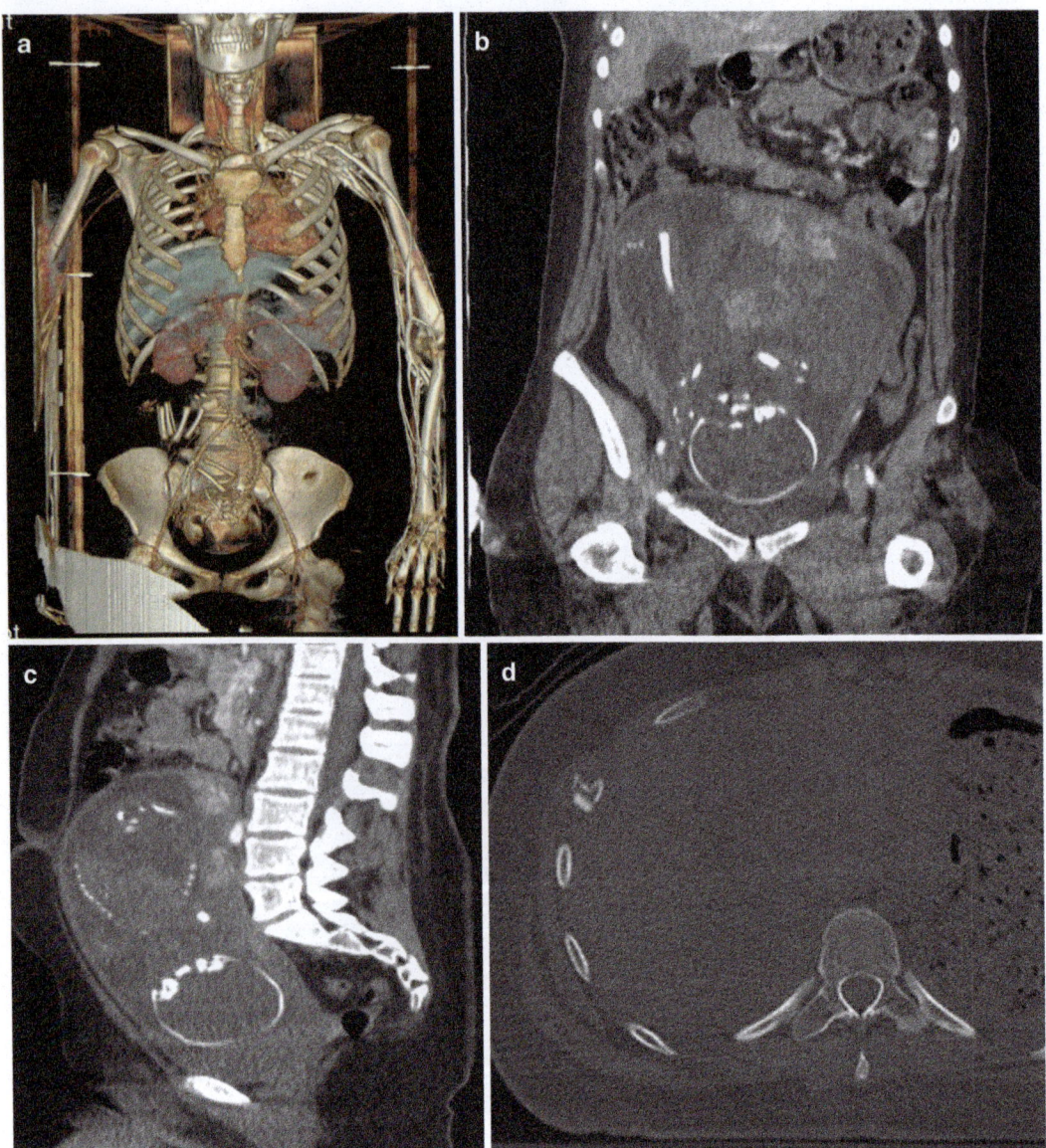

Fig. 7.5 A 19-year-old patient in the final weeks of pregnancy after a motor vehicle collision. Volume-rendered reconstruction (**a**) as well as coronal and sagittal contrast-enhanced images (**b, c**), show a gravid uterus as well as a fetus. Apart from a single rib fracture on the right (**d**), no other maternal injuries were diagnosed

For a non-emergency examination, the diagnosis and treatment are on less time pressure, which means that ultrasound and MR become valid and important alternatives. However, the correct diagnosis is still more important than radiation dose, so if MR or ultrasound is not available, or if those two technologies are not able to solve the problem, CT remains indicated, and it is all about the risk versus the benefit.

If we look at the priorities of various emergency patients like polytrauma, extremity injuries, etc., there are lots of factors that make the CT the technology of choice. As the first priority is diagnosis and treatment, CT plays an important role in trauma settings, especially with 3D data gathering—especially when it becomes more complex, it can help us make the right treatment decisions.

An example of CT use in a trauma setting is presented in Fig. 7.6.

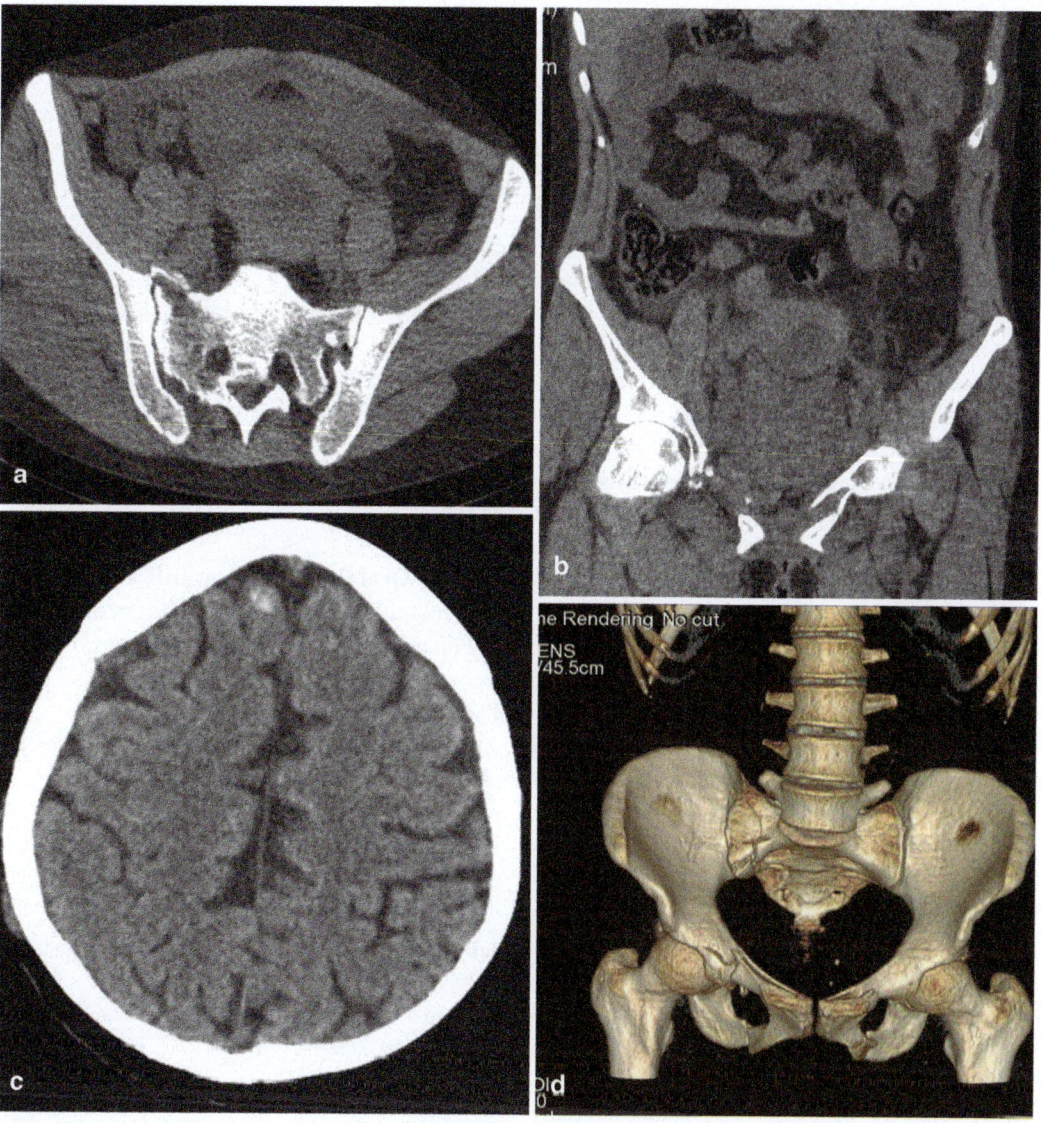

Fig. 7.6 A 33-year-old patient—unaware of her pregnancy—was admitted after motor vehicle collision. On axial (**a**) and coronal (**b**) CT images, a gravid uterus as well as blood in the pelvis is present. The patient sustained also minor brain injury with small cerebral hemorrhagic contusion in the right frontal lobe (**c**). On volume-rendered 3D reconstruction image (**d**), bilateral pelvic ring fractures are well depicted

7.2.2.2 Radiation Risks in Pregnant Patients

The main risk is actually not so much to the fetus but the radiation exposure to breast tissue. This is because breast tissue is rapidlly proliferating and is more radiosensitive [10].

Although radiation doses to a fetus tend to be lower than doses to the mother, due to protection from the uterus and surrounding tissues, the human embryo and fetus are sensitive to ionizing radiation at doses greater than 0.1 gray (Gy). Depending on the stage of fetal development, the health consequences of exposure at doses greater than 0.5 Gy can be severe, even if such a dose is too low to cause an immediate effect for the mother. The health consequences can include growth restriction, malformations, impaired brain function, and childhood cancer [13].

If the uterus is positioned outside the field of view, the conceptus is exposed to scattered radiation only, and the conceptus dose is minimal [14].

What is negligible is the risk of radiation-induced malformation in the fetus.

It is accepted practice to protect the patient and the fetus by shielding areas most susceptible to the effects of radiation, limiting the time of exposure, and using alternative modalities to evaluate areas closest to the developing fetus whenever possible [15].

Fetal Risks

Health effects to a fetus from radiation exposure depend largely on the radiation dose. Up to 50 mGy, there are NO known detectable noncancer health effects.

Within 50–500 mGy range, we have to keep in mind that the dosage of 50 mGy is something that we hardly ever reach in our population—even in setting of severe trauma. The dose of 500 mGy or greater, on the other hand, is excessive, and is only possible to achieve with substantial repeated exposures for one person over time [16].

Depending on the gestational age, we see different types of problems that can potentially occur:

- up to 2 weeks: slightly more failure to implant, but probably not significant (noncancer) health effect.
- 2–7 weeks: possible growth retardation, incidence of major malformation may increase slightly.
- 8–15 weeks: possible growth retardation, dose-dependent IQ reduction (up to 15 points), severe retardation in <20%.
- >15 weeks: noncancer health effects not detectable [16].

The problems mentioned above are considered highly dose dependent, and occur mostly towards the end of the spectrum 50–500 mGy [10].

If we look at the absolute numbers of cancer probability, the cancer risk of someone who has not received extra radiation (just the background radiation), although controversial, the estimated childhood risk is 0.3% and the lifetime cancer risk is about 38%. In the range from 0 to 50 mGy—which is the range that is usually administered in polytrauma for instance—this can go up to 1% in childhood, and the lifetime cancer possibility is just slightly increased up to 40%. That changes very rapidly when the dose goes up, to dosages that we do not normally use, as summarized in Table 7.1 [16].

7.2.2.3 Oral Contrast Administration

Oral contrast agents are not absorbed by the patient, and do not cause real or theoretical harm [10].

7.2.2.4 Iodinated Contrast Media

Although iodinated contrast media can cross the placenta and either enter the fetal circulation or pass directly into the amniotic fluid, animal studies have reported no teratogenic or mutagenic effects from its use. Therefore, IV iodinated CT

Table 7.1 Carcinogenic effects of prenatal radiation exposure

Radiation	Childhood cancer	Lifetime cancer
No radiation	0.3%	38%
0–50 mGy	0.3–1%	38–40%
50–500 mGy	1–6%	40–55%
>500 mGy	>6%	>55%

contrast material is considered a Food and Drug Administration (FDA) category B agent with no known adverse effects during pregnancy. Despite this lack of known harm, it generally is recommended that contrast only be used if absolutely required to obtain additional diagnostic information that will affect the care of the fetus or woman during the pregnancy [13].

Traditionally, lactating women who receive intravascular iodinated contrast have been advised to discontinue breastfeeding for 24 h. However, because of its water solubility, less than 1% of iodinated contrast administered to a lactating woman is excreted into the breast milk, and less than 1% of this amount of contrast will be absorbed through the infant's gastrointestinal tract. Therefore, breastfeeding can be continued without interruption after the use of iodinated contrast [10].

An example of CT use in a trauma setting is presented in Fig. 7.7.

7.2.2.5 Effect of Iodine Contrast on Thyroid of the Fetus

The fetal thyroid is highly sensitive to acute iodine overload. Maternal administration of iodide (sodium iodide) or exposure to iodine-containing medications has been shown to induce changes in neonatal thyroid function in both animals and humans [17].

A potential adverse effect on the fetal thyroid from maternal intravenous administration of iodinated contrast agent resulting in neonatal hypothyroidism has been postulated, but has not been systematically studied, to our knowledge [18].

In the summary document of the Contrast Media Safety Committee of ESUR, it was stated that fetal exposure to iodinated contrast media and iodide is likely to be short lived and that all infants born to mothers who received iodinated contrast during pregnancy should have their thyroid function checked in the first week of life [19].

As discussed previously, in pregnant patients, it is recommended to use an iodinated contrast agent without hesitation, as a nonenhanced CT examination may be nondiagnostic and necessitate a repeat examination, increasing the radiation dose [7].

An example of CT use in a trauma setting is presented in Fig. 7.8.

7.2.3 MRI

MRI is preferable to CT during pregnancy as it provides soft-tissue imaging without the risk of ionizing radiation. However, magnetic resonance imaging is rarely performed in acute trauma because requires separation of a patient from emergency personnel, is a difficult setting to monitor the patient, and is time intensive.

After the initial evaluation, MR imaging can be an excellent choice in specific situations, including spinal, complex neurologic, and soft-tissue injuries. MR imaging protocols for pregnant patients should be tailored to include the minimum number of sequences required to answer the particular clinical question. MR imaging may also have a role in reducing radiation exposure in patients who require follow-up imaging of injuries diagnosed at initial presentation, or in stable patients who develop new pain or warning symptoms after an initial negative evaluation [6].

An example of MRI use in a trauma setting is presented in Fig. 7.9.

7.2.3.1 Magnetic Resonance Imaging Safety

The principal advantage of MRI over ultrasonography and computed tomography is the ability to image deep soft tissue structures in a manner that is not operator dependent and does not use ionizing radiation.

The American College of Radiology states that MR imaging is a useful problem-solving technique. MRI at 1.5 T or less has been shown to be safe in all trimesters of pregnancy. Pregnant women should, therefore, be imaged at 1.5 T or less. The safety of MRI at 3 T for pregnant women has not yet been proven [13].

Intravenous gadolinium, the contrast medium used for MRI, is a US Food and Drug Administration class C agent which can cross the placenta and circulate indefinitely in fetal circulation. Studies in animals have shown that these agents have the potential of inducing congenital anomalies. Although there is no such significant evidence in humans, intravenous gadolinium is preferably avoided during pregnancy, and used

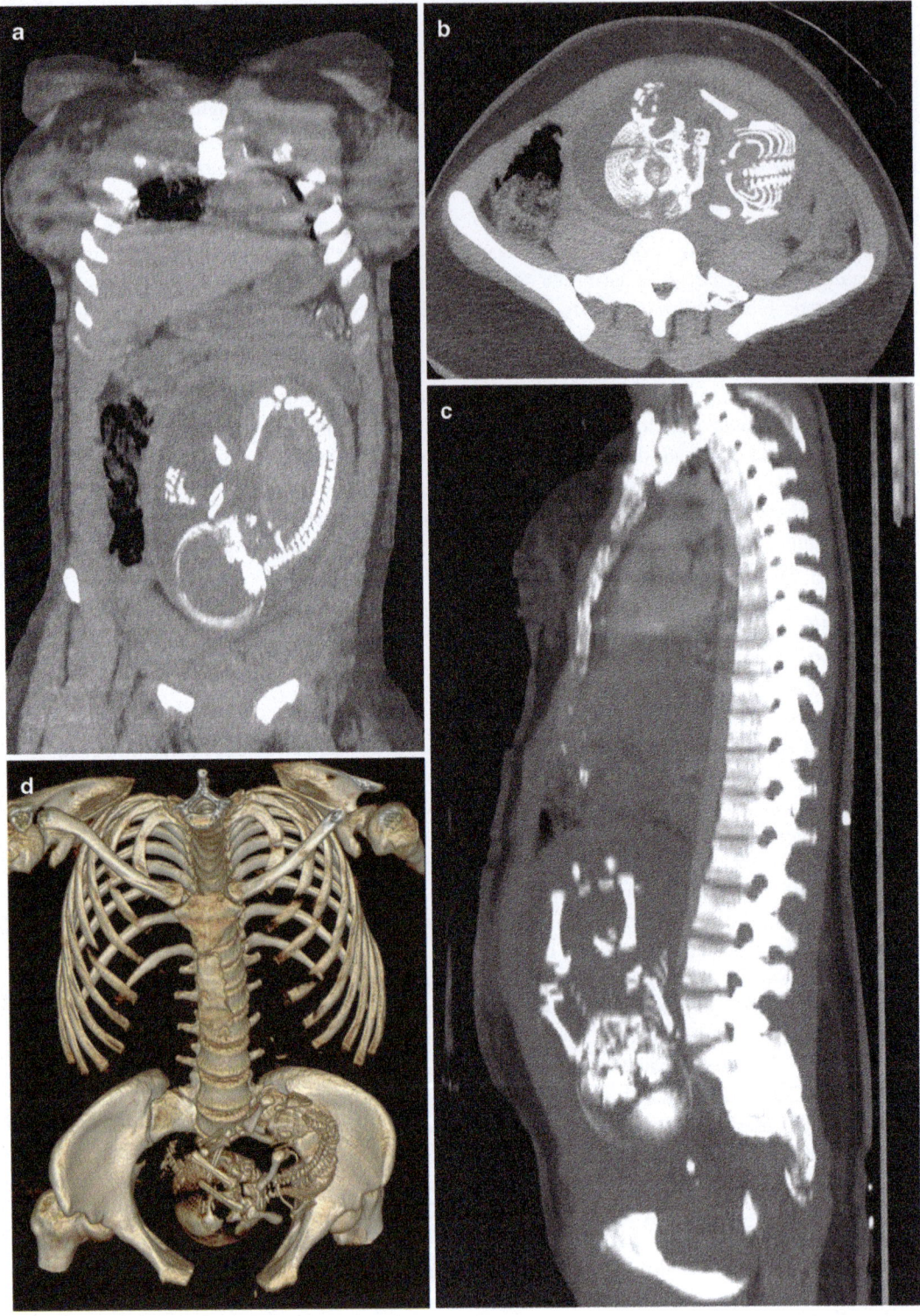

Fig. 7.7 A 23-year-old patient at 38 weeks of gestational age admitted after high-velocity motor vehicle collision. The fetus was pronounced dead in utero. On coronal (**a**) and axial (**b**) and sagittal MIP CT images (**c**), the fetal skeleton in the uterine cavity is well depicted. The 3D reconstruction image (**d**) shows extensive injury to patient's pelvis bones, with "open-book" fracture and traumatic diastasis of the pubic symphysis

Fig. 7.8 A 32-year-old patient at 36 weeks of gestational age (**a**) after motor vehicle collision. On axial (**b**) and sagittal (**c**) non-enhanced CT images, an advanced pregnancy with gravid uterus and fetal skeleton was clearly visible. On sagittal (**d**) and axial (**e**) images in a bone window setting, an L3 vertebral body burst fracture is evident

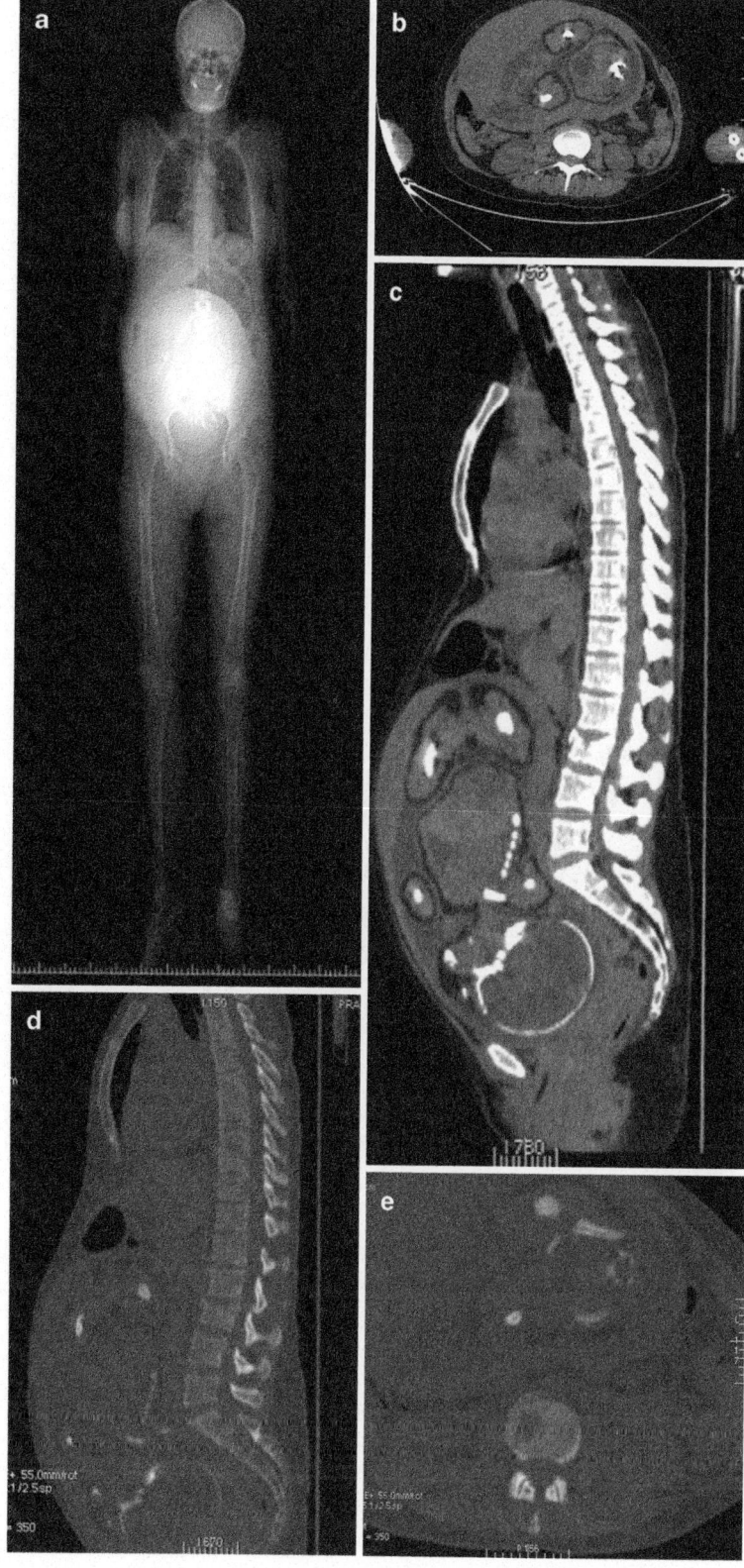

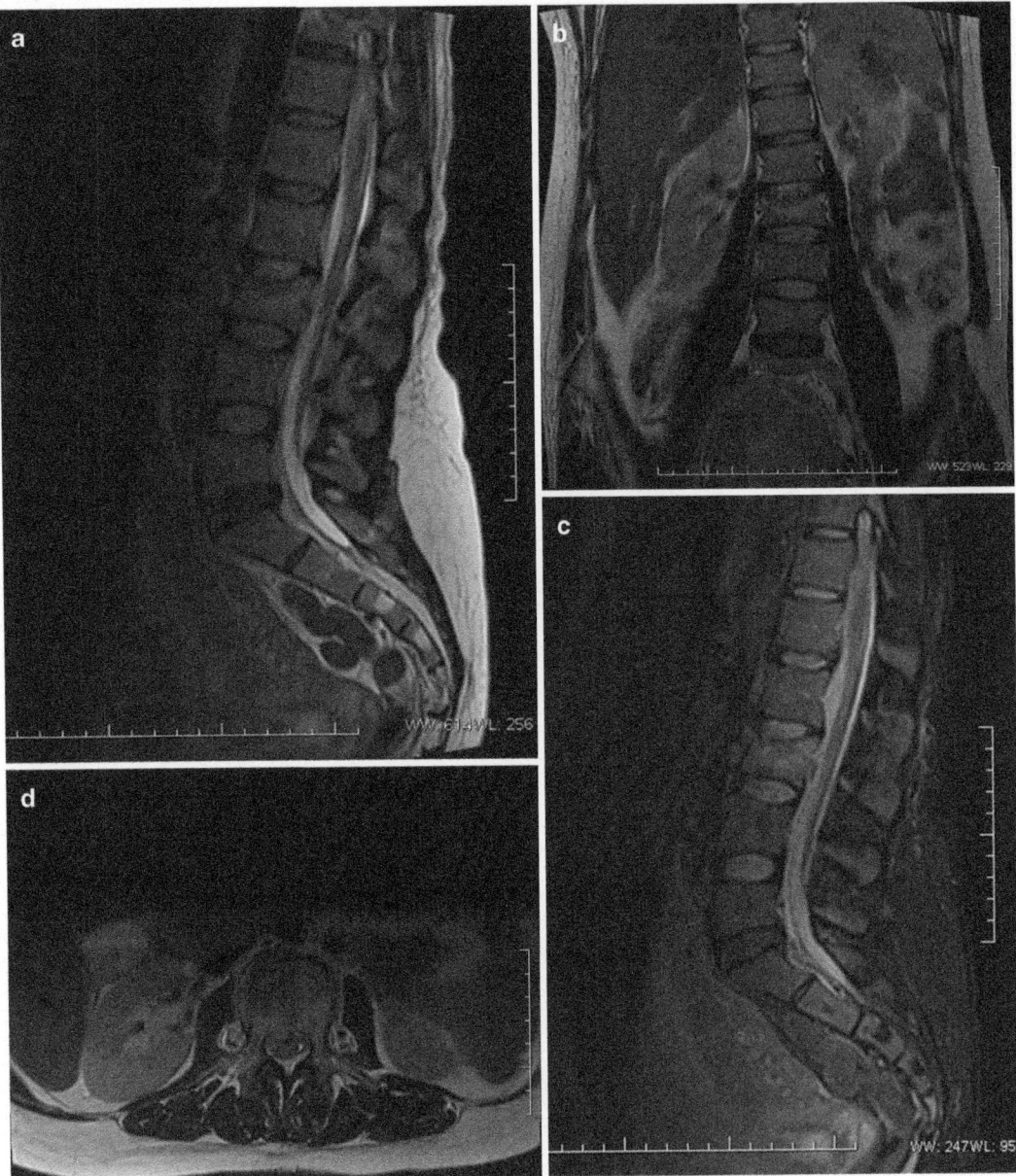

Fig. 7.9 Same patient presented in Fig. 7.8. After an emergency cesarean section, she was sent for MRI for further L3 fracture spine assessment. On sagittal (**a**) and coronal (**b**) T2-weighted MR images, loss of vertebral body height is well depicted. Sagittal STIR image (**c**) shows bone marrow edema in the superior aspect of L3 vertebrae suggesting bone contusions. On an axial T2-weighted image (**d**), note that the posterior aspect of the vertebral body is displaced backward into the spinal canal, resulting in post-traumatic stenosis

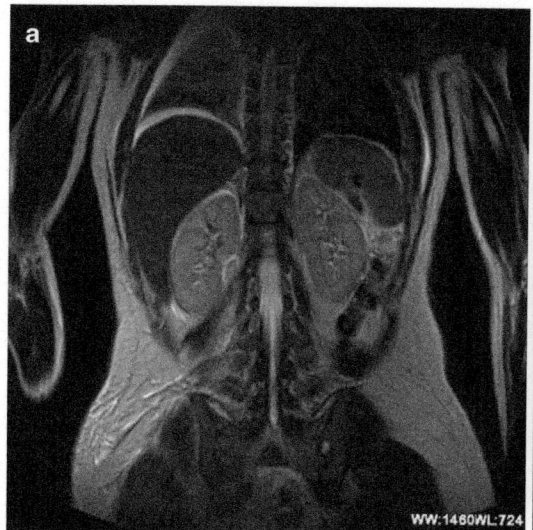
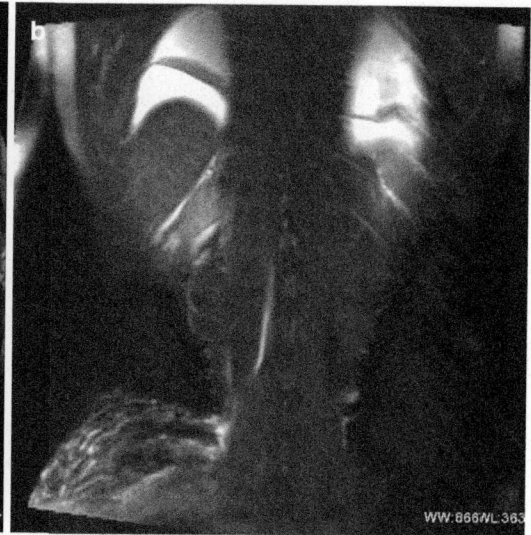

Fig. 7.10 A 30-year-old patient in the first trimester of her second pregnancy following a motor vehicle collision. On coronal T2-weighted image, a small amount of free intraperitoneal fluid and fluid in the right pleural cavity is visible (**a**). On coronal T2 fat-sat image, soft-tissue edema of the right pelvis is also seen (**b**)

only in situations in which the potential benefits clearly outweigh the possible risks [16].

An example of MRI use in a trauma setting is presented in Fig. 7.10.

Rapid sequence MRI is preferable to conventional MRI breath-hold multi-planar T2-weighted sequences based on the half-Fourier reconstruction technique (HASTE), the balanced gradient-echo sequences (such as FIESTA, true FISP, BSSFP), and axial and sagittal T1-weighted GRE images, and diffusion sequences should be used as a basic protocol. The time required for the mentioned protocol usually does not exceed 20 min [12].

The water solubility of gadolinium-based agents limits their excretion into breast milk. Less than 0.04% of an intravascular dose of gadolinium contrast is excreted into the breast milk within the first 24 h. Of this amount, the infant will absorb less than 1% from his or her gastrointestinal tract. Although theoretically any unchelated gadolinium excreted into breast milk could reach the infant, there have been no reports of harm. Therefore, breastfeeding should not be interrupted after gadolinium administration.

An example of MRI use in a trauma setting is presented in Fig. 7.11.

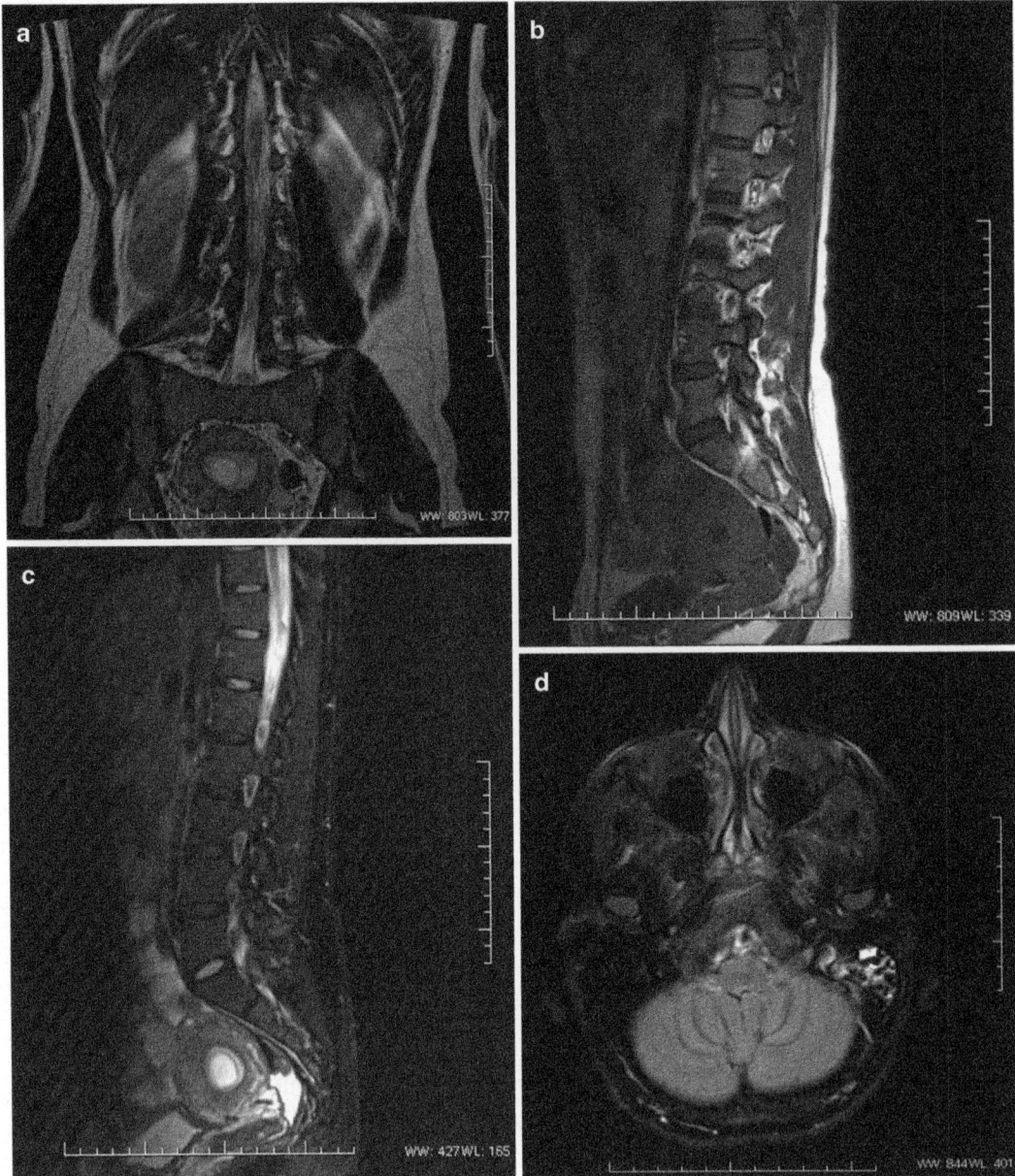

Fig. 7.11 A 19-year-old patient after a motor vehicle collision with lumbar spine and head injury. On coronal T2-weighted and on sagittal T1-weighted as well STIR images (**a–c**), no obvious spine or soft tissue injuries were diagnosed. However, an anembryonic pregnancy with a gestational sac and no visible embryo was suspected. A small amount of free fluid can be noted in Morison's pouch. Head MRI shows on axial FLAIR (**d**) and axial T1-weighted image (**e**); high intensity content of the mastoid cells on the left consistent with blood due to longitudinal temporal bone fracture. Axial T2-weighted MR image (**f**) shows a right temporal lobe contusion with cortical edema with associated accompanied hyperintense signal from blood in cerebrospinal fluid at the level of injury visible on coronal T1-weighted MR image (**g**)

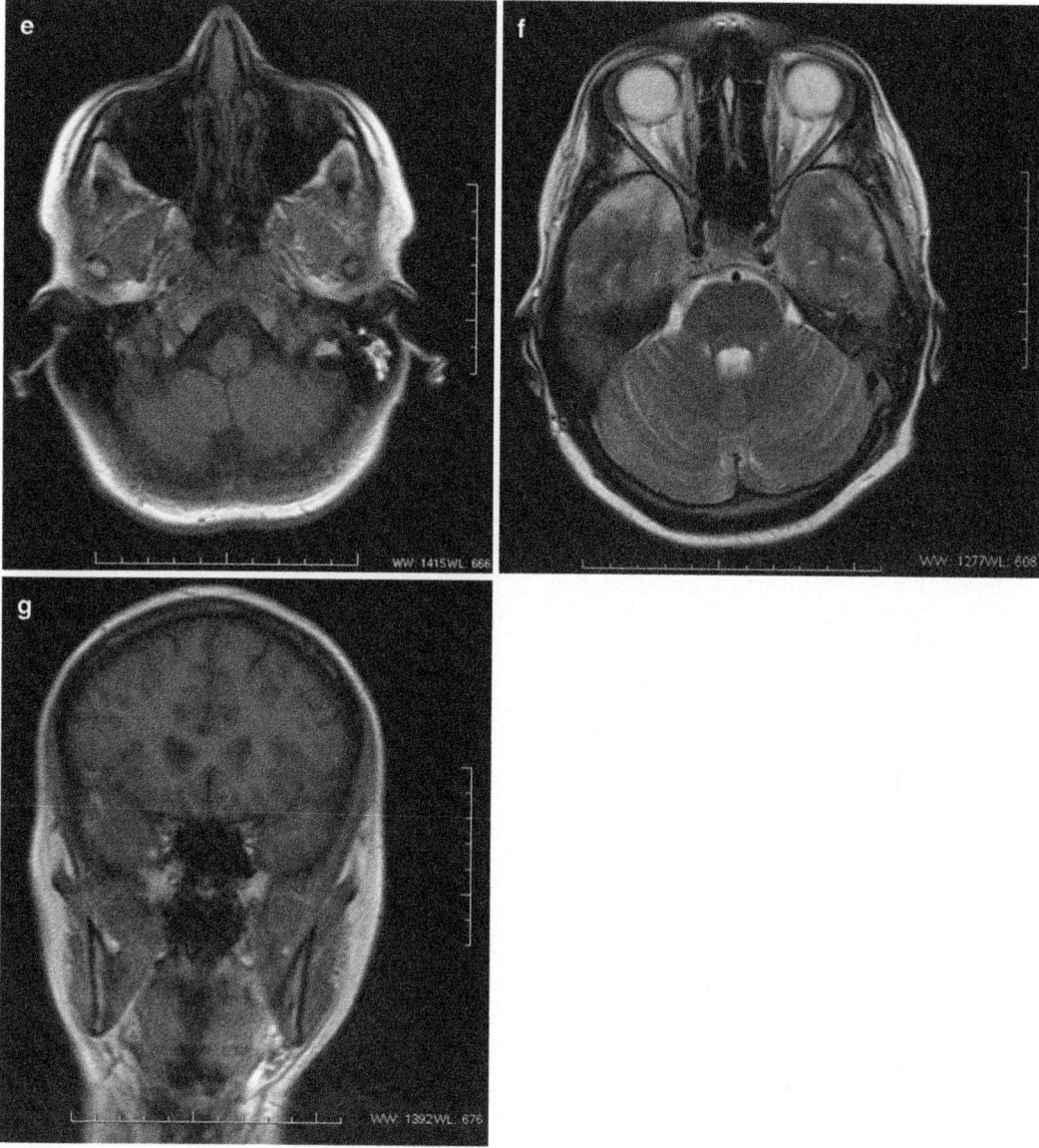

Fig. 7.11 (continued)

7.3 Conclusions

Pregnant patients may experience nonobstetrical emergencies over the course of their pregnancy such as trauma—being the leading cause of maternal mortality and a significant cause of fetal loss. A healthy pregnancy requires a healthy mother, and delayed diagnosis of emergencies in pregnancy threatens the mother and her fetus. Concerns about fetal radiation exposure should neither deter nor delay radiologic evaluation.

Managing the pregnant trauma patient requires a multidisciplinary approach. In the acute setting, US is frequently used to evaluate the pregnant trauma patient; however, it is important to remember that US is not a substitute for a clinically needed diagnostic computed tomographic

(CT) examination. Magnetic resonance imaging is rarely performed in acute trauma due to technical difficulties and time required; however, it can be an excellent choice for follow-up, especially in spinal, complex neurologic, and soft-tissue injuries.

References

1. Petrone P, Talving P, Browder T, Teixeira PG, Fisher O, Lozornio A, Chan LS. Abdominal injuries in pregnancy: a 155-month study at two level 1 trauma centers. Injury. 2011;42(1):47–9.

2. Brookfield KF, Gonzalez-Quintero VH, Davis JS, Schulman CI. Maternal death in the emergency department from trauma. Arch Gynecol Obstet. 2013;288:507–12.

3. El-Kady D, Gilbert WM, Anderson J, Danielsen B, Towner D, et al. Trauma during pregnancy: an analysis of maternal and fetal outcomes in a large population. Am J Obstet Gynecol. 2004;190:1661–8.

4. Gazmararian JA, Lazorick S, Spitz AM, Ballard TJ, Saltzman LE, et al. Prevalence of violence against pregnant women. JAMA. 1996;275:1915–20.

5. Garg N, Sharma A, Khanna P, Goel V. Trauma in pregnancy – a brief review. Trauma Emerg Care. 2017;2(3):1–4.

6. Raptis C, Mellnick V, Raptis D. Imaging of trauma in the pregnant patient. Radiographics. 2014;34:748–63.

7. Sadro C, Bernstein M, Kanal K. Imaging of trauma: Part 2, Abdominal trauma and pregnancy— a radiologist's guide to doing what is best for the mother and baby. AJR Am J Roentgenol. 2012a;199:1207–19.

8. Leggon RE, Wood GC, Indeck MC. Pelvic fractures in pregnancy: factors influencing maternal and fetal outcomes. J Trauma. 2002;53:796–804.

9. Sadro CT, Zins AM, Debiec K, Robinson J. Case report: lethal fetal head injury and placental abruption in a pregnant trauma patient. Emerg Radiol. 2012b;19:175–80.

10. Tirada N. Imaging pregnant and lactating patients. Radiographics. 2015;35:1751–65.

11. ACOG Committee the American College of Obstetricians and Gynecologists. ACOG committee opinion. Obstet Gynecol. 2017;130:e210–6.

12. Masselli G, Brunelli R, Monti R. Imaging for acute pelvic pain in pregnancy. Insights Imaging. 2014;5(2):165–81.

13. Zachariah S, Fenn M, Jacob K, et al. Management of acute abdomen in pregnancy: current perspectives. Int J Womens Health. 2019;11:119–34.

14. McCollough C, Schueler B, Atwell T. Radiation exposure and pregnancy: when should we be concerned? Radiographics. 2007;27:909–18.

15. Shaw P, Duncan A, Vouyouka A. Radiation exposure and pregnancy. J Vasc Surg. 2011;53:28S–34S.

16. Centers for Disease Control and Prevention Radiation and Pregnancy: A Fact Sheet for Clinicians. 2019. Retrieved from http://emergency.cdc.gov/radiation/prenatalphysician.asp.

17. Atwell T, Lteif A, Brown D. Neonatal thyroid function after administration of IV iodinated contrast agent to 21 pregnant patients. AJR Am J Roentgenol. 2008;191:268–71.

18. Bourjeily G, Chalhoub M, Phornphutkul C. Neonatal thyroid function: effect of a single exposure to iodinated contrast medium in utero. Radiology. 2010;256(3):744–50.

19. Rajaram S, Exley CE, Fairlie F, et al. Effect of antenatal iodinated contrast agent on neonatal thyroid function. Br J Radiol. 2012;85:238–42.

Imaging of Early Obstetric Emergencies

Margarita V. Revzin and Mariam Moshiri

Contents

M. V. Revzin (✉)
Department of Radiology and Biomedical Imaging,
Yale School of Medicine, New Haven, CT, USA
e-mail: margarita.revzin@yale.edu

M. Moshiri
Department of Radiology, University of Washington
School of Medicine, Seattle, WA, USA
e-mail: Moshiri@uw.edu

8.1   Introduction

Early pregnancy-related emergencies account for approximately 1–1.3% of all visits to the emergency department (ED) and over 1,000,000 ED visits annually in the United States [2]. Common presenting symptoms include abdominal pelvic pain and vaginal bleeding, for which a variable range of etiologies exist. These include benign etiologies such as hemorrhagic ovarian cysts, to potentially life-threatening conditions such as ruptured ectopic pregnancy. Despite the availability of many diagnostic tools such as clinical assessment, laboratory evaluation, and imaging, accurate diagnosis of early pregnancy-related emergencies can be challenging due to non-specific imaging findings and vague symptomatology at presentation. It is therefore imperative for the radiologist to be familiar with normal and abnormal imaging appearances that may be seen in early pregnancy, as well as the current accepted terminology of early pregnancy complications and their treatment and management options. This knowledge will empower the radiologist to provide rapid recognition of pregnancy complications, and allow for accurate and efficient communication with referring physicians, which will in turn allow prompt management of these conditions (Fig. 8.1). This chapter will provide a review of normal embryologic stages that are seen in early pregnancy, an algorithm for how to assess early pregnancy, and will highlight characteristic and pathognomonic findings in order to

improve pattern recognition and help distinguish pathological processes encountered in the first trimester.

8.2 Early Embryo Development with Sonographic Correlation and Viability Assessment

During ovulation, the oocyte is released from the ovary and traverses the fallopian tube, where it can be viable for up to a few days. Conception occurs if a spermatocyte fertilizes the oocyte, a process in which genetic material is combined (fused). In a successful pregnancy, the fertilized oocyte travels into the uterus and implants within the uterine wall. At this stage, it is called a blastocyst. This process usually occurs on day 8–10 following ovulation. Rapid cell division of the blastocyst continues with the development of an embryo and production of human chorionic gonadotropin (HCG), which influences progesterone production and maintenance of the corpus luteum. At this time, no significant changes are seen on ultrasound except for mild thickening of the endometrium.

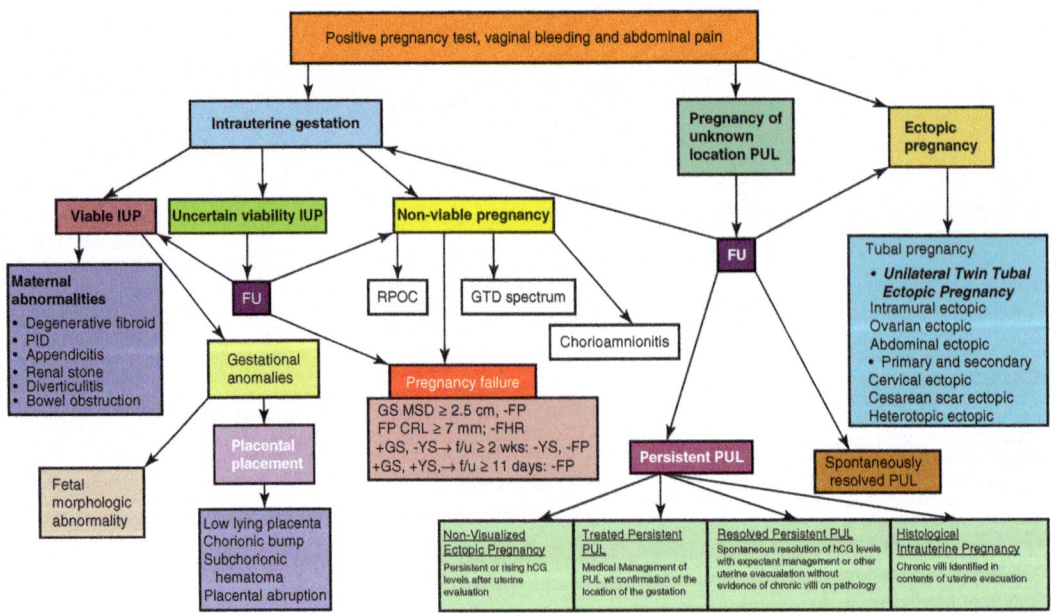

Fig. 8.1 Algorithm for assessment of early pregnancy and appropriate management of patients presenting with positive pregnancy test

It is important to establish a clear understanding of how gestational age is calculated. By convention, gestational age is calculated from the first day of a woman's last menstrual period. However, since conception does not take place until after ovulation, approximately 14 days (or 2 weeks) after the last menstrual period, note should be made of the 2-week discrepancy between the clinical and histologic gestational ages. For the sake of clarity and convenience, we will refer to clinical gestational age of the embryo and fetus in this chapter. The gestational sac (GS) becomes apparent on sonographic evaluation at approximately 4.5–5 weeks of gestation (or approximately 2.5–3 weeks post-ovulation), appearing as an anechoic 2–3 mm cystic space that is eccentrically located within the endometrium (Fig. 8.2). Any cystic space or collection that is identified within the endometrial canal in a pregnant woman should be assumed to represent an early gestation or IUP. Slightly later in the development, two characteristic signs can be recognized associated with a gestational sac: the *intradecidual sign* and the *double sac* sign. The intradecidual sign refers to an eccentrically positioned GS within the echogenic decidua, adjacent to the collapsed intrauterine cavity that is visualized as a thin echogenic line (Fig. 8.3). The double sac sign is more definitive for diagnosis of an intrauterine pregnancy (IUP), and is characterized by the presence of two concentric echogenic rings (decidua capsularis around the chorion—inner ring, and decidua parietalis—outer ring) with the inner ring surrounding the small fluid collection. The echogenic rings are separated by a thin crescent of endometrial fluid (Fig. 8.3) [3]. The intradecidual sign can be seen earlier in pregnancy and is not associated with uterine contour disruption, whereas the double decidual sign is seen at a later time and results in protrusion of the GS into the cavity with distortion of the endometrial contour. The yolk sac (YS) supports the developing embryo by providing nutrients, and becomes distinguishable at approximately 5.5 weeks of gestation, seen on ultrasound as a round anechoic structure with a thin wall. The yolk sac increases in size until tenth week of gestation, measuring up to 5–6 mm, then subsequently regresses, and is no longer visible on US by 12–15 weeks [4]. In general, by 6 weeks of gestation, the fetal pole is visible, with a measurable crown-rump length (CRL) and a detectable heart rate (Fig. 8.2).

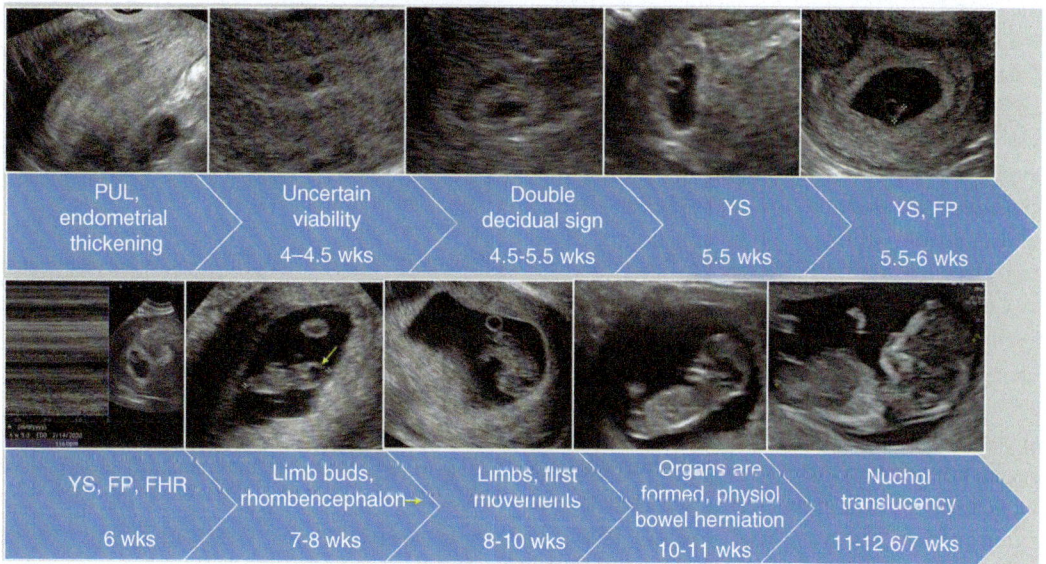

Fig. 8.2 Time line diagram of the fetal development in the first trimester with imaging correlation

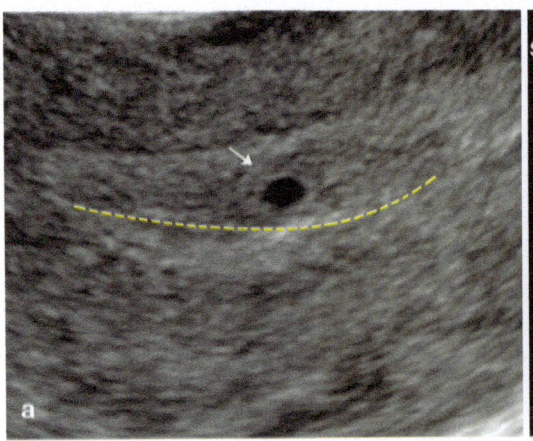

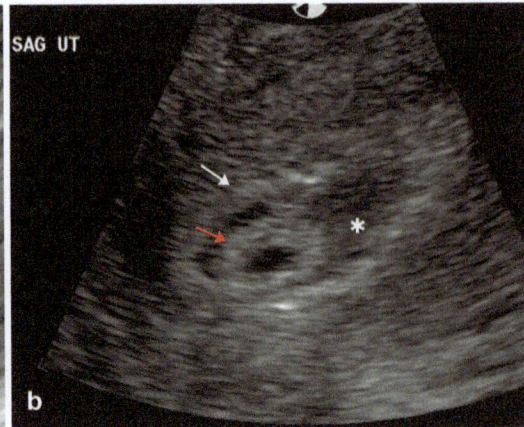

Fig. 8.3 (**a**) Intradecidual sign. Intradecidual sign refers to an eccentrically positioned gestational sac (GS) (arrow) within the echogenic decidua, adjacent to the collapsed intrauterine cavity that is visualized as a thin echogenic line (yellow dashed line in **a**). (**b**) Double decidual sign. A 28-year-old pregnant woman with abdominal pain with last menstrual period (LMP) 5 weeks ago. Gray-scale transvaginal ultrasound demonstrates a cystic space surrounded by two concentric echogenic rings with the inner ring representing decidua capsularis around the chorion (red arrow in **b**) and the outside ring corresponding to decidua parietalis (white arrow in **b**). The echogenic rings are separated by hypoechoic crescent of endometrial fluid (asterisk)

Ultrasound assessment allows measurement of the gestational sac and calculation of the mean sac diameter (MSD). Although the mean sac diameter growth rate is variable, in general, it grows approximately 1.13 mm/day [5]. The embryo resides within the amniotic cavity and the YS within the chorionic cavity. In the period of gestational development between 6.5 and 10 weeks, there is a linear relationship between the diameter of the amniotic cavity and the CRL, with 10% larger amniotic cavity mean diameter than CRL [6]. Amniotic and chorionic cavities and the CRL proportionally enlarge until tenth week of gestation. After the tenth week, the amniotic cavity expands at a higher rate than the chorionic cavity due to urine production by the fetus, resulting in fusion of the amnion and chorion at 14–16 weeks (Fig. 8.4) [7].

In normal pregnancies, the fetal pole should become apparent at a mean sac diameter of less than 2.5 cm. Fetal heart rate is assessed on ultrasound utilizing motion mode (M-mode), and should be present in all embryos with a CRL of 7 mm or larger [3, 8]. Cardiac activity can usually be demonstrated as early as 6–6.5 weeks of gestation within embryos measuring as little as 1–2 mm [9]. A normal heart rate in early pregnancy before 8 weeks of gestation should be

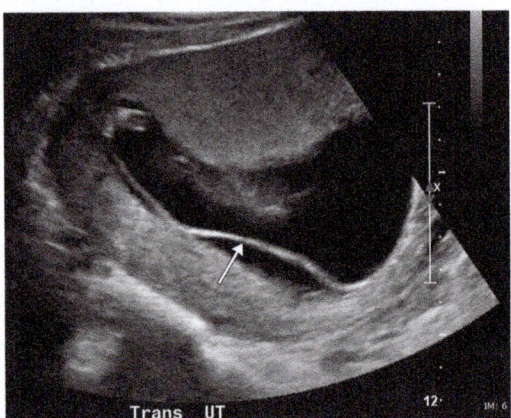

Fig. 8.4 Partial chorioamniotic fusion in a 37-year-old pregnant woman at 12 weeks of gestation who presented with abdominal pain and cramping. Gray-scale transverse image of the uterus via a transabdominal approach demonstrates partial fusion of the amniotic and chorionic membranes (arrow) due to disproportionally rapid growth of the amniotic cavity and relatively slow growth of the chorionic cavity. Chorioamniotic separation should be suspected if discernible amniotic and chorionic membranes are seen after 14 weeks of gestation. Chorioamniotic separation is associated with aneuploidy and chromosomal abnormalities; therefore, careful morphological assessment at 18 weeks of gestation should be performed

greater than 100 bpm (beats per minute). After 8 weeks of gestation, the normal fetal heart rate (FHR) is expected to be in the range of 120–

180 bpm. Episodic variability is commonly seen at this gestational age, and should be differentiated from sustained bradycardia or persistent tachycardia [8]. By the seventh to eighth weeks of gestation, the cephalad and caudal poles of the embryo become apparent, and the rhombencephalon (a landmark for the hindbrain) can be seen as an anechoic (cystic) space in the cephalad pole. The four limb buds of the embryo develop around 8–9 weeks of gestation, and the first movement is seen as early as 8–8.5 weeks. A timeline of the sonographic features of normal early pregnancy development is listed in Fig. 8.2.

8.2.1 Human Chorionic Hormone

The developing pregnancy is supported by serum chorionic gonadotropic hormone (hCG), which is produced by the syncytiotrophoblasts of the developing placenta. The concentration of the hCG hormone in the mother's serum correlates very closely with the size and development of the gestational sac and embryo [10]. In a normal IUP, the hCG levels doubles approximately every 48 h, whereas in ectopic or failed pregnancies, the hCG levels either rise at a slower rate, plateau, or drop [11]. The hCG levels in viable intrauterine pregnancies, non-viable intrauterine pregnancies, and ectopic pregnancies have considerable overlap, so a single hCG measurement does not distinguish reliably among them [12–14]. Extensive research has been performed with the goal of identifying a range, or discriminatory zone or level—defined as the hCG value above which an intrauterine gestational sac is consistently seen on ultrasonography in normal pregnancies—of serum hCG levels that can be used as a prognostic factor for viability of early pregnancy, as a predictor of pregnancy failure, or a predictor of ectopic pregnancy. However, based on current investigations and research, a discriminatory level is not reliable. Doubilet et al. in their research found that the hCG discriminatory level is not reliable for excluding a normal intrauterine pregnancy, and concluded that the likelihood of a fetus surviving the first trimester and developing into a viable pregnancy with resultant live-born baby was unrelated to the initial ultrasound scan results [10]. Therefore, as per guidelines and recommendations of the SRU consensus article, an early pregnancy with a non-visualized IUP should be closely monitored and followed with repeat transvaginal ultrasound (TVUs) and serial hCG levels to confirm the status and site of the pregnancy. Once again it should be stressed that assessment based on hCG levels is not considered a definitive assessment, and therefore neither medical treatment with methotrexate (MTX) nor surgical management should be undertaken in a hemodynamically stable patient with a pregnancy of unknown location, if sonography demonstrates no findings of intrauterine or ectopic pregnancy [10].

8.2.2 Pregnancy of Unknown Location

Pregnancy of unknown location (PUL) refers to a condition in which a woman has a positive pregnancy test result but no evidence of intrauterine or extrauterine pregnancy on transvaginal sonography [15]. The reported incidence of PUL in women during early pregnancy assessment varies from 7% to 30% [16]. The wide range of reported PUL incidence can be partially explained by a number of factors, including differing levels of expertise of the performing sonographers, uterine or pelvic disease that affects visualization of an early pregnancy, obesity, or the presence of intrauterine devices [17]. There are four main outcomes of PUL: failed PUL, a visualized intrauterine pregnancy (IUP) regardless of viability, a visualized ectopic pregnancy (EP), or persisting PUL (Fig. 8.1) [15]. As per the consensus statements published by the Society of Radiologists in Ultrasound in 2013 and the International Society of Ultrasound in Obstetrics and Gynecology (ISUOG) in 2006, women with a PUL should be followed with serial hCG levels and transvaginal ultrasound until a final diagnosis can be made [18]. The detailed classification and reporting system as well as clinical management options are listed in Fig. 8.1; important terminology is listed in Table 8.1 [15].

Table 8.1 Terminology

Viable pregnancy	Pregnancy that can result in a live-born fetus
Non-viable pregnancy	Pregnancy that cannot result in a live-born fetus (includes ectopic and failed pregnancy)
Intrauterine pregnancy (IUP) of uncertain viability	IUP with no definite sign of failure or survival (i.e., no fetal pole or heartbeat)
Pregnancy of unknown location (PUL)	Positive biochemical pregnancy test, but no visible pregnancy on imaging
Positive biochemical pregnancy test	Serum human chorionic gonadotropin (hCG) concentration is above a positive threshold (5 mIU/ml)

8.2.3 Pregnancy Failure

Early pregnancy failure refers to loss of an intrauterine pregnancy in the first trimester, and is defined as a non-viable intrauterine pregnancy with either an empty gestational sac or a gestational sac containing a fetus without fetal heart activity within the first 12 6/7 weeks of gestation [19, 20]. Early pregnancy failure is common, occurring in 10% of all clinically diagnosed pregnancies. Approximately 80% of all pregnancy failures occur within the first trimester [21–23]. Early pregnancy failures significantly increase with age, with a rate of 9–17% in women between the ages of 20 and 30, over 40% by the age of 40, and over 80% at the age of 45 years [24]. Up to 70% of spontaneous miscarriages exhibit an abnormal karyotype. In the absence of karyotypic abnormality, pregnancy failures can be associated with luteal phase defects, immunological factors, infection, alcohol, smoking, or lethal genetic abnormalities [25, 26].

When symptomatic, patients with early pregnancy failure may present with vaginal bleeding and/or abdominal pain. The methods of diagnosis and management of this condition have changed markedly in the recent past, with treatment now most often consisting of medical or expectant management in outpatient clinics.

Women in early pregnancy who present to the emergency department with vaginal bleeding and pain are at risk for early pregnancy failure, with

miscarriage being the most common complication. Another very dangerous complication of early pregnancy is ectopic pregnancy.

There are a number of sonographic findings that are diagnostic of pregnancy failure (Fig. 8.1). In 2012, the Society of Radiologists in Ultrasound (SRU) published a consensus article that provided recommendations on how to definitively diagnose pregnancy failure, with the goal of eradicating any possibility of misdiagnosis and mismanagement of an early IUP [27]. There are four primary findings diagnostic of pregnancy failure that are recognized, and every emergency and general radiologist should be well acquainted with them and their role in evaluating a first-trimester pregnancy. These consist of the following:

1. *Absent cardiac activity* in an embryo with a **crown-rump measurement of equal or greater than 7 mm** is considered diagnostic of pregnancy failure, with a specificity and positive predictive value of 100% (Fig. 8.5).
2. *Absent embryo* with a **mean gestational sac diameter equal to or greater than 25 mm**, with a specificity of 100% for the diagnosis of pregnancy failure (Fig. 8.6).
3. *Absent embryo or no cardiac activity* on the current examination, with a prior US obtained at least 2 weeks earlier that documented a gestational sac **without yolk sac**.
4. *Absent embryo or no cardiac activity* on the current examination, with a prior US obtained at least 11 days earlier that documented a gestational sac **with a yolk sac** (Fig. 8.7).

In addition to the primary ultrasound criteria listed above, which ensure absolute certainty in the diagnosis of pregnancy failure, there are additional findings which carry a poor prognostic value for the development of a normal IUP. These include small ratio of GS size to the size of the embryo (less than 5 mm difference between the MSD and the CRL of an embryo) [28] (Fig. 8.8), large YS (greater than 7 mm) [29, 30], small size of the amnion in relation to the fetus/embryo, heart rate less than 85–90 bpm, irregular GS (irregular contour and/or distorted sac shape)

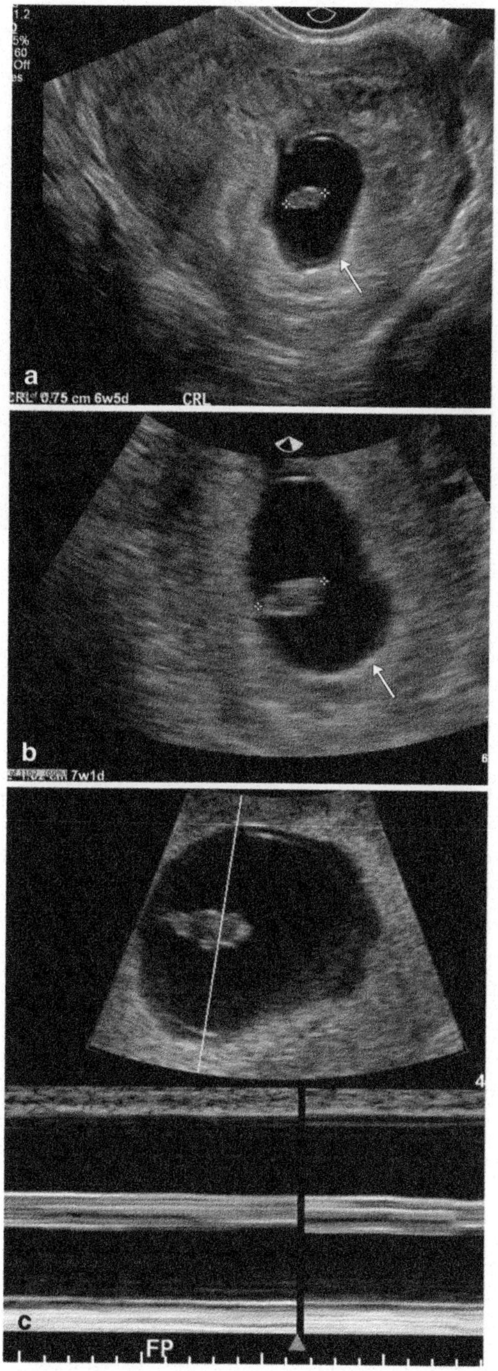

Fig. 8.5 Pregnancy failure in a 32-year-old pregnant woman with vaginal bleeding and a positive pregnancy test. (**a**, **b**) Gray-scale transvaginal ultrasound demonstrates an intrauterine gestational sac (arrow) with a fetal pole within it (FP). The crown-rump length (CRL) of the fetal pole measures 10 mm. (**c**) No cardiac activity is detected on M-mode

(Figs. 8.9 and 8.10), relatively large amniotic cavity, calcified YS, interval passage of a gestational sac from the fundal endometrial canal to the mid or lower uterine segment or the cervix (Fig. 8.11), and degenerative hydropic changes of the chorionic villi (Tables 8.2 and 8.3). Although these are all predictors of poor outcome, they do not definitely exclude the possibility of normal pregnancy development [9, 31–34]. The possibility of incorrect dates based on the provided LMP should also be considered [8].

8.2.3.1 Septic Spontaneous Pregnancy Failure

A septic abortion refers to an infection of the placenta and/or fetus, or products of conception. Although infection is localized primarily in the placenta, it can spread to the surrounding uterus, pelvis, and solid organs, which is more commonly seen with prolonged or potent toxin-producing bacteria. The main cause of septic abortions is unsafe abortion techniques, defined as *"procedures for terminating an unintended pregnancy either by individuals without the necessary skills or in an environment that does not conform to minimum medical standards, or both"* [35, 36]. Persistent IUDs in pregnant patients have also been implicated in the development of septic abortion. There is a tendency of this group of patients to present initially to the emergency department instead of an outpatient facility [37]. Delay in diagnosis may lead to devastating consequences, including infertility, septic shock, or death. The total number of unsafe pregnancy termination procedures is relatively large, for example, just in 2008 worldwide, over 21 million pregnancies were terminated unsafely. Complications from these terminations accounted for 13% of all maternal deaths and were second only to maternal hemorrhage [38]. Improper or inadequate removal of retained products of conception was the cause of septic pregnancy failures, with subsequent infiltration of the placental tissue by the bacteria and continuous spread of the infection into the uterus and bloodstream, resulting in bacteremia. Although most of the causative bacteria are derived from the vaginal flora, a high rate of anaerobic bacteria have also been isolated,

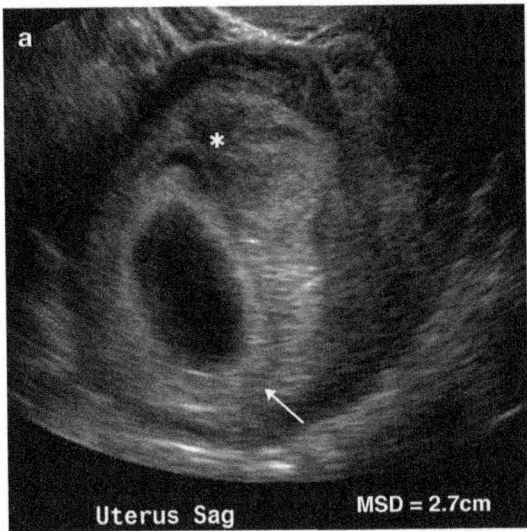

Fig. 8.6 Pregnancy failure in a 35-year-old woman who presented to the emergency department with abdominal pain, and was found to have positive pregnancy test with hCG of 680 mIU/ml. (**a**, **b**) Gray-scale transvaginal images demonstrate a gestational sac (GS) (arrows in **a**, **b**) with a mean sac diameter (MSD) = 2.7 cm, corresponding to an estimated gestational age of 7 weeks and 6 days. No fetal pole, cardiac activity, or yolk sac is identified within the GS. Note the small subchorionic hemorrhage (asterisk)

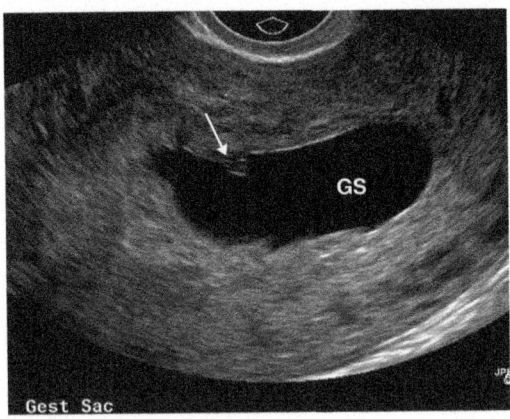

Fig. 8.7 Pregnancy failure in a 42-year-old pregnant woman who presented with pelvic pain and vaginal spotting. Transvaginal gray-scale ultrasound image reveals a disproportionally large gestational sac (GS) and a very small yolk sac (arrow). The fetal pole was not seen, and no cardiac activity was detected. The mean sac diameter (MSD) measured 3.73 cm, corresponding to a gestational age of 9 weeks and 2 days. Prior ultrasound obtained 12 days before demonstrated a GS with a yolk sac and no fetal pole (not shown)

such as *Peptostreptococcus* [39]. Some toxin-producing organisms, such as *Clostridium perfringens*, group A streptococcus, and some strains of *E. coli*, proliferate rapidly within dead tissue and become isolated from the vasculature.

Clinically, patients present with fever, bleeding, abdominal and pelvic pain, and declining hCG levels. Spontaneous abortion with endometritis and incomplete abortion are part of the differential considerations. Ultrasound is obtained to assess for presence of retained products of conception or the spectrum of pregnancy failures. Increased vascular flow to the myometrium and endometrium is observed on color Doppler ultrasound (Fig. 8.12). Management with resuscitation with intravenous fluids and extended coverage antibiotics is the mainstay of treatment in the emergency department [20, 40].

8.2.4 Subchorionic Hematoma

Subchorionic hematoma (SH) refers to hemorrhage around a portion of the gestational sac, and represents the most common type of intrauterine hematoma during pregnancy [4]. SH is thought to result from partial detachment of the trophoblast from the uterine wall, with blood dissecting between the chorion and the decidual layer of the endometrium [41]. The reported incidence is 18–22% in first-trimester pregnancies, which usually presents with vaginal bleeding [42, 43].

The most common sonographic finding associated with subchorionic hematoma is a crescentic, oval, or linear/curvilinear fluid collection enveloping part of the gestational sac which is situated at the outer aspect of the chorion (Fig. 8.13). The location of the fluid collection and its size should be reported, with the size of the collection graded into small, moderate, and large. Large-sized sub-

chorionic hematomas are associated with a significantly poorer prognosis, with a doubling of the risk of failed pregnancy when compared to small and moderate size. It is estimated that up to 18.8% of patients who present with large intrauterine hematomas in the first trimester of pregnancy develop subsequent failed pregnancy [44, 45]. If found, in addition to the size of the hema-

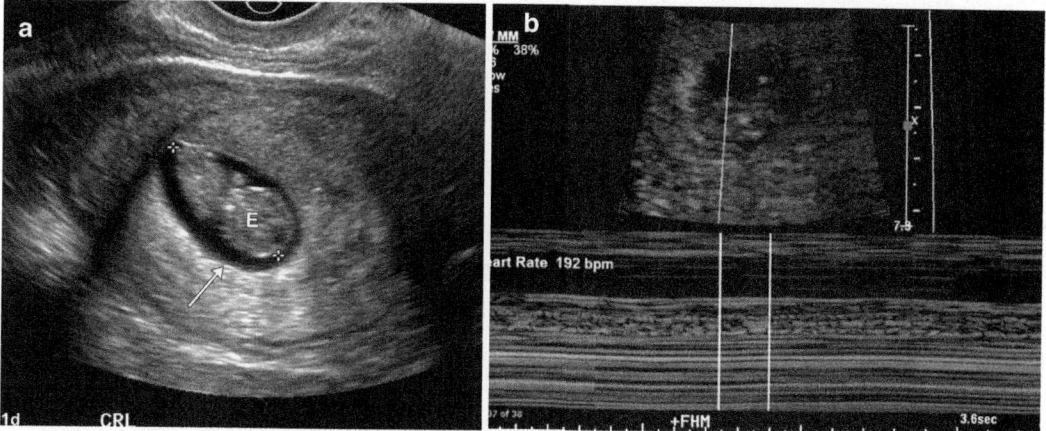

Fig. 8.8 Pregnancy failure in a 34-year-old pregnant woman who presented with vaginal bleeding and pelvic pain. (a) Gray-scale transvaginal ultrasound image demonstrates a relatively small gestational sac (arrow in a) with mean sac diameter (**MSD**) measuring 1.9 cm, which corresponds to the approximate gestational age of *6 weeks and 4 days*. The embryo (E) is present with a crown-rump length (*CRL*) of 2.37 cm, which corresponds to the gestational age of **9 weeks and 1 day**. (b) Persistent tachycardia was observed on M-mode imaging

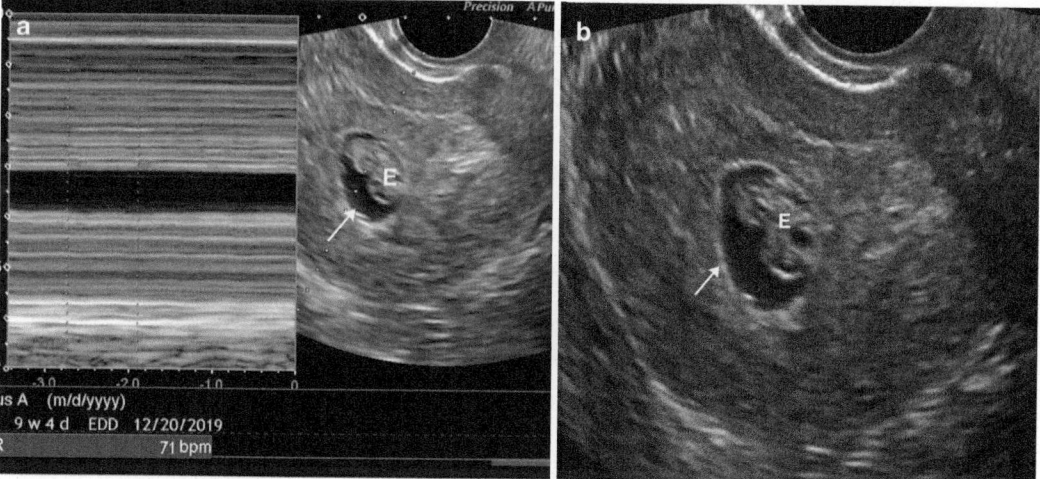

Fig. 8.9 Persistent bradycardia as a poor prognostic factor of a viable IUP. (a) M-mode and (b) associated gray-scale image of the uterus obtained via a transvaginal approach demonstrates persistent bradycardia (FHR = 71 bpm) in a 9-week 4-day gestation. Note abnormal ratio between the relatively large embryo (E) and the relatively small size of the gestational sac (GS) (arrow). The MSD corresponded to a gestational age of 6 weeks and 6 days, and the CRL measurements corresponded to the gestational age of 9 weeks and 4 days. (c) Pregnancy loss was documented on a subsequent follow-up visit several days later. M-mode demonstrated absent cardiac activity

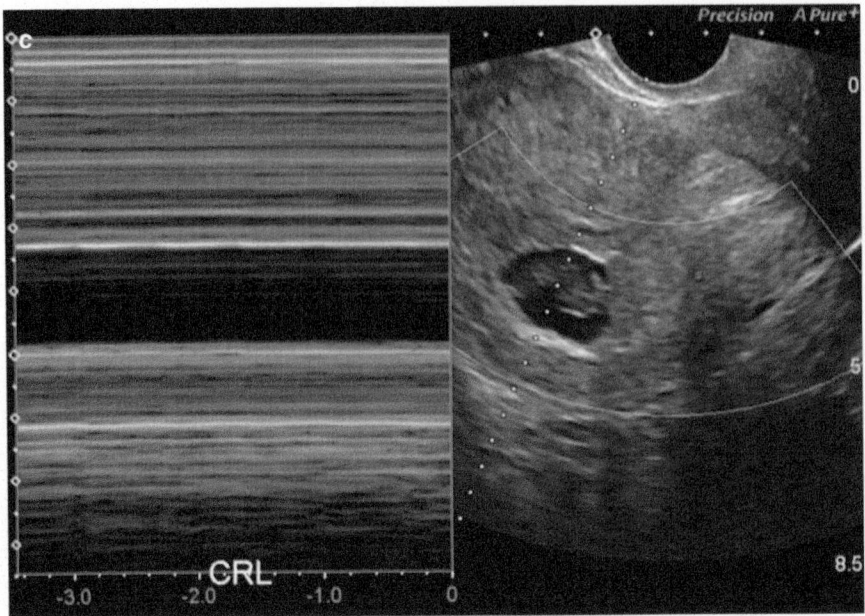

Fig. 8.9 (continued)

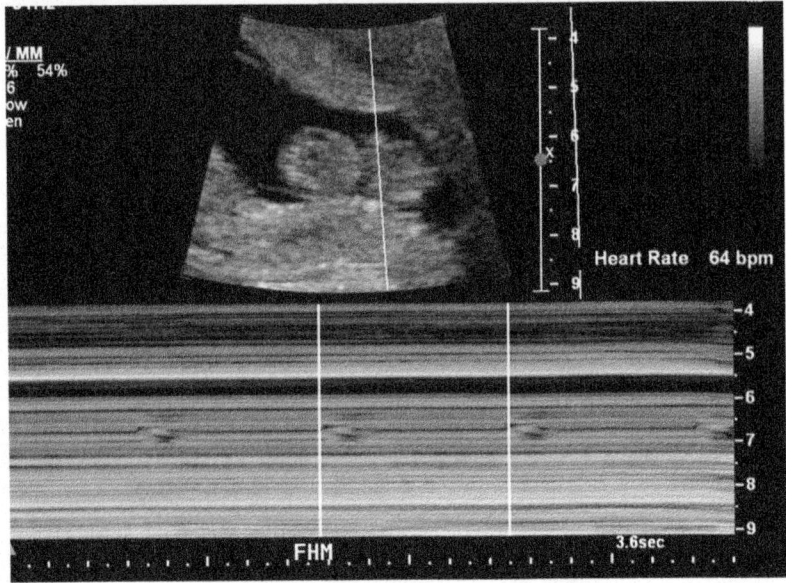

Fig. 8.10 Bradycardia. Intrauterine gestation ectopically positioned in the lower uterine segment in a 26-year-old pregnant woman presented with abdominal cramps. Transvaginal ultrasound was performed that revealed a gestational sac (GS) positioned in the lower uterine seg- ment just superior to the cervical junction (not shown). Based on CRL measurements, the embryo's gestational age was approximately 10 weeks and 2 days. Persistent bradycardia was detected (FHR = 64 bpm)

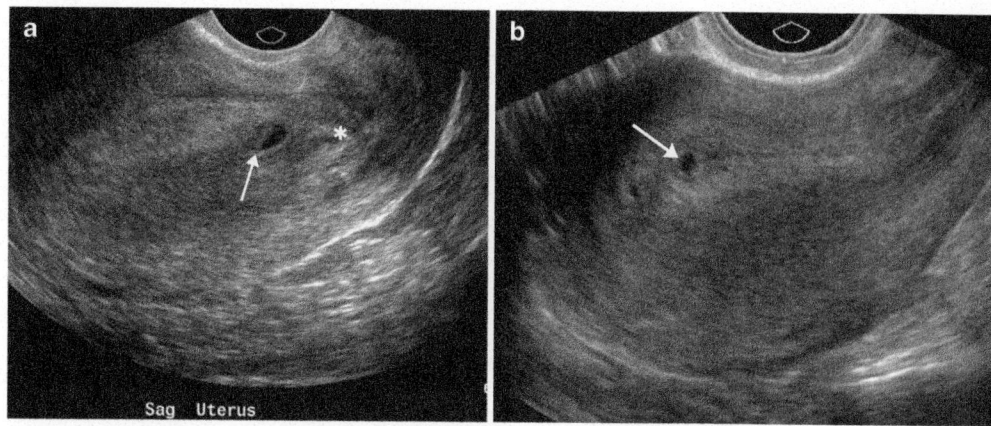

Fig. 8.11 Pregnancy failure in a 23-year-old woman who presented with bleeding and abdominal cramping. (**a**) Sagittal gray-scale transvaginal US image of the uterus demonstrates a cystic space with a small yolk sac within the lower uterine segment (arrow in **a**). No fetal pole or cardiac activity is detected. Complex fluid, likely hemorrhage, is noted within the endometrial canal (asterisk). (**b**) Prior ultrasound obtained 3 days before revealed a intrauterine cystic space in the fundal portion of the endometrial cavity (arrow in **b**). Findings are compatible with passage of a non-viable pregnancy

Table 8.2 Early pregnancy indicators of poor prognosis

Morphological appearance of indicators	Imaging findings of indicators
Gestational sac	Irregular contour, low-lying, mobile on real-time imaging; large size (MSD-GS <5 mm, MSD >2.5 cm)
Yolk sac	Calcified, large (>7 mm)
Amnion	Empty, enlarged
Embryo	Amorphous shape, hydropic change
Cardiac activity	Sustained bradycardia of ≤85 bpm
Chorionic villi	Hydropic change
Subchorionic hemorrhage (SCH)	Large, specifically if encircles greater than 2/3 of the GS circumference. SCH and persistently low fetal cardiac activity (<100 bpm at age of 6 weeks, or <120 bpm at a gestation age of greater than 6.5 weeks)

MSD mean sac diameter, *GS* gestational sac

Table 8.3 Intrauterine pregnancy (IUP) of unknown viability and imaging signs

Intrauterine pregnancy (IUP) of unknown viability	CRL < 7 mm
	MSD 16–24 mm, no embryo (−FP)
	+GS, −YS → follow-up US 7–13 days after a scan shows no embryo (−FP)
	+GS, +YS → follow-up US 7–10 days after a scan shows no embryo (−FP)
	Empty amnion (+YS, −FP), amnion is adjacent to YS
	LMP ≥ 6 weeks before a scan and no embryo (−FP)
	Large yolk sac (>7 mm)
	Sustained bradycardia (<80 bpm)
	Small GS in relation to size of embryo (MSD-CRL < 5 mm)

Note: adapted from Refs. [3, 8]
FP fetal pole, *CRL* crown-rump length, *GS* gestational sac, *MSD* mean sac diameter, *YS* yolk sac, *LMP* last menstrual period

toma, embryonic cardiac activity should also be reported since there is a higher chance of pregnancy failure in those with subchorionic hematoma and low heart rate. Furthermore, large hematomas with the highest rates of failure generally encase at least two-thirds of the GS circumference [45]. The echogenicity of the collection on ultrasound imaging variable depending on the acuity of the hematoma, with more hyperacute or chronic hematomas nearly anechoic, and more acute/subacute hematomas hyperechoic to mixed echogenicity (Fig. 8.14). Patients with a large SH should be closely followed with serial hCG levels and transvaginal ultrasound examinations. Differential diagnosis includes first-trimester incomplete chorioamniotic fusion, intrauterine mass, slow venous flow, and a vanishing twin.

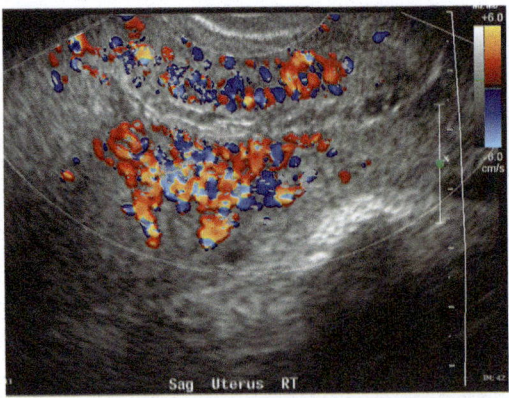

Fig. 8.12 Septic abortion in a 32-year-old woman following dilatation and curettage (D&C) for retained products of conception (RPOC) after elective termination of pregnancy at 11 weeks, who presented with pelvic pain, spotting, fever, and leukocytosis. Color Doppler transvaginal ultrasound image demonstrates marked hyperemia of the endometrium and myometrium. No evidence of retained products of conception is noted. A small amount of a complex fluid is seen within the endometrial cavity. Findings are compatible with septic abortion and endometritis–myometritis

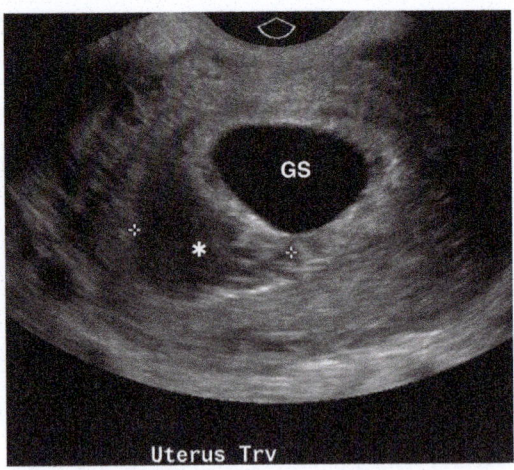

Fig. 8.13 Endovaginal US image shows a large subchorionic hemorrhage (SCH) in a 7-week 0-day gestation in a 37-year-old woman. A large hypoechoic collection (asterisk) separates the chorion from the echogenic decidua, and encircles almost 1/3 of the circumference of the gestational sac (GS). Normal cardiac activity was detected with a FHR of 119 bpm (not shown)

8.2.5 The Chorionic Bump

The chorionic bump is a focal protuberance or solid mass-like structure that bulges from the choriodecidual surface into the GS (Fig. 8.15). It was previously considered a risk factor for nonviability during the first trimester, and had been reported to be associated with a high rate of pregnancy loss of up to 50% [46]. Based on the evolution of sonographic findings associated with this diagnosis, it was postulated that the chorionic bump likely represented sequelae of a small subchorionic bleed, and is thought to be associated with a guarded prognosis [46, 47]. Currently, although it still remains a risk factor for nonviability in pregnancy, most cases are reported to result in a live birth as long as the pregnancy is otherwise normal [48, 49].

8.2.6 Gestational Trophoblastic Disease

Gestational trophoblastic disease (GTD) results from the abnormal proliferation of trophoblastic tissue, and encompasses a wide spectrum of diseases ranging from benign hydatidiform moles

(partial and complete), to malignant invasive moles (10%), placental site trophoblastic tumor, choriocarcinoma, and the rare epithelioid trophoblastic tumor (ETT) (less than 1%) [50].

Although GTD is an uncommon cause of first-trimester bleeding, vaginal bleeding is the most common clinical presentation of early pregnancy [51]. The diagnosis of GTD in the first trimester can be a challenge, as the maternal serum hCG levels may remain within normal limits and the patient may be asymptomatic, with the exception of non-specific vaginal bleeding. It is important to note that only 50% of patients with GTD will develop very high levels of maternal serum hCG levels (>100,000 mIU/ml), and therefore, the absence of this factor does not exclude the diagnosis. It is possible that later in the second trimester, new symptoms develop which are related to excessive uterine growth such as hyperemesis and hypertension. GTD can have somewhat of a variable appearance on ultrasound, depending on the chromosomal composition and anomaly; however, the findings generally overlap between various forms of the disease, and a definitive diagnosis can only be made by pathological assessment. In a *complete molar pregnancy*, a large heterogeneous echogenic mass with multiple tiny cystic channels,

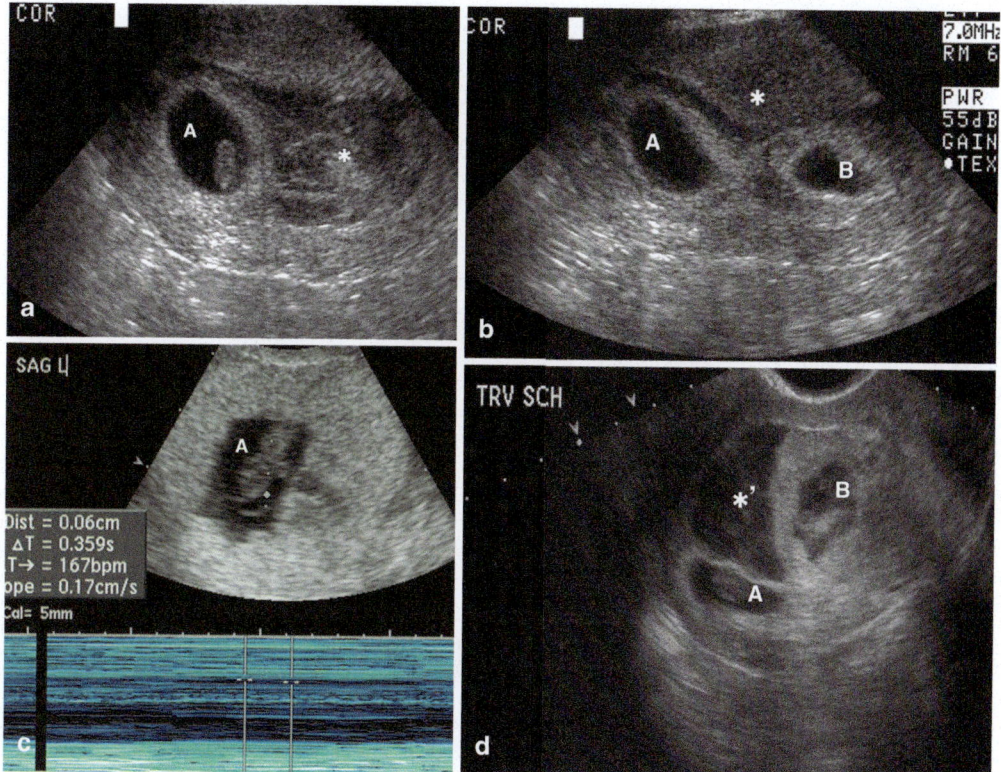

Fig. 8.14 Evolution of the subchorionic hemorrhage in a twin pregnancy. (**a**, **b**) Endovaginal US image shows a large early subacute subchorionic hemorrhage (SCH) in a 6-week 5-day twin gestation. A large iso- to hypoechoic collection (∗ in **a**, **b**) is seen between two gestations, which separates the chorions from the echogenic deciduae, and encircles almost 1/3 of the circumference of each gestational sac (twin A, twin B). (**c**) M-mode image showed tachycardia in both A and B embryos with FHRs of 167 bpm in twin A and 171 bpm in twin B (not shown). (**d**) Follow-up endovaginal ultrasound demonstrated the evolution of the blood products within the SCH, with subacute and chronic blood products appearing more hypoechoic on ultrasound (∗')

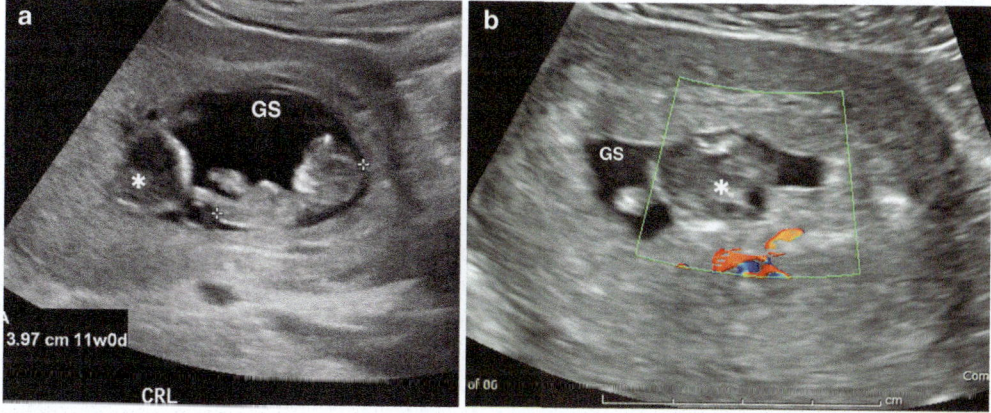

Fig. 8.15 Chorionic bump in a 31-year-old pregnant woman who presented with positive hCG and vaginal bleeding. (**a**) Gray-scale transvaginal ultrasound image demonstrates a single IUP with the CRL of the fetus measuring 3.97 cm, which corresponds to an approximate gestational age of 11 weeks and 0 days. Adjacent to the fetus, there is a convex hypoechoic bulge (asterisk) protruding into the gestational sac (GS) compatible with chorionic bump. (**b**) Color Doppler image demonstrates no vascular flow within the chorionic bump (asterisk)

Fig. 8.16 Complete molar pregnancy in a 24-year-old woman who presented with abdominal pain, and a positive pregnancy test with a hCG levels of greater than 100,000 mIU/ml. (**a**) Gray-scale transvaginal ultrasound image demonstrates an enlarged uterus containing a complex vascular heterogeneous, predominantly hyperechoic, mass with multiple cystic areas expending the endometrial canal (M). Note the cervix is closed (Cx). (**b**) Spectral Doppler shows high-amplitude low-resistance waveforms (PSV = 78.6 cm/s) that usually are associated with placental flow

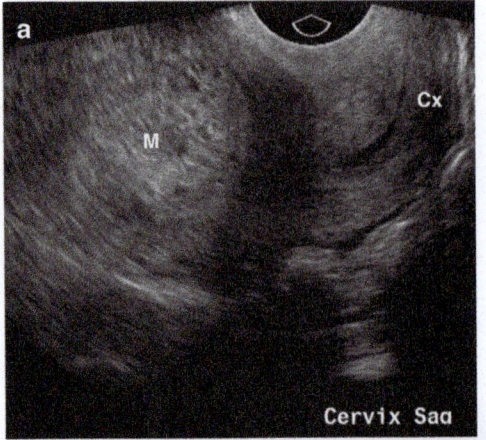

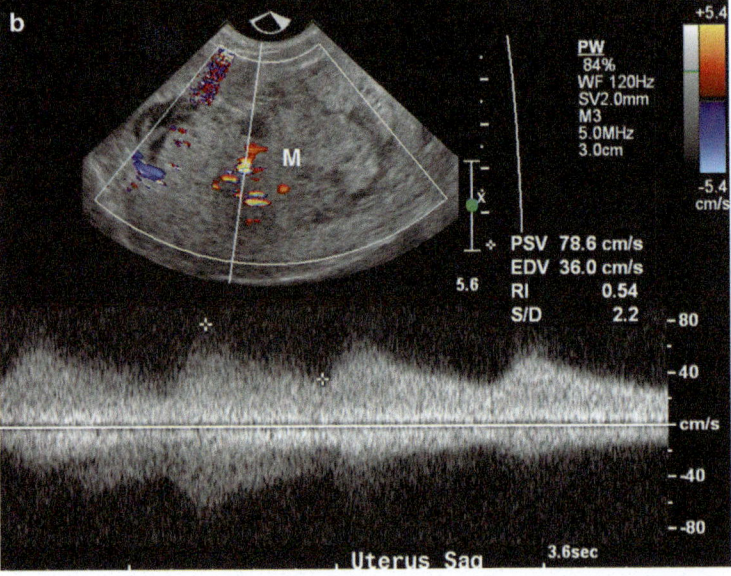

representing hydropic chorionic villa (a.k.a. a "snowstorm appearance" or "cluster of grapes" appearance), is seen on gray-scale. Vascular flow is usually detected on color and spectral Doppler ultrasound, in association with the absence of any fetal parts (unless twin pregnancy) and the presence of high levels of maternal serum hCG levels (Fig. 8.16). Theca-lutein ovarian cysts are a hallmark of molar pregnancy on ultrasound; however, they are identified in fewer than 50% of cases. They present as enlarged overstimulated ovaries, due to high levels of circulating hormones. In cases of a *partial mole*, the sonographic characteristics of the mass include larger cysts and a "Swiss cheese" appearance. In these instances, the fetus has triploidy, which is manifested by growth restriction and fetal malformations (Fig. 8.17) [51,

52]. Partial molar pregnancy may be difficult to differentiate from hydropic degeneration of placenta, which is characterized by intrauterine fetal demise and cystic changes within the degenerating placenta. These two pathologic processes may only be distinguishable on pathological assessment. Patients with an *invasive mole* often demonstrate distortion of the uterine zonal structures, irregularity of the boundary between the tumor and myometrium, and possibly parametrial tissue invasion. However, distant metastases are rare. Theca lutein cysts are also observed (Fig. 8.18). *Gestational choriocarcinoma* may be indistinguishable from a complete mole and may arise from a known molar pregnancy (50%), a failed pregnancy (30%), or a term or ectopic pregnancy (20%) [53]. They can often demonstrate hemor-

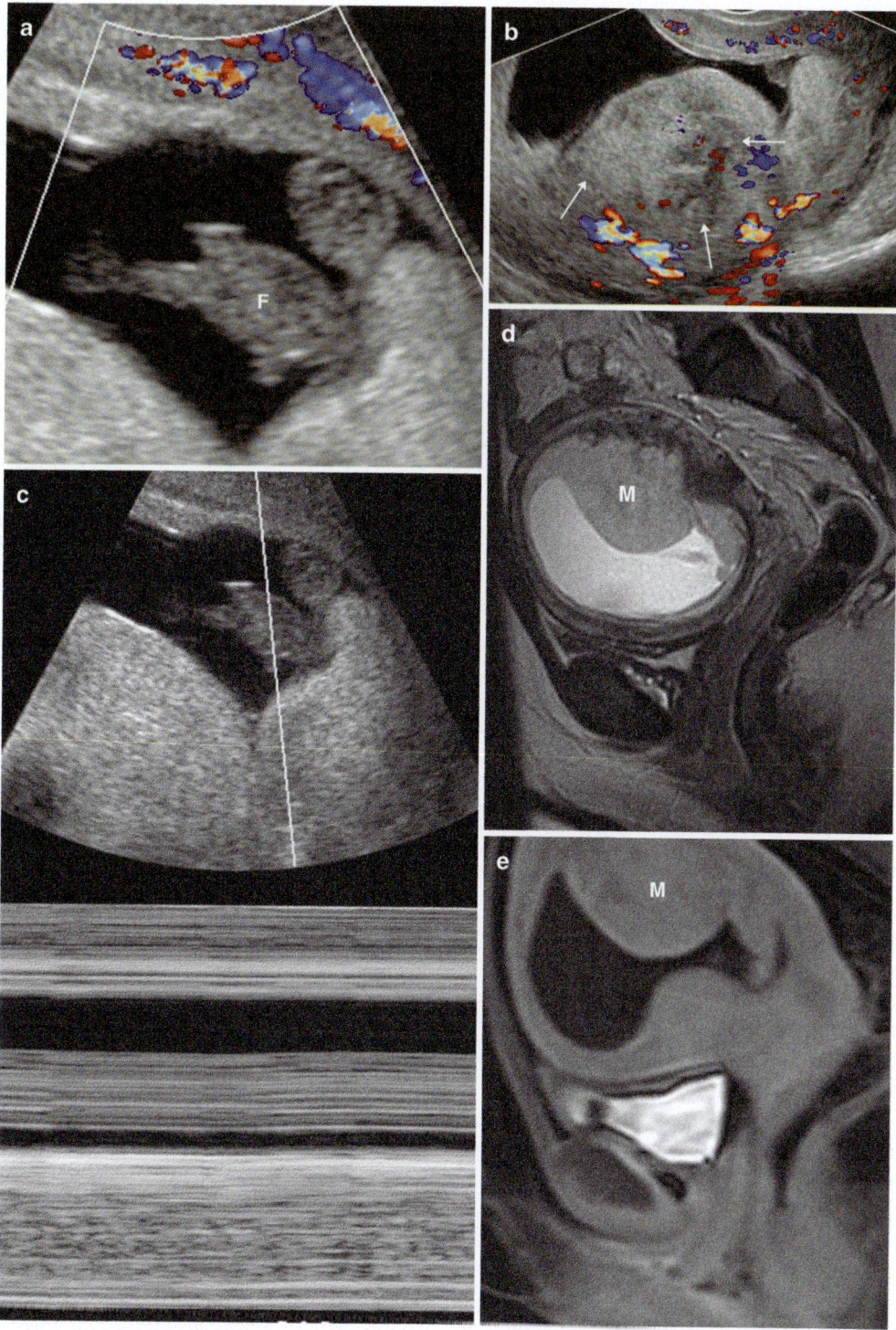

Fig. 8.17 Partial molar pregnancy in a woman presenting with positive pregnancy test. (**a, b**) Transabdominal color Doppler pelvic US images show a dysmorphic fetus (F in **a**) and an enlarged heterogeneous placenta (white arrows in **b**). (**c**) No cardiac activity was detected, compatible with non-viable pregnancy. (**d**) T2-weighted and (**e**) IV contrast-enhanced T1-weighted MRI images obtained in the sagittal plane confirm the diagnosis of a partial molar pregnancy (M in **d, e**). Please note that hydropic degeneration of placenta may have a very similar appearance

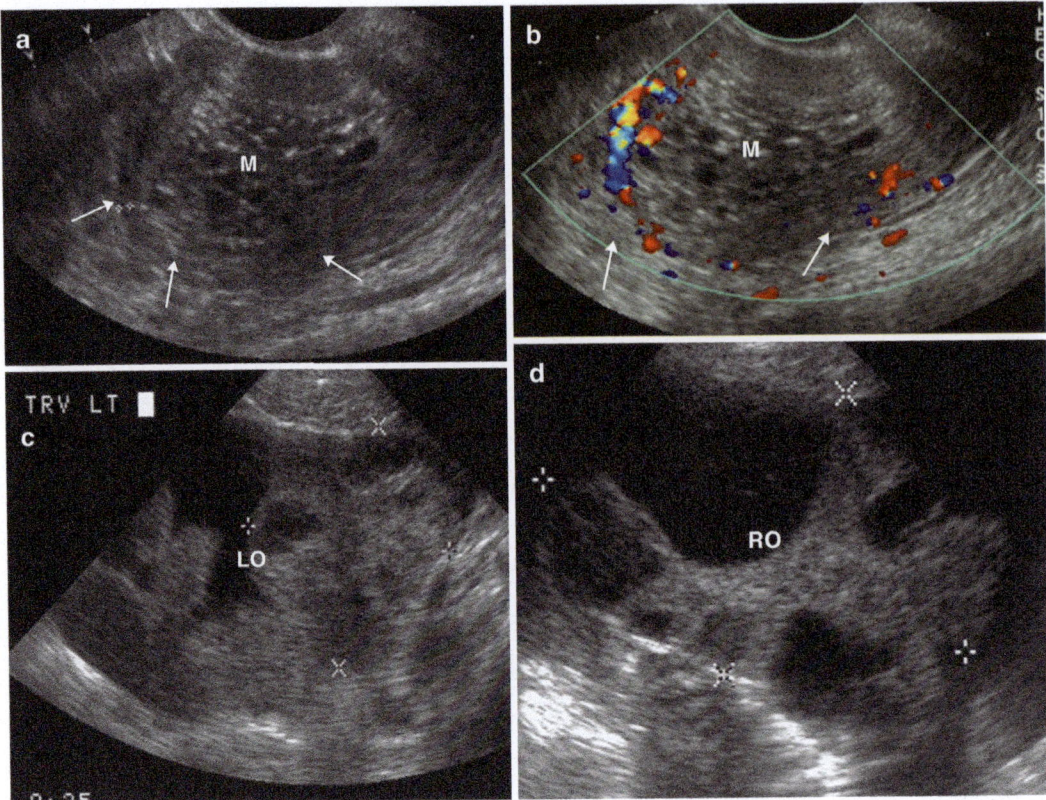

Fig. 8.18 Invasive molar pregnancy in a 35-year-old pregnant woman who presented with vaginal bleeding. (**a**, **b**) Transvaginal gray-scale and color Doppler images show an enlarged uterus containing a vascular complex echogenic mass (M in **a**, **b**) containing multiple cystic areas. The mass is extending into the myometrium with thinning of the myometrium (arrow in **a**, **b**). (**c**, **d**) Gray-scale transvaginal ultrasound images show bilateral enlarged ovaries with multiple theca lutein cysts (*RO* right ovary, *LO* left ovary)

rhagic or necrotic components (Fig. 8.19). Epithelioid tumors can also arise either from term pregnancies or from failed or molar pregnancies, and tend to metastasize locally [4].

Management of these tumors depends on a scoring system developed by the Federation of Gynecology and Obstetrics. Chemotherapy, curettage, and/or hysterectomy are the mainstreams of therapy.

8.2.7 Chorioamnionitis

Chorioamnionitis or intraamniotic infection is an acute inflammation of the membranes and chorion of the placenta, which is typically caused by ascending polymicrobial bacterial infection in the setting of membrane rupture [54]. Although chorioamnionitis more commonly occurs in the second or third trimester, it may also be seen during the first trimester. Causative agents usually represent ascending bacteria from the vaginal tract and may include *Ureaplasma* species and *Mycoplasma hominis*, found in the lower genital tract of over 70% of women. Overall, 1–4% of all births in the US are complicated by chorioamnionitis; [55] however, the frequency of chorioamnionitis varies markedly by diagnostic criteria, specific risk factors, and gestational age [56].

Chorioamnionitis that develops in the first trimester of pregnancy is commonly associated with such risk factors as nulliparity, retained intrauterine devices, African American ethnicity, multiple vaginal examinations, chorionic villous sampling (CVS), amniocentesis, smoking, alcohol and/or drug abuse, immunocompromised states, bacterial vaginosis, sexually transmissible genital infections, and vaginal colonization with ureaplasma [54].

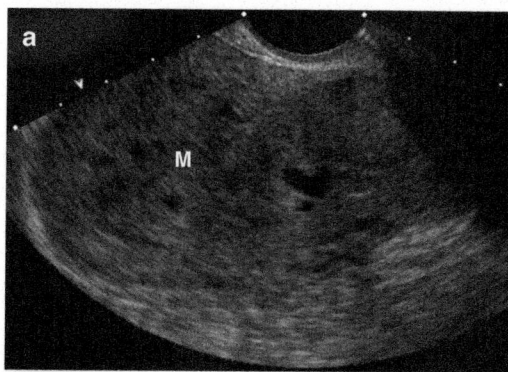

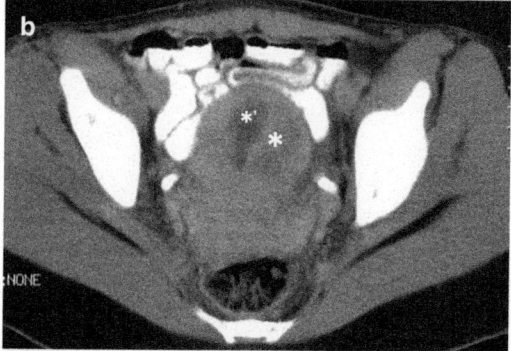

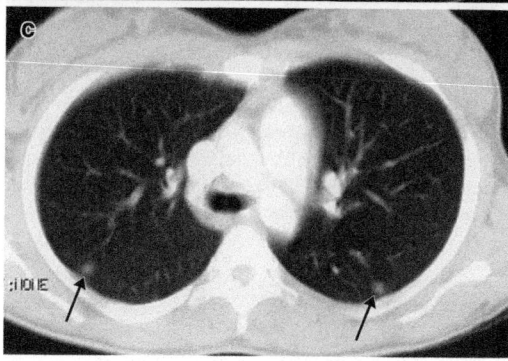

Fig. 8.19 Choriocarcinoma in a woman with positive hCG and shortness of breath. (**a**) Gray-scale transvaginal ultrasound image obtained in the sagittal plane demonstrates a complex heterogeneous uterine mass (M in **a**) that distends the uterine cavity and extends into the myometrium reaching the serosal surface (not shown). Myometrial extension was also confirmed on pathology. (**b**, **c**) IV contrast-enhanced CT images of the pelvis and chest obtained in the axial plane demonstrate thickened heterogeneous uterine myometrium (∗ in **b**) and distended endometrium (∗'). Multiple pulmonary metastases are seen on chest CT (arrows in **c**)

The inflammatory response to the ascending or retrograde passage of the infection to the chorion and umbilical cord of the fetus may produce clinical chorioamnionitis and/or lead to prostaglandin release, ripening of the cervix, membrane injury, and labor at term or premature birth at earlier gestational ages. Aside from the risk of direct fetal infection and sepsis, the fetal inflammatory response may induce cerebral white matter injury. The key clinical findings associated with clinical chorioamnionitis include fever (>100.4 °F) (seen in 95–100% of patients), uterine fundal tenderness (seen in <20%), maternal tachycardia (>100/min) (seen in 50–80%), fetal tachycardia (>160/min) (seen in 40–70%), and purulent or foul amniotic fluid (seen in <25%) [55, 57, 58].

Amniotic cultures demonstrate microbial growth, which is the diagnostic reference standard.

Maternal leukocytosis, defined as WBC greater than 12,000/mm³, is seen in 70–90% of cases of clinical chorioamnionitis. Ultrasound findings include cervical length shortening, presence of debris (or sludge) in the amniotic fluid, oligohydramnios, and increased fetal heart rate of more than 160 bpm. Hyperemia of the uterus may be present, but is non-specific. Prompt initiation of antibiotic therapy is essential to prevent both maternal and fetal complications in the setting of clinical chorioamnionitis.

8.2.8 IUD Failure

Intrauterine devices are commonly used as a means of contraception by women of childbearing age. It is reported that the failure rate of all IUDs is estimated at approximately 1%, with patients becoming pregnant despite an appropriately situated IUD. Patients with an indwelling IUD who become pregnant are prone to a number of complications, including a higher rate of spontaneous pregnancy failure of up to 16% [59, 60], vaginal bleeding, placental abruption, low birth weight fetuses, chorioamnionitis, and pre-term delivery (Fig. 8.20) [59, 61]. Removal of the IUD early in pregnancy is associated with better outcomes. The decision to remove an IUD in the second trimester depends on its association with the placental location or the gestational sac. High risk of spontaneous miscarriage precludes removal of the IUD in the third trimester. Therefore, early assessment of IUD location may have a significant impact on the successful outcome of the pregnancy (Figs. 8.21 and 8.22) [60–62].

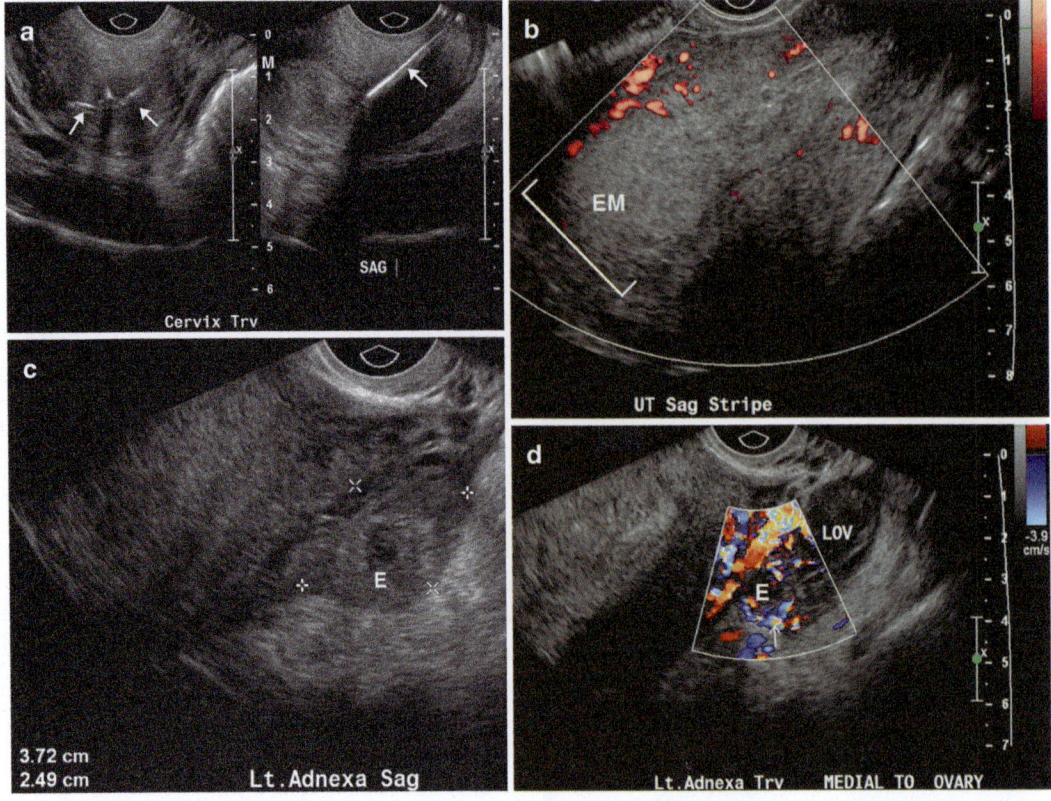

Fig. 8.20 IUD failure with adnexal ectopic pregnancy. (a) Transvaginal US gray-scale image of the uterus obtained in the sagittal and transverse planes demonstrates abnormally low positioning of the IUD in the lower uterine segment, with both limbs embedded within the myometrium (arrows).

(b) Power Doppler image of the uterus in the sagittal plane shows thickening of the fundal endometrium (EM) with no evidence of a gestational sac. (c, d) Gray-scale and color Doppler images of the left adnexa show ectopic pregnancy (E) adjacent to the left ovary (LOV) with peripheral flow

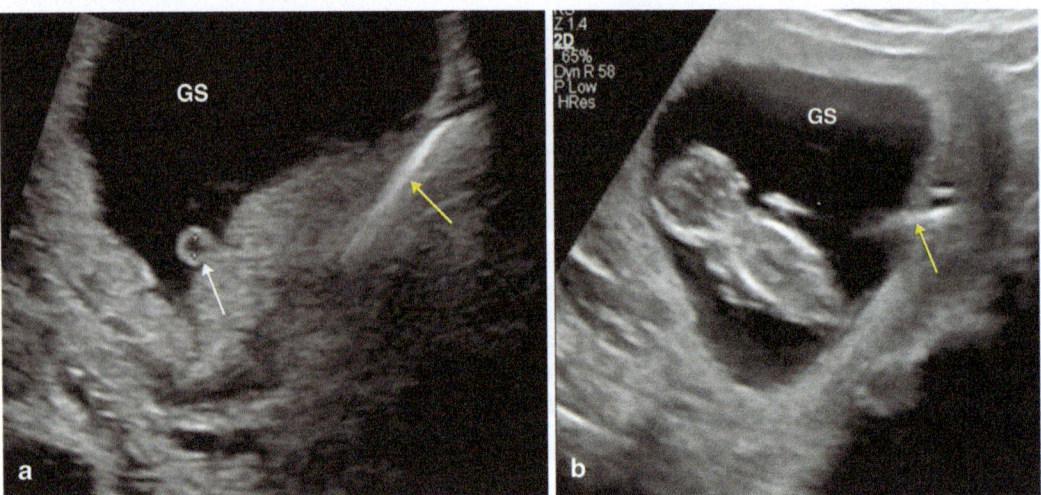

Fig. 8.21 IUD failure with viable IUP. (a) Gray-scale transabdominal US of the pelvis demonstrates IUD within the endometrial canal (yellow arrow in a) adjacent to a gestational sac (GS). A yolk sac is noted (white arrow in a). (b) Part of the

IUD is protruding into the gestational sac, containing a viable fetus (yellow arrow in b). Cardiac activity with a FHR of 144 bpm in this 11-week 5-day gestation was present (not shown). *IUD* intrauterine device, *FHR* fetal heart rate

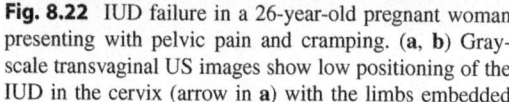

Fig. 8.22 IUD failure in a 26-year-old pregnant woman presenting with pelvic pain and cramping. (**a, b**) Grayscale transvaginal US images show low positioning of the IUD in the cervix (arrow in **a**) with the limbs embedded within the lower uterine segment myometrium (not shown) and an early gestational sac (GS) of approximate gestational age of 5 weeks in the fundal endometrium (arrow in **b**). No yolk sac, fetal pole, or cardiac activity was yet seen

8.2.9   RPOC and AVM

In a first-trimester pregnancy, retained products of conception (RPOC) refer to the persistence of fetal tissue following either a failed pregnancy or an elective/emergent pregnancy termination. The concern for RPOC can be raised if a patient with first-trimester pregnancy failure presents with prolonged abnormal vaginal bleeding and absent or abnormal decline of maternal serum hCG levels. Pathologically, RPOC are characterized by the presence of chorionic villi, representing embryonic tissue that attaches to the decidua basalis of the endometrium and contains placental tissue as well as fetal capillaries. The incidence rate of RPOC is 3–5% following spontaneous vaginal deliveries [63]. Clinically, first-trimester patients usually present with abdominal pain and cramping as well as substantial vaginal bleeding. On occasion, RPOC may serve as a nidus of infection resulting in the development of fever. On ultrasound, RPOC can be diagnosed based on the presence of an echogenic or heterogeneous focal endometrial mass, or an area of endometrial thickening, demonstrating internal vascularity (Fig. 8.23). Spectral Doppler ultrasound can be helpful to differentiate placental flow within the RPOC from myometrial flow, with RPOC demonstrating peak systolic velocities over 21 cm/s (placental flow) when compared to lower peak systolic

velocity flow in the myometrium [64]. Kamaya et al. graded the presence or absence of vascularity within the suspected RPOC in order to differentiate this potentially harmful entity from a more benign blood clot [65]. They found that type 3 and type 4 vascularity were more commonly associated with RPOC than with a blood clot. Real-time evaluation with adjusting patient position during scanning may also help to differentiate mobile clot and intraluminal endometrial debris from RPOC [66]. Additional diagnostic considerations include increased flow in the myometrial tissue as a response to a developing fetus and the life-threatening condition of an arteriovenous fistula or malformation (AVM).

A diagnosis of RPOC can be accurately achieved when a combination of findings is utilized, including clinical presentation and history, laboratory results, and sonographic findings. RPOC are managed either medically, via the administration of a prostaglandin E1 analog, or surgically by means of curettage or hysteroscopic removal [4].

AVMs are usually associated with the presence of multiple enlarged serpentine vascular channels within the myometrium that may extend into the endometrium, without a large soft-tissue component. AVMs demonstrate low-resistance high-amplitude waveforms, with occasionally identifiable feeding arteries and draining veins (Fig. 8.24). AVMs are most commonly associated

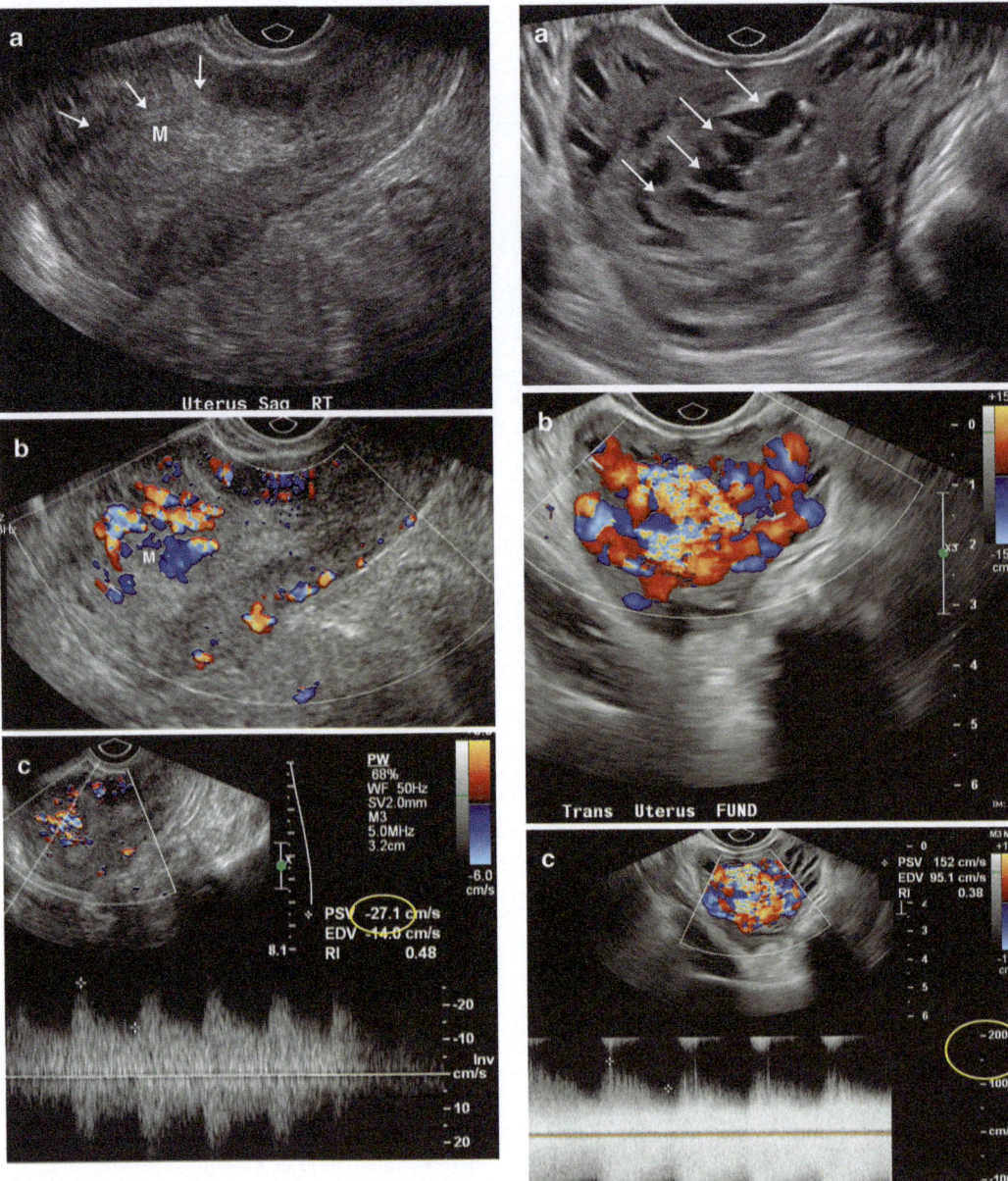

Fig. 8.23 Retained products of conception (RPOC) in a 41-year-old woman presenting with abdominal pain, cramping and massive vaginal bleeding, and positive hCG of 300 mIU/ml. (**a, b**) Gray-scale and color Doppler transvaginal ultrasound images obtained in the sagittal plane show an echogenic vascular mass (M) within the fundal endometrium. Substantial flow is noted within the anterior fundal endometrium. Note the irregular endometrial junction (arrows in **a**). (**c**) Spectral Doppler interrogation of the RPOC demonstrates a PSV of 27 cm/s (yellow circle) compatible with placental flow

Fig. 8.24 Arteriovenous malformation (AVM) in a 36-year-old woman following dilation and curettage (D&C) who presented with massive vaginal bleeding for 3 days. (**a, b**) Gray-scale and color Doppler transvaginal US images obtained in the sagittal (**a**) and transverse (**b**) planes demonstrate multiple serpiginous anechoic spaces in the endometrium and myometrium (arrows in **a**) that fill with color on color Doppler. (**c**) Spectral Doppler image of the uterus shows low-resistance very high amplitude waveforms compatible with arteriovenous shunting (PSV = 152 cm/s, yellow circle)

with a history of prior dilatation and curettage (D&C). If an AVM is suspected, management typically involves either confirmation with MRI or administration of a longer course of uterotonics with possible embolization.

8.3 Ectopic Pregnancy

Ectopic pregnancy (EP) is defined as implantation of a fertilized oocyte outside of the body of the uterus. Ectopic pregnancies account for 1–2% of spontaneous conceptions and 2–5% of pregnancies achieved through assisted reproductive technology [12, 67]. Despite the significant decline in maternal mortality rates over the last five decades, ectopic pregnancy continues to be the leading cause of maternal death during the first trimester, with approximately 2.6 deaths per 10,000 pregnancies. In 2011–2013, ruptured ectopic pregnancy accounted for 2.7% of all pregnancy-related deaths, and was the leading cause of hemorrhage-related mortality [68–72].

Several risk factors increase the likelihood of developing an ectopic pregnancy, including a prior history of pelvic inflammatory disease, prior surgery, endometriosis, use of intrauterine devices, history of prior ectopic gestations, assisted reproductive technology, infertility, smoking, congenital uterine anomalies, and advanced maternal age [68]. Clinical presentation is variable, with the classic signs of amenorrhea, pelvic pain, and vaginal bleeding seen in

less than 50% of patients with confirmed EP [12, 73, 74]. The extent of vaginal bleeding is variable and may be confused with fetal loss. Clinical presentation, laboratory tests including maternal serum hCG levels, and transvaginal ultrasound all play crucial roles in the initial evaluation and diagnosis of this condition. Ectopic pregnancies are classified according to the location of the implanted blastocyst (see Fig. 8.25).

8.3.1 Tubal Pregnancy

The fallopian tubes are the most common site of an ectopic pregnancy. They account for 93–98% of all ectopics, of which 13% are isthmic, 75% ampullary, and 12% fimbrial [75–77]. Although the etiology of tubal ectopic pregnancy is not entirely clear, it has been proposed that this pathological process results from a combination of impaired embryo-tubal transport and environmental changes within the tube that result in early implantation [78, 79]. Tubal damage following surgery and/or prior tubal infection, especially with *Chlamydia trachomatis*, are the main risk factors of tubal pregnancy [77, 78]. However, the aforementioned risk factors do not always correlate with an ectopic pregnancy; many women without risk factors develop tubal ectopics, and many women with risk factors do not develop EP. Clinical presentation may be variable, ranging from asymptomatic to the classic presentation described above, to other less frequently

Fig. 8.25 Diagram of uterus with demonstration of various sites of ectopic pregnancies and statistics of occurrence

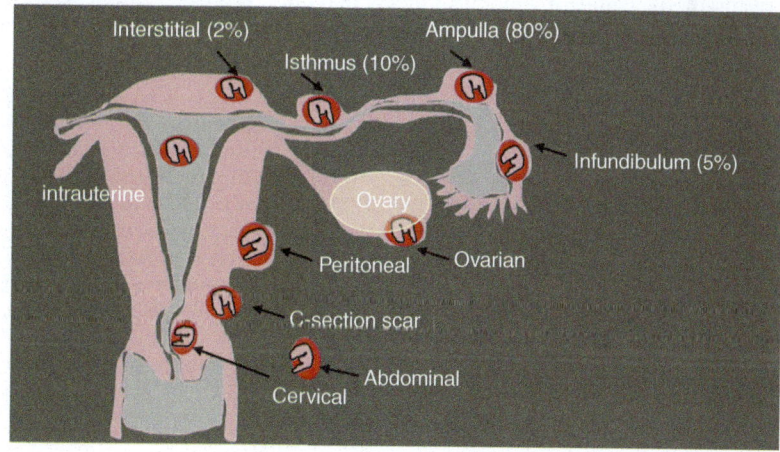

seen clinical signs including nausea, vomiting, and diarrhea. Therefore, the diagnosis of EP should be considered in all women of reproductive age presenting with a sudden onset of abdominal pain or gastrointestinal symptoms [80].

Sonographic features of a tubal ectopic pregnancy include a tubal ring-shaped focus with an echogenic thick wall and an internal cystic space that may or may not contain a yolk sac and/or embryo that may or may not demonstrate cardiac activity. The presence of a yolk sac, cardiac activity, and/or an embryo definitively establishes a diagnosis of ectopic pregnancy (Fig. 8.26). Other sonographic appearances may be slightly atypical, and are characterized by the presence of a solid adnexal hyperechoic or heterogeneous mass, making the diagnosis more challenging. Free fluid is often associated with EP, either in the adnexa or the cul-de-sac. Differential considerations should include hemorrhagic or an enlarged corpus luteum (Fig. 8.27). A key to establishing the correct diagnosis is the real-time transvaginal assessment of a suspicious adnexal mass, with the employment of a compression technique to mobilize the ovary. This determines if the mass moves together with or independent from the ovary when pressure is applied, thereby allowing distinction of an adnexal mass from one originating from the ovary [4]. Although both tubal ectopic pregnancies and corpus lutea usually demonstrate a peripheral "ring-of-fire" pattern of flow on color Doppler ultrasound, vascularity is substantially more apparent in a corpus luteum [81]. The positive predictive value of a mobile adnexal mass in a symptomatic patient with a positive serum hCG levels and no intrauterine pregnancy is over 90% [82, 83]. With improving expertise and equipment, the sensitivity of transvaginal ultrasound has become substantially greater than ultrasound using a transabdominal approach [84]. The management of tubal ectopic pregnancy either involves the use of systemic MTX therapy or laparoscopic resection of the EP. MTX treatment is a more cost-effective therapy, and offers preservation of fertility in most affected patients.

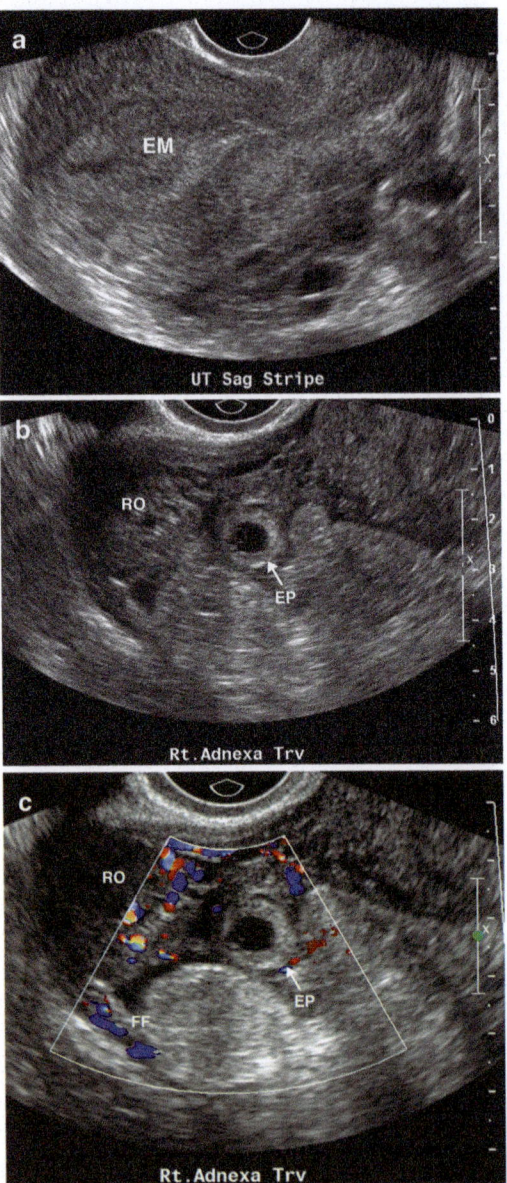

Fig. 8.26 Tubal ectopic pregnancy in a 28-year-old woman who presented with pelvic pain and a positive pregnancy test. (**a**) Gray-scale transvaginal ultrasound image obtained in the sagittal plane demonstrates a thickened endometrium with no evidence of intrauterine pregnancy (EM in **a**). (**b**, **c**) Gray-scale and color Doppler transvaginal ultrasound image of the right adnexa demonstrates a cystic space surrounded by an echogenic ring, compatible with tubal ectopic pregnancy (EP in **b**, **c**). Note that the right ovary (RO in **b**, **c**) is separated by echogenic fat from the ectopically located gestational sac (EP). No fetal pole or yolk sac is seen within. A trace of complex fluid (FF in **c**) is seen in the right adnexa

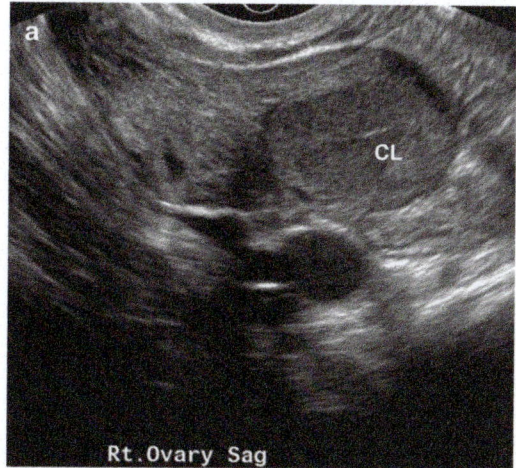

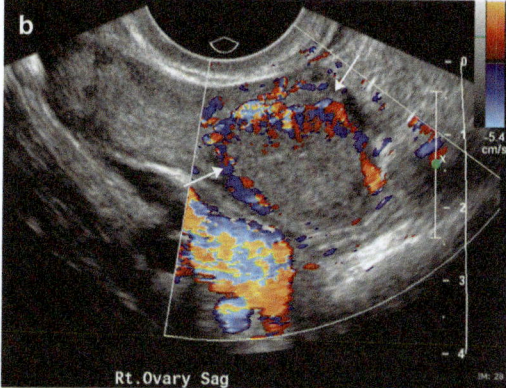

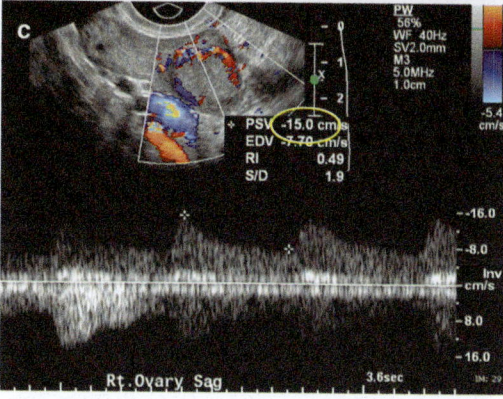

8.3.1.1 Unilateral Twin Tubal Ectopic Pregnancy

Unilateral twin tubal ectopic pregnancy is characterized by presence of two gestational sacs ectopically positioned within a fallopian tube. This type of ectopic pregnancy is very rare, with an incidence rate of less than 0.5% [85]. Patients undergoing *in vitro* fertilization have a higher rate of developing twin ectopic pregnancy, and therefore, the level of suspicion should be high. On ultrasound, two adjacent echogenic-walled rings are identified with or without fetal embryos, yolk sacs, or cardiac activity.

8.3.2 Other Locations of Ectopic Pregnancies

Other types of ectopic pregnancies account for fewer than 10% of all ectopic gestations, and can be divided into five main subcategories: interstitial, heterotopic, cervical, C-section scar, ovarian, and abdominal ectopic. Both abdominal and ovarian ectopic pregnancies are extremely rare.

8.3.3 Heterotopic Pregnancy

Heterotopic pregnancy is defined as the coexistence of intrauterine and extrauterine pregnancies (Fig. 8.28). The incidence depends on whether the pregnancy was a result of assisted reproductive techniques or developed by natural conception. In the former, the incidence rate can be as high as 1 in 100 [86], with the risk increasing in proportion to the number of embryos transferred by *in vitro* fertilization (IVF). If more than four embryos are transferred, the risk has been reported to be as high as 1 in 45 [87]. If the pregnancy is a result of natural conception, the incidence is much lower, approximately 1 in 30,000 pregnancies. Management consists of minimally invasive procedures including the intracardiac injection of minimally invasive procedures including the potassium chloride (KCl) and/or local injection of MTX for selective termination of the ectopic pregnancy and preservation of the IUP. It is

Fig. 8.27 Hemorrhagic corpus luteum in a 24-year-old pregnant woman who presented with abdominal pain. (**a**) Gray-scale and (**b**) color Doppler transvaginal US images show a complex solid-appearing corpus luteum (CL in **a**) that resembles and ovarian ectopic pregnancy. Peripheral flow is seen on color Doppler (arrow in **b**). (**c**) Spectral Doppler interrogation of the corpus luteum periphery shows low-resistance waveforms with PSV of 15 cm/s (yellow circle)

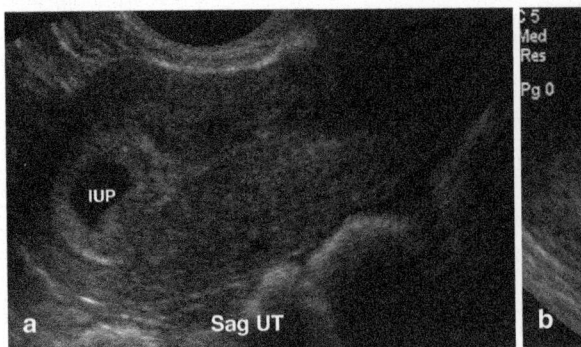
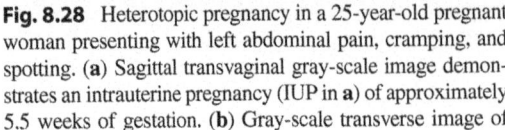
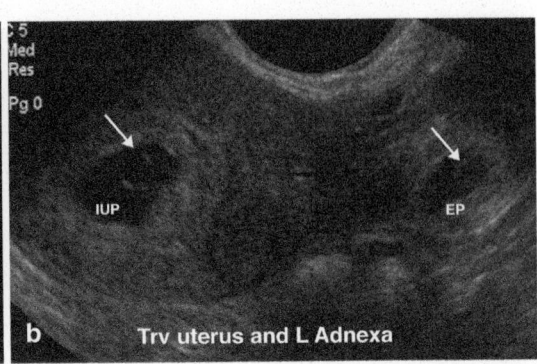

Fig. 8.28 Heterotopic pregnancy in a 25-year-old pregnant woman presenting with left abdominal pain, cramping, and spotting. (**a**) Sagittal transvaginal gray-scale image demonstrates an intrauterine pregnancy (IUP in **a**) of approximately 5.5 weeks of gestation. (**b**) Gray-scale transverse image of the uterus demonstrates an IUP containing a yolk sac (arrow in **b**). No fetal pole or fetal heart rate is yet seen. An additional gestational sac is also seen in the left adnexa, compatible with a tubal ectopic pregnancy (EP) of similar gestational age with only the yolk sac seen (arrow)

important to remember that visualizing an IUP does not exclude the presence of an additional pregnancy elsewhere in the pelvis, especially if the pregnancy is the result of an IVF [88].

8.3.4 Interstitial Ectopic Pregnancy

Interstitial ectopic pregnancies (IEP) account for 2–4% of all ectopics, and represent the most common site of non-tubal pregnancies. In these instances, the implantation of the gestational sac occurs in the interstitial (intra-myometrial) portion of the fallopian tube as it traverses the uterus at the level of the muscular wall of the uterine cornu, a.k.a. at the junction of the fallopian tube with the uterus. This area can accommodate the growth of an ectopic pregnancy more than any other location due to the ability of the tissues at this location to expand or stretch. Additionally, since the GS is located in the close proximity to the intra-myometrial arcuate vasculature, rupture of the ectopic sac can result in massive hemorrhage with a consequent maternal mortality rate 15 times higher than in other tubal ectopic pregnancies [89]. Specifically, the mortality rate associated with IEP is 2.5%, compared to 0.4% with other EPs. The main risk factor for developing an IEP is a history of prior intrauterine instrumentation.

On ultrasound examination, it is important to correctly identify the interstitial segment of the fallopian tube, which is best seen in transverse plane at the fundus of the uterus as a thin echogenic line extending from the endometrial canal through the myometrium to the uterine serosa. In IEP, the GS is implanted at and within this echogenic line with minimal surrounding myometrium (less than 5 mm thickness) in all imaging planes around the GS (aka the "myometrial mantle"). The "interstitial line sign" refers to a line that extends from the ectopically positioned GS to the endometrial canal, with a reported sensitivity of (80%) and specificity of (98%) [90]. The location of the GS outside of the endometrial cavity (extra-endometrial) is the key imaging finding (Fig. 8.29). 3D ultrasound performed in the coronal plane may be particularly helpful for accurately assessing the location of the GS and establishing the correct diagnosis.

There has been some confusion with the terminology applied to ectopic pregnancies, specifically with regard to cornual, interstitial, and angular EPs. A *cornual ectopic* pregnancy usually refers to a pregnancy that arises in a cornua of a morphologically abnormal uterus, such as in case of unicornuate, bicornuate, or septate uterus (Fig. 8.30). An *interstitial ectopic* pregnancy is located lateral to the round ligament in the interstitial segment of the fallopian tube. An *angular ectopic pregnancy* is located very high in the uterine cavity but technically still remains within the endometrium, medial to the uterotubal junction, which at laparoscopy is shown to result in upward and outward displacement of the round ligament reflection [91]. Angular pregnancies are

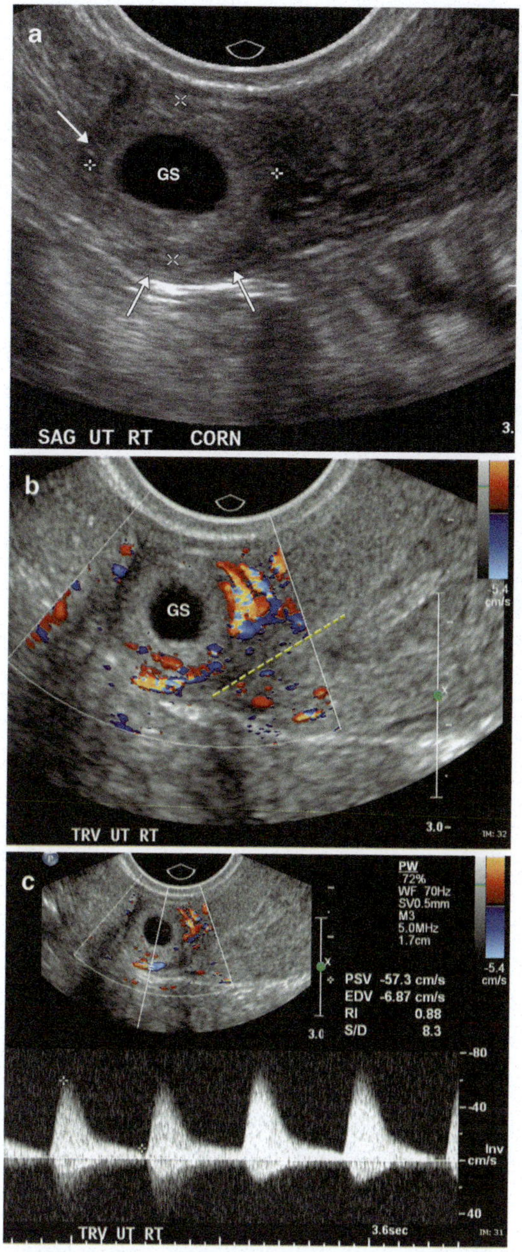

Fig. 8.29 Interstitial ectopic pregnancy in a 37-year-old woman with abdominal pain and positive hCG. (**a**) Gray-scale transvaginal ultrasound image demonstrates a gestational sac (GS) located high in the fundus of the uterus which is completely surrounded by myometrium (myometrial mantle sign, arrows in **a**) with associated abnormal protrusion of the uterine contour (bulging sing). (**b**) Color Doppler image shows peritrophoblastic flow around the GS and the "interstitial line sign", manifested by an echogenic line extending from the endometrium to the interstitial ectopic pregnancy (dashed yellow line). (**c**) Spectral Doppler reveals placental high amplitude blood flow (PSV = 57 cm/s)

considered on a spectrum between normally positioned pregnancies and interstitial pregnancies, and therefore require serial follow-up ultrasound examinations to ensure the correct diagnosis. The majority of suspected angular pregnancies will declare themselves to be normal in location on subsequent US examinations [91]. In practice, very few true angular pregnancies will continue to survive, and there is a high risk of maternal mortality as well [92].

Management of an interstitial ectopic pregnancy includes the use of MTX (either systemic or local), KCl injection into the sac, conservative laparoscopic surgery, uterine artery embolization, cornuectomy, or hysterectomy. The latter two treatment options are usually reserved for emergent situations or when other less invasive methods have failed. Uterine rupture is the most dangerous complication of an IEP, usually occurring by the second trimester, and is associated with an increased likelihood of massive hemorrhage.

8.3.5 C-Section Scar Ectopic Pregnancy

Cesarean scar ectopic pregnancy occurs when a blastocyst implants at the anterior wall in the lower uterine segment at the site of a cesarean scar. It is one of the rare forms of ectopic pregnancy with an incidence rate of less than <1% [93–96]. The main risk factor for a cesarean scar pregnancy is a history of prior C-section, with over 72% of cases seen in women who have had two or more cesarean deliveries [93, 95, 97]. The predisposing cause is thought to be due to the poor vascular supply to the lower uterine segment, leading to incomplete wound healing and resultant formation of focal dehiscent tracts, allowing an opportunity for the GS to implant improperly [98]. There are a number of devastating complications that are associated with this type of ectopic pregnancy, such as development of placenta previa/accreta, uterine rupture, and massive hemorrhage, all of which are responsible for the very high morbidity and mortality associated with this pathology [99]. Uterine rupture and hemorrhage are due to anterior growth of the intramural GS, which can lead to further

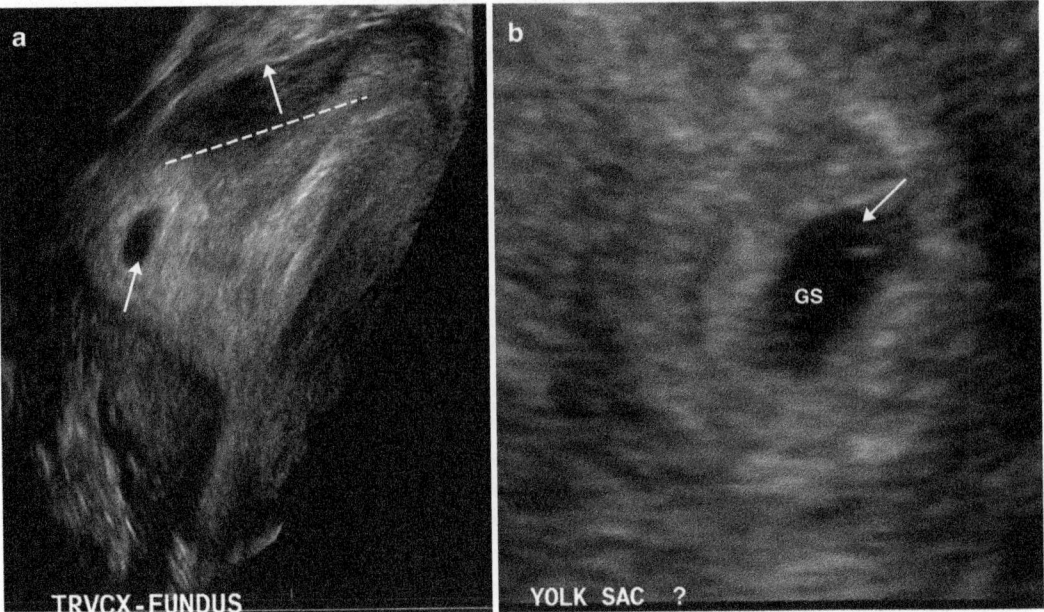

Fig. 8.30 Cornual ectopic pregnancy in a 40-year-old pregnant woman with partially septate uterus. (**a**) Coronal 3D transvaginal ultrasound images demonstrate an isoechoic muscular septum extending from the fundal portion of the uterus to the mid-uterus. The apex of the fundal contour of the uterus is convex (>5 mm above a dashed line drawn between the tubal ostia, arrow above the dashed line). A 5.5-week gestational sac (GS) is located in the right cornua of the uterus (arrow). (**b**) Magnified gray-scale image of the gestational sac (GS) shows a small yolk sac within it (arrow in **b**). The double decidual sign is noted in (**b**)

dehiscence of the hysterotomy scar. Posterior growth of the GS results in intraluminal extension of the GS, thus challenging the ability of the radiologist to establish an accurate diagnosis. Up to 40% of cesarean pregnancies present with vague non-specific symptoms [100]. C-section scar ectopic pregnancies may therefore go undiagnosed and present at a later stage of pregnancy or due to arising complications. Early recognition as well as prompt medical or surgical management is the key to reducing maternal complications and mortality. Although these types of pregnancies can present at any time from implantation and very rarely even to term, they most commonly present in the first trimester. Patients with this condition may be asymptomatic, with the diagnosis made while performing an ultrasound in the provider's office, or if symptomatic, may present with vaginal bleeding and/or abdominal pain and cramping.

On sonography, cesarean scar pregnancies can be recognized when a GS is noted at the level of the C-section scar. The sagittal plane of imaging is best for visualizing the lower uterine segment scar. A characteristic triangu-

lar shape of the GS and its extension to the anterior serosa surface of the uterus are the commonly noted findings (Fig. 8.31) [4, 96]. The presence of peritrophoblastic flow and echogenic margins of the GS may also be evident. Depending on the gestational age, the GS may be empty or contain a yolk sac and/or embryo with possible cardiac activity. Apparent thinning of the myometrium is seen anterior to the sac. In the cases of cesarean scar ectopic, the intracardiac injection of KCl or intracardiac and/or systemic injection of MTX are the preferred methods of treatment.

8.3.6 Cervical Ectopic Pregnancy

Cervical ectopic pregnancy, which occurs due to implantation of the blastocyst within the endocervical canal, is quite rare, and accounts for fewer than 1% of all ectopic pregnancies. The risk factors for this diagnosis include prior D&C, prior interventions, and the presence of an IUD [68, 101–103]. The clinical presentation is similar to

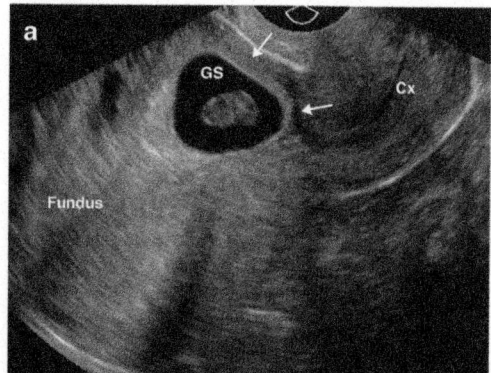

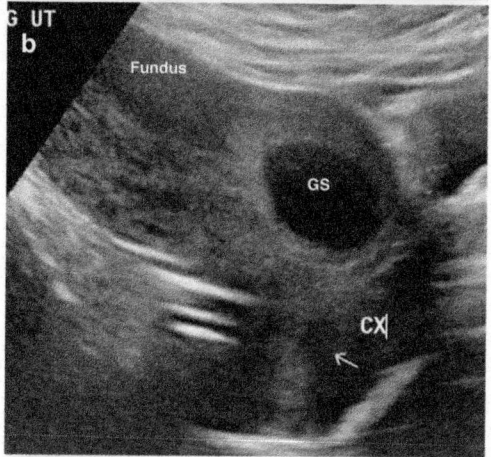

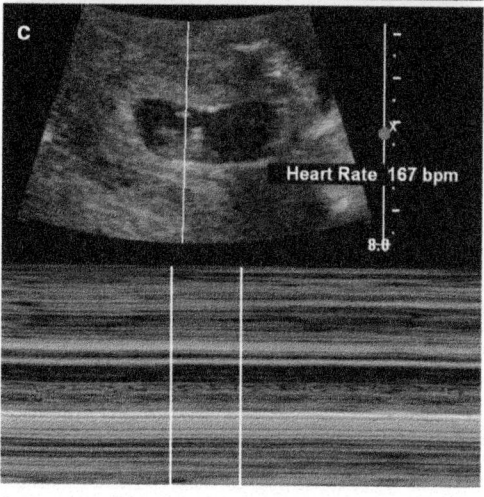

other types of ectopic pregnancies, with patients presenting to the emergency department with the complaints of vaginal bleeding, pain, and a positive pregnancy test. Sonographic assessment is the key to diagnosis of a GS within the endocervical canal (Fig. 8.32). It is important to differentiate a cervical ectopic pregnancy from an on-going spontaneous abortion, which relies on the availability of prior imaging demonstrating an IUP. In addition, fetal cardiac activity and vascular flow around the GS may only be detected in a cervical ectopic pregnancy and not associated with a miscarriage. In the case of a cervical ectopic, the GS is usually well formed with a smooth contour, whereas in abortion in progress, the gestational sac is typically deformed and mobile within the endometrial canal. This phenomenon can be observed on real-time transvaginal imaging when gentle pressure is applied by the US probe. Echogenic blood products distending the endometrial canal may also be evident (Fig. 8.33). The internal and external cervical os are usually closed with a cervical ectopic, whereas the internal cervical os is usually opened to allow passage of the aborted gestation. If the diagnosis is uncertain in a hemodynamically stable patient, a limited and directed close interval follow-up ultrasound examination can be performed in 24–48 h. Hemodynamically stable patients may undergo medical treatment; however, unstable patients are usually treated with surgery [4]. It is important to understand that misdiagnosis of a cervical ectopic pregnancy as an abortion in progress may be devastating as incorrect diagnosis may lead to wrong choice in management, such as D&C, resulting in massive life-threatening hemorrhage secondary to trophoblastic invasion of the cervix and lack of musculature in the cervical wall to allow hemostasis [103].

Fig. 8.31 Cesarean scar in a 32-year-old woman with history of prior cesarean section now with positive pregnancy test. (**a**) Gray-scale sagittal transvaginal ultrasound image shows a viable gestational sac (GS) of approximate gestational age of 7 weeks and 4 days located in the anterior lower uterine segment, with thinning of the overlying anterior myometrium (arrows) representing a cesarean section scar. Fetal heart rate was 167 bpm (not shown). (**b**) Gray-scale transabdominal US shows an empty uterine fundus and the cervical canal (arrow, Cx). (**c**) Magnified image with M-mode shows fetal heart rate of 147 bpm

8.3.7 Intramural Ectopic Pregnancy

Intramural ectopic pregnancy refers to implantation of the GS within the uterine myometrium. It is surrounded by myometrium in all imaging planes, and lies separately from the endometrial canal and fallopian tubes. The incidence rate is less than 1% of all ectopic pregnancies. Just as

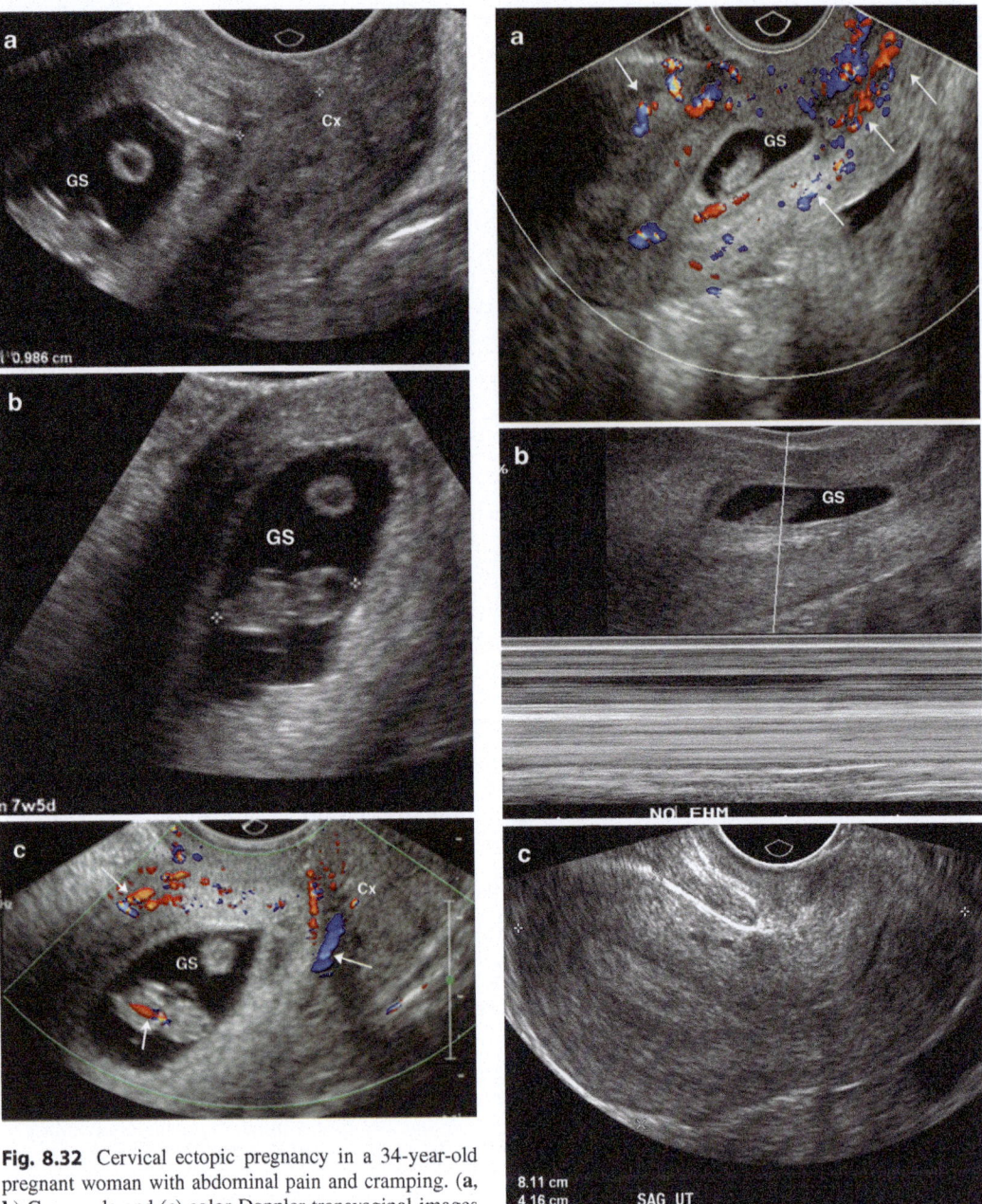

Fig. 8.32 Cervical ectopic pregnancy in a 34-year-old pregnant woman with abdominal pain and cramping. (**a**, **b**) Gray-scale and (**c**) color Doppler transvaginal images demonstrate an ectopically-located gestational sac (GS in **a**–**c**) situated within the endocervical canal (Cx in **a**) with a viable fetus of approximate gestational age of 7 weeks and 5 days. Color Doppler image demonstrates vascular flow within the fetal aorta and peritrophoblastic vascular flow (arrows in **c**)

Fig. 8.33 Cervical ectopic pregnancy versus spontaneous miscarriage in progress in a 19-year-old woman presenting with cramping and vaginal bleeding. (**a**) Color Doppler transvaginal US image in the sagittal plane demonstrates a somewhat deformed and irregular gestational sac (GS in **a**, **b**) containing a fetus. Vascular flow is seen in the uterine myometrium and cervical stroma (arrows in **a**), but no peritrophoblastic vascular flow or flow within the fetus is seen. (**b**) M-Mode image shows the absence of cardiac activity in the fetus. (**c**) Follow-up gray-scale transvaginal US image in the sagittal plane obtained 3 days later shows an empty uterus compatible with a completed miscarriage

with other ectopic pregnancies, intramural ectopic pregnancy presents with abdominal pain, bloating, and a positive maternal serum hCG levels. Factors that predispose to development of intramural pregnancy include adenomyosis, *in vitro* fertilization, defective trophoblastic activity, and previous uterine trauma such as dilation and curettage or myomectomy [104].

8.3.8 Ovarian Pregnancy

An ovarian pregnancy refers to an ectopic pregnancy within an ovary. In this type of EP, the oocyte is not released at ovulation, but becomes fertilized within the ovary which is where the pregnancy then implants. *In vitro* fertilization (IVF), prior ectopic pregnancies, the presence of an IUD, and prior pelvic infections are a few recognized risk factors [101, 105, 106]. The incidence rate of ovarian ectopic has been reported at approximately 0.15–3% [107, 108]. The incidence of ovarian ectopic pregnancy has been increasing, possibly due to a higher awareness of this condition and improved diagnostic techniques. An untreated ovarian pregnancy may cause potentially fatal intra-abdominal bleeding. Clinically, patients may present with unilateral abdominal pain or light vaginal bleeding. Signs of this condition may include hypovolemia and circulatory shock due to internal bleeding [109]. Ultrasound is the first-line diagnostic modality that ensures identification and localization of this type of ectopic pregnancy. However, a major dilemma in establishing the diagnosis relates to distinguishing an ovarian ectopic pregnancy from a corpus luteum or hemorrhagic corpus luteum, which can have a variable appearance on ultrasound, and can also present as a mass in the ovary. Peripheral vascular flow is associated with both diagnostic considerations. Identification of a yolk sac and/or embryo with possible cardiac activity are the only truly distinguishing features of an intraovarian ectopic. In addition, follow-up ultrasound examinations may help to differentiate a growing ectopic pregnancy from an involuting corpus luteum with progressively crenulated margins (Fig. 8.34). Another diagnostic challenge is to distinguish an ovarian ectopic preg-

nancy from a tubal ectopic, particularly in the case of a fimbrial EP. This challenge can be solved by demonstrating displacement of a tubal ectopic pregnancy from the ovary when transvaginal probe pressure is applied. When both gestational sac and ovary move as a single unit, a diagnosis of ovarian ectopic is more favorable. Management of an ovarian ectopic is mostly surgical with conservative ovarian wedge resection; however, successful medical treatment with systemic MTX has also been reported [110–112].

8.3.9 Abdominal Pregnancy

An abdominal ectopic pregnancy results from implantation of the gestational sac outside the uterus but within the peritoneal cavity, most commonly in the anterior or posterior uterine pouches or the uterine serosa. Other implantation sites including the liver, omentum, bowel, and spleen are even rarer [101, 113, 114]. Risk factors include pelvic inflammatory disease, prior pelvic and/or fallopian tube surgeries, prior ectopic pregnancies, endometriosis, and assisted reproductive technologies [12]. Abdominal ectopic pregnancies are very rare, representing 0.9–1.4% of all ectopic pregnancies [77, 115]. They can be classified as primary or secondary [77] depending on the location of fertilization. Fertilization in the peritoneal cavity results in primary abdominal pregnancy. The secondary type is the result of rupture of a previously undetected tubal or ovarian ectopic pregnancy which subsequently becomes intraperitoneal.

Abdominal ectopic pregnancies are associated with higher risk of maternal mortality as well as perinatal mortality and morbidity when compared to both normal and other types of ectopic pregnancy. Maternal mortality is 7.7 times higher than that of tubal ectopic pregnancies, and 90 times higher than that of a normal intrauterine pregnancy [114, 115]. This is one of the few ectopic sites in which delivery of a healthy viable infant is possible, although not without high risk of developing a serious complication. If the diagnosis is made after the 20th week of gestation, no morphologic fetal abnormalities are found, and the mother is hemody-

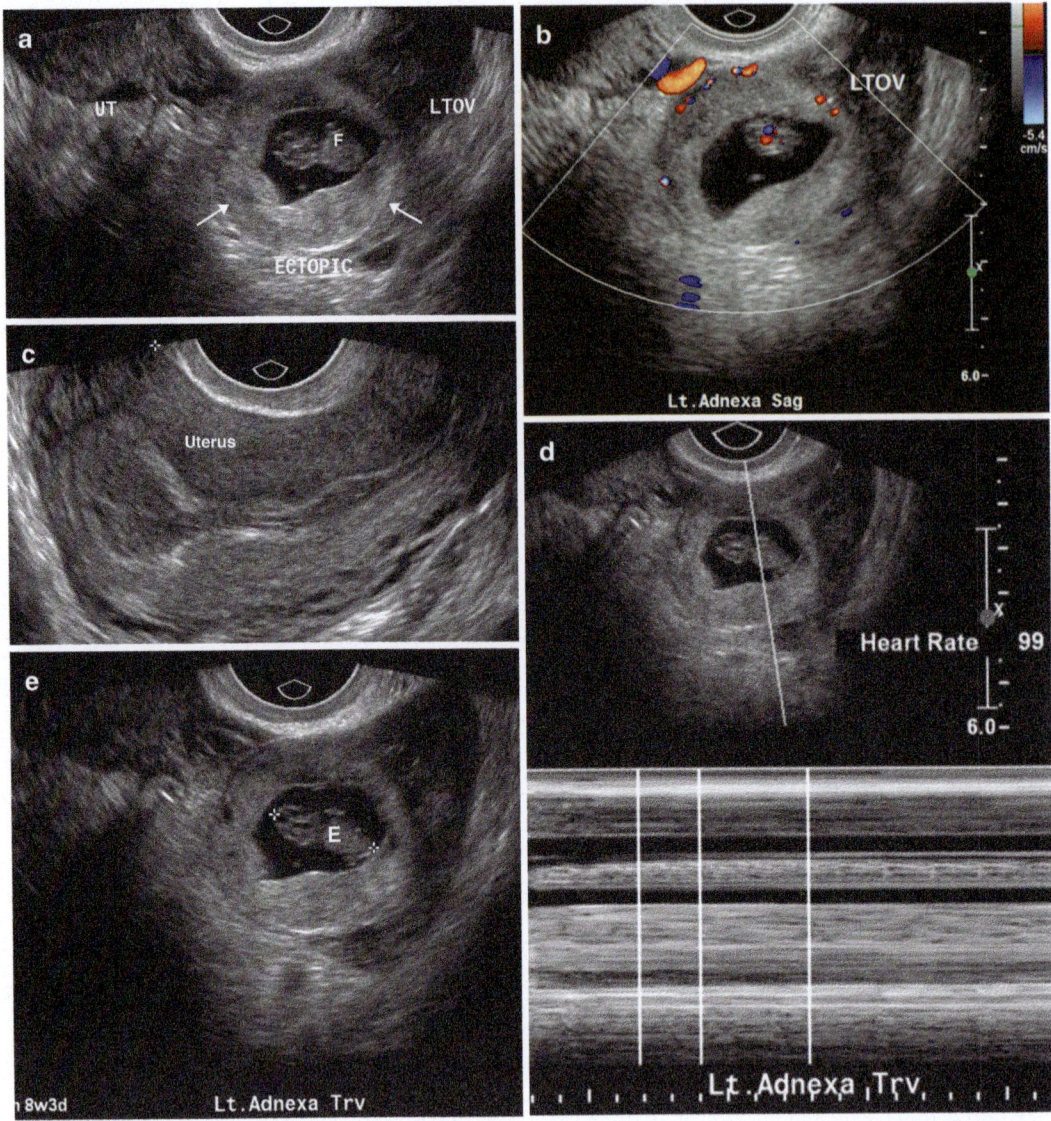

Fig. 8.34 Ovarian ectopic pregnancy in a 28-year-old woman with abdominal pain and a positive pregnancy test. (**a**) Gray-scale and (**b**) color Doppler transvaginal US images demonstrate an ectopic viable intra-ovarian gestational sac inseparable from the left ovary (LTOV) with a thick echogenic margin (arrows in **a**) and containing a fetus (F in **a**). Note fetal cardiac and trophoblastic flow in (**b**). (**c**) Gray-scale transvaginal US of the ectopic pregnancy shows that by CRL measurements the approximate gestational age of ectopic pregnancy was 8 weeks and 3 days. (**d**) M-mode image of the ovarian ectopic pregnancy shows a fetal heart rate of 99 bpm. (**e**) Gray-scale of the uterus obtained in the sagittal plane shows no intrauterine pregnancy

namically stable, then expectant management can be offered. However, the delivery is advised to take place at 35 weeks of gestation, and the placenta can be left *in situ* in order to decrease the risk of intraperitoneal bleeding [4]. Diagnosis of an abdominal ectopic pregnancy is usually made by transabdominal ultrasound. The gesta-tional sac may be found between loops of bowel demonstrating echogenic thick margin and peri-trophoblastic flow on Doppler US or can be attached to the serosal/capsular surface of vital organs. There is an associated empty uterine cavity with no other ectopic pregnancies found (Fig. 8.35).

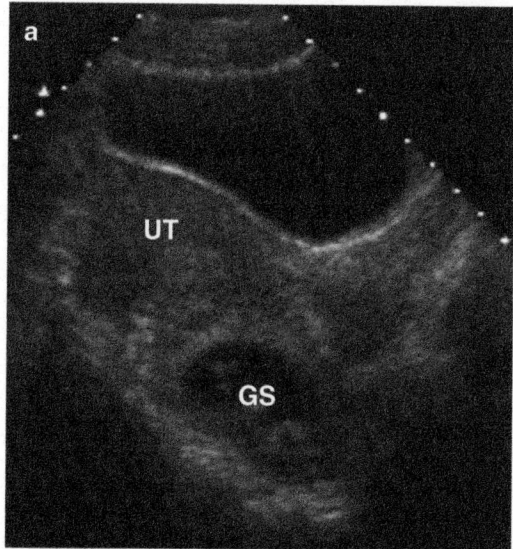

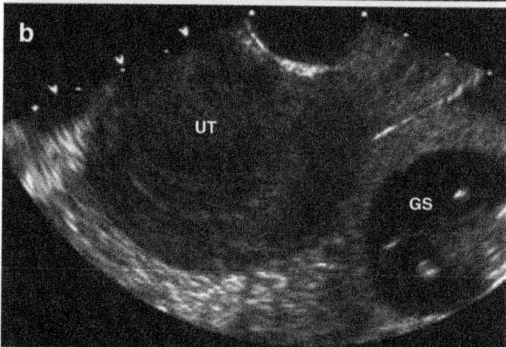

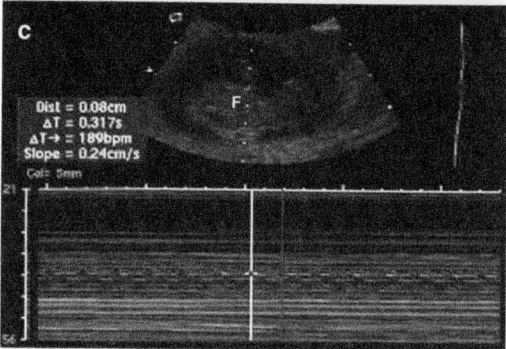

Fig. 8.35 Abdominal ectopic pregnancy in a woman patient with a positive pregnancy test and abdominal pain. (**a**) Gray-scale transabdominal and (**b**) transvaginal images show a viable abdominal intraperitoneal ectopic gestational sac (GS) in the left adnexa separate from the left ovary and the fallopian tube. The uterus (UT) is empty with mild thickening of the endometrium. (**c**) Cardiac activity is seen within the fetus (F) on the M-mode image with the FHR = 189 bpm

8.4 Conclusion

Early pregnancy complications requiring visit to the emergency department are relatively common, and present with vague symptomatology and non-specific laboratory findings resulting in long differential diagnoses. Ultrasound is the initial imaging modality of choice for evaluation, characterization, and management recommendation of various obstetrical pathologies during the first-trimester pregnancy. The familiarity of radiologists with the characteristic appearance and differentiating characteristics and feature of such diseases is paramount in establishment of correct diagnosis to ensure prompts medical, surgical, or expectant management.

Acknowledgments The authors thank Henry Douglas for his help with images.

Grant Funding and Financial Support Related to the topic: None.

Disclosures: Margarita V Revzin: none. Mariam Moshiri: none.

References

1. Expert Panel on Women's Imaging, Brown DL, Packard A, et al. ACR Appropriateness Criteria((R)) first trimester vaginal bleeding. J Am Coll Radiol. 2018;15(5S):S69–77.
2. Wittels KA, Pelletier AJ, Brown DF, Camargo CA Jr. United States emergency department visits for vaginal bleeding during early pregnancy, 1993–2003. Am J Obstet Gynecol. 2008;198(5):523.e1–6.
3. Rodgers SK, Chang C, DeBardeleben JT, Horrow MM. Normal and abnormal US findings in early first-trimester pregnancy: review of the Society of Radiologists in Ultrasound 2012 Consensus Panel Recommendations. Radiographics. 2015;35(7):2135–48.
4. Phillips CH, Wortman JR, Ginsburg ES, Sodickson AD, Doubilet PM, Khurana B. First-trimester emergencies: a radiologist's perspective. Emerg Radiol. 2018;25(1):61–72.
5. Nyberg DA, Mack LA, Laing FC, Patten RM. Distinguishing normal from abnormal gestational sac growth in early pregnancy. J Ultrasound Med. 1987;6(1):23–7.
6. Horrow MM. Enlarged amniotic cavity: a new sonographic sign of early embryonic death. AJR Am J Roentgenol. 1992;158(2):359–62.

7. Yeh HC, Rabinowitz JG. Amniotic sac development: ultrasound features of early pregnancy—the double bleb sign. Radiology. 1988;166(1 Pt 1):97–103.

8. Doubilet PM, Benson CB, Bourne T, Blaivas M, Society of Radiologists in Ultrasound Multispecialty Panel on Early First Trimester Diagnosis of Miscarriage, Exclusion of a Viable Intrauterine Pregnancy. Diagnostic criteria for nonviable pregnancy early in the first trimester. Ultrasound Q. 2014;30(1):3–9.

9. Levi CS, Lyons EA, Zheng XH, Lindsay DJ, Holt SC. Endovaginal US: demonstration of cardiac activity in embryos of less than 5.0 mm in crown-rump length. Radiology. 1990;176(1):71–4.

10. Doubilet PM, Benson CB. Further evidence against the reliability of the human chorionic gonadotropin discriminatory level. J Ultrasound Med. 2011;30(12):1637–42.

11. Levine A, Zagoory-Sharon O, Feldman R, Weller A. Oxytocin during pregnancy and early postpartum: individual patterns and maternal-fetal attachment. Peptides. 2007;28(6):1162–9.

12. Barnhart KT. Clinical practice. Ectopic pregnancy. N Engl J Med. 2009;361(4):379–87.

13. Barnhart KT. Early pregnancy failure: beware of the pitfalls of modern management. Fertil Steril. 2012;98(5):1061–5.

14. Condous G, Kirk E, Lu C, et al. Diagnostic accuracy of varying discriminatory zones for the prediction of ectopic pregnancy in women with a pregnancy of unknown location. Ultrasound Obstet Gynecol. 2005;26(7):770–5.

15. Barnhart K, van Mello NM, Bourne T, et al. Pregnancy of unknown location: a consensus statement of nomenclature, definitions, and outcome. Fertil Steril. 2011;95(3):857–66.

16. Kirk E, Condous G, Bourne T. Pregnancies of unknown location. Best Pract Res Clin Obstet Gynaecol. 2009;23(4):493–9.

17. Ko JK, Cheung VY. Time to revisit the human chorionic gonadotropin discriminatory level in the management of pregnancy of unknown location. J Ultrasound Med. 2014;33(3):465–71.

18. Condous G, Timmerman D, Goldstein S, Valentin L, Jurkovic D, Bourne T. Pregnancies of unknown location: consensus statement. Ultrasound Obstet Gynecol. 2006;28(2):121–2.

19. National Institute for Health Care Excellence. Ectopic pregnancy and miscarriage: diagnosis and initial management in early pregnancy of ectopic pregnancy and miscarriage. London; 2012.

20. ACOG Practice Bulletin No. 200: early pregnancy loss. Obstet Gynecol. 2018;132(5):e197–207.

21. Wang X, Chen C, Wang L, Chen D, Guang W, French J. Conception, early pregnancy loss, and time to clinical pregnancy: a population-based prospective study. Fertil Steril. 2003;79(3):577–84.

22. Zinaman MJ, Clegg ED, Brown CC, O'Connor J, Selevan SG. Estimates of human fertility and pregnancy loss. Fertil Steril. 1996;65(3):503–9.

23. Wilcox AJ, Weinberg CR, O'Connor JF, et al. Incidence of early loss of pregnancy. N Engl J Med. 1988;319(4):189–94.

24. Practice Committee of the American Society for Reproductive Medicine. Evaluation and treatment of recurrent pregnancy loss: a committee opinion. Fertil Steril. 2012;98(5):1103–11.

25. Morin L, Cargill YM, Glanc P. Ultrasound evaluation of first trimester complications of pregnancy. J Obstet Gynaecol Can. 2016;38(10):982–8.

26. Casciani E, Masselli G, Luciani ML, Polidori NF, Piccioni MG, Gualdi G. Errors in imaging of emergencies in pregnancy. Semin Ultrasound CT MR. 2012;33(4):347–70.

27. Hu M, Poder L, Filly RA. Impact of new society of radiologists in ultrasound early first-trimester diagnostic criteria for nonviable pregnancy. J Ultrasound Med. 2014;33(9):1585–8.

28. Bromley B, Harlow BL, Laboda LA, Benacerraf BR. Small sac size in the first trimester: a predictor of poor fetal outcome. Radiology. 1991;178(2):375–7.

29. Lindsay DJ, Lovett IS, Lyons EA, et al. Yolk sac diameter and shape at endovaginal US: predictors of pregnancy outcome in the first trimester. Radiology. 1992;183(1):115–8.

30. Levi CS, Lyons EA, Dashefsky SM, Lindsay DJ, Holt SC. Yolk sac number, size and morphologic features in monochorionic monoamniotic twin pregnancy. Can Assoc Radiol J. 1996;47(2):98–100.

31. Rowling SE, Coleman BG, Langer JE, Arger PH, Nisenbaum HL, Horii SC. First-trimester US parameters of failed pregnancy. Radiology. 1997;203(1):211–7.

32. Levi CS, Lyons EA, Lindsay DJ. Early diagnosis of nonviable pregnancy with endovaginal US. Radiology. 1988;167(2):383–5.

33. Pexsters A, Luts J, Van Schoubroeck D, et al. Clinical implications of intra- and interobserver reproducibility of transvaginal sonographic measurement of gestational sac and crown-rump length at 6–9 weeks' gestation. Ultrasound Obstet Gynecol. 2011;38(5):510–5.

34. Levi CS, Lyons EA, Lindsay DJ. Ultrasound in the first trimester of pregnancy. Radiol Clin N Am. 1990;28(1):19–38.

35. World Health Organization. The prevention and management of unsafe abortion: report of a technical working group, Geneva, 12–15 April 1992. Geneva: World Health Organization; 1993.

36. World Health Organization. Unsafe abortion: global and regional estimates of the incidence of unsafe abortion and associated mortality in 2008. 6th ed. Geneva: World Health Organization; 2011.

37. Septic abortion and IUDs. Br Med J. 1978;1(6114):719.

38. Kassebaum NJ, Bertozzi-Villa A, Coggeshall MS, et al. Global, regional, and national levels and causes of maternal mortality during 1990–2013: a systematic analysis for the Global Burden of Disease Study 2013. Lancet. 2014;384(9947):980–1004.

39. Rotheram EB Jr, Schick SF. Nonclostridial anaerobic bacteria in septic abortion. Am J Med. 1969;46(1):80–9.
40. Finkielman JD. Management of septic abortion. N Engl J Med. 1994;331(25):1717.
41. Maso G, D'Ottavio G, De Seta F, Sartore A, Piccoli M, Mandruzzato G. First-trimester intrauterine hematoma and outcome of pregnancy. Obstet Gynecol. 2005;105(2):339–44.
42. Leite J, Ross P, Rossi AC, Jeanty P. Prognosis of very large first-trimester hematomas. J Ultrasound Med. 2006;25(11):1441–5.
43. Pedersen JF, Mantoni M. Prevalence and significance of subchorionic hemorrhage in threatened abortion: a sonographic study. AJR Am J Roentgenol. 1990;154(3):535–7.
44. Trop I, Levine D. Hemorrhage during pregnancy: sonography and MR imaging. AJR Am J Roentgenol. 2001;176(3):607–15.
45. Bennett GL, Bromley B, Lieberman E, Benacerraf BR. Subchorionic hemorrhage in first-trimester pregnancies: prediction of pregnancy outcome with sonography. Radiology. 1996;200(3):803–6.
46. Harris RD, Couto C, Karpovsky C, Porter MM, Ouhilal S. The chorionic bump: a first-trimester pregnancy sonographic finding associated with a guarded prognosis. J Ultrasound Med. 2006;25(6):757–63.
47. Tan S, Ipek A, Akin Sivaslioglu A, Sungu N, Sarici OU, Karaoglanoglu M. The chorionic bump: radiologic and pathologic correlation. J Clin Ultrasound. 2011;39(1):35–7.
48. Arleo EK, Dunning A, Troiano RN. Chorionic bump in pregnant patients and associated live birth rate: a systematic review and meta-analysis. J Ultrasound Med. 2015;34(4):553–7.
49. Arleo EK, Troiano RN. Chorionic bump on first-trimester sonography: not necessarily a poor prognostic indicator for pregnancy. J Ultrasound Med. 2015;34(1):137–42.
50. Shaaban AM, Rezvani M, Haroun RR, et al. Gestational trophoblastic disease: clinical and imaging features. Radiographics. 2017;37(2):681–700.
51. Lazarus E, Hulka C, Siewert B, Levine D. Sonographic appearance of early complete molar pregnancies. J Ultrasound Med. 1999;18(9):589–594; quiz 595–6.
52. Alazzam M, Young T, Coleman R, et al. Predicting gestational trophoblastic neoplasia (GTN): is urine hCG the answer? Gynecol Oncol. 2011;122(3):595–9.
53. Dhanda S, Ramani S, Thakur M. Gestational trophoblastic disease: a multimodality imaging approach with impact on diagnosis and management. Radiol Res Pract. 2014;2014:842751.
54. Tita AT, Andrews WW. Diagnosis and management of clinical chorioamnionitis. Clin Perinatol. 2010;37(2):339–54.
55. Gibbs RS, Duff P. Progress in pathogenesis and management of clinical intraamniotic infection. Am J Obstet Gynecol. 1991;164(5 Pt 1):1317–26.
56. Soper DE, Mayhall CG, Dalton HP. Risk factors for intraamniotic infection: a prospective epidemiologic study. Am J Obstet Gynecol. 1989;161(3):562–566; discussion 566–8.
57. Newton ER. Chorioamnionitis and intraamniotic infection. Clin Obstet Gynecol. 1993;36(4):795–808.
58. Riggs JW, Blanco JD. Pathophysiology, diagnosis, and management of intraamniotic infection. Semin Perinatol. 1998;22(4):251–9.
59. Brahmi D, Steenland MW, Renner RM, Gaffield ME, Curtis KM. Pregnancy outcomes with an IUD in situ: a systematic review. Contraception. 2012;85(2):131–9.
60. Kim SK, Romero R, Kusanovic JP, et al. The prognosis of pregnancy conceived despite the presence of an intrauterine device (IUD). J Perinat Med. 2010;38(1):45–53.
61. Thonneau PF, Almont T. Contraceptive efficacy of intrauterine devices. Am J Obstet Gynecol. 2008;198(3):248–53.
62. Ganer H, Levy A, Ohel I, Sheiner E. Pregnancy outcome in women with an intrauterine contraceptive device. Am J Obstet Gynecol. 2009;201(4):381. e1–5.
63. Epperly TD, Fogarty JP, Hodges SG. Efficacy of routine postpartum uterine exploration and manual sponge curettage. J Fam Pract. 1989;28(2):172–6.
64. Pellerito JS, Troiano RN, Quedens-Case C, Taylor KJ. Common pitfalls of endovaginal color Doppler flow imaging. Radiographics. 1995;15(1):37–47.
65. Kamaya A, Krishnarao PM, Folkins AK, Jeffrey RB, Desser TS, Maturen KE. Variable color Doppler sonographic appearances of retained products of conception: radiologic-pathologic correlation. Abdom Imaging. 2015;40(7):2683–9.
66. Kamaya A, Krishnarao PM, Nayak N, Jeffrey RB, Maturen KE. Clinical and imaging predictors of management in retained products of conception. Abdom Radiol (NY). 2016;41(12):2429–34.
67. Practice Committee of American Society for Reproductive Medicine. Medical treatment of ectopic pregnancy: a committee opinion. Fertil Steril. 2013;100(3):638–44.
68. Lin EP, Bhatt S, Dogra VS. Diagnostic clues to ectopic pregnancy. Radiographics. 2008;28(6):1661–71.
69. Creanga AA, Callaghan WM. Recent increases in the U.S. maternal mortality rate: disentangling trends from measurement issues. Obstet Gynecol. 2017;129(1):206–7.
70. Creanga AA, Shapiro-Mendoza CK, Bish CL, Zane S, Berg CJ, Callaghan WM. Trends in ectopic pregnancy mortality in the United States: 1980–2007. Obstet Gynecol. 2011;117(4):837–43.
71. Cantwell R, Clutton-Brock T, Cooper G, et al. Saving mothers' lives: reviewing maternal deaths to make motherhood safer: 2006–2008. The Eighth Report of the Confidential Enquiries into Maternal Deaths in the United Kingdom. BJOG. 2011;118(Suppl 1):1–203.

72. Centers for Disease Control and Prevention. Ectopic pregnancy—United States, 1990–1992. MMWR Morb Mortal Wkly Rep. 1995;44(3):46.

73. Weckstein LN. Current perspective on ectopic pregnancy. Obstet Gynecol Surv. 1985;40(5):259–72.

74. Weckstein LN, Boucher AR, Tucker H, Gibson D, Rettenmaier MA. Accurate diagnosis of early ectopic pregnancy. Obstet Gynecol. 1985;65(3):393–7.

75. Varma R, Gupta J. Tubal ectopic pregnancy. BMJ Clin Evid. 2009;2009:1406.

76. Walker JJ. Ectopic pregnancy. Clin Obstet Gynecol. 2007;50(1):89–99.

77. Bouyer J, Coste J, Fernandez H, Pouly JL, Job-Spira N. Sites of ectopic pregnancy: a 10 year population-based study of 1800 cases. Hum Reprod. 2002;17(12):3224–30.

78. Shaw JL, Dey SK, Critchley HO, Horne AW. Current knowledge of the aetiology of human tubal ectopic pregnancy. Hum Reprod Update. 2010;16(4):432–44.

79. Shaw JL, Oliver E, Lee KF, et al. Cotinine exposure increases Fallopian tube PROKR1 expression via nicotinic AChRalpha-7: a potential mechanism explaining the link between smoking and tubal ectopic pregnancy. Am J Pathol. 2010;177(5):2509–15.

80. Bacci A, Lewis G, Baltag V, Betran AP. The introduction of confidential enquiries into maternal deaths and near-miss case reviews in the WHO European Region. Reprod Health Matters. 2007;15(30):145–52.

81. Atri M. Ectopic pregnancy versus corpus luteum cyst revisited: best Doppler predictors. J Ultrasound Med. 2003;22(11):1181–4.

82. Doubilet PM. Ultrasound evaluation of the first trimester. Radiol Clin N Am. 2014;52(6):1191–9.

83. Frates MC, Doubilet PM, Peters HE, Benson CB. Adnexal sonographic findings in ectopic pregnancy and their correlation with tubal rupture and human chorionic gonadotropin levels. J Ultrasound Med. 2014;33(4):697–703.

84. Kirk E, Papageorghiou AT, Condous G, Bottomley C, Bourne T. The accuracy of first trimester ultrasound in the diagnosis of hydatidiform mole. Ultrasound Obstet Gynecol. 2007;29(1):70–5.

85. Eddib A, Olawaiye A, Withiam-Leitch M, Rodgers B, Yeh J. Live twin tubal ectopic pregnancy. Int J Gynaecol Obstet. 2006;93(2):154–5.

86. Fernandez H, Gervaise A. Ectopic pregnancies after infertility treatment: modern diagnosis and therapeutic strategy. Hum Reprod Update. 2004;10(6):503–13.

87. Dor J, Seidman DS, Levran D, Ben-Rafael Z, Ben-Shlomo I, Mashiach S. The incidence of combined intrauterine and extrauterine pregnancy after in vitro fertilization and embryo transfer. Fertil Steril. 1991;55(4):833–4.

88. Kirk E, Bottomley C, Bourne T. Diagnosing ectopic pregnancy and current concepts in the management of pregnancy of unknown location. Hum Reprod Update. 2014;20(2):250–61.

89. Lau S, Tulandi T. Conservative medical and surgical management of interstitial ectopic pregnancy. Fertil Steril. 1999;72(2):207–15.

90. Ackerman TE, Levi CS, Dashefsky SM, Holt SC, Lindsay DJ. Interstitial line: sonographic finding in interstitial (cornual) ectopic pregnancy. Radiology. 1993;189(1):83–7.

91. Arleo EK, DeFilippis EM. Cornual, interstitial, and angular pregnancies: clarifying the terms and a review of the literature. Clin Imaging. 2014;38(6):763–70.

92. Alanbay I, Ozturk M, Karasahin KE, Yenen MC. Angular pregnancy. Turk J Obstet Gynecol. 2016;13(4):218–20.

93. Ash A, Smith A, Maxwell D. Caesarean scar pregnancy. BJOG. 2007;114(3):253–63.

94. Wang CB, Tseng CJ. Primary evacuation therapy for Cesarean scar pregnancy: three new cases and review. Ultrasound Obstet Gynecol. 2006;27(2):222–6.

95. Jurkovic D, Hillaby K, Woelfer B, Lawrence A, Salim R, Elson CJ. First-trimester diagnosis and management of pregnancies implanted into the lower uterine segment Cesarean section scar. Ultrasound Obstet Gynecol. 2003;21(3):220–7.

96. McKenna DA, Poder L, Goldman M, Goldstein RB. Role of sonography in the recognition, assessment, and treatment of cesarean scar ectopic pregnancies. J Ultrasound Med. 2008;27(5):779–83.

97. Maymon R, Halperin R, Mendlovic S, Schneider D, Herman A. Ectopic pregnancies in a Caesarean scar: review of the medical approach to an iatrogenic complication. Hum Reprod Update. 2004;10(6):515–23.

98. Godin PA, Bassil S, Donnez J. An ectopic pregnancy developing in a previous caesarian section scar. Fertil Steril. 1997;67(2):398–400.

99. Ben Nagi J, Ofili-Yebovi D, Marsh M, Jurkovic D. First-trimester cesarean scar pregnancy evolving into placenta previa/accreta at term. J Ultrasound Med. 2005;24(11):1569–73.

100. Wu R, Klein MA, Mahboob S, Gupta M, Katz DS. Magnetic resonance imaging as an adjunct to ultrasound in evaluating cesarean scar ectopic pregnancy. J Clin Imaging Sci. 2013;3:16.

101. Panelli DM, Phillips CH, Brady PC. Incidence, diagnosis and management of tubal and nontubal ectopic pregnancies: a review. Fertil Res Pract. 2015;1:15.

102. Hofmann HM, Urdl W, Hofler H, Honigl W, Tamussino K. Cervical pregnancy: case reports and current concepts in diagnosis and treatment. Arch Gynecol Obstet. 1987;241(1):63–9.

103. Chukus A, Tirada N, Restrepo R, Reddy NI. Uncommon implantation sites of ectopic pregnancy: thinking beyond the complex adnexal mass. Radiographics. 2015;35(3):946–59.

104. Memtsa M, Jamil A, Sebire N, Jauniaux E, Jurkovic D. Diagnosis and management of intramural ectopic pregnancy. Ultrasound Obstet Gynecol. 2013;42(3):359–62.

105. A multinational case-control study of ectopic pregnancy. The World Health Organization's Special Programme of Research, Development and Research

Training in Human Reproduction: Task Force on Intrauterine Devices for Fertility Regulation. Clin Reprod Fertil. 1985;3(2):131–43.

106. Ko PC, Lo LM, Hsieh TT, Cheng PJ. Twenty-one years of experience with ovarian ectopic pregnancy at one institution in Taiwan. Int J Gynaecol Obstet. 2012;119(2):154–8.

107. Nwanodi O, Khulpateea N. The preoperative diagnosis of primary ovarian pregnancy. J Natl Med Assoc. 2006;98(5):796–8.

108. Raziel A, Mordechai E, Schachter M, Friedler S, Pansky M, Ron-El R. A comparison of the incidence, presentation, and management of ovarian pregnancies between two periods of time. J Am Assoc Gynecol Laparosc. 2004;11(2):191–4.

109. Raziel A, Schachter M, Mordechai E, Friedler S, Panski M, Ron-El R. Ovarian pregnancy-a 12-year experience of 19 cases in one institution. Eur J Obstet Gynecol Reprod Biol. 2004; 114(1):92–6.

110. Habbu J, Read MD. Ovarian pregnancy successfully treated with methotrexate. J Obstet Gynaecol. 2006;26(6):587–8.

111. Di Luigi G, Patacchiola F, La Posta V, Bonitatibus A, Ruggeri G, Carta G. Early ovarian pregnancy diagnosed by ultrasound and successfully treated with multidose methotrexate. A case report. Clin Exp Obstet Gynecol. 2012;39(3):390–3.

112. Kiran G, Guven AM, Kostu B. Systemic medical management of ovarian pregnancy. Int J Gynaecol Obstet. 2005;91(2):177–8.

113. Yagil Y, Beck-Razi N, Amit A, Kerner H, Gaitini D. Splenic pregnancy: the role of abdominal imaging. J Ultrasound Med. 2007;26(11):1629–32.

114. Poole A, Haas D, Magann EF. Early abdominal ectopic pregnancies: a systematic review of the literature. Gynecol Obstet Investig. 2012;74(4):249–60.

115. Atrash HK, Friede A, Hogue CJ. Abdominal pregnancy in the United States: frequency and maternal mortality. Obstet Gynecol. 1987;69(3 Pt 1):333–7.

Imaging of Late Obstetrical and Post-partum Emergencies

9

Richard Tsai, Kristina Sondgeroth,
Daniel R. Ludwig, and Vincent M. Mellnick

Contents

9.1 Introduction

Maternal mortality is rare in the developed world, but has increased in the early 2000s, with pregnancy-related mortality rising from 7.2 deaths per 100,000 live births in 1987 to 17.8 deaths per 100,000 live births in 2009 [1]. Although the majority of these deaths are due to chronic medical conditions in the mother, a small but substantial proportion of these deaths are caused by acute emergencies or urgencies secondary to an obstetrical cause, including those related to the uterus or the placenta [2–5]. In the late obstetrical and in the post-partum periods, multiple technical factors and anatomic and physiologic changes introduce unique diagnostic dilemmas.

Imaging of the pregnant and post-partum patient poses many technical challenges, as there is a need to balance the benefits of obtaining diagnostic information with the potential risks of ionizing radiation to the mother and fetus. Because computed tomography (CT), the usual

R. Tsai (✉)
Advanced Radiology Consultants,
Leawood, KS, USA

K. Sondgeroth
Department of Maternal Fetal Medicine, Southern
Illinois University, School of Medicine,
Springfield, IL, USA
e-mail: ksondgeroth86@siumed.edu

D. R. Ludwig · V. M. Mellnick
Mallinckrodt Institute of Radiology, Washington
University School of Medicine in St. Louis,
Saint Louis, MO, USA
e-mail: Ludwigd@wustl.edu; mellnickv@wustl.edu

© Springer Nature Switzerland AG 2020
M. N. Patlas et al. (eds.), *Emergency Imaging of Pregnant Patients*,
https://doi.org/10.1007/978-3-030-42722-1_9

185

workhorse in acute abdominal and pelvic imaging, uses ionizing radiation, the use of CT caries a theoretical risk of fetal anomalies and malignancy. Fetal radiation doses of less than 50 mGy are not believed to be associated with fetal loss or anomalies, and most abdomen and pelvis CT examinations can be performed using doses around 25 mGy or less [6, 7]. However, stochastic effects from radiation, particularly cancer, do not have a threshold limit [8]. Therefore, sonography and magnetic resonance imaging (MRI), which do not use ionizing radiation, are strongly preferred in the pregnant patient. The use of CT should be reserved for the setting of trauma or in those situations in which other imaging modalities are not readily available, and in which a delay in diagnosis may increase the risk of fetal loss or maternal morbidity [9–15]. Iodinated contrast agents are not contraindicated during pregnancy and should be used as otherwise are indicated with CT examinations. Because gadolinium crosses the placenta, the use of IV gadolinium-based contrast agents should only be used in the pregnant patient if it potentially substantially improves diagnostic performance, which may then lead to improved fetal or maternal outcome [6].

Unfortunately, the perinatal period also poses many diagnostic challenges to the radiologist and the clinician. Many laboratory tests and physical examination findings are muddied by the normal physiologic alterations during pregnancy [14]. Several anatomic factors can also make diagnosis of obstetrical conditions difficult for the radiologist. The enlarging gravid uterus causes anatomic distortion of many adjacent pelvic organs, and the CT or MRI appearance of the uterus or placenta may be confusing to less experienced radiologists.

In this chapter, we describe key imaging findings of late obstetric and immediate post-partum emergencies.

9.2 Late Obstetrical Emergencies

9.2.1 Placental Emergencies

The placenta has both fetal and maternal components, and functions to support the normal growth and development of the fetus [16]. The placenta is most commonly located along the anterior or posterior uterine wall, with extension to the lateral uterine walls. The umbilical cord typically inserts centrally within the placenta, but may have eccentric locations [17]. Often times, the placenta is overlooked during cross-sectional imaging, and varying levels of experience make the placenta difficult to evaluate on modalities which are uncommonly used in the pregnant patient, namely, CT and MRI. At MRI, the placenta appears as a T2 hyperintense, T1 isointense (relative to skeletal muscle) discoid structure. The placental-myometrial–decidua interface is seen as low-signal-intensity line on T2-weighted images (Fig. 9.1). IV contrast-enhanced CT will demonstrate homogeneously avidly enhancing discoid soft tissue (Fig. 9.2).

Abnormal placental implantation or cord insertions may result in placenta previa or vasa previa. These conditions may complicate delivery, and thus constitute obstetrical urgencies. Furthermore, the attachment of the placenta to the uterine wall may be compromised by multiple factors, leading to premature separation of the placenta, resulting in placental abruption. On the other end of the spectrum, abnormal adherence or penetration of the chorionic villi into or through the uterine wall may lead to placenta accreta, increta, or percreta. These conditions are important causes of hemorrhage in the second half of pregnancy and during labor.

9.2.1.1 Placenta and Vasa Previa

The placenta normally implants in the upper uterine segment, greater than 2 cm from the internal cervical os. If the edge of the placenta is located within 2 cm from the internal os, but does not directly cover it, it should be referred to as low lying. If the placental edge covers the internal cervical os, it should be referred to as placenta previa (Fig. 9.3) [18]. The reported incidence of placenta previa is approximately 1.3% of pregnancies, and is associated with advanced maternal age, prior cesarean delivery (CD), infertility treatments, and recurrent miscarriage [19, 20]. Classically, placenta previa presents as painless bleeding in the late second

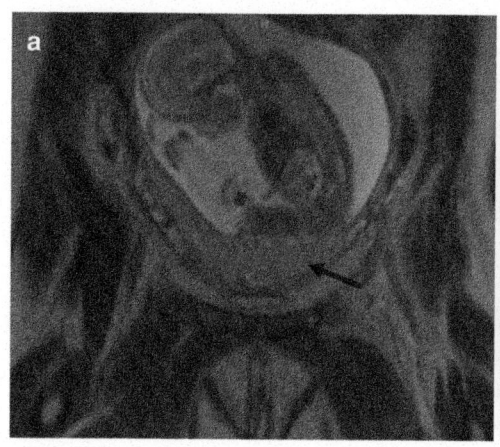 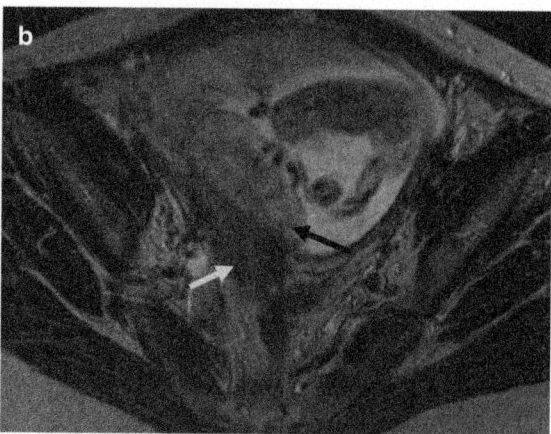

Fig. 9.1 Twenty-eight-year-old woman, 25 weeks estimated gestational age, presented for evaluation for evaluation of suspected acute appendicitis. Coronal (**a**) and axial (**b**) T2-weighted MR images demonstrate normal appearance of the placenta (black arrows), with abnormal location completely covering the cervical os (white arrow). Findings are diagnostic of placenta previa

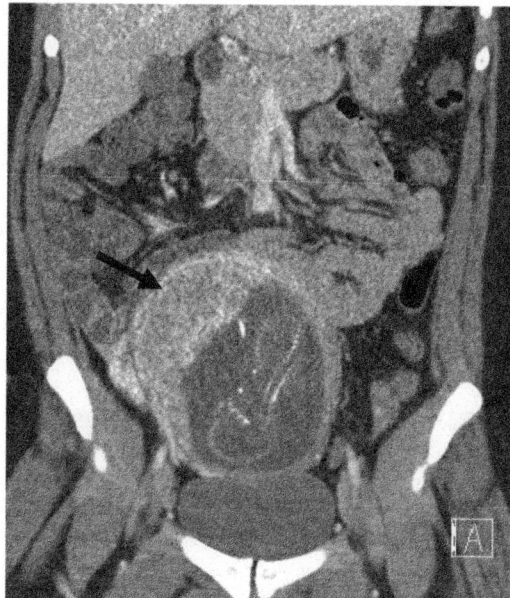

Fig. 9.2 Twenty-two-year-old woman, 22 weeks estimated gestational age, who presented after a motor vehicle collision. Coronal CT image with IV contrast demonstrates relatively homogenously enhancing, normal placenta (arrow), with a single intrauterine gestation

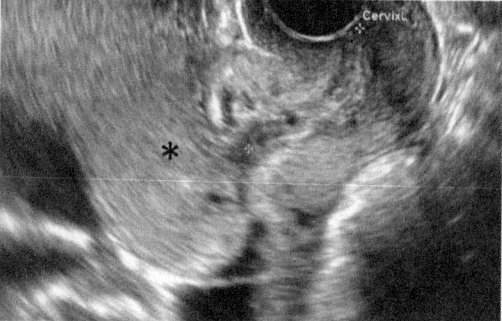

Fig. 9.3 Thirty-year-old woman, 18 weeks gestation, presented for an anatomy sonogram. Transvaginal longitudinal ultrasound demonstrates the placenta (black asterisk) extending completely over the cervical os (yellow calipers). Findings are diagnostic of placenta previa

or early third trimester. Complications of placenta previa include malpresentation, hemorrhage, and intrauterine growth restriction [21]. It is important to note that the diagnosis of placenta previa should not be given before 16 weeks gestation, as growth of the uterus may pull the placenta upwards away from the cervical os, and prior to 16 weeks the diagnosis would otherwise be overestimated [17].

The diagnosis of placenta previa is often made with routine transvaginal ultrasound, although translabial approaches have also been described [22]. Transabdominal ultrasound is less accurate in the diagnosis of placenta previa, because frequently the internal cervical os and the lower placental edge cannot be imaged adequately [23]. Care must be taken with a transvaginal approach in advanced pregnancies, as the risk of infection or premature rupture of the membranes is increased. The transvaginal probe does not lead to an increase in bleeding, as the angle of the probe places the tip against the anterior aspect of the cervix, and the optimal imaging of the cervix is often performed 2–3 cm away from the cervix [24]. Although MRI can be used to readily detect placenta previa, it is less specific than ultrasound with color Doppler [25].

On the other hand, vasa previa refers to the condition in which fetal vessels run through the membranes over the cervical os, unprotected by the placenta or umbilical cord [26]. The incidence of vasa previa is 1 in 2500 deliveries [26]. Risk factors include placenta previa, accessory placental lobes, multiple gestations, and in vitro fertilization [27]. When undiagnosed, vasa previa has a perinatal mortality of 60% if delivered vaginally, underlining the importance of accurate and prospective radiologic diagnosis. Fetal demise occurs when these vessels are torn, leading to hemorrhage, or when the unprotected fetal vessels become compressed, leading to decreased fetal perfusion [28].

The diagnosis of vasa previa can be made using ultrasound (Fig. 9.4). Ultrasound images demonstrate a tubular echoic structure crossing the cervical os, often associated with placenta previa and/or an accessory placental lobe. The use of Doppler ultrasound will demonstrate that this structure is vascular, with fetal umbilical arterial and venous waveforms. Care must be taken to differentiate vasa previa from cord presentation, the latter of which will move with Trendelenburg positioning. In the setting of vasa previa, cesarean delivery is typically performed preterm to avoid the onset of spontaneous labor [29].

9.2.1.2 Placenta Accreta, Increta, and Percreta

Abnormalities in increased placental adherence to the uterine wall are called placenta accreta. Placenta accreta is usually the general term used to describe all forms of abnormally increased adherence of the placenta. More specifically, placenta increta is used when the placenta invades the myometrium, and placenta percreta refers to invasion past the myometrium, involving the uterine serosa or adjacent organs.

Diagnosis of placenta accreta is paramount, as massive obstetric hemorrhage may be associated with these conditions, necessitating a cesarean hysterectomy. The incidence of placenta accreta has increased by tenfold in the past 50 years, and is now estimated at 1 in 2500 deliveries, due to the increased rate of cesarean deliveries [30, 31].

Ultrasound remains the most effective way of detecting placenta accreta, with MRI serving as a supplemental diagnostic test [32]. Sonographic features include loss of the normal retroplacental clear space, irregularity of the interface, increased

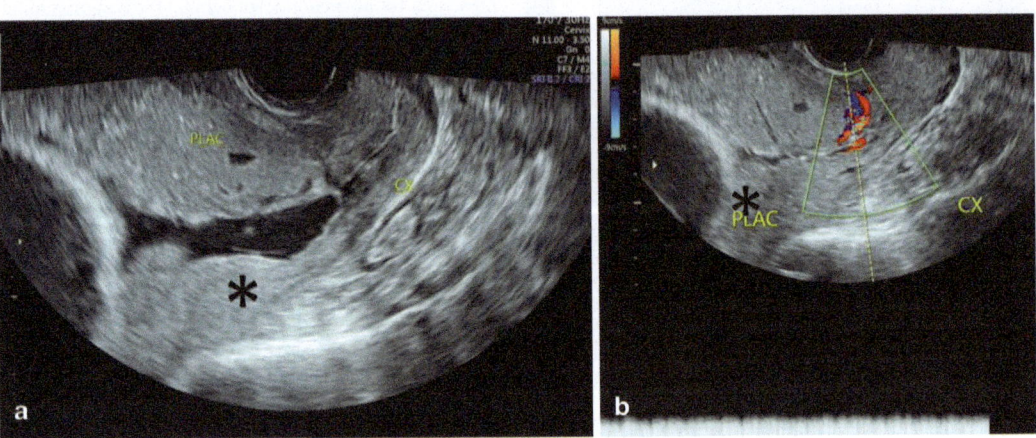

Fig. 9.4 Forty-two-year-old woman, 28 weeks estimated gestational age, presents with known anterior placenta previa and a posterior succenturiate lobe. Ultrasound was performed for evaluation of suspected vasa previa. Transvaginal longitudinal gray scale (**a**) and Doppler (**b**) images demonstrate the anterior placenta previa and posterior succenturiate lobe (black asterisk). Color Doppler overlay demonstrates vascular flow and placental venous signal, indicating concurrent vasa previa

vascularity at the interface between the uterus and bladder, and prominent placental lacunae, the latter of which has the highest positive predictive value (Fig. 9.5) [33, 34].

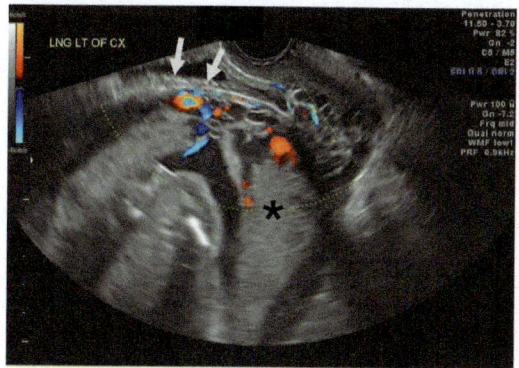

Fig. 9.5 Thirty-seven-year-old woman referred for known placenta previa and history of multiple cesarean deliveries. Transvaginal longitudinal ultrasound image demonstrates a low-lying placenta (black asterisk) with complete coverage of the cervical os, indicating placenta previa. In addition, there are serpentine anechoic structures low in the pelvis which demonstrate vascularity with Doppler (white arrows). These represent prominent, increased placental lacunae, and are highly suggestive of placenta accreta. Placenta accreta was confirmed at the time of cesarean hysterectomy

Typically, MRI is performed as a supplemental examination when percreta is suspected, or when the diagnosis of placenta accreta by ultrasound is unclear. MRI evaluation should include single-shot T2-weighted imaging and T1-weighted fat-suppressed imaging in multiple planes, in relation to the placental-myometrial junction. Gadolinium-based IV contrast agents are typically not administered for the evaluation of placenta accreta due to the unclear benefit in diagnosis, compared with the potential/theoretical risks of administration [34]. On MRI, placenta accreta can be seen as intraplacental bands and increased vascularity at the placental-myometrial junction (Fig. 9.6). The differentiation of the depth of myometrial invasion can be challenging on MRI, and findings of percreta are only suggested when placental vascularity, distortion, or frank invasion of adjacent structures are present. IV contrast may be given in select patients where the diagnosis is uncertain on non-contrast MRI, or in cases of fetal demise or fetal conditions incompatible with life (Fig. 9.7).

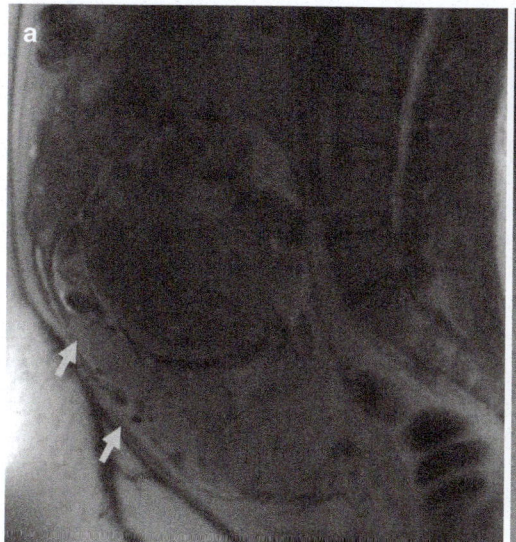
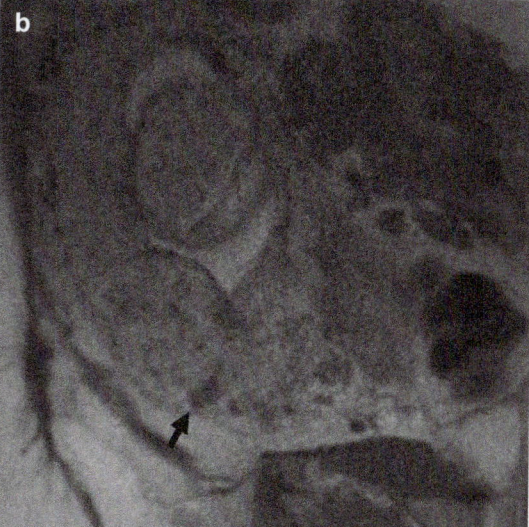
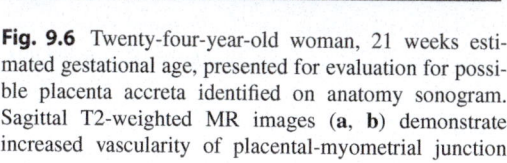

Fig. 9.6 Twenty-four-year-old woman, 21 weeks estimated gestational age, presented for evaluation for possible placenta accreta identified on anatomy sonogram. Sagittal T2-weighted MR images (**a**, **b**) demonstrate increased vascularity of placental-myometrial junction (white arrows). Intraplacental bands (black arrow) are also seen. Findings are strongly suggestive of placenta accreta, which was confirmed at the time of cesarean delivery

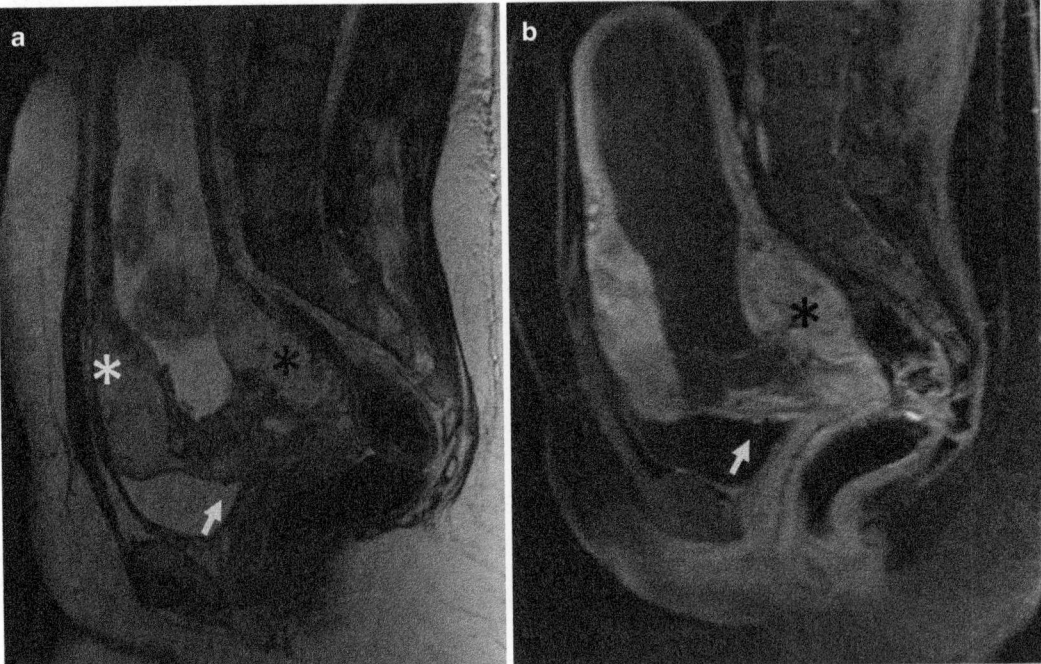

Fig. 9.7 Thirty-two-year-old woman, at 20 weeks estimated gestational age, with greater than five prior cesarean deliveries, presents for evaluation of suspected accreta. The fetus was anencephalic on prior ultrasound, and so IV gadolinium contrast was administered. Sagittal T2 (**a**) and post-contrast T1 (**b**) weighted MR images demonstrate an accessory placental lobe (black asterisks).

Note the increased vascularity at the placental-myometrial junction (white asterisk, image **a**). Vascularity along the dome of the bladder on this MR examination (white arrows) raised high suspicion for placenta percreta with involvement of the bladder. All of these findings were confirmed at the time of cesarean hysterectomy

9.2.1.3 Placental Abruption

Premature separation of the placenta from the implantation site is known as placental abruption. Placental abruption complicates approximately 1% of pregnancies, occurring in 6.5 per 1000 births, and is the leading cause of vaginal bleeding in the second half of pregnancy [35, 36]. Although rare, there is a relatively high associated perinatal mortality, with an estimated 119 deaths per 1000, and is the most common cause of fetal death in cases where the mother survives [35]. Risk factors include chronic hypertension, advanced maternal age, trauma, cocaine use, smoking, intrauterine infections, preterm premature rupture of the membranes, and polyhydramnios [36].

Placental abruption is a clinical diagnosis presenting with abdominal pain and vaginal bleeding. Ultrasound is poor in this diagnosis, with sensitivities as low as 25%; however, when diagnosed on ultrasound, abruption has a poorer prognosis, which is likely due to the relatively larger size of the retroplacental hematoma when it is visible [37]. MRI has been shown to be much superior for the diagnosis of placental abruption, with a sensitivity of 100% in one prospective study [38]. The degree of uteroplacental separation has a direct correlation with poor fetal outcome [39]. Nonetheless, because the management and diagnosis of abruption is often on a clinical basis, so imaging is usually not necessary.

Abruption can be unexpected identified if pain from abruption presents as gastrointestinal in origin. On MRI, abruption presents as retroplacental (between the placenta and uterine wall) or marginal retroplacental hemorrhage. MR signal characteristics will vary depending on acuity of the placental abruption. Acute hemorrhage will be

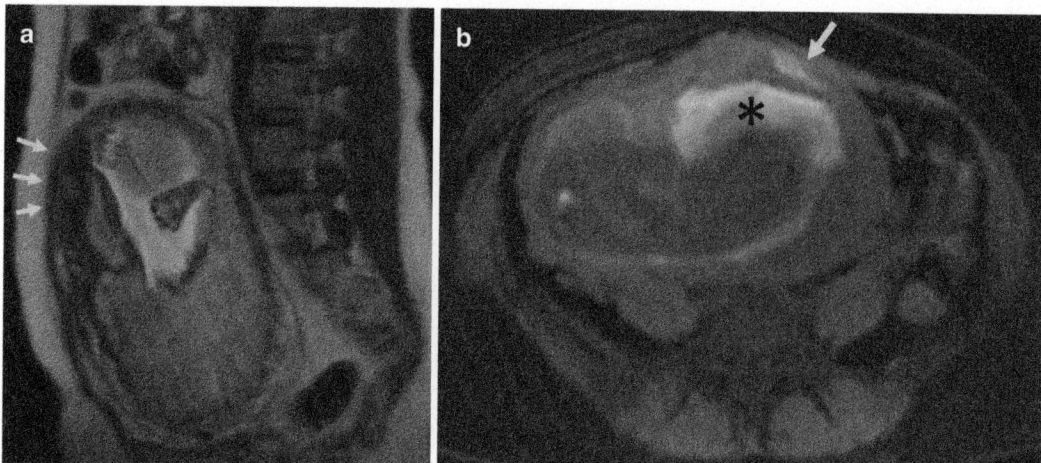

Fig. 9.8 Thirty-nine-year-old woman, 22 weeks estimated gestational age, with the history of chronic hypertension and cocaine use presented with abdominal pain and vaginal bleeding. Sagittal T2-weighted (**a**) and axial fat-suppressed T1-weighted gradient echo (**b**) non-contrast MR images demonstrate increased T1 signal within the amniotic sac, indicating subacute hemorrhage (black asterisk, image **b**). In addition, a T1 hyperintense, T2 hypointense retroplacental collection (white arrows) is present, representing subacute placental abruption

T1 isointense to hypointense and T2 hypointense, subacute hemorrhage is T1 hyperintense, and chronic hemorrhage is T1 and T2 hypointense (Fig. 9.8) [38, 40, 41].

As discussed previously, CT with iodinated contrast is the mainstay of imaging the pregnant patient in the setting of trauma. Placental abruption complicates 1–5% of minor and 20–50% of major traumas [42]. The performance of CT in this diagnosis is in the range of 86–100% for sensitivity and 80–98% for specificity [43]. On CT, placental abruption presents as a contiguous retroplacental or marginal retroplacental, full-thickness region of decreased enhancement which forms acute angles with the myometrium. The retroplacental hematoma itself may be difficult to detect, as it often has the same attenuation as adjacent myometrium (Fig. 9.9) [10, 43]. Placental abruption may be associated with uterine rupture.

When evaluating the placenta for abnormalities on MRI, it is important to be aware of the appearance of a focal myometrial contraction which may be misconstrued as a uterine mass or collection. Focal myometrial contractions can appear mass-like, and often have a low signal on T2-weighted images; this is thought to be due to blood squeezed out of the contracted areas, leading to decreased signal intensity [44]. Diagnosis is more straightforward when they are transient, but sustained uterine contractions have also been described, and may persist throughout the entirety of the MR examination. MR images will demonstrate a focal region of T2 hypointensity centered within the myometrium which may bulge into the endometrium, or placenta that may resolve on later pulse sequences (Fig. 9.10). This finding can be differentiated from masses or collections, by noting its somewhat indistinct margins and transient nature.

9.2.1.4 Uterine Rupture

Uterine rupture is one of the most feared obstetrical emergencies, which may result in peripartum hemorrhagic shock, hysterectomy during CD, and maternal and fetal death [45–47]. The incidence of uterine rupture is fewer than 1 in 1000 deliveries, and has been reported to increase to up to 1.7% in patients with a history of CD [48, 49]. Other risk factors for uterine rupture include prior uterine surgery, malpresentation, and labor dystocia [50]. Uterine rupture may occur during a trial of labor after prior CD, and is thus most commonly diagnosed by the obstetrician, followed by emergent CD for maternal or fetal instability. Therefore, uterine rupture during the laboring process is rarely seen by the radiologist.

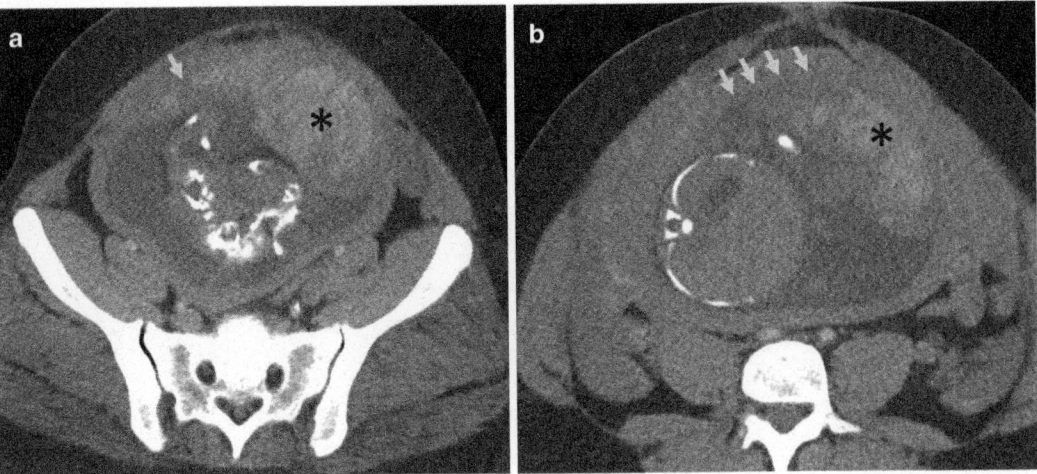

Fig. 9.9 Thirty-nine-year-old woman, 30 weeks estimated gestational age, presented after a severe motor vehicle collision with abdominal pain. Axial CT images with IV contrast at the level of the sacrum and L3 (**a** and **b**, respectively) demonstrate portions of the placenta, with normal, homogenous enhancement (black asterisk). However, there are also areas of full-thickness hypoattenuation along the marginal aspect of the placenta (white arrows), which raised substantial concern for placental abruption. The patient also had bright red vaginal bleeding, and these findings were confirmed on emergent cesarean delivery

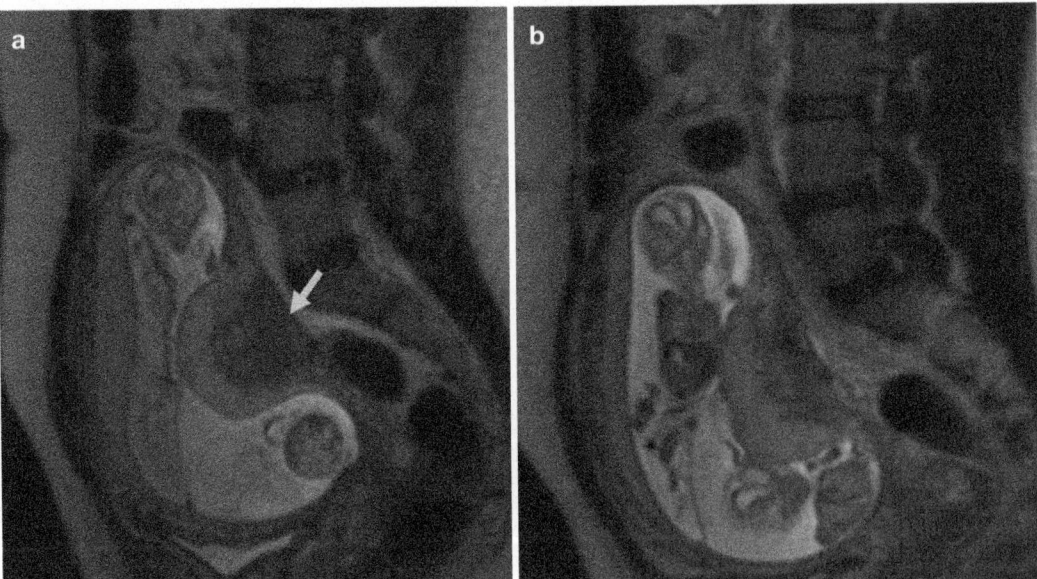

Fig. 9.10 Thirty-two-year-old woman, 15 weeks estimated gestation age, presented with right lower quadrant pain and clinical concern for acute appendicitis. Earlier (**a**) and later (**b**) sagittal T2-weighted MR images obtained 15 min apart, through the uterus, demonstrate a focal, mass-like region of T2 hypointensity (arrow) centered in the posterior uterine myometrium, which bulges into the placenta. The later image (**b**) demonstrates near resolution of this finding, indicating a transient, focal myometrial contraction

However, traumatic uterine rupture is a diagnosis readily made by the radiologist. Traumatic uterine rupture occurs in fewer than 1% of pregnant trauma patients, and unlike nontraumatic uterine rupture, almost always results in fetal mortality [51, 52]. Maternal mortality after traumatic uterine rupture approaches 10%, and prompt diagnosis is of the utmost importance [52].

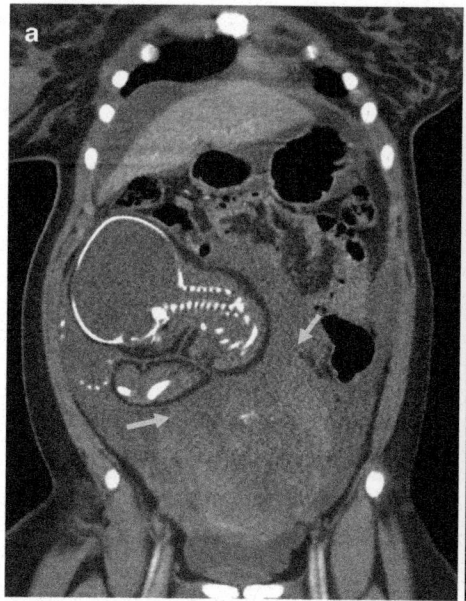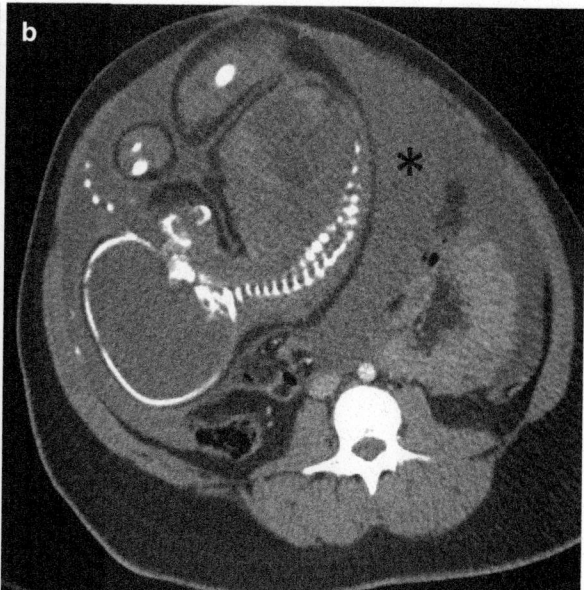

Fig. 9.11 Eighteen-year-old woman, unknown gestation age, presented after a severe motor vehicle collision. Coronal (**a**) and axial (**b**) CT images with IV contrast demonstrate a free-floating fetus outside of the margins of the uterus (arrows, **a**), indicating uterine rupture. Note that there is no enhancing tissue corresponding to the placenta, which represents complete placental abruption, which was confirmed at the time of surgery. A large amount of hemoperitoneum (asterisk, **b**) is also present

In the setting of trauma, IV contrast-enhanced CT is the recommended modality. Traumatic uterine rupture can have many associated findings including hemoperitoneum, focal lacerations, or even complete focal defects within the uterus, which present as full or partial-thickness regions of hypoattenuation within the myometrium. A variable degree of herniated fetal contents may occur (Fig. 9.11). The intense forces that lead to traumatic uterine rupture also may lead to placental abruption, the findings of which have been previously discussed.

9.2.1.5 Uterine Incarceration

Uterine incarceration is a rare, but potentially devastating complication of pregnancy [53–55]. Risk factors for uterine incarcerations include posterior or fundal fibroids, adhesions (including from endometriosis), variant uterine morphology, and variant pelvic anatomy which retains the uterine fundus within the pelvis [54, 56]. Uterine incarceration occurs when a retroverted or flexed gravid uterus becomes entrapped within the pelvis by the sacral promontory and pubic symphysis, with the gravid uterus failing to ascend [54]. Growth of the uterus causes compression of the bladder between the growing uterus and pubic symphysis. Later, posterior growth of the uterus may cause mass effect on the rectum, and may lead to rectal ischemia. Presenting symptoms include urinary retention and vague abdominal and pelvic pain [54]. Because of its nonspecific clinical symptoms, uterine incarceration is difficult to diagnose clinically. Complications of delayed or missed diagnosis of uterine incarceration include intrauterine fetal demise, uterine ischemia, premature labor and deliver, and decreased intrauterine growth [57].

Uterine incarceration is a difficult diagnosis to make on ultrasound, but can be suggested when the cervix is difficult to identify in the second or third trimester, and/or if there is an appearance of an extrauterine pregnancy [58]. In uterine incarceration, the cervix extends upward and superior to the bladder with a long, stretched course. Associated findings include a compressed and

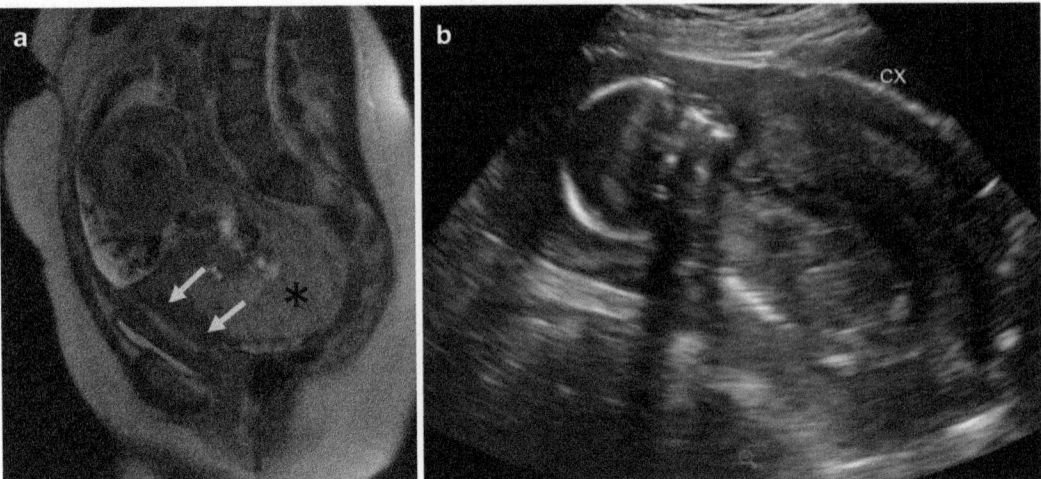

Fig. 9.12 Thirty-two-year-old woman in the third trimester of pregnancy presented with vague abdominal pain. Sagittal T2-weighted MR image (**a**), and transabdominal ultrasound (**b**) image, demonstrate a retroverted and retroflexed uterus, with the fundus of the uterus located below the pelvic brim (black asterisk). This resulted in elongation of the cervix (white arrows), which caused mass effect on the pubic symphysis. These findings are diagnostic of uterine incarceration, which was confirmed at the time of caesarian delivery

elongated bladder. Care should be taken not to mistake the cervix for an empty uterus, and the posterior location of the fetus as an extrauterine pregnancy.

Uterine incarceration suspected on ultrasound or physical examination may be confirmed by pelvic MRI. Pelvic MRI allows a larger field of view of the pelvis, and thus a more comprehensive analysis of the pelvic anatomy, which may aid in the diagnosis of uterine incarceration. The same correlative findings at the time of ultrasound are seen on MRI, include a retropositioned uterus, a stretched and elongated cervix, and an abnormally located uterine fundus which is trapped under the sacral promontory (Fig. 9.12).

9.3 Immediate Post-partum Emergencies

The post-partum period is defined as immediately after birth of a newborn and subsequent delivery of the placenta, to 6–8 weeks after birth [59]. Many unique pathologic entities occur in this period of time, primarily due to the involution of the uterus and pelvic vascularity, as well from a multitude of physiologic changes. In addition, many diagnostic challenges arise as a result of an atypical but normal appearance of the uterus. Post-partum hemorrhage (PPH), vascular thrombosis, infections, and genitourinary injuries are some of the complications seen in this period.

9.3.1 Post-partum Hemorrhage

The American College of Obstetricians and Gynecologists has newly defined post-partum hemorrhage (PPH) as cumulative blood loss greater than or equal to 1000 mL of blood, with accompanying signs or symptoms of hypovolemia within 24 h of delivery, regardless of route [60]. PPH is the leading cause of maternal mortality worldwide [61, 62]. Clinical symptoms of blood loss in the pregnant patient are not usually present until blood loss is substantial, and thus, those patients with tachypnea, tachycardia, and hypotension should have a low index of suspicion for imaging [63]. The management of PPH is complicated by the broad etiologies which may lead to PPH, include uterine atony, lacerations, retained and/or adherent placenta, defects of coagulation, vascular injury, and uterine inversion [64]. Most of these diagnoses are not radiologically apparent, but imaging can play a role in the diagnosis of retained products of conception (RPOC) and uterine pseudoaneursym, as well as for characterization of the hemolysis, elevated liver enzymes, and low platelets (HELLP) syndrome.

9.3.1.1 Retained Products of Conception

Retained products of conception is a common and treatable complication following both vaginal delivery (VD) and CD, and occurs in an estimated 3% of pregnancies [65]. Risk factors include placenta accreta, failure to progress during labor, and delivery requiring instrumentation. Patients present with vaginal bleeding, and may also have abdominal pain or febrile illness. Early diagnosis is paramount in the treatment of RPOC, and consists of surgical/manual intervention and/or uterotonic medications [61]. Complications of RPOC include PPH, infection, perforation, and potential future obstetrical complications. Imaging plays a critical role in the diagnosis of RPOC, as elevated white blood cell count and human chorionic gonadotropin may not be helpful in the immediate post-partum setting [66].

Ultrasound is an accurate tool for the diagnosis of RPOC, and combined gray scale and color Doppler has shown the highest sensitivity and specificity [65, 67–70]. Gray-scale ultrasound demonstrates thickening of the endometrial echo complex (ECC) and may demonstrate an endometrial or intrauterine mass; however, thickening of the ECC is reported to have the highest sensitivity [68]. Doppler ultrasound should be used to demonstrate increased vascularity within an endometrial or intrauterine mass, which may otherwise represent an organized intrauterine blood clot (Fig. 9.13) [70]. Vascularity within the thickened ECC or a mass demonstrated at the time of Doppler imaging increases the PPV to 96%. Blood flow should be visible, and bridge both the endometrial region and myometrium. If present, large vessels should be reported, and avoided to prevent inadvertent unroofing during dilation and curettage [68]. Large vascular structures which only reside within the myometrium should raise suspicion for an arteriovenous malformation rather than RPOC. On the other hand, one important caveat is that relatively avascular RPOC may not demonstrate flow on Doppler imaging [71]. Thus, in the presence of a thickened ECC and clinical history supportive of RPOC, the radiologist may still suggest the presence of RPOC.

Although not the preferred imaging modalities, the radiologist should also be aware of the imaging appearance of RPOC on CT and MRI. CT will demonstrate an avidly enhancing mass within the uterus (Fig. 9.13), which sometimes can be difficult to differentiate from blood clot without the presence of an initial non-contrast scan. MRI shows similar findings, with a mass within the endometrial canal that demonstrates enhancement on post-contrast images; T2-weighted images show variable signal intensity depending on the degree of tissue necrosis (Fig. 9.14).

9.3.1.2 HELLP Syndrome

The clinical presentation of hemolysis, elevated liver enzymes, and low platelets (HELLP) syndrome is one extreme point on the spectrum of pre-ecclampsia. This syndrome is associated with increased rates of maternal and fetal morbidity and mortality [72]. Once the diagnosis of HELLP syndrome has been made, the clinician should move towards delivery. Pathogenesis includes a maternal immunological maladaptation to the invading trophoblast, which triggers an inflammatory cascade, and induces thrombotic microangiopathy [73]. Thus, even though these patients experience low platelets, they are prone to thrombosis including pulmonary emboli. The imaging manifestations of HELLP syndrome are, therefore, a result of this thrombosis. One potentially life-threatening complication of HELLP syndrome is hepatic hemorrhage and rupture. Findings at the time of CT and ultrasound include wedge-shaped hepatic hypoattenuation representing infarcts, with perihepatic hemorrhage representing hepatic rupture (Fig. 9.15).

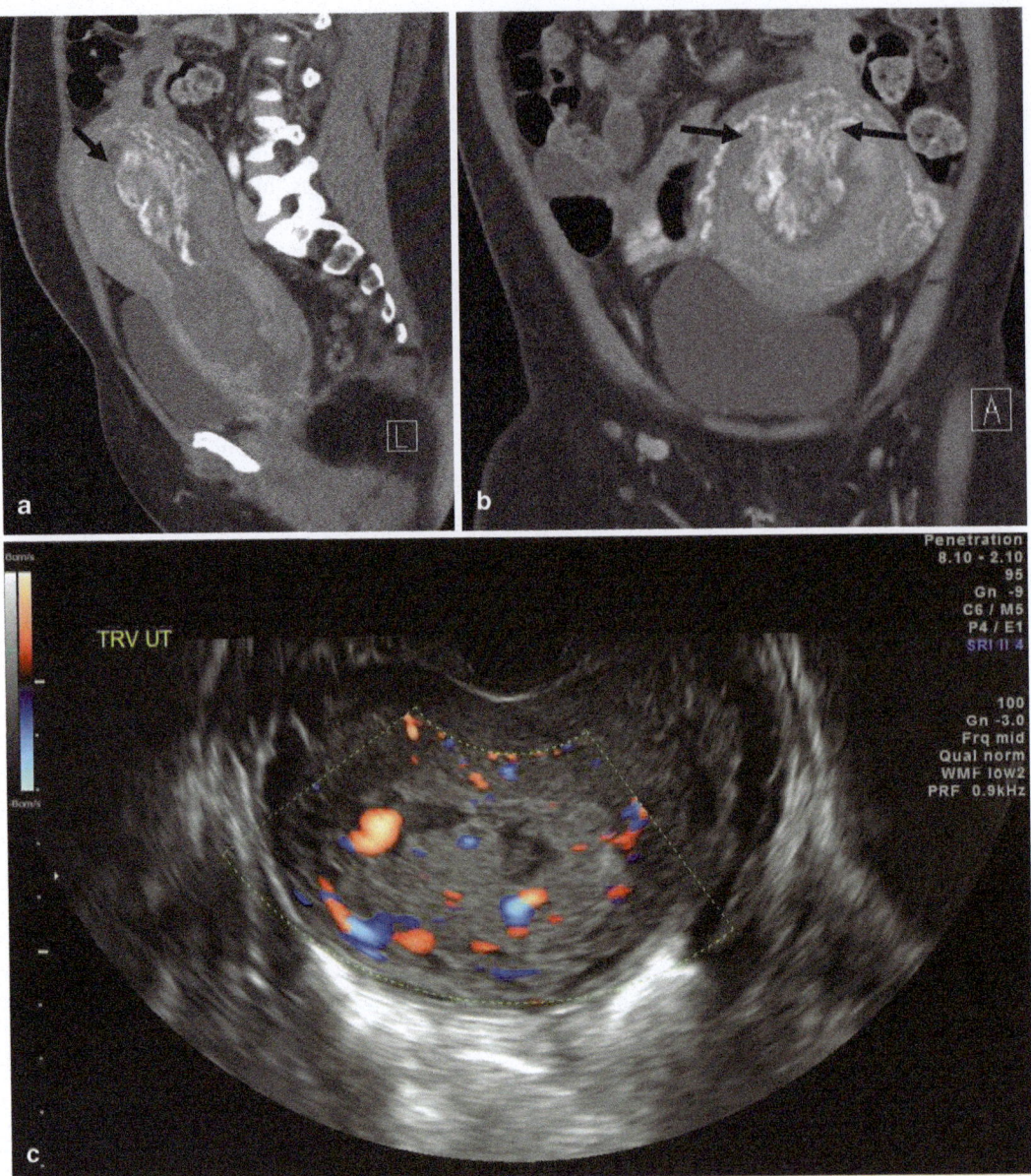

Fig. 9.13 Twenty-eight-year-old woman postoperative day 1 after cesarean delivery at an outside hospital, presented with persistent vaginal bleeding. Sagittal (**a**) and coronal (**b**) IV contrast-enhanced CT images demonstrate a hyperenhancing mass at the uterine fundus (arrows). Transabdominal transverse ultrasound image (**c**) demonstrates an echogenic endometrial mass with color flow, which is highly consistent with retained products of conception

9.3.1.3 Uterine Artery Injury

The uterine artery is a branch of the anterior division of the internal iliac artery and supplies the uterus; its course is highly variable, and as such is predisposed to injury during pelvic surgery [74]. Certainly, the uterine artery is most commonly injured during CD, with one series demonstrating 27/57 patients with uterine artery injury secondary to CD [75]. Uterine artery injury and subsequent pseudoaneurysm formation can present in the immediate post-partum setting, but most commonly has a delayed presentation of 14.5 days; because of

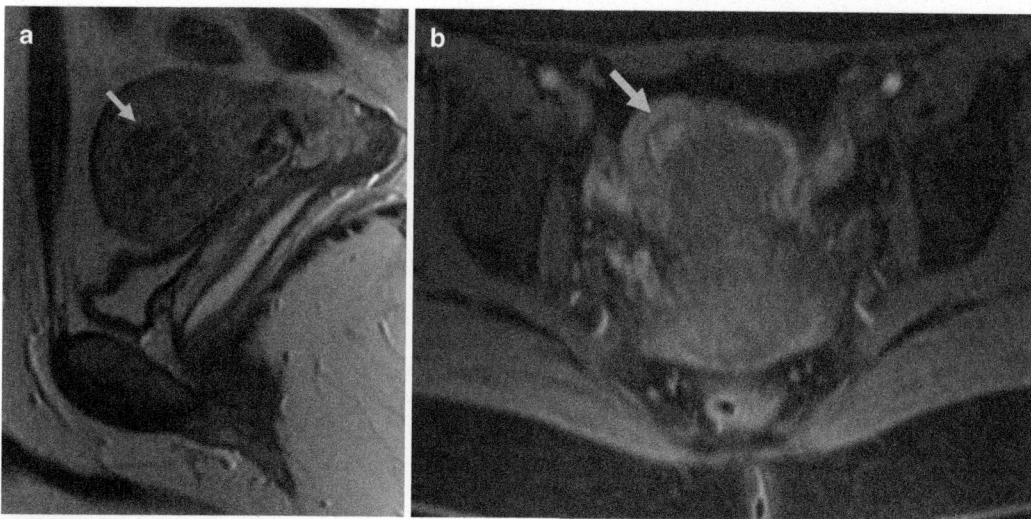

Fig. 9.14 Twenty-five-year-old woman presented from an outside hospital with continued vaginal bleeding after vaginal delivery. Sagittal T2-weighted (**a**) and axial post-contrast T1-weighted (**b**) MR images demonstrate a mass along the right cornua, which has heterogeneous T2 signal (arrows). The contrast-enhanced image demonstrates enhancement of this mass. Findings are compatible with retained products of conception, which was confirmed at subsequent dilation and curretage

this delayed presentation, uterine artery pseudoaneurysm is not commonly thought of when evaluating for post-partum hemorrhage [75]. Embolization and treatment of these pseudoaneurysms can be performed by interventional radiology.

Uterine artery pseudoaneurysms have an imaging appearance very similar to pseudoaneurysms elsewhere in the body, and appear as focal collections of contrast which mirror arterial enhancement on post-contrast imaging. Importantly, there may be non-visualization of the aneurysm due to mass effect from adjacent hematoma, and the radiologist should have a continued index of suspicion for uterine artery injury should even if one is not visualized, in the presence of unexplained large-volume vaginal bleeding (Fig. 9.16).

9.3.2 Ovarian Vein Thrombosis and Thrombophlebitis

In the post-partum period, the differential for puerperal fevers is broad, including those of gastrointestinal, genitourinary, and infectious etiologies [76]. Ovarian vein thrombosis can occur after any gynecologic surgery, but is particularly increased after CD, reaching an incidence of almost 2% [77]. Superimposed infection of the ovarian vein thrombosis leads to thrombophlebitis, and patients may present with lower quadrant pain, fever, nausea, and vomiting. Thrombosis of the ovarian vein is thought to be due to incompetent venous valves, stasis of blood flow, and the increased thrombotic state associated with the post-partum period [78]. The mainstay of management for ovarian vein thrombophlebitis is low-molecular-weight heparin and broad-spectrum antibiotics [79].

The most sensitive imaging modality has been reported to be CT, although ultrasound and MRI can also reveal ovarian vein thrombophlebitis, with reported sensitivities of 100%, 52%, and 92%, respectively [80]. Due to the dependence of blood clot age on ultrasound appearance, thrombus can appear hypoechoic, hyperechoic, or isoechoic. MRI appearance is also variable, with the T1 signal dependent on the age of the thrombus. On non-contrast MRI, thrombus can be suggested as decreased signal on balanced steady-state free-procession images, as well as a loss of normal flow voids on T2-weighted images. CT will demonstrate low-attenuation filling defect(s) within the ovarian vein(s). Interestingly,

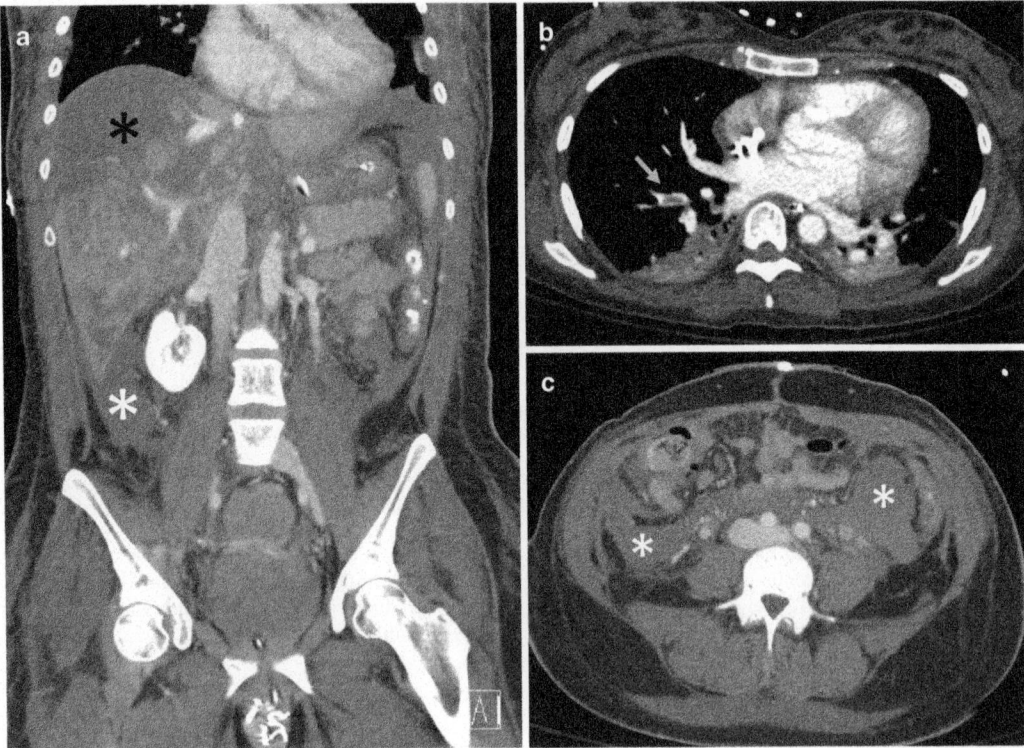

Fig. 9.15 Twenty-nine-year-old post-partum woman after urgent cesarean delivery with severe pre-eclampsia, low platelets, and elevated liver enzymes, indicating the HELLP syndrome. Coronal and axial CT images of the abdomen (**a, c**). The axial CT image of the mid chest (**b**) demonstrate wedge-shaped regions of hypoattenuation in the liver (black asterisk), with associated perihepatic and abdominal hemoperitoneum (white asterisks). The axial CT image of the lower chest (**c**) shows a right lower lobe segmental pulmonary embolism (arrow), which can be seen due to the hypercoagulable state which occurs in HELLP syndrome. Note is made of bibasilar atelectasis, with relative hypoenhancement of the atelectatic right lower lobe, likely indicative of superimposed pneumonia or infarction. A gastric catheter and central venous catheter are partially visualized on the above images. Diffuse anasarca, a common finding in HELLP syndrome, is present in this patient

the right ovarian vein is more commonly affected, in up to 90% of patients. Knowledge of the normal course of the ovarian veins is critical—the left ovarian vein empties into the left renal vein, whereas the right ovarian vein directly empties into the inferior vena cava. Therefore, right ovarian vein thrombus may more readily extend into the inferior vena cava (Fig. 9.17), and the left ovarian vein can lead to secondary thrombosis of the left renal vein. Careful search for pulmonary embolism at the lung bases on CT (or MRI) should be performed after ovarian vein thrombus has been identified. Stranding surrounding and inflammatory changes of the ovarian vein suggests superimposed infection and the diagnosis of ovarian vein thrombophlebitis; this distinction is important, as the thrombus may be a source of septic emboli (Fig. 9.18).

9.3.3 Post-partum Infection and Endometritis

Endometritis is the infection of the uterine decidua and represents the most common cause of post-partum fever. Patients typically present within the first 24 h after VD or CD, with low-grade fevers and abdominal pain [81]. The strongest risk factor for endometritis is CD, specifically emergent CD, with rates of endometritis in CD of up to 30 times those occurring with VD [82]. Although the diagnosis of endometritis is typically a clinical one,

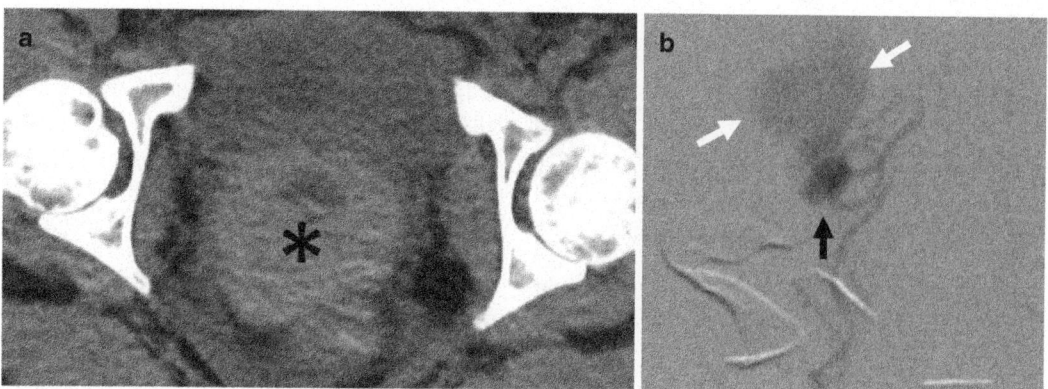

Fig. 9.16 Thirty-nine-year-old woman postoperative day 2 from cesarean delivery presented with persistent bright red vaginal bleeding. Non-contrast axial CT image (**a**) demonstrates large amounts of blood (asterisk) within the vaginal canal. Given the high clinical suspicion for vascular injury, the patient underwent conventional pelvic angiography (**b**), which demonstrated a focal saccular outpouching (black arrow) arising from the left uterine artery with surrounding extravasation (white arrows), indicating with a bleeding pseudoaneurysm

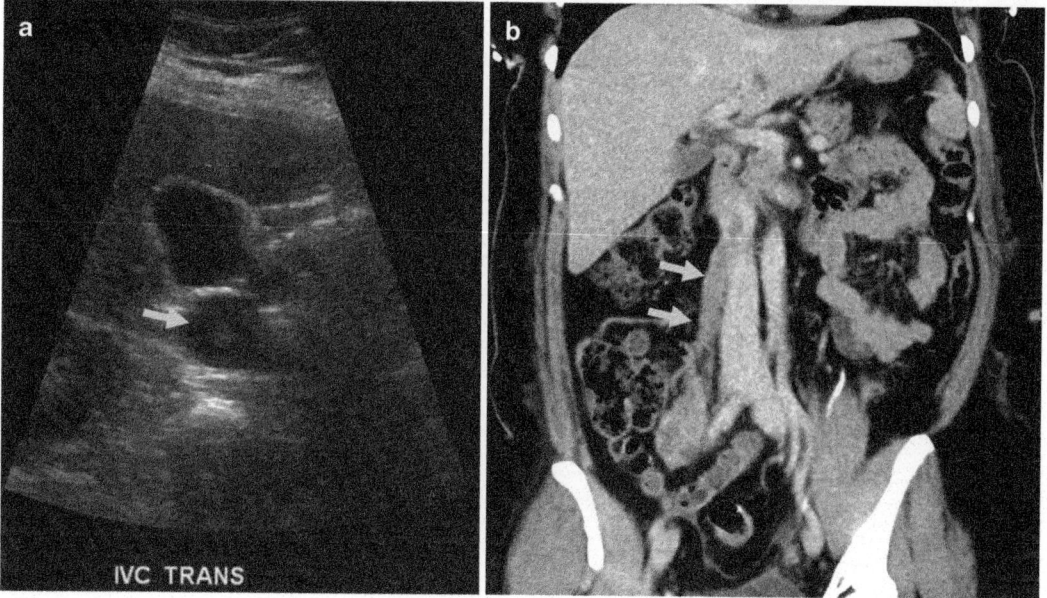

Fig. 9.17 Twenty-eight-year-old woman postoperative day 6 from cesarean delivery, who presented with right lower quadrant pain. Initial transverse ultrasound image (**a**) demonstrated an echogenic free-floating filling defect (arrow) within the inferior vena cava. Subsequent coronal CT image with IV contrast, obtained to evaluate the extent of the clot (**b**), demonstrates the thrombus (arrows) occupying almost the whole length of the right ovarian vein, and extending into the inferior vena cava

imaging may play a role in management. Organized fluid collections representing abscesses, infected hematomas, and uterine dehiscence all can be diagnosed or at least suggested on post-partum cross-sectional imaging.

Although seemingly straightforward, in the immediate post-partum period there are often blood products, gas, and even soft tissue within the uterus and/or pelvis in the case of CD; full-thickness hypoattenuating defects through the uterine wall are expected after CD, and should

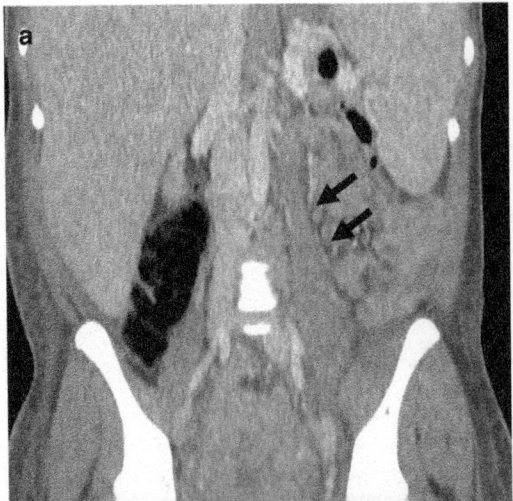

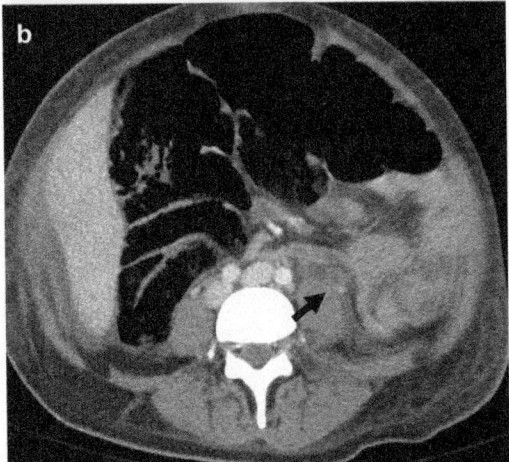

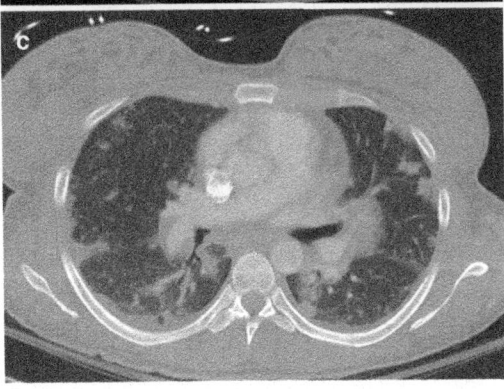

Fig. 9.18 Thirty-year-old woman postoperative day 5 from cesarean delivery, who presented with sepsis and left lower quadrant pain. Coronal and axial CT images with IV contrast through the abdomen (**a, b**), and axial CT image through the chest from the same examination (**c**), demonstrate a thrombus within the left gonadal vein (arrows), with surrounding stranding, indicating thrombophlebitis. Multiple peripheral nodules and wedge-shaped air-space opacities (**c**) are seen within the lungs, which represent septic emboli

not be misconstrued as dehiscence (Fig. 9.19). Furthermore, post-partum gas within the endometrium may be seen as late as 3 weeks after delivery, and itself is not an accurate indicator of infection [83]. The post-gravid-uterus may also appear hypervascular, and less experienced radiologists may mistake this appearance for an underlying pathology.

Ultimately, the diagnosis of endometritis is a clinical one, and the value added by radiology comes in identifying complications that may alter patient management. The diagnosis of endometritis should be suggested when a greater amount of tissue and gas is seen either within the endometrium than is usually expected, or extending through a uterine dehiscence leading to an abscess (Fig. 9.20). Peritoneal thickening and enhancement is suggestive of peritonitis, and rim-enhancing fluid collections on CT or MRI should raise suspicion of an abscess or infected hematoma.

9.3.4   Urinary Tract Injuries

The ureters have a long, retroperitoneal course, and cross along the medial aspect of the psoas muscles and posterior to the uterine artery, residing in the lateral aspect of the uterosacral ligaments. Their location is in close proximity to pelvic structures, and injury to the ureters is a well described complication of pelvic surgery. The risk of injury to the ureter after CD is 0.3–0.9%, with the most common location occurring at the suspensory ligament of the ovary [84, 85]. The left ureter is thought to be predisposed to injury due to the anterior displacement by the sigmoid colon [86]. Intraoperatively, patients with suspected ureteral injury can be identified by a lack of ureteral jet at icystoscopy, or evidence of urinary leak after injection of methylene blue or indigo carmine. Patients may be asymptomatic or can present with peritonitis, vague abdominal pain, or flank pain, as well as a rising serum creatinine level [87].

Ideally, this complication would be found while the patient is in the operating room. After closure, suspected ureteral injury is best evaluated on imaging with CT urography. Images are

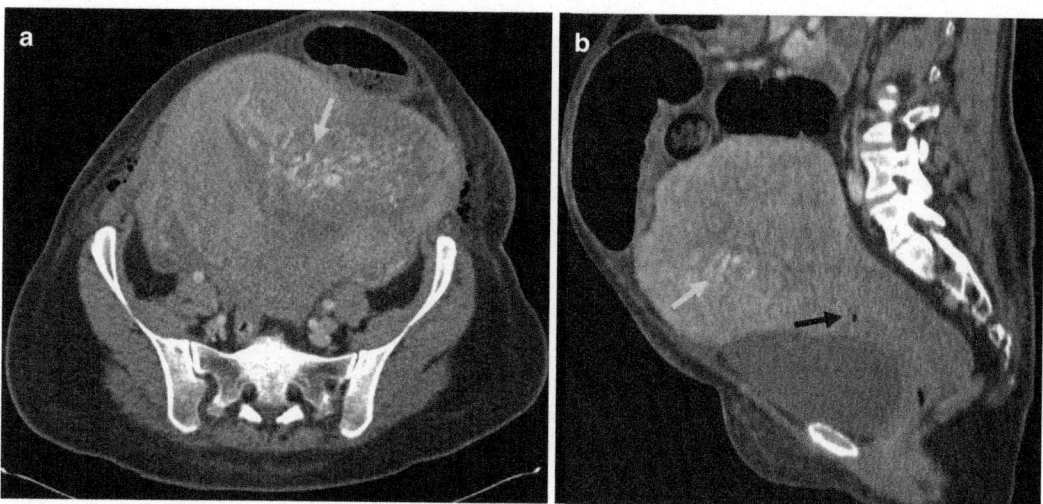

Fig. 9.19 Forty-year-old woman postoperative day 2 from cesarean delivery, with increasing abdominal pain. Axial (**a**) and sagittal (**b**) CT images with IV contrast through the abdomen and pelvis demonstrate the normal appearance of a post-gravid uterus. A small fleck of gas (black arrow) is seen in the region of the low-transverse uterine incision. Prominent vascularity in the anterior uterine wall (white arrows), represent a normal finding after cesarean delivery, and should not be confused with a uterine arteriovenous malformation

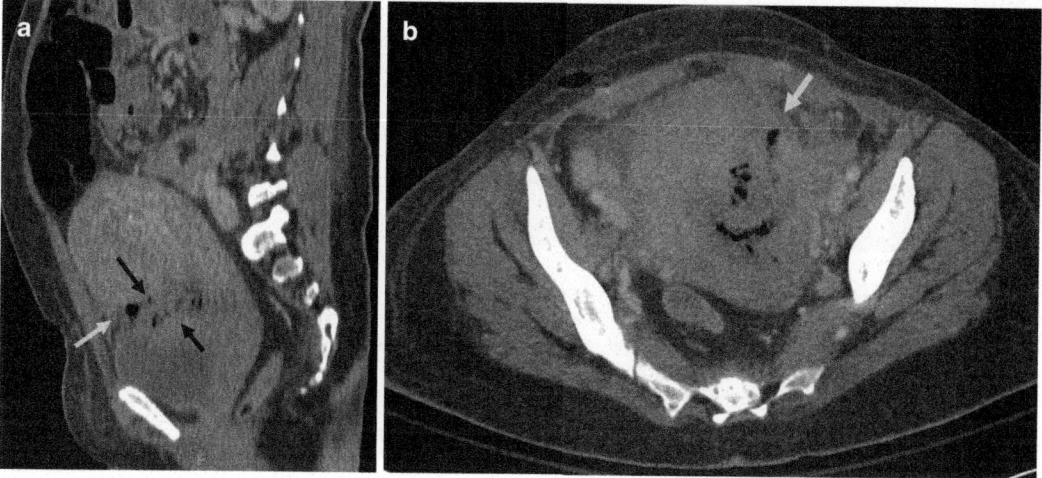

Fig. 9.20 Thirty-year-old woman postoperative day 3 from cesarean delivery, presented with abdominal pain and fevers. Sagittal (**a**) and axial (**b**) CT images with IV contrast demonstrate a gas and fluid collection emanating from the low-transverse uterine incision (white arrows). In addition, there is a large defect through the lower uterine segment (black arrows). These findings indicate an abscess and uterine dehiscence, with associated endometritis, and were confirmed with growth from positive cultures after placement of a percutaneous drainage catheter

obtained in both portal venous and excretory phases (the latter approximately 10 min after injection of intravenous contrast). The examination can be tailored to the patient, and more delayed images may be necessary. Obvious cases of ureteral injury are seen by free leakage of opacified urine into a urinoma with possible hydronephrosis; however, if the ureter is transected, hydronephrosis with an abrupt cutoff should also raise suspicion for ureteral injury (Fig. 9.21). It is important to note that ureteral injury may rarely occur spontaneously during normal vaginal delivery, and is thought to be due to the increased pressure secondary to ureteral

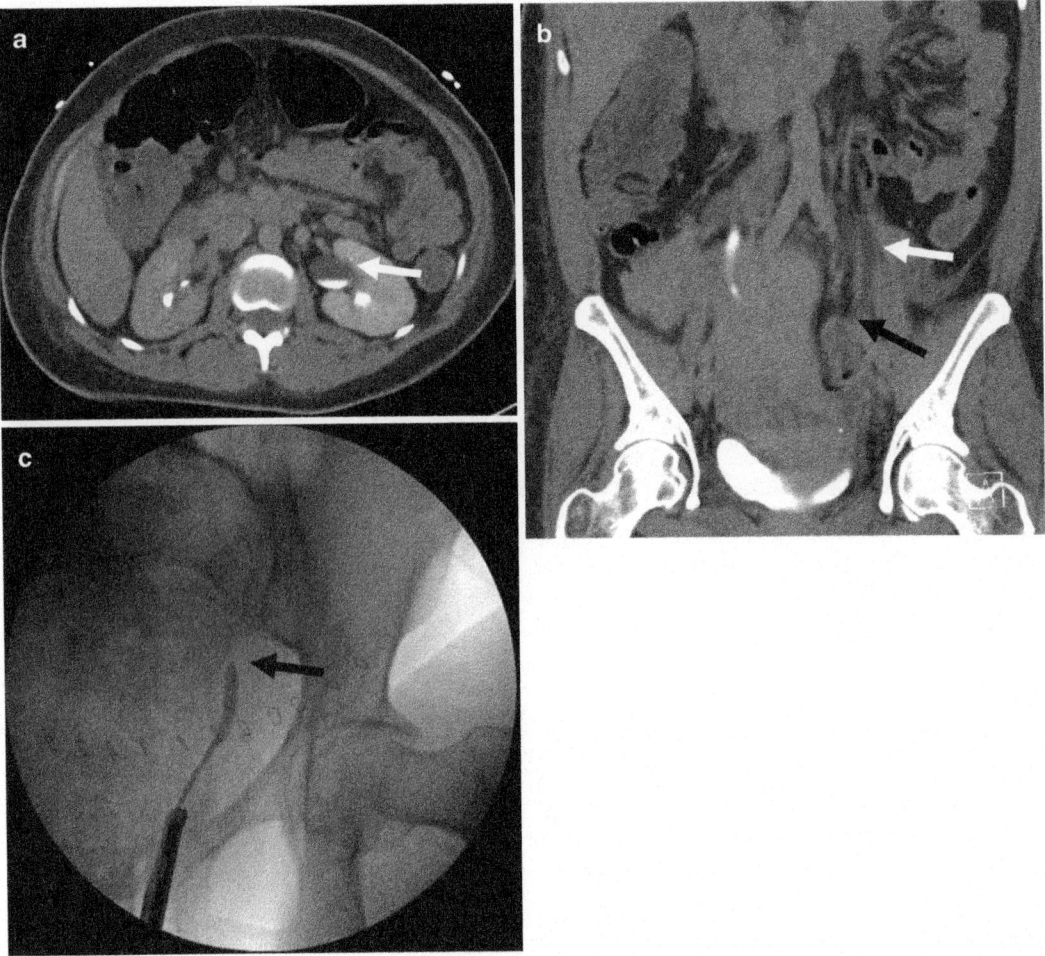

Fig. 9.21 Thirty-three-year-old woman undergoing evaluation 2 days after cesarean delivery, with increasing serum creatinine level, and left flank pain. Axial (**a**) and coronal (**b**) CT urography images demonstrate mild left hydronephrosis (white arrow) to the level of an abrupt cutoff at the distal left ureter (black arrow). Note that the left ureter is not opacified with contrast, even on the imaging obtained after a 70-min delay (image **b**). The CT findings raised a high suspicion for complete ligation of the distal left ureter. Retrograde pyelogram (image **c**) demonstrates abrupt cutoff of the distal ureter (black arrow) 6 cm from the ureterovesical junction, confirming the findings at CT urography. The patient was managed by ureteral reimplantation

compression and increased traction placed on the ureter during active labor (Fig. 9.22) [88].

The most commonly injured organ during pelvic surgery is the bladder, with an incidence approaching 1% following CD [84, 89–91]. The most common location of bladder injury is at dome, and an intraperitoneal bladder rupture is the most common type of injury [89]. The imaging appearance of bladder injury is similar to that of ureteral injury, with high-attenuation urine on CT cystography or conventional cystography seen in the abdominal cavity. An intraperitoneal bladder injury would present as contrast surrounding bowel loops, mesentery, or along the paracolic gutters, while an extraperitoneal bladder injury would be seen infiltrating along the space of Retzius, soft tissues of the lower extremity, or retroperitoneum. It is important to note that the diagnostic modality of choice is CT cystography or conventional cystography, as a CT urogram may not generate the intravesical pressure needed to reveal a bladder injury (Fig. 9.23).

Another described complication in the region of the bladder is the bladder flap hematoma. This

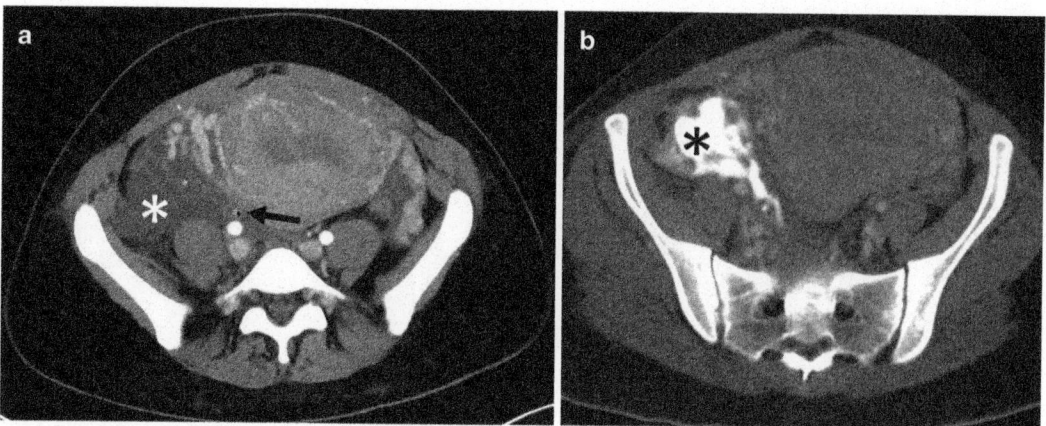

Fig. 9.22 Eighteen-year-old woman, 1 day after sponta-neous vaginal delivery, presented with increasing abdomi-nal pain. Axial portal venous phase (**a**) CT image demonstrates water attenuation fluid tracking along the retroperitoneum (white asterisk) with an associated fleck of gas next to the left ureter (black arrow). The findings raised suspicion for ureteral injury, which was confirmed with active opacified urine extravasation from the ureter (black asterisk) on the excretory image (**b**)

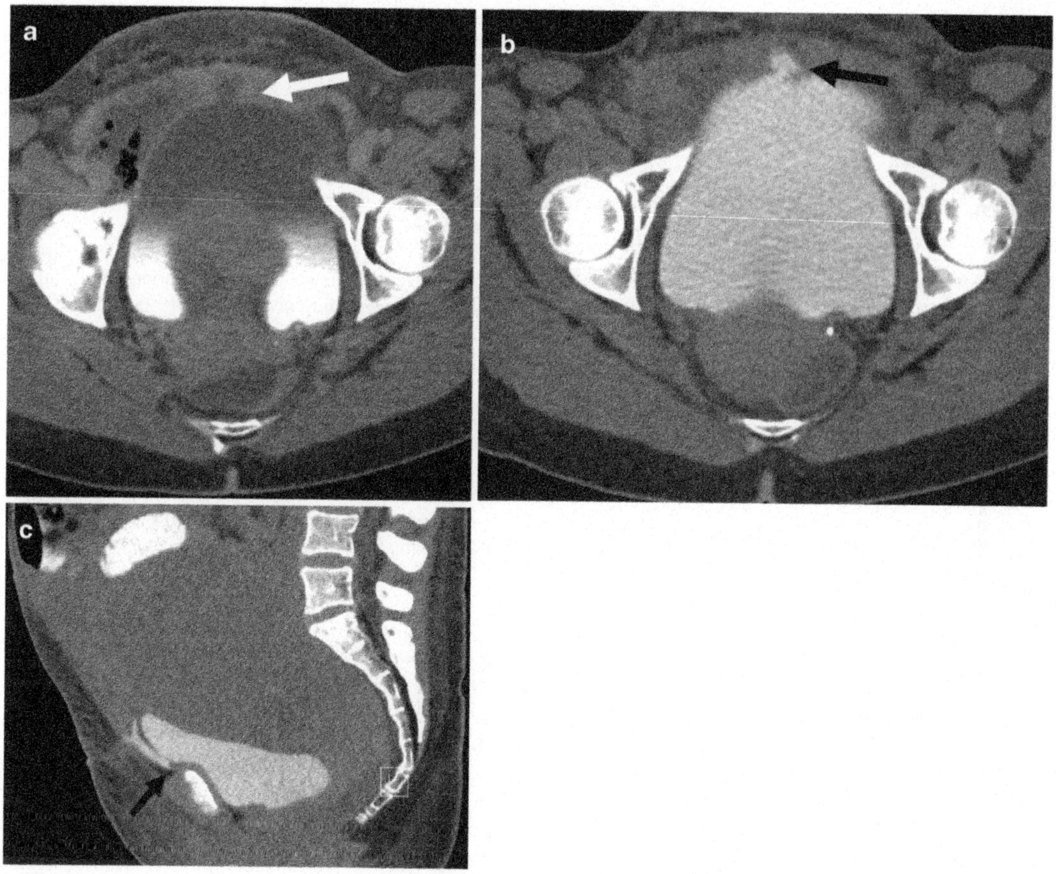

Fig. 9.23 Thirty-five-year-old woman undergoing evalu-ation 1 day after cesarean delivery for increasing abdomi-nal distension. Excretory-phase axial CT image (**a**) demonstrates contrast opacification in the bladder, but no obvious signs of a bladder leak. However, a large amount of fluid was seen in the abdomen, which prompted CT cystography. Axial (**b**) and sagittal (**c**) images from CT cystography demonstrate an intraperitoneal bladder leak near the dome (black arrow). In retrospect, this is seen on the excretory-phase image (white arrow)

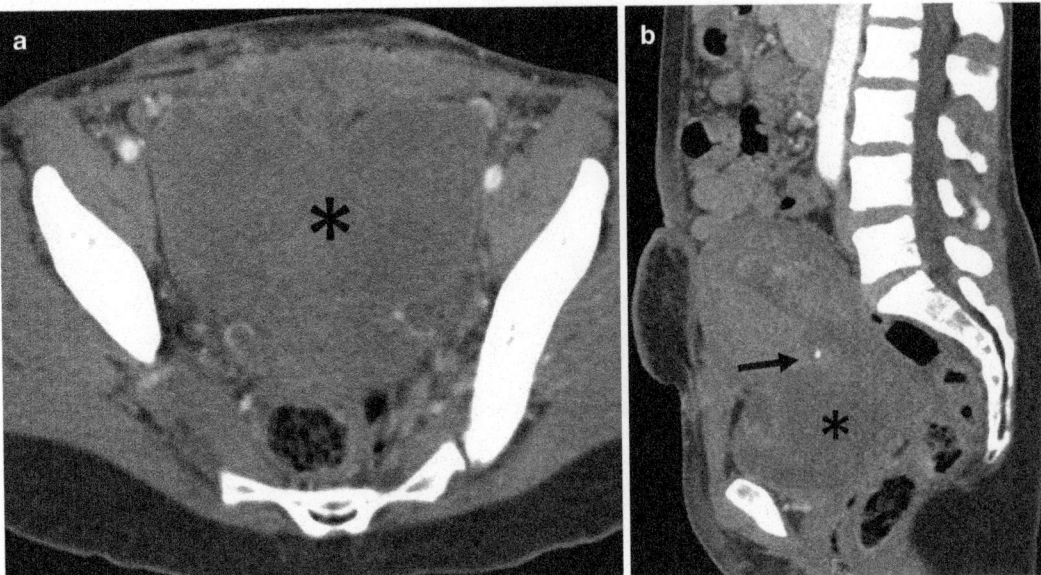

Fig. 9.24 Thirty-six-year-old woman postoperative day 2 from cesarean delivery presented with suprapubic pain. Axial (**a**) and sagittal (**b**) CT images with IV contrast demonstrate a large high-attenuation collection (black asterisk) between the bladder and the uterus (i.e., the vesi-couterine space). Note the small uterine defect (black arrow) in the lower uterine segment compatible with the uterine incision. The findings are compatible with a bladder flap hematoma, which was managed conservatively

misnomer represents a hematoma that develops in a potential space between the bladder and the uterus (i.e., the vesicouterine space), and occurs after a low uterine transverse incision. Small bladder flap hematomas are common after CD, and occur in up to 50% of patients [92]. Larger bladder flap hematomas may cause pain or mass effect on adjacent structures. On CT, a bladder flap hematoma presents as a relatively high-attenuation collection in the vesicoureterine space (Fig. 9.24). Patients are usually managed conservatively, with consideration of surgical evacuation or percutaneous drainage if the hematoma becomes infected or very symptomatic.

Disclosures The authors have no relevant financial disclosures.

References

1. Creanga AA, Berg CJ, Ko JY, Farr SL, Tong VT, Bruce FC, et al. Maternal mortality and morbidity in the United States: where are we now? J Womens Health (Larchmt). 2014;23(1):3–9.
2. Campbell KH, Savitz D, Werner EF, Pettker CM, Goffman D, Chazotte C, et al. Maternal morbidity and risk fo death at delivery hospitalization. Obstet Gynecol. 2013;122(3):627–33.
3. Kuklina E, Callaghan W. Chronic heart disease and severe obstetric morbidity among hospitalisations for pregnancy in the USA: 1995–2006. BJOG. 2011;118(3):345–52.
4. Bateman BT, Bansil P, Hernandez-Diaz S, Mhyre JM, Callaghan WM, Kuklina EV. Prevalence, trends, and outcomes of chronic hypertension: a nationwide sample of delivery admissions. Am J Obstet Gynecol. 2012;206(2):134.e1–8.
5. Cantwell R, Clutton-Brock T, Cooper G, Dawson A, Drife J, Garrod D, et al. Saving mothers' lives: reviewing maternal deaths to make motherhood safer: 2006–2008. BJOG. 2011;118:1–203.
6. American College of Obstetricians and Gynecologists' Committee on Obstetric Practice. Committee opinion No. 656: guidelines for diagnostic imaging during pregnancy and lactation. Obstet Gynecol. 2016;127(2):e75–80.
7. McCollough CH, Schueler BA, Atwell TD, Braun NN, Regner DM, Brown DL, et al. Radiation exposure and pregnancy: when should we be concerned? Radiographics. 2007;27(4):909–17.
8. Mettler FA. Medical effects and risks of exposure to ionising radiation. J Radiol Prot. 2012;32(1):N9–13.
9. Tsai R, Raptis D, Raptis C, Mellnick VM. Complications after gynecologic and obstetric procedures: a pictorial review. Curr Probl Diagn Radiol. 2018;47(3):189–99.

10. Raptis CA, Mellnick VM, Raptis DA, Kitchin D, Fowler KJ, Lubner M, et al. Imaging of trauma in the pregnant patient. Radiographics. 2014;34(3):748–63.

11. Khandelwal A, Fasih N, Kielar A. Imaging of acute abdomen in pregnancy. Radiol Clin N Am. 2013;51(6):1005–22.

12. Andersen B, Nielsen TF. Appendicitis in pregnancy: diagnosis, management and complications. Acta Obstet Gynecol Scand. 1999;78(9):758–62.

13. Sharp HT. The acute abdomen during pregnancy. Clin Obstet Gynecol. 2002;45(2):405–13.

14. Cappell MS, Friedel D. Abdominal pain during pregnancy. Gastroenterol Clin N Am. 2003;32(1):1–58.

15. Woodfield CA, Lazarus E, Chen KC, Mayo-Smith WW, et al. Am J Roentgenol. 2010;194(6_Suppl):WS14–30.

16. Gude NM, Roberts CT, Kalionis B, King RG. Growth and function of the normal human placenta. Thromb Res. 2004;114(5–6):397–407.

17. Elsayes KM, Trout AT, Friedkin AM, Liu PS, Bude RO, Platt JF, et al. Imaging of the placenta: a multimodality pictorial review. Radiographics. 2009;29(5):1371–91.

18. Reddy UM, Abuhamad AZ, Levine D, Saade GR. Fetal imaging workshop invited participants. Fetal imaging. J Ultrasound Med. 2014;33(5):745–57.

19. Grobman WA, Gersnoviez R, Landon MB, Spong CY, Leveno KJ, Rouse DJ, et al. Pregnancy outcomes for women with placenta previa in relation to the number of prior cesarean deliveries. Obstet Gynecol. 2007;110(6):1249–55.

20. Sheiner E, Shoham-Vardi I, Hallak M, Hershkowitz R, Katz M, Mazor M. Placenta previa: obstetric risk factors and pregnancy outcome. J Matern Neonatal Med. 2001;10(6):414–9.

21. Miller DA, Chollet JA, Goodwin TM. Clinical risk factors for placenta previa–placenta accreta. Am J Obstet Gynecol. 1997;177(1):210–4.

22. Dawson WB, Dumas MD, Romano WM, Gagnon R, Gratton RJ, Mowbray RD. Translabial ultrasonography and placenta previa: does measurement of the os-placenta distance predict outcome? J Ultrasound Med. 1996;15(6):441–6.

23. Smith RS, Lauria MR, Comstock CH, Treadwell MC, Kirk JS, Lee W, et al. Transvaginal ultrasonography for all placentas that appear to be low-lying or over the internal cervical os. Ultrasound Obstet Gynecol. 1997;9(1):22–4.

24. Oyelese Y, Smulian JC. Placenta previa, placenta accreta, and vasa previa. Obstet Gynecol. 2006;107(4):927–41.

25. Moodley J, Ngambu N, Corr P. Imaging techniques to identify morbidly adherent placenta praevia: a prospective study. J Obstet Gynaecol (Lahore). 2004;24(7):742–4.

26. Oyelese KO, Turner M, Lees C, Campbell S. Vasa previa: an avoidable obstetric tragedy. Obstet Gynecol Surv. 1999;54(2):138–45.

27. Schachter M, Tovbin Y, Arieli S, Friedler S, Ron-El R, Sherman D. In vitro fertilization is a risk factor for vasa previa. Fertil Steril. 2002;78(3):642–3.

28. Oyelese Y, Catanzarite V, Prefumo F, Lashley S, Schachter M, Tovbin Y, et al. Vasa previa: the impact of prenatal diagnosis on outcomes. Obstet Gynecol. 2004;103(5, Part 1):937–42.

29. Swank ML, Garite TJ, Maurel K, Das A, Perlow JH, Combs CA, et al. Vasa previa: diagnosis and management. Am J Obstet Gynecol. 2016;215(2):223. e1–6.

30. Riteau A-S, Tassin M, Chambon G, Le Vaillant C, de Laveaucoupet J, Quéré M-P, et al. Accuracy of ultrasonography and magnetic resonance imaging in the diagnosis of placenta accreta. PLoS One. 2014;9(4):e94866.

31. Committee on Obstetric Practice. ACOG Committee Opinion. Placenta accreta. Number 266, January 2002. American College of Obstetricians and Gynecologists. Int J Gynaecol Obstet. 2002;77(1):77–8.

32. Dwyer BK, Belogolovkin V, Tran L, Rao A, Carroll I, Barth R, et al. Prenatal diagnosis of placenta accreta: sonography or magnetic resonance imaging? J Ultrasound Med. 2008;27(9):1275–81.

33. Comstock CH, Love JJ, Bronsteen RA, Lee W, Vettraino IM, Huang RR, et al. Sonographic detection of placenta accreta in the second and third trimesters of pregnancy. Am J Obstet Gynecol. 2004;190(4):1135–40.

34. Warshak CR, Eskander R, Hull AD, Scioscia AL, Mattrey RF, Benirschke K, et al. Accuracy of ultrasonography and magnetic resonance imaging in the diagnosis of placenta accreta. Obstet Gynecol. 2006;108(3, Part 1):573–81.

35. Ananth CV, Wilcox AJ. Placental abruption and perinatal mortality in the United States. Am J Epidemiol. 2001;153(4):332–7.

36. Oyelese Y, Ananth CV. Placental abruption. Obstet Gynecol. 2006;108(4):1005–16.

37. Glantz C, Purnell L. Clinical utility of sonography in the diagnosis and treatment of placental abruption. J Ultrasound Med. 2002;21(8):837–40.

38. Masselli G, Brunelli R, Di Tola M, Anceschi M, Gualdi G. MR imaging in the evaluation of placental abruption: correlation with sonographic findings. Radiology. 2011;259(1):222–30.

39. Ananth CV, Berkowitz GS, Savitz DA, Lapinski RH. Placental abruption and adverse perinatal outcomes. JAMA. 1999;282(17):1646–51.

40. Trop I, Levine D. Hemorrhage during pregnancy. Am J Roentgenol. 2001;176(3):607–15.

41. Fadl SA, Linnau KF, Dighe MK. Placental abruption and hemorrhage—review of imaging appearance. Emerg Radiol. 2019;26(1):87–97.

42. Desforges JF, Pearlman MD, Tintinalli JE, Lorenz RP. Blunt trauma during pregnancy. N Engl J Med. 1990;323(23):1609–13.

43. Wei SH, Helmy M, Cohen AJ. CT evaluation of placental abruption in pregnant trauma patients. Emerg Radiol. 2009;16(5):365–73.

44. Fujiwara T, Togashi K, Yamaoka T, Nakai A, Kido A, Nishio S, et al. Kinematics of the uterus: cine mode MR imaging. Radiographics. 2004;24(1):e19.

45. Farmer RM, Kirschbaum T, Potter D, Strong TH, Medearis AL. Uterine rupture during trial of labor after previous cesarean section. Am J Obstet Gynecol. 1991;165(4):996–1001.

46. Yap OWS, Kim ES, Laros RK. Maternal and neonatal outcomes after uterine rupture in labor. Am J Obstet Gynecol. 2001;184(7):1576–81.

47. Gardeil F, Daly S, Turner MJ. Uterine rupture in pregnancy reviewed. Eur J Obstet Gynecol Reprod Biol. 1994;56(2):107–10.

48. Turner MJ. Uterine rupture. Best Pract Res Clin Obstet Gynaecol. 2002;16(1):69–79.

49. Motomura K, Ganchimeg T, Nagata C, Ota E, Vogel JP, Betran AP, et al. Incidence and outcomes of uterine rupture among women with prior caesarean section: WHO multicountry survey on maternal and newborn health. Sci Rep. 2017;7:44093.

50. Ofir K, Sheiner E, Levy A, Katz M, Mazor M. Uterine rupture: risk factors and pregnancy outcome. Am J Obstet Gynecol. 2003;189(4):1042–6.

51. Brown HL. Trauma in pregnancy. Obstet Gynecol. 2009;114(1):147–60.

52. El Kady D, Gilbert WM, Anderson J, Danielsen B, Towner D, Smith LH. Trauma during pregnancy: an analysis of maternal and fetal outcomes in a large population. Am J Obstet Gynecol. 2004;190(6):1661–8.

53. Gibbons JM, Paley WB. The incarcerated gravid uterus. Obstet Gynecol. 1969;33(6):842–5.

54. Van Winter JT, Ogburn PL, Ney JA, Hetzel DJ. Uterine incarceration during the third trimester: a rare complication of pregnancy. Mayo Clin Proc. 1991;66(6):608–13.

55. Barton-Smith P, Kent A. Asymptomatic incarcerated retroverted uterus with anterior sacculation at term. Int J Gynecol Obstet. 2007;96(2):128.

56. van Beekhuizen HJ, Bodewes HW, Tepe EM, Oosterbaan HP, Kruitwagen R, Nijland R. Role of magnetic resonance imaging in the diagnosis of incarceration of the gravid uterus. Obstet Gynecol. 2003;102(5 Pt 2):1134–7.

57. Gardner CS, Jaffe TA, Hertzberg BS, Javan R, Ho LM. The incarcerated uterus: a review of MRI and ultrasound imaging appearances. Am J Roentgenol. 2013;201(1):223–9.

58. Fernandes DD, Sadow CA, Economy KE, Benson CB. Sonographic and magnetic resonance imaging findings in uterine incarceration. J Ultrasound Med. 2012;31(4):645–50.

59. Plunk M, Lee JH, Kani K, Dighe M. Imaging of postpartum complications: a multimodality review. Am J Roentgenol. 2013;200(2):W143–54.

60. Menard MK, Main EK, Currigan SM. Executive summary of the reVITALize initiative. Obstet Gynecol. 2014;124(1):150–3.

61. Committee on Practice Bulletins-Obstetrics. Practice bulletin No. 183. Obstet Gynecol. 2017;130(4):e168–86.

62. Say L, Chou D, Gemmill A, Tunçalp Ö, Moller A-B, Daniels J, et al. Global causes of maternal death: a WHO systematic analysis. Lancet Glob Health. 2014;2(6):e323–33.

63. Pacagnella RC, Souza JP, Durocher J, Perel P, Blum J, Winikoff B, et al. A systematic review of the relationship between blood loss and clinical signs. PLoS One. 2013;8(3):e57594.

64. Dahlke JD, Mendez-Figueroa H, Maggio L, Hauspurg AK, Sperling JD, Chauhan SP, et al. Prevention and management of postpartum hemorrhage: a comparison of 4 national guidelines. Am J Obstet Gynecol. 2015;213(1):76.e1–76.e10.

65. van den Bosch T, Daemen A, Van Schoubroeck D, Pochet N, De Moor B, Timmerman D. Occurrence and outcome of residual trophoblastic tissue: a prospective study. J Ultrasound Med. 2008;27(3):357–61.

66. Malvern J, Campbell S, May P. Ultrasonic scanning of the puerperal uterus following secondary postpartum haemorrhage. J Obstet Gynaecol Br Commonw. 1973;80(4):320–4.

67. Atri M, Rao A, Boylan C, Rasty G, Gerber D. Best predictors of grayscale ultrasound combined with color Doppler in the diagnosis of retained products of conception. J Clin Ultrasound. 2011;39(3):122–7.

68. Sellmyer MA, Desser TS, Maturen KE, Jeffrey RB, Kamaya A. Physiologic, histologic, and imaging features of retained products of conception. Radiographics. 2013;33(3):781–96.

69. Alcázar JL, Baldonado C, Laparte C. The reliability of transvaginal ultrasonography to detect retained tissue after spontaneous first-trimester abortion, clinically thought to be complete. Ultrasound Obstet Gynecol. 1995;6(2):126–9.

70. Matijevic R, Knezevic M, Grgic O, Zlodi-Hrsak L. Diagnostic accuracy of sonographic and clinical parameters in the prediction of retained products of conception. J Ultrasound Med. 2009;28(3):295–9.

71. Kamaya A, Petrovitch I, Chen B, Frederick CE, Jeffrey RB. Retained products of conception: spectrum of color Doppler findings. J Ultrasound Med. 2009;28(8):1031–41.

72. Sibai BM. Diagnosis, controversies, and management of the syndrome of hemolysis, elevated liver enzymes, and low platelet count. Obstet Gynecol. 2004;103(5, Part 1):981–91.

73. Abildgaard U, Heimdal K. Pathogenesis of the syndrome of hemolysis, elevated liver enzymes, and low platelet count (HELLP): a review. Eur J Obstet Gynecol Reprod Biol. 2013;166(2):117–23.

74. Pelage JP, Le Dref O, Soyer P, Jacob D, Kardache M, Dahan H, et al. Arterial anatomy of the female genital tract: variations and relevance to transcatheter embolization of the uterus. AJR Am J Roentgenol. 1999;172(4):989–94.

75. Isono W, Tsutsumi R, Wada-Hiraike O, Fujimoto A, Osuga Y, Yano T, et al. Uterine artery pseudoaneurysm after cesarean section: case report and literature review. J Minim Invasive Gynecol. 2010;17(6):687–91.

76. Prieto-Nieto MI, Perez-Robledo JP, Rodriguez-Montes JA, Garci-Sancho-Martin L. Acute appendicitis-like symptoms as initial presentation of ovarian vein thrombosis. Ann Vasc Surg. 2004;18(4):481–3.

77. Ortín X, Ugarriza A, Espax RM, Boixadera J, Llorente A, Escoda L, et al. Postpartum ovarian vein thrombosis. Thromb Haemost. 2005;93(5):1004–5.
78. Kominiarek MA, Hibbard JU. Postpartum ovarian vein thrombosis: an update. Obstet Gynecol Surv. 2006;61(5):337–56. 8p
79. Själander A, Jansson J-H, Bergqvist D, Eriksson H, Carlberg B, Svensson P. Efficacy and safety of anticoagulant prophylaxis to prevent venous thromboembolism in acutely ill medical inpatients: a meta-analysis. J Intern Med. 2008;263(1):52–60.
80. Mwickier D, Setiawan AT, Evans RS, Erdman WA, William Stettier R, Brown CEL, et al. Imaging of puerperal septic thrombophlebitis: prospective comparison of MR imaging, CT, and sonography. Am J Roentgenol. 1997;169(4):1039–43.
81. Maharaj D. Puerperal pyrexia: a review. Part I. Obstet Gynecol Surv. 2007;62(6):393–9.
82. Menacker F, Hamilton BE. Recent trends in cesarean delivery in the United States. NCHS Data Brief. 2010;35:1–8.
83. Zuckerman J, Levine D, McNicholas MM, Konopka S, Goldstein A, Edelman RR, et al. Imaging of pelvic postpartum complications. AJR Am J Roentgenol. 1997;168(3):663–8.
84. Eisenkop SM, Richman R, Platt LD, Paul RH. Urinary tract injury during cesarean section. Obstet Gynecol. 1982;60(5):591–6.
85. Yossepowitch O, Baniel J, Livne PM. Urological injuries during cesarean section: intraoperative diagnosis and management. J Urol. 2004;172(1):196–9.
86. Obarisiagbon EO, Olagbuji BN, Onuora VC, Oguike TC, Ande ABA. Iatrogenic urological injuries complicating obstetric and gynaecological procedures. Singap Med J. 2011;52(10):738–41.
87. Chan JK, Morrow J, Manetta A. Prevention of ureteral injuries in gynecologic surgery. Am J Obstet Gynecol. 2003;188(5):1273–7.
88. Narasimhulu DM, Egbert NM, Matthew S. Intrapartum spontaneous ureteral rupture. Obstet Gynecol. 2015;126(3):610–2.
89. Phipps MG, Watabe B, Clemons JL, Weitzen S, Myers DL. Risk factors for bladder injury during cesarean delivery. Obstet Gynecol. 2005;105(1):156–60.
90. Rajasekar D, Hall M. Urinary tract injuries during obstetric intervention. Br J Obstet Gynaecol. 1997;104(6):731–4.
91. Lee JS, Choe JH, Lee HS, Seo JT. Urologic complications following obstetric and gynecologic surgery. Korean J Urol. 2012;53(11):795.
92. Rodgers SK, Kirby CL, Smith RJ, Horrow MM. Imaging after cesarean delivery: acute and chronic complications. Radiographics. 2012;32(6):1693–712.

The manufacturer's authorised representative in the EU is Springer
Nature Customer Service Centre GmbH, Europaplatz 3, 69115 Heidelberg,
Germany. If you have any concerns regarding our products, please
contact ProductSafety@springernature.com

Printed and bound by CPI Group (UK) Ltd, Croydon, CR0 4YY
29/04/2026
02099454-0007